Seventh Edition

EFFECTIVE DENTAL ASSISTING

Seventh Edition

EFFECTIVE DENTAL ASSISTING

Shirley Pratt Schwarzrock, Ph.D.
Formerly Assistant Professor,
faculty of School of Dentistry,
University of Minnesota

•

James R. Jensen, D.D.S., M.S.
Associate Dean,
School of Dentistry,
University of Minnesota

•

Kay L. Schwarzrock, B.A.

•

Lorraine Schwarzrock, M.A., CCC - SP

WCB Wm. C. Brown Publishers

Book Team

Project Editor *Colin H. Wheatley*
Production Editor *Anne E. Gardiner*
Designer *Heidi J. Baughman*
Art Editor *Janice M. Roerig*
Photo Editor *Carrie Burger*
Visuals Processor *Kenneth E. Ley*

 Wm. C. Brown Publishers

President *G. Franklin Lewis*
Vice President, Publisher *George Wm. Bergquist*
Vice President, Publisher *Thomas E. Doran*
Vice President, Operations and Production *Beverly Kolz*
National Sales Manager *Virginia S. Moffat*
Advertising Manager *Ann M. Knepper*
Marketing Manager *Craig S. Marty*
Editor in Chief *Edward G. Jaffe*
Production Editorial Manager *Colleen A. Yonda*
Production Editorial Manager *Julie A. Kennedy*
Publishing Services Manager *Karen J. Slaght*
Manager of Visuals and Design *Faye M. Schilling*

The credits section for this book begins on page 604, and is considered
an extension of the copyright page.

Library of Congress Catalog Card Number: 89–063270

ISBN 0–697–11315–9

Printed in the United States of America by Wm. C. Brown Publishers,
2460 Kerper Boulevard, Dubuque, IA 52001

10 9 8 7 6 5 4 3 2 1

Table of Contents

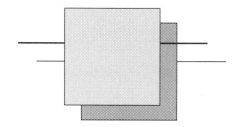

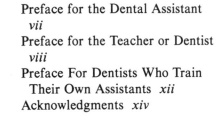

Preface for the Dental Assistant
vii
Preface for the Teacher or Dentist
viii
Preface For Dentists Who Train
Their Own Assistants xii
Acknowledgments xiv

Part 1 *The Practice of Dentistry 1*

1   The Profession of Dentistry: A
    Team Approach 2
2   The Profession of Dentistry: Past
    18
3   Dental-Medical Terminology
    (Nomenclature) 28
4   Dental Jurisprudence 32

Part 2 *People and Personnel: The Human Element 52*

5   Fundamental Principles of Human
    Relations 53
6   Communicating and Interacting
    with People 68
7   Reception Procedures 79

Part 3 *Administration of the Business Office 91*

8   Administrative Planning 92
9   Time Control: The Appointment
     Book 107
10   Mail Service and Care 119
11   Supplies and Their Control 125
12   Preservation of Written Records:
     Filing 132
13   Written Communications 141
14   Arrangements for the Meeting-
     minded Dentist 151

Part 4 *Professional and Business Records 156*

15   Clinical Records 157
16   Financial Records: Part One,
     Receipts 166
17   Financial Records: Part Two,
     Disbursements 177
18   Records for Taxes, Insurance, and
     Prepaid Care Programs 198
19   Credit and Collections 212

Part 5   *Elementary Dental Knowledge 224*

20   The Systems of the Body *225*
21   Anatomy of the Head, and Anesthesia *254*
22   Identification of Teeth and Cavity Classification *278*
23   Diet and Nutrition *285*
24   Microbiology and Sterilization *297*
25   Oral Pathology and Dental Caries *309*
26   Drugs, First Aid and Emergency Care *323*
27   Preventive Dentistry and Personal Oral Hygiene *338*
28   Dental Specialties *348*

Part 6   *The Dental Office: Its Armamentarium and Maintenance 369*

29   The Dental Office: Its Atmosphere, Housekeeping, Equipment, and Maintenance *370*
30   Dental Instruments: Their Use, Care, and Identification *379*

Part 7   *Dental Materials and Laboratory Procedures 413*

31   Restorative Materials *414*
32   Impression Materials *432*
33   Casts and Dies *437*
34   Basic Principles of Casting to Dimension *459*

Part 8   *Radiography 477*

35   Radiography: Elementary Knowledge *478*
36   Radiographic Techniques *494*

Part 9   *Operatory Procedures 511*

37   The Chairside Dental Health Team *512*
38   Applying Principles of Four-handed Dentistry in Daily Practice *520*
39   Chairside Assisting *538*

Appendices: *563*
    Tables of Weights and Measures *564*
    Table of the More Common Latin or Greek Terms and Abbreviations Used in Prescription Writing *567*
    Table of Thermometric Equivalents *568*
    Table of Certain Diseases *570*
    Improving Your Speaking Ability *574*

Glossary *577*
Word Element Glossary *599*
Notes by Chapter *602*
Photo Credits *604*
Line Art Credits *606*
Bibliography *608*
Index of Instruments *610*
Index *612*

Preface

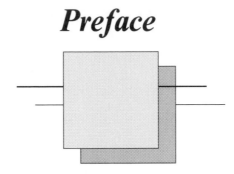

For the Dental Assistant

A career as a dental assistant can be a most rewarding way of life. In this capacity you become an integral part of a professional team dedicated to the oral health care and welfare of people. Dental assistants are intelligent, effective, and personable health professionals.

The profession requires the learning of a vast amount of detail about dentistry and people. *Effective Dental Assisting* attempts to start you on your career with a mastery of fundamentals. The *Workbook,* which accompanies the text, has a "Preface for the Prospective Dental Assistant" which will help you learn how to study, accomplish your goals, take examinations, and be interviewed by a prospective employer. It will also help you organize your study habits and use of time.

Effective Dental Assisting is written simply, attempting to present the technical material in terms which can be understood. There may be many ways to reach a given goal. We attempt to teach *one* way, acknowledging the facts that others may use a different approach, and that the dentist who employs the assistant may not perform dental routines exactly as described in this text. However, once the dental assistant *learns* the objectives of any given routine and is familiar with dental instruments, the adjustment to differing routines is easy.

This text is equally well adapted for use by the individual pursuing a course of study in dental assisting in a school and by the individual who is already employed or is being trained by the dentist-employer.

The close association the dental team enjoys with patients is one of the assets of the profession. Patients confide in their dental health team. The strict code of ethics is not only essential, it is mandatory. The patients' trust and confidence in the dentist and the dental team *must never be violated.* **What you see here, what you hear here, what you do here, stays here when you leave here.** The philosophy expressed in this statement must be the rule by which the dental health team members live.

Shirley Schwarzrock
James Jensen

Preface

For the Teacher or Dentist

Major advances in materials and techniques of delivering oral health care have drastically changed the practice of dentistry. The team concept has become a requirement; dental assisting is now a necessity. Preferably more than one assistant can and should be utilized.

Effective Dental Assisting, the *Workbook for Effective Dental Assisting,* and the *Manual* for the *Workbook* have been written to aid in training (1) dental assistants in formal training courses and (2) dental assistants in the office of the individual dentist who is faced with the problems of training a new employee. Even the dentist who hires a certified dental assistant will find *Effective Dental Assisting* helpful for purposes of review and clarification of office routine, provided the office is organized in the manner suggested.

Since dental assistants will find armamentarium of many ages, this edition of *Effective Dental Assisting* continues to provide an opportunity for familiarity with the old as well as the new. It is our goal to illustrate as many techniques of assisting with materials and processes as possible, older methods as well as new techniques.

As in previous editions, the authors have attempted to provide specific and detailed routines commonly used in a dental office.

Insofar as the space limitation imposed by one volume permits, the illustrations present typical samples of each item with which a dental assistant should be familiar. The manufacturer may vary, the form may be slightly different, but the illustrations, including instruments, equipment, and business records, are intended to help the student learn by recognition from photographs when actual specimens are not available.

Some Important Considerations for the Seventh Edition

This text presents *every phase of dental assisting.* No other text is necessary to train any assistant in the dental office. It is all here: an overview of the profession of dentistry; the various roles of the team members; dental vocabulary, ethical and legal considerations; working with people; communication skills for dentistry; all business office practices including bookkeeping, collection procedures, a study of professional and clinical records; followed by a careful study of the elementary dental knowledge that team members need, the armamentarium, dental materials, radiography, and operatory procedures for the chair assistant. When students have mastered the material in this text, they are ready to serve in any capacity as an assistant in the dental office.

Dentistry has undergone drastic changes which are reflected in the revisions in this text. The classic basic knowledge has remained while new material reflects those changes.

1. The dental specialties have been thoroughly revised and expanded. Each specialty discussion details specifics for the dental assistant in that specialty. Illustrations have been added.
   a. Endodontics has been expanded, and added illustrations are utilized to clarify procedures for the assistant. Duties of the assistant are explained.
   b. Oral and Maxillofacial Surgery reflects the expansion of this specialty, both in text and illustrations. Detailed duties of the assistant from the moment the

patient calls until the patient is dismissed are carefully stated in exact language. In addition, materials for patient education and instruction are also given.

  c. Orthodontics has been updated to reflect the prepackaged materials and new approaches. Illustrations have been added.

  d. Carefully prepared lists of duties are found in each of the specialties. Also, each specialty has been updated.

2. While obsolete illustrations have been deleted, new illustrations reflecting today's method of practicing dentistry have been added. Note that all dental operations involving patients now require gloves, masks, and glasses for both the dentist and chair assistant. These requirements are shown in the illustrations for four-handed dentistry. A number of illustrations have been added to the chapters on specialties (chap. 28) and instrument identification (chap. 30). The illustrations in chapter 38 on four-handed dentistry have all been updated to reflect the required gloves, glasses, and masks.

   The illustrations are not used to glamorize the dental assistant but rather to permit the assistant to understand more easily some aspect of a subject not readily understood without a visual image. The student will appreciate the illustrations of the passing of instruments, and the instrument identification photographs as well as illustrations of the steps of the many detailed processes that must be accurately performed in the dental office. For studies of anatomy the illustrations clarify the relationship between the structures and also permit identification of the structures.

3. The computer has become an important addition to some dental practices. Our section on computers in the dental office has been expanded to reflect this change.

4. Vocabulary lists are found at the end of some chapters. These words refer to material studied in that specific chapter.

5. The fifth edition introduced a unique way of developing a dental vocabulary: the study of word elements. That remains the same in this seventh edition. This technique of studying word elements expands the approaches to learning a professional vocabulary. Each word element is defined and then used in an example. A definition of the example is also given. Thus, the word element, the kind of element, and its definition are combined with a dental-medical vocabulary word using that word element, followed by a definition of that word. The following is an example of the format used to present each word element.

Word Elements	
Word Element	*Example*
dent combining form meaning: tooth	*edentulous* without teeth

   Only ten such elements are defined in chapter 3, the dental terminology chapter. Ten is a small enough list to memorize. All ten of the word elements in chapter 3 refer to quantities one through ten, making the memorization of the ten somewhat easier.

   No student can be expected to memorize 270 word elements in one chapter, but divided into units of ten word elements, spread out over twenty-seven chapters, the task is no longer overwhelming. With the acquisition of this word element knowledge, the student can easily build an excellent dental vocabulary. Thus, ten word elements will be found at the end of chapters 4 through 30. They are not necessarily appropriate to the discussion contained in the chapter, but the ten are usually related to each other insofar as possible, making the memorization easier. By the time the student is prepared to study clinical assistant duties, the dental-medical word element vocabulary has been assimilated.

6. Eye-catching boxes alert the reader to important facts in certain sections of the book. Each emergency technique is summarized in a box with a boldface title. The steps to be taken in a specific emergency are listed in the box. The emergencies are alphabetized so the assistant can quickly refer to any emergency that occurs and have an enumeration of the necessary actions at hand.

Some summaries of important facts or processes have also been boxed to aid the student in review and memorization.

7. The section on Dental Materials has been revised to reflect the new materials and techniques. The chapter on restorative materials (chap. 31) now includes discussions of the materials in use today. Obsolete materials have been eliminated. Chapter 33 has been completely rewritten and reorganized. It now teaches clearly, step by step, the processes in making casts, dies, and restorations.

8. A new index of instrument illustrations follows the text. If the dentist asks for an instrument by name (a Cryer elevator, for example), a neophyte dental assistant can look it up in the Index of Instrument Illustrations, quickly turn to the illustration, and with a picture for comparison, find the instrument in the office armamentarium.

9. We have included the summaries and study questions that were so well-received in the past editions.

10. We believe that we have organized the text in a logical sequence for teaching. However, many may wish to teach differently. *The order of the text should present no problems because the topics are clearly separated and can be arranged in any order the teacher desires.*

Our rationale for the order of this text is that we believe a beginning dental assistant should have a body of basic knowledge prior to being exposed to patients. We also believe that the learning process is facilitated if the assistant acquires that knowledge in a specific order.

The overview of dentistry—its history, organization, ethics, the oral health team, and where the dental assistant belongs in that total picture—should be understood first. Then the dental assistant should learn the basics for acquiring a professional vocabulary. Next, with the legal problems dentists are experiencing today, we believe that *no one should ever work with a patient until the reasonable actions to protect the office from unjustified claims are understood.* Thus, we included dental jurisprudence in the first part of the book.

Since dentistry is based on providing service, our second section is devoted to the human element—the psychology of working with people, communicating and interacting with patients and staff, and reception procedures.

We believe the dental assistant must understand the business side of dentistry, including practice administration, appointment-making, and financial and clinical records. It is highly important that this knowledge be acquired before the dental assistant attempts to serve as a clinical assistant because it is necessary to know all the records utilized and to be able to respond to written requests.

Elementary dental knowledge—the systems of the body, anatomy of the head and neck, anesthesia, identification of teeth, cavity classification, diet and its relation to dental health, microbiology, sterilization, oral pathology, dental caries, drugs, first aid and emergency care, preventive dentistry and certain dental specialties—is studied before the assistant is introduced to the operatory.

The understanding of the office equipment, its value and care as well as the armamentarium of dentistry that the assistant must recognize, care for, and often use is now presented, followed by a discussion and understanding of dental materials and laboratory procedures. Next, the radiography basics are presented. Some assistants may use this section extensively, others may not be involved in either the care or the use of radiographs.

The last three chapters are devoted to the chairside dental health team and the assistant's performance on that team. Without the preceding chapters, the assistant's performance in the operatory would be less effective. Therefore, we placed this very important section at the end of the text.

The last chapter (chap. 39) is a series of reminder lists of armamentarium for each dental operation. Since not all dentists practice alike, space is provided with each list to accommodate the need for adding materials used in a specific office. It is possible for the dentist to delete items not used and add others that are used. The assistant can refer to this chapter whenever there is a question about the necessary equipment for a specific operation. (Perhaps some operation is infrequently performed, and there is uncertainty about the necessary armamentarium.)

11. There is some variance in the length of chapters, but we believe that to pad a chapter with unnecessary words to keep all the chapters equally long is not performing a service for education. To combine some unrelated subjects just to make the chapters of similar length also seems unwise. Thus, you will find that there are a few shorter chapters but *the title of each chapter is indicative of the content of that chapter.*

12. We have included the personal speech improvement materials from the fourth edition in the Appendix for the benefit of the individual who wishes to practice speech skills. Formerly this material was part of the communication chapter, but most schools teach full courses in speech. Therefore, we have retained in the Appendix these few pages for the interested student.

    The Appendix also includes valuable tables of weights and measures, Latin and Greek abbreviations used in prescription writing, thermometric equivalents, and a table of certain diseases.

13. Metric conversion tables have been supplied inside the front cover for easy accessibility.

14. Our Glossary is a compilation of words found in the text rather than an attempt to include a medical dictionary. The guide for pronunciation is based on the Schwarzrock technique for teaching pronunciation, using a minimum of diacritical markings and a maximum of sound combinations that do not require reference to a pronunciation marking list. This technique was developed in 1954 and has been utilized frequently since then.

    Each definition in our Glossary is an attempt to assist the student to better understand the technical definition found in a medical dictionary. All the definitions have been carefully researched and checked against the leading medical dictionaries for accuracy.

15. We have studied the guidelines teachers use in preparing students to take the accreditation examination for certification by the American Dental Assistants Association. Insofar as humanly possible, without knowledge of the actual examination, we have included the materials that are listed as areas of knowledge necessary for passing examinations. It is our belief that our text satisfies these requirements insofar as the written word can accomplish the task. Certainly, application of the principles will require actual performance of tasks.

    We hope that the additions and changes to this, the seventh edition, will provide teachers and dentists with worthwhile materials for their dental assistants.

    Shirley Schwarzrock
    James Jensen

Preface

For Dentists Who Train Their Own Assistants

The dentists who undertake to train their own assistants can profit from organizing a training program. The new assistant will appreciate an orderly approach to training. The time and effort required to teach the assistant to work in the manner the dentist prefers can be reduced and the production level raised.

You, the dentist, should be familiar with the complete text. Wherever necessary, adapt the instructions to your particular methods of operating and administering your office. It is recommended that you indicate the order in which you wish your assistant to learn the various procedures and duties. The new assistant should then be expected to know only those sections or procedures which have been assigned until all the techniques you require have been mastered.

Use of the *Workbook* will aid materially in helping the neophyte understand the textbook. You can ask your new assistant to answer the questions in the *Workbook* for the section you have assigned in the text.

The *Manual* for the *Workbook* is a publication designed for the dentist or teacher. Part One contains suggestions about effective teaching procedures. Part Two states the correct answer and the page number of *Effective Dental Assisting* where the correct answer will be found.

Dentistry is a self-limiting profession. With the exception of the dental hygienist's work and that performed by a laboratory technician, every operation for which the dentist receives remuneration is one the dentist must personally perform during the number of hours spent in the dental office. The use of dental assistants to perform all tasks which are interruptions of the dentist's chair time and to increase production through chairside assisting is the best solution to a difficult problem in economics and personal health.

Any task that a dental assistant can be taught to do for the dentist should be delegated to an assistant. The degree to which this delegation of tasks is successfully carried in various dental offices often accounts for the variation in production and, as a direct result, in the amount of time the dentist must work.

There are a number of sources of lost productive time that apply to any office, regardless of the fact that not all dentists produce at the same rate. *One important cause of lost productive time is disorganization of the dentist's work habits at the chair.* In order to produce efficiently, the dentist's operative procedures must always be the same in sequence of procedure and instrumentation for each type of operation. The use of diamond and/or carbide instruments for operative procedures at the higher operating speeds requires a systematic procedure, together with the use of a well-trained assistant, to achieve maximum benefits.

Any dentist who has worked alone is thoroughly aware of production-disturbing factors in the dental office. Answering the telephone, making appointments, collecting fees, processing X rays, purchasing supplies, talking with salespeople, cleaning up after operative work, sterilizing instruments—these are but a few of the production-disturbing factors. Hiring an assistant to assume these duties, when the patient load warrants, creates an increase in services rendered that is very apparent. The dentist's output of energy and degree of strain become less when the benefits of office efficiency are secured.

The dental assistant's primary job is to keep the dentist at the chair providing dental care which no one else in the office can provide. To do so requires control of, or elimination of, production-disturbing factors while serving the public graciously and assisting in the production of dentistry at the chair.

To be successful in this primary task, the dental assistant must be trained to exercise control of the office by the best means possible. The dentist must be cooperative in the exercise of such control by the staff.

Dental assisting is a complex job. It requires a high level of intelligence, social adjustment, emotional stability, speech ability, manual dexterity, and personal drive to be a success. Good health and the personal habits of good grooming are also essential. With these tangible and intangible qualifications, a trainee has an excellent chance of becoming a good assistant if the training is well organized.

Through long practice, the dentist has become familiar with his or her preferred office procedures; the details are a simple routine. To a new employee these are a thousand-and-one confusing details. Responsibility for but one new idea at a time gives the trainee an orderly approach to these details. A better trained employee will be the result if concentration on one idea at a time is permitted.

In order to facilitate the use of this text in the individual dental office, the dentist should take time to accomplish the following:

1. Organize instrumentation and sequence in all dental operations.
2. Make the necessary changes or additions in the text, especially in the operative section, to conform to the dentist's personal work habits.

    Chapter 39 lists armamentarium for many dental procedures. Add or delete instruments in these lists to reflect your preferences. Your dental assistant can then be certain to provide you with those instruments necessary for each operation.

3. Indicate to the assistant the order in which the various duties and operations are to be learned. Carefully verify the answers in the neophyte's *Workbook* and be certain that the materials studied are understood.
4. Make a list of the time required for typical operations, from the average number of surfaces of amalgam restorations per hour to the time required for denture work and its associated laboratory requirements—for all routine procedures performed in your practice—to be typed and mounted inside the back cover of the appointment book or placed in a permanent location at the desk where appointments are made.
5. Turn to chapter 39 and fill in the exposure time for X rays as used in your office.
6. As the dental assistant grows in ability, be cooperative in delegating authority. Any indication of lack of confidence on the part of the employer-dentist can seriously impair the self-confidence of an employee.

The procedures outlined in this text are not assumed to apply to all dental offices, nor to include all dental procedures. They are presented with the sole purpose of providing a starting point in training for the neophyte. If no outline of procedure for a specific duty were used, only generalities would remain. The dental assistant, regardless of training or experience, *must always learn the procedures as used in the office in which she or he is employed.*

Shirley Schwarzrock
James R. Jensen

Acknowledgments

We wish to express our deep appreciation to those who through their kindness, generosity, and friendship have continued to provide information and support for this seventh edition. Many will remain anonymous. To those we can only say, "Thank you."

Members of the University of Minnesota Dental School faculty deserve a special mention for contributing so much that is current and viable for dentistry today. They are (in alphabetical order):

Mrs. Joan Dako, Director, Art Studio, Dental Audio Visual Department for all the drawings in this edition;

Anthony DiAngeles, D.D.S., M.P.H., Clinical Professor Operative Dentistry for his chapter on four-handed dentistry;

William P. Frantzich, D.D.S., M.S.D., Clinical Associate Professor, Division of Oral and Maxillofacial Surgery for the oral surgery materials;

Anna Hampel, D.D.S., M.S.D., Dr. Med. Dent., Professor of Biomaterials for her work on Dental Materials; and

Mary Schwind, B.A., Librarian School of Dentistry, for her assistance with the reference lists.

We are also grateful to:

Kay Schwarzrock, B.A., Project Manager, HEMAR Service Corporation of America for her section on use of computers in the dental office; and

Hugh Silkensen, D.D.S., M.S.D., orthodontist, Russellville, Arkansas for the sections on orthodontia.

Without the team approach this volume could not be as accurate and effective as it is, since knowledge has become so specialized that experts from many fields are necessary to produce the required materials. The quality of the text is enhanced by the decades of private practice experience of its dental contributors.

In addition to the above-mentioned persons, we appreciate the continued efforts of Marcus Dental Supply Company, Minneapolis, Minnesota for their supply of illustrations of equipment and instruments and to Spillane's, Inc. for the special printings designed especially for this text.

Donald Hauptfeuhrer, Department of Radiology, University of Illinois, College of Dentistry, made a unique contribution to the radiography section for the fifth edition. We are still indebted to him for that input.

Shirley Schwarzrock
James R. Jensen

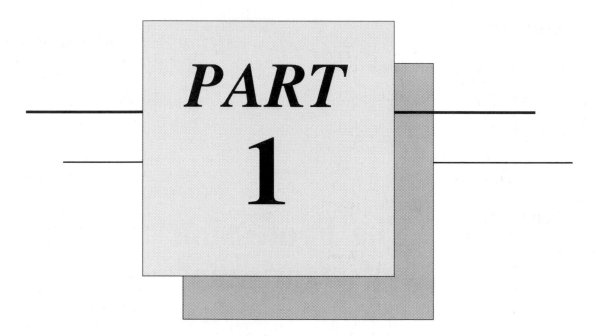

PART 1

The Practice of Dentistry

The practice of dentistry is constantly undergoing change. The changes occur as a result of (1) the increased knowledge acquired by the continuing research programs and (2) the constant pressure on the dental profession created by increasing numbers of people to be treated. Team dentistry is now the accepted method of providing dental care. The aim of Part One of this text is to alert the *neophyte* (beginner or a newcomer to a group) dental assistant to the factors that are encountered in the practice of dentistry today. Included in this section are explanations of dentistry as it exists today, its history, technical vocabulary, and *jurisprudence* (law governing dentistry).

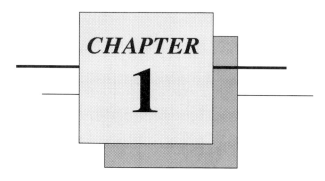

The Profession
of Dentistry:
A Team Approach

Dentistry Today
   Service to the Public
   Need and Demand for Dental Services
The Role of the Dentist
   General Dentistry
   Dental Specialties
   Types of Practice
   Principles of Ethics
The Dental Health Team
The Role of the Dental Assistant
   Duties in the Dental Office
   The Professional Dental Assistant
   Ethics for the Dental Assistant
     Objectives
     Principles of Ethics
   Personal Impression Created by the Dental
      Assistant
     Grooming
     Inadvertent Communication
The Desirable Team Member
Cooperating with the Team

Dentistry Today

The rapid changes that are occurring today due to our increasing knowledge cause changes in the dental profession. Dental services today are being delivered differently from the style of twenty—ten—or even five years ago; but regardless of the changing form of delivery of dental services, we must remember a few very basic unchanging facts.

A dentist strives to achieve a healthy and aesthetically pleasing mouth for each patient and then assist the patient to maintain that condition. The dentist is responsible for the work of all persons employed to assist him or her in reaching that goal.

The profession of dentistry in the United States has successfully led the way in implementing effective preventive measures and reduced the incidence and severity of dental caries and periodontal disease. Thus, dentistry has been responsible for improving the oral health of the individual, and in turn, the oral health of the nation. In addition, all over the world people are benefiting from the dental research in prevention that has been conducted in the United States.

Although disease incidence and patterns have changed dramatically for younger patients, the life expectancy of the population has been extended. Thus, the needs of the elderly are requiring more attention by the dental team, not only in the area of prevention, but in treatment of their special needs.

The dental assistant, as a part of the oral health care delivery team, plays a very important role in Patient Education and Prevention.

Today, *team* is the important concept in dentistry. A group of trained specialists, under the supervision and control of the dentist, assist in the performance of dentistry. Each team member contributes the skills of his or her specialty—dental hygienist, dental chair assistant, extended duties assistant, laboratory technician, receptionist, secretary, accountant, office administrator. Whatever his or her training, the individual performs a service that, together with the contributions of the other team members under the direction of the dentist, attains the goal of a healthy mouth for every patient willing to accept the treatment.

The team concept, then, creates the necessity for cooperation and rapport among the team members: each must appreciate the contributions of others; each must be aware of the responsibilities and limitations of his or her own contributions to the overall objectives.

In addition to understanding their own responsibilities, all team members should have an understanding of these important concepts:

1. An overall perspective of the dental profession including the roles of the dentist and all auxiliaries
2. Dentistry's purpose and service to the public
3. Ethical standards set by the dental profession
4. The history and background of dentistry as we know it today
5. Dental vocabulary and nomenclature
6. Legal regulations (jurisprudence) governing the practice of dentistry

These subjects are all presented in the chapters in the first section of this text.

Service to the Public

Access to good health—including a healthy mouth—is the right of every person in today's world. More people are comprehending that good *oral health* (mouth health) is essential to good general health.

"The beginning of preventive medicine is care of the mouth" is a widely quoted statement made by one of the Mayo brothers who founded the Mayo Clinic in Rochester, Minnesota.

In the 1930s, Dr. Weston A. Price conducted investigations of dental deformities and dental decay among various racial groups all over the world. His report on the South Sea Islanders was typical of his reports on other groups studied.

When the Islanders retained their primitive ways of life and existed on native foods, they did not develop dental deformities nor dental decay; yet such deformities and decay were common among the Islanders who lived on imported foods.[1] Dental deformities and dental decay are therefore often called *diseases of civilization.*

Dentistry is performed because patients seek care. If nothing else motivates the patient, pain does. Anyone who does not have regular dental checkups may develop a toothache and thus seek care. Patients who have more knowledge about dentistry and good health usually seek dental care on a regular basis—to prevent pain if for no other reason. For many patients, personal appearance may be the most important reason for seeking dental care. The person who has lost a front tooth usually desires a replacement immediately.

Members of the dental profession are well aware that personal appearance and prevention of pain are not the only reasons for regularly scheduled dental care. Good health requires a healthy mouth. The oral cavity is the portal through which all nourishment enters the body. The first step in the digestion of food occurs in the mouth. The action of ptyalin in the saliva begins the conversion of starches to sugars. The teeth are used to break up the larger food particles by a grinding action, making it easier for the ptyalin to begin its work. The ability to masticate food properly is important for the entire process of digestion. This ability also enhances the pleasure we experience from eating.

Oral health and general health are very closely related. Many systemic diseases have oral manifestations; a high percentage of cancer originates in the mouth area. Thus, maintaining oral health is one of the basic functions of the dental profession.

The purpose of dentistry, then, is to serve the public by:

1. Assisting patients to maintain good oral health
2. Assisting patients to maintain the ability to masticate (chew) food throughout life
3. Assisting patients to maintain or to improve personal appearance
4. Assisting patients to avoid oral diseases and pain by practicing preventive dentistry
5. Assisting patients by providing relief from oral pain

Need and Demand for Dental Services

The need for dental care is different from the demand for such care. That is, people need the care but may not ask for it. Since dental caries affects most of our population, and periodontal disease and malocclusions are nearly as rampant, a universal need for dental treatment of some kind exists.

However often potential patients do not seek dental care. It is true that some areas of the country are without enough dentists to care adequately for the demand for services. Other reasons for dental neglect are that some persons are afraid of dentistry, others may be ignorant of dentistry's contributions to comfort, appearance, and improved ability to masticate food, unaware of the importance to general health of the condition of the mouth, unable to afford dentistry, or do not believe they can afford dentistry. For any one of these reasons potential patients fail to seek the care they need.

Other potential patients do seek care. Although caries and periodontal disease are under better control, patients' appreciation and demand for good dental care has increased; thus, more demand for dental care exists today.

In addition, oral health care is now receiving attention from state, local, and federal government agencies. Attempts are being made to broaden health care coverage to include dentistry. The intention seems to be that complete health care should be available to citizens from birth to death. Currently, many citizens have health care benefits through governmental programs, private insurance carriers, union contracts, employer's fringe benefits, and dental service plans. Payments for these services are referred to as third-party payments. Someone who does not receive the service makes all or part of the payment. Examples are government agencies, unions, employers, or insurance carriers. Thus, people who have not had dental care because they couldn't (or wouldn't) pay for such care may now receive care as part of their benefits from employment. The economic barrier to dental care has been removed for many. Therefore, we find increased numbers of patients to be treated due to third-party payment.

The Role of the Dentist

Dentistry is performed by the dentist who alone is responsible for the diagnosis and care plan for each patient, regardless of the amount of assistance he or she decides to utilize. The dentist is required to be highly trained and qualified before being allowed to practice dentistry.

In order to be accepted in a dental school today an applicant must have spent three or four years studying cultural and scientific subjects at an undergraduate college.

After acceptance into a dental school, a student studies dental subjects. In addition, the student must take extensive course work in clinical and basic sciences in order to allow the future dentist to develop the basic clinical judgment necessary to the effective practice of dentistry. A dental education requires a sound foundation in biochemistry, pharmacology, pathology, microbiology, physiology, and anatomy with special emphasis on the head and neck. Anatomy includes neuroanatomy (study of the nervous system), gross anatomy (study of the complete body and its parts), microscopic anatomy (microscopic study of normal tissues), embryology (study of growth and development of the body before birth), and dental anatomy (study of teeth, their relationship to each other in the dental arch, and the surrounding oral tissues). The student must also pass examinations in preclinical and clinical dental topics and related areas.

General Dentistry

It is easy to understand that every dentist must be highly trained in the many disciplines of dentistry. "General dentistry" encompasses all these disciplines; thus, the general dentist must be capable of providing services in all these areas: oral diagnosis and treatment, pedodontics, operative dentistry, fixed and removable prostheses, endodontics, periodontics, oral and maxillofacial surgery, and orthodontics. If you are employed in a general dentist's office, all of the chapters of this text (including the specialties) are necessary for your education and use. *This text presents all of the subjects that are required for work in the general dentist's office.*

Most dentists are engaged in the general practice of dentistry; that is, the dental procedures that they accomplish for their patients may be in any field of dentistry. In rural or isolated areas, the dentist is more likely to engage in most of the types of work that comprise the total dental field. In metropolitan areas where specialists are more readily available, the "general" dentist may frequently refer patients with particularly difficult problems to specialists for treatments requiring a high degree of skill in a limited dental field.

Dental Specialties

Increase in knowledge in various fields in dentistry, as in medicine, that require advanced training and special skills has created the need for specialists. The growth of urban centers of population and the development of transportation facilities have provided the opportunity for specialists to serve.

A *specialist* in dentistry is a dentist who limits a practice to one type of work, in contrast to the *general* dentist who practices in more than one field of dentistry. In dentistry there are eight specialties recognized by the American Dental Association. Each specialty has qualifications and examinations to be met before a dentist can announce himself or herself a specialist. These eight specialties are as follows:

1. **Endodontics** is restricted to working with the *etiology* (causative factors), diagnosis, prevention, and treatment of diseases of the dental pulp; and with the effects of these diseases on the various structures that compose the pulp and periapical tissues.
2. **Dental Public Health** is confined to working with public education in dental health, prevention, and treatment programs for any department of health, whether it is supported by federal, state, county, or local governments.
3. **Oral and Maxillofacial Surgery** is restricted to the diagnosis of diseases, injuries, and defects of the human jaws and associated structures and treatment by surgical techniques.
4. **Oral Pathology** is restricted to the study of oral diseases, their diagnosis or identification, their causes, how they proceed, and what effect they produce, as well as their relationships to the rest of the body.
5. **Orthodontics** is restricted to correcting dental *anomalies,* which usually means improving the appearance and the ability to masticate of patients whose dental arches and/or jaws are malformed. The public generally refers to this process as "straightening teeth," but a much more complicated process is involved. This specialist must be skillful in understanding functions and aesthetics of teeth within the jaws and in correcting the relationships of upper and lower arches to create a pleasing outward appearance while providing the ability to masticate food effectively.
6. **Pedodontics** is restricted to dentistry for children. "It includes training the child to accept dentistry; restoring and maintaining the primary, mixed, and permanent dentitions; applying preventive measures for dental caries and periodontal disease; and preventing, intercepting, and correcting various problems of occlusion."[2]
7. **Periodontics** is restricted to the diagnosis, treatment, and prevention of diseases of the supporting structures of the teeth, including deviations from normal anatomy and physiology. The public commonly refers to all these diseases and problems under one misleading word, "pyorrhea."
8. **Prosthodontics** is restricted to the restoration and maintenance of oral function by the replacement of missing teeth and structures by artificial devices. It includes diagnosing, planning, preparing, and inserting suitable substitutes for one or more teeth and the associated tissues. Some of the devices are referred to as "fixed" because they are cemented permanently to existing teeth, but some replacements are removable. A full denture is the replacement for all the teeth in one arch; it restores aesthetics and function. The prosthetic replacement of part of the teeth in one arch is called a partial denture. An improper term for a denture is "plate." The three main branches of prosthodontics are fixed prosthodontics, removable prosthodontics, and maxillofacial prosthetics.

The dentist in general practice may refer patients to a specialist in the aforementioned fields, may ask for consultation regarding a particular case, or may ask for assistance from a specialist in a particular field in the normal conduct of dental practice.

Types of Practice

Whether general practitioners or specialists, dentists may have a private (solo) practice or belong to a group of dentists in what is called a group practice.

In a **solo practice,** as the name implies, a dentist is the only dentist in the office. The dentist owns the building or rents the space and alone is responsible for the dentistry performed in that office. The reception room may be shared with another dentist or a physician, but the practice is private—the dentist's own. Assistants may or may not be hired as the dentist chooses.

A **group practice** means a group of dentists work together under some plan on which they have agreed. It may be a group of specialists and generalists or it may be a group of general practitioners. Any agreement that is satisfactory to them is acceptable. They may share their reception room, office expenses, employees, a working code, and even their office space and/ or income. In this situation, several different group options are utilized. The group may be an association, a corporation, or a partnership, or one dentist may hire all the others. It is also possible that a group practice may include all kinds of health care treatment: physicians, dentists, etc. However, the laws for dentists forbid them to enter into a partnership for the practice of dentistry with anyone but a dentist. If the group practice includes physicians, it usually is an arrangement concerning the office space with each person practicing separately.

Some group practices have been established to provide dental care to a particular group of patients; that is, a union may establish a dental clinic to care for the needs of all union members.

One advantage of group practice is the ease of sharing off-hour emergency work. Each member of the group takes a turn at providing the evening or weekend emergency care that is necessary in any practice. (You may be called upon to assist during emergency service some evening or weekend.) Each dentist can more easily arrange time away from the office for personal improvement and vacations because his or her patients can receive care from other dentists in the group during his or her absence. Another advantage is the economic stability that occurs when a group shares the economic burden of the office overhead.

Perhaps of most importance to employees are the tax advantages accorded corporations and partnerships that permit the establishment of employee and employer fringe benefits; this awarding of benefits is quite impossible in a solo practice.

With each passing year there are more prepaid dental plans. These programs affect the type of dental practice because more patients request care. (It is free or less expensive.) Therefore, to meet the increased demand for dental care, more team dentistry is practiced. Since teams work together to provide the service, it is imperative that all team members understand and abide by the code of ethics that governs the practice of dentistry. The dentist is responsible for the actions of all team members who must also abide by the code of ethics for dentistry.

Principles of Ethics

A code of ethics is a statement of moral obligation. Most professions have developed some code of ethics. The health sciences policy in general applies to pharmacy, nursing, public health, dentistry, and medicine. Each profession is dedicated to the care of its area of responsibility in the overall health of the patient.

The code of ethics of the dental profession is a statement of the high principles by which dentists are expected to practice. The code has been developed by the ADA and regulates the conduct of dentists who are members of the organization.

The code of ethics is not to be confused with any legal regulations placed on dentistry by the communities in which dentistry is practiced. These laws are made by legislators and enforced by the community. The profession of dentistry imposes a stricter code of ethical conduct on dentists than the legal regulations imposed by communities.

The dentist is responsible for the actions of his or her employees. Therefore, the code of ethics is just as important for the employees to understand as for the dentist. Every employee must abide by these regulations just as the dentist must.

The practice of dentistry achieved the stature of a profession in the United States and acquired the three unfailing characteristics of a profession: education beyond the usual level, the primary duty of service to the public, and the right to self-government.

It is important that all dentists abide by *The Principles of Ethics* of the American Dental Association.

1. Education beyond the usual level is required. All dentists have the obligation of keeping their knowledge and skill current by continuing education throughout their professional lives.

2. Service to the public requires dentists to give the best service of which they are capable, and to avoid conduct which lowers the esteem of dentistry. They must not deny any patient service solely on the basis of the patient's race, creed, color, or national origin.
3. Government of a profession requires that all members of the profession participate in the organization of its society and abide by the society's rules of ethics.
4. The dentist should be a leader in the community in efforts to improve the dental health of the public, in addition to being a leader in other areas of service.
5. The dentist is obliged to provide emergency service for anyone requiring care; to then return the patient to his or her regular dentist and to provide that dentist with a report of the emergency treatment.
6. In the use of auxiliary personnel, the dentist has an obligation to protect the health of the patient by not delegating to anyone less qualified any service that requires the competence of the dentist. He or she must further prescribe and supervise the work of all auxiliary personnel.
7. The dentist has the obligation to seek consultation whenever the welfare of the patient will be advanced by such consultation. Treatment will not be undertaken by the consultant without the consent of the attending dentist.
8. The dentist may not criticize the work of another dentist orally or in writing to a member of the public. Lack of knowledge of the conditions under which the service was performed preclude judging the work. The dentist has an obligation to provide corrective treatment, but in such a way as to avoid reflection on the previous dentist or the dental profession. He or she is also required to cooperate with public officials and to provide expert testimony on request.
9. The dentist may not accept or tender rebates or split fees.
10. The dentist may not prescribe, dispense, or promote the use of drugs or other agents whose formulas are not available to all dentists—nor can he or she hold out as exclusive any agent, method, or technique.
11. Patents and copyrights may be secured, provided that they and the remuneration derived from them are not used to restrict research, practice, or benefits of the patented or copyrighted material.
12. Advertising should not be used.
13. Cards, letterheads, and announcements must be appropriate to the profession.
14. Office door lettering and signs should be of the size and style consistent with the dignity of the profession and the custom of the community.
15. A dentist may use his or her titles or degrees in connection with the practice of dentistry, but not in promotion of any commercial endeavor.
16. The dentist may participate in a program of health education of the public, providing it is in keeping with the dignity of the profession.
17. A dentist may contract with individuals and organizations to provide dental health care if the agreement is not in violation of *The Principles of Ethics.*
18. Only a dentist who limits practice exclusively to one of the special areas provided by the ADA can include a statement of this limitation on stationary, letterheads, cards, and directory listings. The phrase "Practice limited to . . ." is the preferred wording.
19. A directory listing must be available to all dentists in similar circumstances, and must be consistent in style with the custom of the dentists in the community.
20. Only when required by law can designations such as "Professional Corporation, Inc." or "Group Clinic" be used as the name of a practice.
21. Problems of ethics should be solved at the local level if possible. Only when absolutely necessary should they be appealed to the constituent society and the Judicial Council of the ADA.

Abiding by *The Principles of Ethics,* which have been evolved by the national and local dental organizations, dentists practice in any number of ways, depending on their modes of operation and choices of specialty. They maintain offices and hire personnel to complete their teams selected with consideration for their individual needs for assistance.

The Dental Health Team

Although a number of dentists still work alone, most dentists hire at least one assistant to provide certain services that relieve the dentist of interruptions at the chair. The concept of team dentistry has more frequently created the need for several assistants. Dentists usually staff their offices with team members who are educated in different specialties and, therefore, are able to make various contributions to the oral health care delivery team.

However many staff members the dentist hires, one fact is important to understand: the dentist alone is responsible for the diagnosis and treatment for each patient. Should any team member fail to perform accurately the work assigned, the dentist is responsible legally for whatever ills the patient experiences.

A team means a number of persons working together. The critical words are *working together*. A team means cooperation, getting a job done. In the dental office it is also necessary to perform this job harmoniously—with each team member carrying his or her responsibilities effectively so other team members can accomplish their parts of the joint effort.

The oral health team attempts to provide excellent care for each patient who enters the office. It is to be expected that a practicing dentist will have the team well organized, and a new assistant who enters the team relationship should be made aware of her or his place within the group. Perhaps nothing will be said about the "team," but it is hoped that the new assistant will feel the team spirit of these oral health care delivery team professionals.

What positions exist on the dental health team? How can one move from one position to another? The dentist is the captain of the team and he or she determines the work to be accomplished by others and then hires the assistants to fulfill these needs. The important factor is that a dentist is privileged to determine the needs to be met and to employ team members to meet those needs.

Many dental offices may have an office administrator who oversees the coordination of the efforts of all employees. Other employees may include the chairside assistant, hygienist, expanded duties assistants, laboratory technicians, and certain business office employees whose titles will vary from office to office. The most common titles in that group will be receptionist, bookkeeper, and patient educator. The office administrator may be the person whose responsibilities are reception of patients and/or bookkeeping and/or patient education. In some offices the office administrator will have separate responsibilities. All or some of these functions will be performed by other staff members. For purposes of clarifying specific tasks, we will consider the separate responsibilities of reception, bookkeeping, and patient education.

When patients enter a dental office, they may encounter members of the oral health care delivery team in this order: receptionist, bookkeeper, hygienist, patient educator, dental assistant or chairside assistant, coordinating assistant, laboratory assistant, expanded duties personnel, and laboratory technician.

The **receptionist** is a most important team member who plans the appointments, scheduling patients carefully so that time is not wasted. The receptionist is also responsible for the telephone—one of the most important instruments in the office since it is often the first contact a patient has with the office. From this first contact, the patient forms an opinion about the dental office and may confuse quality of dental care with the degree of friendliness experienced in the telephone contact. Through the use of the telephone, patients can be lost or gained, service can be rendered, or people turned away in frustration and anger.

The receptionist also greets patients and cares for anyone who enters the reception room, including salespersons and professional colleagues of the dentist.

Effective reception means that excellent communication techniques are developed so that patients enjoy coming to this particular office. The receptionist may also be responsible for making the financial arrangements during case presentations.

The **bookkeeper** may be the receptionist, or a full-time bookkeeper with no other responsibilities, or the dentist may utilize the services of an accounting firm. Some employee in the dental office will record and verify records of service and payments due and received.

The **secretarial assistant** performs all duties concerning the business side of dentistry. Often the receptionist and secretarial assistant are combined.

The **hygienist** is a certified and licensed employee of the dentist, permitted by state law to perform certain specific tasks under the direction of the dentist. Prophylaxis, taking dental X rays, and patient education are tasks that a hygienist may perform under the supervision of the dentist-employer. A minimum two-year course of study is necessary prior to certification or licensing.

The **patient educator** teaches home oral hygiene—preventive care of the mouth. The patient educator shows patients how to care for their mouths and how to keep them clean and well exercised at home so that the excellent restorations that are placed by the dentist receive proper maintenance between recalls.

Although treatment of disease is necessary, prevention is the first consideration for all diseases affecting the human body. Oral diseases are no exception.

If a disease can be prevented, treatment will not be necessary. If a disease is treated, the patient should be told how to avoid a recurrence. Oral health needs far exceed the ability of the dental profession to provide adequate treatment. It is the goal of the dental profession, therefore, not only to provide the necessary corrective treatment, but to prevent occurrence and recurrence by teaching good preventive dental care. Such preventive educational programs need professional guidance, a responsibility usually assigned to the auxiliaries on the team: the dental assistant, the dental hygienist, or, in many offices, the patient educator.

The **chairside assistant** sits beside the patient and is the dentist's second pair of hands—thus the common term "four-handed dentistry." The clinical assistant makes it possible for the dentist to maintain concentration in the patient's mouth by eliminating the need to reach for instruments or look away from the site of concentration. This assistant will anticipate the dentist's needs, will be ready to supply the materials as needed, and knows the routines as well as the dentist. Usually the dentist and clinical assistant develop a private communication system utilizing the turn of the hand, movement of the head, or even a short word such as "Now" to indicate the change in instrumentation or procedure.

A group practice may also employ a coordinating assistant and a laboratory assistant. The **coordinating assistant,** another chairside specialist, is an additional pair of hands to serve the clinical assistant who serves the dentist. The coordinating assistant learns to recognize the routines so well that the materials needed by the chair assistant are anticipated. The chair assistant never leaves the patient. The coordinating assistant is expected to supply anything not already at the chair. These two assistants in conjunction with the dentist provide what is known as "six-handed dentistry."

The **laboratory assistant** may spend the day in the dental laboratory, preparing impressions, waxing restorations, pouring models—doing any of the many tasks that are necessary to complete restorations the dentist is designing for patients.

New team members are being added as recognition of the need for their services develops. The new team members are referred to as **expanded duties personnel.** These assistants may perform some tasks for which they have been trained and certified as able to perform under the direction of the dentist. Dental assistants who take required courses and pass registration examinations are called **certified dental assistants.**

Formerly, an assistant was not permitted to work inside the mouth. Now the assistant can be trained in certain intraoral procedures to further expand the production capabilities of the dental team. There are several levels of expanded duties. It is conceivable that a good dental assistant can return to school from time to time to develop more skills. Given the desire, capacity, and determination, and by continuing to acquire education, such an assistant could become a dentist.

The **laboratory technician** may or may not be part of the office staff. If the dentist employs a laboratory technician and provides space in the office for laboratory work, then the laboratory technician is a member of that team. If the dentist prefers to utilize the services of a commercial laboratory, the team relationship may not be as evident, but nevertheless, cooperation and goodwill must exist.

The technician is trained to perform laboratory operations primarily concerned with the fabrication of appliances such as fixed and removable prostheses.

The oral health care delivery team may consist of the office administrator, the hygienist, the chair assistant, the coordinating assistant, expanded duties personnel, the patient educator, the receptionist, the bookkeeper, the secretarial assistant, and the laboratory technician—all directed by the dentist.

Not members of the office team, but closely associated with the team, are persons who assist the team.

Dental supply salespersons call on the office regularly and can ease the ordering of supplies.

Detail persons are special dental supply employees who frequently visit the offices with the salespersons. These specialists are informed about new products or instruments that the supply house is promoting.

Manufacturers of dental equipment are not as likely to visit the dental office, but their representatives often show new equipment. Sometimes the dental supply salesperson is also a representative of equipment manufacturers. These firms often do extensive research for dentistry and aid in the promotion of new methods of doing dentistry.

The Role of the Dental Assistant

Dental assistants most certainly play an important role and assume ever-increasing responsibilities on the team. This book is written for the beginning dental assistant who must experience training either in school or in the dental office.

The individual whose interests indicate that a career in dental assisting would be desirable is likely to find dental assisting a career of intense personal satisfaction.

Let us look at the role of the beginning dental assistant.

A dental assistant is usually a person with a constitution of steel, a good sense of humor, a pleasant personality, and a sense of enjoyment in serving people.

Do you feel happy when you help someone with a problem that he or she cannot solve alone? When another human being looks at you, smiles, and says, "Thanks! That was a big help to me!" do you feel personal satisfaction?

That's the way a good dental assistant can feel every day because the daily routine includes helping people to be more comfortable and healthier even though they may not always smile their appreciation.

Work opportunities: Where can you find a position as a dental assistant? You will readily think of working for a dentist in either solo or group practice, but there are other fields for your consideration.

Federal agencies offer jobs in clinics and hospitals where dental assistants are employed.

The armed services employ dental assistants. Often these jobs are assigned to members of the armed services, so that to be eligible one must join the specific service.

Children's hospitals may maintain dental clinics for their patients.

University dental schools employ dental assistants in TEAM (Training in Expanded Auxiliary Management) and DAU (Dental Auxiliary Utilization) clinics to assist in training dental students in four- and six-handed dentistry.

Further education can lead to a position as an educator who trains dental assistants in dental assistant teaching programs.

Duties in the Dental Office

Should your decision be to work in a private office, what duties can you expect? The dental assistant may be the only employee in the office

assisting at the chair,
receiving patients,
attending to the secretarial duties,
keeping the financial records, and
making appointments.

In an office where there are more employees, one may be a chair assistant who assists only at the chair and perhaps performs some laboratory work.

If there are two or more assistants, the second assistant may be a receptionist and office administrator, caring for the business routines of the office.

If multiple assistants are used, the assignment usually will be specific at the time the assistant is hired, such as chair assistant, coordinating assistant, or receptionist. The assignment will be made on the basis of the education and certification of the individual employee.

The job of the dental assistant is primarily to save the dentist's time; to do for the dentist those things which do not require professional dental training and would interrupt the actual production of dental work for patients. Secondarily, the dental assistant aids directly in the production of dental services at the chair. There are hundreds of duties, operations, techniques, instruments, medications, and other details to learn. No single operation is an exact replication of another; no two patients are just alike in their reactions or needs. Remember that, in spite of its complexity, learning this work can become confusing only if you let it become so.

No matter how complete your education, the dentist for whom you work may perform dentistry differently from the way it is performed in your school. Your job will be easier to learn if you take one operation at a time and learn thoroughly what is required for it and what it is meant to accomplish. Then, and only then, learn a new operation. Aim for the ability to anticipate the needs of the dentist in your preparations in the office. Learn to work in close harmony with the dentist. If you first understand just what a particular job is meant to accomplish, you will approach your part of it with more confidence and understanding. Consequently, you will be able to assist more successfully.

While no single dental service is an exact repetition when performed for different patients, there are certain basic details that will be repeated routinely. You can learn these basic points for any given operation. Experience will teach you how to take care of the variable elements of all operations. That phase of the work will come with time and intelligent observation on your part. Always prepare everything that is normally required for an operation. Be prepared to handle the unusual quickly on request, or, if possible, before such request—upon observing its need.

The outlines of routine dental operations in the text are given as examples to aid in breaking down your particular office routine. It is not possible to write outlines of procedure that will satisfy all dentists. Nearly all dental offices have differences in procedure to some extent in the way patients are treated, in the way an inlay preparation or an amalgam preparation is made, or in the manner the practice is conducted. It is your duty to fit into an office, not to revolutionize it—unless you are specifically invited to reorganize some phase. There are many paths to the same goal. There are many ways, for example, to construct full upper and lower dentures. Adapt yourself to the routines your dentist desires.

Memorize one basic routine at a time. Learn by name the instruments, materials, or medications required for that routine; learn the sequence of their use and where each belongs in the cabinet or laboratory before proceeding to another routine. Ask all the questions you feel are necessary, but cultivate the note-taking habit so that you will not find it necessary to ask the same question twice.

To repeat, *the object in having a dental assistant in the first place is to save time*. The more time you save your dentist, the better assistant you are. You are there to help the dentist; the more quickly you learn the various routines and the more rapidly you perform each one, the better you are doing your job. Whatever your work of the moment, learn to do it rapidly and thoroughly.

Make it your objective to know your work to the last detail, to maintain a constant interest in the patient as an individual, to do each job quietly and efficiently, and to be part of a smooth-running organization.

The Professional Dental Assistant

A profession requires that the person received education beyond the usual level, that the primary duty is service to the public, and that the profession as a whole has the right to govern itself. Dentistry is a profession. The dental assistants who are part of the oral health care team are also professionals. The organization that has helped most to elevate dental assisting to the status of a profession is the American Dental Assistants Association.

This organization, formed in 1924, has established educational requirements whereby a dental assistant can become a *Certified Dental Assistant*. The rise in status of the dental assistant can be largely attributed to the dedicated individuals who have worked diligently as members of the American Dental Assistants Association. In 1960 the goal of certification and educational requirements for the dental assistant was established by action of the American Dental Association.

Since then a Certified Dental Assistant must have completed an accredited educational program prior to taking the certification examination. A Certified Dental Assistant must enroll in continuing educational programs to remain currently certified.

The Dental Assistant, the journal of the American Dental Assistants Association, is a most helpful publication that you can read regularly. When you have become eligible for membership and actually join the American Dental Assistants Association, you receive this periodical. Reading the journal, attending meetings, and continuing to study all help one to improve professional skills.

Good professionals continue to read current literature concerning their profession. The library of the American Dental Association provides such services. This library is one of the finest in the nation, and books are regularly loaned through mail services. It is not possible to exhaust your opportunities to know more about your work.

Join your Dental Assistants Association and take an active part in its programs and functions. Cultivate a feeling of enthusiasm about your work and about the dental profession.

Know that you have an important part in providing a very necessary service to humanity.

Ethics for the Dental Assistant

Regardless of the size of the office staff with which you work, there are certain principles of behavior to be observed. A standard of professional conduct in keeping with the high principles of dental ethics is required.

The American Dental Assistants Association has formulated this Code of Ethics:

Objectives

The objectives of this Association shall be to continue to share in the responsibility for quality dental health care delivery to all Americans, to ensure the professional welfare of American Dental Assistants Association members and all dental assistants, to advance the practice of dental assisting toward the highest standards of performance attainable, to provide quality continuing education which will enhance the knowledge, skills, and professional growth of the dental assistant, and to communicate effectively with all members of health related professions and the consumer public.

Principles of Ethics

1. Conduct of Members. The conduct of every member shall be governed by the Principles of Ethics of the American Dental Assistants Association and of the constituent association and component society within which jurisdiction the member is located. The member shall maintain honesty in all things, obedience to the dental practice act of the state in which employed, and adherence to the professional ethics required by the employer.
2. Obligations. Every member of this Association shall have the obligation to:
   A. Hold in confidence the details of professional services rendered by any employer and the confidences of any patient.
   B. Increase abilities and skills by seeking additional education in the dental assisting field.
   C. Refrain from performing any service which requires the professional competence of a dentist or is prohibited by the dental practice act of the state in which the member is employed.

D. Participate actively in the efforts of this Association and the constituent associations and component societies to improve the educational status of the dental assistant.

E. Support these Principles of Ethics and the Pledge.

3. Use of the Title, "Certified Dental Assistant." Those dental assistants who hold certificates issued for the current year by the Certifying Board for the Dental Assisting Professions may use the title "Certified Dental Assistant" in connection with employment and Association activities.

4. Dental Assistants' Pledge. The following shall be the official pledge of the American Dental Assistants Association as written by Dr. Charles Nelson Johnson of Chicago, Illinois, first advisor to the Association:

"I solemnly pledge that, in the practice of my profession I will always be loyal to the welfare of the patients who come under my care, and to the interest of the practitioner whom I serve. I will be just and generous to the members of my profession, aiding them and lending them encouragement to be loyal, to be just, to be studious. I hereby pledge to devote my best energies to the service of humanity in that relationship of life to which I consecrated myself when I elected to become a dental assistant."

In providing a service to the public, as in the dental office, it is inevitable that you will come into contact with much information that is to be treated with the strictest confidence. The personal records that the office keeps of the dental work, physical history, and details of the patient are the property of the dentist, not of the patient. This does not imply freedom to use such information for any purpose other than that for which it is intended. There is no justification ever for reporting outside the office the slightest bit of information you have learned while in the office. It is confidential information. Treat it as such.

Records should not be left where a patient might see and (with a natural curiosity) read them, whether they are those of that patient or of another patient. Always place them in such a position as to make it inconvenient for the patient to see the records.

A nationally syndicated columnist published a letter in which the writer expressed anger. She was employed in the downtown area of a city. At lunch the dental assistants, lawyers' secretaries, medical assistants, a minister's secretary, and nurses with whom she ate were always discussing over the luncheon table the personal business of patients and clients. She was angry because she felt that there was nowhere she could go for care of her personal health problems, religious problems, or legal problems, and feel that the matter would be treated confidentially. From the points of view of the dentist who is pledged to confidential care and the patient who is at the mercy of the dentist and staff, this accusation could not be more serious. Be certain that you do not fall into this category of thoughtless assistants. Remember, *what you see here, what you hear here, what you do here, stays here when you leave here.*

Being a dental assistant is somewhat like being an ambassador in a foreign country. An ambassador attempts to create an excellent impression so that people who meet him or her will think highly of his or her country. Ask yourself, What kind of impression am I creating for my dentist? What kind of impression am I creating for my profession of dentistry?

Before dentists can practice dentistry they must have patients. What brings patients to the dentist? What causes them to return to that particular dental office?

You yourself become one of the personal advertisements of the office for which you work. In your contacts outside that office, you can do much to bring patients into it; your conduct inside the office can do much to keep those patients who do come. Psychology applied to working with people is of prime importance in all walks of life; and under the conditions of the dental office, it cannot be overemphasized. In Part 2 you will find practical guides for your work with patients.

The dental team members will learn much about the dentist for whom they work. Every phase of the dentist's life becomes known to them to some degree. It is never wise to indicate that you know any of these details. They are not subjects for comment. The dentist knows that you will learn many of these details, but also prefers that you ignore the information. The dental assistant who lives with others (family or friends) sometimes finds it difficult to resist the curiosity expressed about patients, office details, and the dentist. Make it a habit to divulge no information. Again, you have no justification ever for reporting outside the office the slightest bit of information you have learned while in that office.

The dentist and dental assistant are necessarily in a closely interdependent relationship for a considerable part of each day. This in itself tends to produce frictions, the severity of which is governed by the adjustment of the personalities involved. It would be unusual to have every day, week after week, month after month, year after year, go by without occasional irritation. If all office relationships are maintained on a plane of harmony and teamwork, and if there is as little interjection of personal elements as possible, the dentist-assistant team has the best opportunity for continuous harmonious association. Should it become evident that the personalities of the dentist and assistant are not compatible, it is far preferable to terminate the association than to continue to work under conditions that are not pleasant. Moreover, any such friction in the office is very soon evident to patients.

Familiarity can breed contempt. It is best to apply the same principle to the relationship of dentist and assistant. For example, the dentist's spouse should always remain "Mrs. Smith" or "Mr. Smith" to the dental assistant unless there is an extremely strong reason for the relationship to reach the familiarity of first names.

However familiar the office staff may be with each other when by themselves, the dentist should be addressed as "Doctor" when in the presence of patients: "This material is ready, Doctor." When speaking about the dentist, refer to him or her as "Doctor Raeywen." "Doctor Raeywen will see you at three o'clock, Mrs. Jones." It is best to retain this terminology at all times in the office.

The patient's impression of the dentist often begins with the patient's contact with the dental assistant—first on the telephone and later in the reception room. If the telephone contact is effective, the patient looks forward to seeing the office. The condition of the reception room affects his or her impression, but the attitude of the dental assistant can reinforce or obliterate that impression. Therefore, the standard of conduct of the dental assistant should be that which is expected in a professional office: dignified, efficient, tactful—but friendly.

Authority on dentistry. Dental assistants become authorities about dentistry the moment they are hired—whether or not they have any dental knowledge. Patients and often friends assume that assistants are authorities on dentistry regardless of the amount of knowledge the assistants may have acquired. People ask assistants questions about dentistry and believe the answers. Dental assistants must, therefore, be very careful to recognize their responsibilities to the community, and to remember their legal limitations in diagnosis and prescription. (For a discussion of the legal problems dental assistants may experience, study chapter 4, "Dental Jurisprudence.")

Personal Impression Created by the Dental Assistant

The impression that we create on others is determined by our personal appearance and our ability to express ourselves bodily and vocally. A good dental assistant creates a favorable impression on the people who enter the office.

In order to create this impression, there are certain matters that must be given careful attention.

Grooming

To create a good impression on patients, scrupulous personal grooming is essential in the dental office.

In dental assisting cleanliness is important. You are in very close contact with humans all day long. A thoroughly clean body to begin the day will help keep you refreshing in your contacts. It would be advisable for every dental assistant to have a soapy shower or tub bath each morning prior to leaving for work. (This, incidentally, is a delightful habit. It is refreshing and leaves one's body feeling wonderful—a luxury we all ought to enjoy.) With the soaps available today, most of the body odor is controlled for a twenty-four-hour period. If your problem is especially difficult, use a good deodorant immediately after your bath, and you will be pleasant to be near for the entire time you are at the office. Of course, a clean body should be put into all clean clothing.

If you have any special problems with body odor, be sure to take extra precautions with special deodorants. Use unscented products because many patients are allergic to perfumes and colognes. No perfume or cologne is best for the dental office where you are in such close proximity to patients. If you must use perfume or cologne, use it sparingly and only perfume with a mild scent. Remember that perfume and cologne never completely masks odors and to some people perfuming the odors only makes them more nauseating.

It is also important to shampoo your hair at least weekly. Some people find it necessary to shampoo every day if they have problems with excessive oil. Our world today is full of smog and dirt; therefore, a weekly shampoo is a must. Needless to say, tidy hair is important. A simple hairstyle is probably most acceptable in the dental office—nothing that would interfere with good assisting. It is difficult to be touching your hair to keep it coiffed and to assist at the chair at the same time. Hair and mouths simply do not go together!

In recapitulation, then, dental assistants must be scrupulously neat about their persons. Their work brings them into close contact with patients throughout the day, and they are always under critical observation. Here are a dozen reminders:

1. Uniform. Color is being used more frequently for dental uniforms. The traditional white uniform for the dental assistant is still preferred by many dentists, but in a number of offices dentists are substituting color. The psychological reason

lies in part in children's association between white and the nurse or physician who has given them a "shot" that has caused pain. It is also possible that some adult patients may subconsciously feel this discomfort with white. Regardless of the color of the uniform that your office requires, cleanliness is of utmost importance. An extra uniform at the office is a necessity in case there should be an accident that makes it desirable to change during the day.

2. If your uniform is a white dress, your slip should be white also, since colored slips under white uniforms are unattractive. Of course it must be of the correct length, ending in the hemline of the uniform so that it does not show above the hem nor hang below the uniform.

3. Hose should be of a light color. White hose, if preferred, are deductible from income tax as a professional expense. One pair per week is allowed.

4. Shoes. If your uniform is white, white shoes, kept white and in good repair, are in order. Whatever color the shoes required in your office, they ought to be of a conservative type and properly groomed. If you have two pair for use on alternate days, they last longer and give your feet a much needed rest. White shoes are deductible from your income tax as a professional expense.

5. Neat hair. If a cap is not part of the uniform, a hairnet should be worn if there is any question of loose strands.

6. Fingernails should be scrupulously clean, neatly trimmed, and not an excessive length. Use only clear or natural polish if you choose to wear polish. Hands should be kept clean throughout the day. Wash before assisting at the chair and before handling instruments that are to be used.

7. Cosmetics should be used sparingly and in good taste. Remember that the dental assistant receives very close scrutiny. Makeup that might be acceptable when viewed from some distance may not look very attractive when seen at twelve or fifteen inches.

8. Avoid perfume and cologne if at all possible. If not, use only mild, faint scented products. Be certain that the deodorant you use is effective. Perfume or cologne is not a substitute for a bath and a good deodorant.

9. Jewelry, except for a wristwatch (preferably with a sweep-second hand), should not be worn. Mercury, used in most dental offices, is extremely detrimental to gold. Dental assistants who are married may wish to wear wedding rings in the office. Considering the problem with mercury, it would be wise to wear an inexpensive substitute during office hours.

10. Avoid chewing gum. It is offensive to many patients.

11. Wear an apron for the initial daily office dusting.

12. Give yourself a double check on your appearance before receiving the first morning patient. The dental assistant should be able to finish the office-opening duties and verify personal grooming before the first patient arrives.

Inadvertent Communication

In addition to grooming, our ability to express ourselves—bodily and vocally—determines the impression we make on others. The way we walk, hold our heads, use our hands, our eyes, and our shoulders gives those we meet emotional impressions that may speak louder than our voices. The tone with which we greet people often implies more than the words we say. It indicates our mental attitude and provokes a similar response from the person we address. If you speak pleasantly, people are inclined to respond pleasantly. It also helps to look directly into the patient's eyes as you speak.

Watch several strangers walk down the street. Some have good posture and carry their bodies easily; some slouch forward, their eyes on the ground; some stride forward, shoulders back, fists clenched, chin out. Each suggests something about his or her mental attitude—from timidity and fear to belligerence.

Good posture, maintained with an appearance of ease, is the foundation for all good public impression. It suggests self-confidence.

The appearance of lightness on the feet may be attained by practicing this one exercise: Imagine that a wire is attached to your sternum (breastbone), lifting you until the soles of your shoes barely touch the floor. Walk around feeling this sense of "lift." Practice several times daily until the walk becomes automatic.

If properly done, the result will be excellent posture, maintained with ease. Add a cheery smile and a friendly eye contact. You express self-confidence and such radiance that people will enjoy being near you. This manner is the basis for pleasant office and patient relationships. Remember, those who listen to us speak learn what kind of persons we are from the tone we use, the formation of our words, the rapidity with which we speak, and our choice of words. Study the chapter on communications to improve your speaking and listening abilities.

From the foregoing discussions of the role of the dental assistant, we can list these ideas as a guide for conduct until the necessary code of behavior becomes a matter of routine. The office assistant:

1. Should be dignified but not pompous or belittling of patients.
2. Should be clean and neat.
3. Should behave in a manner befitting the principles laid down in Dental Ethics.
4. Must be accurate in the performance of any services requested.
5. Should maintain dignified, courteous relationships with all patients, and with the oral health care delivery team.
6. Has a responsibility to the community because the community considers the dental assistant an authority on dentistry. People will ask questions about dentistry and believe the answers. The assistant must remember the legal limitations in diagnosis and prescription, the responsibilities to the community, and avoid any detrimental comments.
7. Never criticize the dentist to a patient.
8. Remembers: What you see here, what you hear here, what you do here, stays here when you leave here. Any information that a dental assistant sees or hears at the office is confidential information and should never be divulged or commented upon anywhere.

The Desirable Team Member

Whenever people work together, it is necessary to observe some courtesies in order to make it possible for each individual to experience the personal satisfactions that make life enjoyable.

In the dental office, one is often forced to be physically close to other team members and to patients. Such closeness can cause irritation because people need a certain amount of space between themselves and others. This personal space varies with the country in which a person has been raised. For example, in South American countries it is customary for people to be very close. In the northern half of the Western Hemisphere more distance between people is customary. If someone moves closer than eighteen inches to a North American, usually the person whose personal space has been invaded finds himself feeling some irritation. Members of the

dental health team need to recognize this characteristic of our society and make allowance for it when working with patients and with each other. Personal space invaded slowly is less offensive than abrupt encroachment (see chap. 6, "Communicating and Interacting with People," for a more detailed discussion of space needs).

It is also desirable for a team member to be alert to signals from other team members. Sometimes the turn of a hand can mean it is time for a new instrument to be placed in the dentist's hand. Sensitivity to these signals makes for effective teamwork.

Cooperating with the Team

The dental health team has a job to do for the patient. The very reason for the existence of the team is that patient . . . that human being. It is necessary to remember this fact instead of considering the patients as so many cases, numbers, or inanimate objects to be pushed hear and there.

In a well-planned and well-run dental office, each staff member will have explicit instructions about his or her particular duties. It is important to have each team member willing to fit into the pattern of the whole and to work with each other instead of against each other. There must, of necessity, be some flexibility in schedules. There are emergencies that need to be properly handled; there are delays that prevent a dentist from remaining on time; there are patients in pain for whom no time was reserved in the original schedule. It takes good teamwork to handle these upsets in the daily routine, otherwise one member of the team will be unduly burdened or unpleasant frictions will occur. One of the best ways to handle the team effort is to have a written schedule for the team as a whole. This schedule or office administration plan will be discussed later in specific detail.

The comfort and security of the patient are to be uppermost in the minds of the office personnel as they receive, care for, and dismiss patients. An atmosphere of harmony will greatly add to the patient's contentment. There are ten suggestions for team members to remember about their teammates and how to make the team effort profitable and satisfying. The general ideas behind these ten points will be discussed at greater length in the chapter on psychology; but briefly, here are ten ideas:

1. Emphasize the competence of the person.
2. Feel pride in team accomplishments—and allow each person an opportunity to share your feelings. People react favorably to a smooth-working team. Praise your teamwork whenever you can.

3. Make it easier for everyone to accept themselves as they are.
4. Make them feel smile-deserving.
5. Encourage others to express their doubts and disagreements about your suggestions. Only by their expressions of these doubts and disagreements will you really understand your differences and be able to help create a harmonious atmosphere.
6. Ask for regularly scheduled staff conferences at which time everyone's satisfactions and discomforts with the working conditions can be discussed calmly. (Even one assistant and one dentist can have a regularly scheduled staff conference.)
7. Be consistent and dependable.
8. Avoid absenteeism.
9. Create a permissive atmosphere— permissive for creative breakthroughs in working out the techniques that will allow you to assist your dentist more effectively.
10. Show and express your appreciation for your teammates.

Summary

The rapid changes that have occurred in the world today have created changes in the delivery of dental services. *Team* is the concept most frequently utilized in dentistry today.

The purpose of dentistry is to serve the public by:

1. Assisting patients to maintain good oral health
2. Assisting patients to maintain the ability to masticate (chew) food throughout life
3. Assisting patients to maintain or to improve personal appearance
4. Assisting patients to avoid oral diseases and pain by practicing preventive dentistry
5. Assisting patients by providing relief from oral pain

There is more demand for dental care today due to changes in education of patients and in economic benefits for certain groups of people through third-party payments.

Both solo and group practices now utilize dental teams. Ethics by which the dentist must abide must be observed by the team members since the dentist is responsible for the actions of all employees.

There are eight dental specialties at present: endodontics, dental public health, oral and maxillofacial surgery, oral pathology, orthodontics, pedodontics, periodontics, and prosthodontics.

The oral health care delivery team may utilize the services of the dentist, hygienist, chairside clinical assistant, coordinating assistant, expanded duties personnel, laboratory assistant, office administrator, receptionist, bookkeeper, patient educator, and secretary. The dentist organizes the team and decides what auxiliaries to hire.

Dental assistants have the responsibilities of professionals and should join the ADAA and continue to upgrade their education.

A dental assistant is thought to be an authority by laypersons and, therefore, must be careful about inadvertently diagnosing or prescribing.

The personal impression created by the dental assistant is a factor that affects patients and therefore must be given consideration. Further, all dental health team members must remember and practice the rule, *what you see here, what you hear here, what you do here, stays here when you leave here.*

Consideration of the fact that patients are human beings is a very important attitude for all dental assistants to possess.

Observing certain standards of conduct and personal habits when in the dental office increases the effectiveness of the service rendered to patients.

Team members need to work together for a harmonious and efficient atmosphere. Ten suggestions are given for better team relationships.

Study Questions

1. What can dentistry do for patients?
2. How can patients be served best?
3. Why does a dentist hire assistants?
4. What is a specialist? What are the dental specialties?
5. What are third-party payments?
6. What is an oral health care delivery team? What positions are found on the team?
7. What are the ethics by which a dentist practices?
8. What future is there for dental assistants?
9. What standards of conduct are important for a dental assistant? Why are they important?
10. Why is grooming important?
11. What are the essentials for good grooming in the dental office?
12. What is *inadvertent communication?* Why is it important?
13. What is a desirable team member?
14. How does one help to make a good team?

Vocabulary

aesthetically   relating to beauty and the beautiful

anamoly   deviation from the normal

diagnosis   the recognition of the diseases present

etiology   causative factors of a disease

group practice   a group of dentists who work together under a plan they have set up

masticate   to chew

oral   refers to mouth

overhead   business expenses for operation of the dental office

ptyalin   an amylase found in saliva; an amylase is an enzyme which helps break down starches and glycogen

third-party payment   payment made by someone who does not receive the service, such as government agencies, unions, employers, or insurance carriers

CHAPTER 2

The Profession of Dentistry: Past

Ancient History
The Middle Ages
The Eighteenth Century
The Nineteenth Century
    Education and Publications
    Innovators and Progression of the Profession
    Anesthesia
The Twentieth Century
    The Profession
    Growth of Preventive Dentistry
    Professional Advances
    Materials and Equipment for Dentistry

Today, dentistry is a profession requiring highly skilled personnel. It has evolved from primitive attempts to alleviate pain in the mouth. Archeological findings indicate that prehistoric man suffered from dental decay, impacted teeth, severe attrition (wearing down by friction), and abscesses. Toothache seems to have been with us since the beginning of humankind.

In very early recorded history, the practice of the healing arts was intermixed and confused with religious activities. Incantations were often a method of treatment. When a person became ill, it was usually assumed that it was punishment because the gods were displeased. Considering that nothing was known about causative factors in disease, this association with the supernatural was to be expected. The priests, therefore, were the first to be associated with treatment for disease. Treatment consisted of incantations and sacrifices, and occasionally the application of some type of remedy that over the years had been helpful either in fact or in fancy.

As records gradually accumulated, the effectiveness of certain methods or materials in the treatment of specific diseases became evident. As information was passed on to succeeding religious leaders, treatments became more and more specific, and eventually they were separated from the religious element. Such work was then carried on entirely by individuals trained for it.

Ancient History

The recorded history of dentistry begins 7000 years ago in the valley of the Euphrates, known now as Iraq.

5000 B.C.

Clay tablets found by archeologists were the written records of dental-medical history and treatment. One such tablet stated that a parasite worm ate the teeth of humans, causing decay and toothache. This, the most ancient theory of the cause of dental decay, continued to be believed for over 6500 years—until A.D. 1504. (In primitive societies today the legend of the worm is still believed.)

The clay tablets also record some form of alleviation or treatment for pain and decay, including incantations to the gods to destroy the tooth-eating worm.

4000–3000 B.C.

Records of dental treatment were written by several peoples: Egyptian, Chinese, Phoenician, Etruscan, and Indian.

India: Frayed twigs were used for tooth brushes. Dental surgeons removed tartar, extracted teeth, treated pyorrhea, and used dental instruments.

2700 B.C.

China: Nine types of toothache and three types of oral disease were described. Treatment included quaint medications and acupuncture. (Twenty-six sites for needle insertions for toothache and six for gum disease were suggested.) Indian hemp (hashish or marijuana) was used as an anesthetic.

754 B.C.

Etruria: (The Etruscans lived in what is known now as Tuscany, in the middle of Italy.)

Twenty-five centuries ago the **Etruscan** dentists practiced a system of bridgework; they had outstanding skill and craftsmanship for their times. They made dental prostheses, using gold wire to hold the replacement teeth together. The dentists used a large ox tooth as the substance from which they carved the replacement teeth. The appliance that has received the greatest notoriety is a prosthesis for four teeth—upper central incisors and a second bicuspid. These four pontics are held together by pure gold bands neatly soldered together. Three additional bands held the appliance in place.

A preventive appliance, apparently made to keep the teeth steady and to prevent their loss, was also found.

The process of replacing teeth was also utilized by the **Phoenicians** and **Egyptians.** Usually the replacements were made of ivory or bone.

460–377 B.C.

Greece: Hippocrates, the father of medicine, described the practice of tooth extraction for alleviation of pain, but cautioned about post-extraction infections that sometimes followed. He placed great importance on the role of unhealthy teeth in disease. He developed appliances to remedy fractures, used forceps, compounded a dentifrice, and developed a mouth wash. Dental ethics began with Hippocrates. The Hippocratic Oath, which he wrote, is the basis for both dental and medical ethics in the United States today.

384–322 B.C.

Aristotle wrote about comparative anatomy. He explained dental anatomy, although some of his ideas were erroneous. (For example, he stated that men had more teeth than women.) He also suggested that soft, sweet figs damage the teeth because particles become lodged in the teeth and gums and cause putrifactive processes to occur.

330–250 B.C.

Forceps for the removal of teeth were mentioned in Greek writings. Before forceps, knocking out teeth was the primary method of removal.

25 B.C.–A.D. 50

Celsus, author of *De Medicine,* included a description of an orthodontic treatment.

A.D. 131

Asia Minor: Claudius Galen, born in Asia Minor in A.D. 131, was one of the great physicians of early times. (There is some dissention among authorities concerning the date of Galen's birth. We have quoted the date according to Vicenzo Guerini.) Galen spoke of nerves in the teeth, of removing caries with files, and of using other dental treatments. He performed successful operations on cleft lips. He wrote of remedies for specific dental problems, including these: "Drill a hole in a tooth if the tooth aches," and "Make a paste of honey and put it in the cavity in a tooth."[1]

Obviously, dental treatment was recorded all over the world in ancient times.

The Middle Ages

The Middle Ages include the sixth to the fifteenth centuries. Dentistry became a separate profession around A.D. 1500. More advances were recorded in Asia than in Europe. References were made to prosthetic replacement, replantation of teeth, and correction of irregular teeth. Beginning references were made to filling materials and use of dental instruments such as scalers. **France:** References occurred to dental specialties and a special practitioner called a *dentista.*

1425–1519

Leonardo da Vinci, a famous Italian artist, engineer, genius, and scientist, accurately drew the skull, teeth, and associated parts, realizing normal occlusion. He also described and pictured the maxillary sinus (a space existing within the cheekbone, directly above the bicuspid and molar area in the head). His description was written more than a hundred years before Nathanial Highmore's description gave the sinus the name of Antrum of Highmore.

1500–1571

Benvenuto Cellini, an Italian sculptor and worker in gold, invented a method of casting gold into molds. The beginning of gold inlay work can be credited to him.

1510–1590

Ambrose Paré, a French surgeon, is known as the father of modern surgery. He described the transplantation of teeth but did not perform this operation himself. He explained that a princess once had an extraction, and one of her ladies supplied an immediate replacement that later took root.

He also described the first known prosthetic appliance to replace the palate bone (for a cleft palate), and another to replace a large part of the tongue.

1602

Pieter van Foreest, a professor in Leyden, Holland, described an endodontic treatment, including method and materials to be used.

1683

Anthony van Leeuwenhoek, who lived in Delft, Holland, described for the first time the presence of minute "animacules" in the debris about the human teeth. He wrote, "The number of these animacules in the scurf of a man's teeth are so many that I believe they exceed the number of men in the kingdom."[2]

The Eighteenth Century

France: The Cradle of Modern Dentistry is the name given to France, the country where major developments occurred, including the first legislation for the practice of dentistry. Thus, dentistry became a more independent profession.

1728

Pierre Fauchard (1690–1761) was called the father of modern scientific dentistry. He authored an outstanding volume on dentistry, written in 1723 and published in 1728, *Le Chirurgien Dentiste ou traité des dents.* Fauchard's most important work was the establishment of dentistry as a specialized branch of medicine and the publication of the backbone of research to uphold this fact. *Le Chirurgien Dentiste ou traité des dents* included boards of examination, dissertations on orthodontia, surgery, implantation of teeth, periodontia, reflex pains due to teeth, dental anatomy, pathology, dental medicines, operative dentistry including a discussion of caries, filling materials, and prosthetic dentistry. He was the founder of modern scientific dentistry, because he created a special department of the healing arts called dentistry.

1771–1778

England: John Hunter developed two texts on dentistry, one in 1771 and the second in 1778. However, he was not a dentist, but a surgeon to the English Army. He described pyorrhea and alveoli. The descriptions are still valid today.

1752

The United States: John Baker, trained in medicine in England, arrived in the United States, began practicing dentistry, and then taught others—including Paul Revere.

1766

The practice of competent dentistry began in the United States. Until this time there were hardly any persons performing dentistry who had been trained to do so, but at this point, those who were skilled were training others in the skills and arts necessary to perform competent dentistry. Some years would pass before most dentists would be educated, but in 1766 the beginning of competency was seen.

1790

John Greenwood (1760–1819) was one of several dentists who served George Washington. Dr. Greenwood was trained by Dr. Baker. He, in turn, taught other dentists, including Horace Hayden in 1800. In 1790 Dr. Greenwood developed the foot drill.

The Nineteenth Century

With the 1800s dentistry in America began to improve markedly. The center of advancement in dentistry was shifting to America. Some dentists were itinerant dentists, traveling from one community to another. The itinerant dentists may have had no training or they may have been taught by some other dentist. If one dentist trained another, it was customary for him to issue a certificate of training to his trainee.

Education and Publications

Soon, however, attention was to be centered on education.

1801

Skinner wrote the first dental book printed in the United States. He titled it *A Treatise on Human Teeth, Concisely Explaining Their Structures and Cause of Disease and Decay.*

1821–1825

Horace Hayden, M.D., D.D.S., lectured at the University of Maryland. He was the first registered dental practitioner in the United States and, with Chapin Harris, he founded the first dental school in the world, The Baltimore College of Dental Surgery. The University of Maryland School of Dentistry proudly states today that they are the oldest dental school in the world because the Baltimore College of Dental Surgery became the Dental School of the University of Maryland, which was founded in 1840.

1839

The first dental magazine, *The American Journal of Dental Science,* was published; and the first dental society in the United States, The American Society of Dental Surgeons, was organized.

1844

Dr. Samuel Stockton White founded the S. S. White Dental Manufacturing Company in Philadelphia and started the *Dental News Letter* soon thereafter. Later, the *Dental News Letter* was united with the *Journal of the American Dental Association* (1937).

1845

The Ohio Dental College opened its doors in Cincinnati and twenty-one years later graduated the first woman dentist, Lucy Hobbs.

1867

Nathan Keep of Boston succeeded in his work to establish the Harvard Dental School—the first dental school to form an integral part of a university. Dr. Keep had taken a degree in medicine from Harvard in 1827 to be better prepared to carry on his dental practice, and thus became interested in a college for dentists.

Innovators and Progression of the Profession

1822

John Cardette received the John Scott Legacy for the Encouragement of Useful Inventions in the Arts and Sciences. He also received twenty dollars for his work with dentures. He was the first to apply the principle of suction to promote denture retention and thus dispense with spiral springs.

1803

Johann Serre introduced a conical screw for the removal of roots. It is still an accepted practice today.

1810

Simon Hullihan (1810–1857) was born in West Virginia. He became known as the father of oral surgery in the United States.

1828

James Garretson (1828–1895) was responsible for the recognition of oral surgery as a specialty by the profession of dentistry. He also introduced the surgical dental engine.

1826

In France, M. Taveau made a silver paste from the filings of five-franc pieces mixed with mercury. Apparently this new material interested the Crawcour brothers.

1833

The Crawcour brothers came to New York from France to establish their dental practice. They introduced the amalgam filling material, which they called "Royal Mineral Succedaneum"—probably because they felt it would replace the use of gold, the only material that had been used to this date for restoring teeth. It has been suggested that the brothers were more intent on returning to France with a fortune than being of service to dental patients. They were rather careless in their use of the amalgam, which resulted in the Amalgam War.

1835

The Amalgam War was a dissension among American dentists that lasted about fifteen years (until 1850). Dentists took sides in the argument over whether amalgam was a safe material to use. Eventually the necessary research was performed by G. V. Black. His results with amalgam still influence the manufacture and use of our present-day silver amalgam filling materials.

1843

At a meeting of the American Society of Dental Surgery, Chapin Harris motioned, "The use of amalgam was declared [sic] to be malpractice"—a motion that was rescinded in 1850, ending the Amalgam War.[3]

1844

Plaster of Paris was introduced for taking impressions.

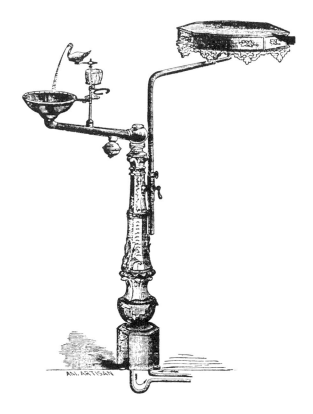

Figure 2.1
Whitcomb fountain spitoon (1866).

1847

Edwin Truman, Queen Victoria's dentist, introduced gutta-percha as a base material for artificial dentures. At this same time, it had become necessary to re-cover the Atlantic cable, its original cover having been seriously corroded by the action of saltwater. Truman suggested the use of gutta-percha for this purpose. Since gutta-percha was highly successful as a covering material, Truman was rewarded. He received an annuity of 1,000 British pounds per year for fifty years.

1848

Thomas W. Evans of Paris began using vulcanized rubber as a base for artificial dentures. In 1854 he constructed a vulcanite denture for Charles Goodyear, Sr., and in 1855 Charles Goodyear, Jr., obtained a patent for the Goodyear Dental Vulcanite Company on the use of this material for denture bases in this country. A fee was charged for license to use the material. Dr. Samuel Stockton White did much to persuade the Goodyear Dental Vulcanite Company to cease this practice.

1852

A rudimentary hypodermic syringe was developed.

Robert Arthur, M.D., D.D.S., Philadelphia, introduced a method he termed "Arthurizing." Dental

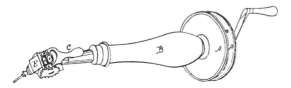

Figure 2.2
Early hand bit and drill.

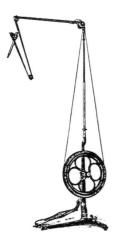

Figure 2.3
Dental foot engine with hand piece attached (1875). The foot engine replaced the early hand bit and drill.

prophylaxis was achieved by separating teeth and filing away coronal portions of the teeth to prevent and/or arrest incipient caries.

Anesthesia

1842–1846

During this period the relief of pain during surgical and dental operations progressed. Ether anesthesia was introduced by two American physicians, Crawford W. Long and Charles T. Jackson and two American dentists, William T. G. Morton and Horace Wells.

Horace Wells, who practiced dentistry in Hartford, Connecticut, first demonstrated (with himself as the patient) the use of nitrous oxide to prevent pain in dental operations. Dr. Wells shouted, "A new era in tooth pulling," as he recovered consciousness from the nitrous oxide.[4]

1859

Neimann isolated cocaine for anesthetic use in Germany.

1884–1886

Koller introduced cocaine as a topical anesthetic.

Hall and Halstead first used cocaine as an injection anesthetic.

1867

Lister initiated the antiseptic era with the idea of antiseptic procedure.

1871

The dental foot-engine, operated with a treadle, was introduced. The same basic mechanism was used throughout most of the armed services in World War II, although it was replaced where feasible before the termination of that war.

1878

Diamond instruments were developed to help reduce tooth structures. Rough chunks of diamonds were pounded into the steel blank, which was shaped like a dental bur or cutting disc. Refinements were continually made until the fine instruments available today were perfected.

1890

Willoughby Miller, D.D.S., an American who was professor of operative dentistry at the dental institute of the University of Berlin, published his discovery of the chemicobacterial cause of dental caries in "Microorganisms of the Human Mouth." He was the first person to demonstrate the essential relationship between mouth bacteria and the decay of teeth.

1891

Greene Vardiman Black (1836–1915), the Grand Old Man of Dentistry, advocated scientific cavity preparation, including extension of the cavity for prevention. He became Professor of Operative Dentistry and Pathology at Northwestern University in 1891 also. His contribution to dentistry probably was most significant in establishing standard cavity preparation and in the design of dental instruments. He contributed to the advancement of every form of dentistry and revolutionized its practice. Today there are Black Study Clubs all over the country, through which dentists advance their knowledge.

1895

Dr. G. V. Black proposed balanced alloys for amalgam.

William K. Roentgen discovered X rays quite by accident, and he immediately published the discovery for the advancement of dental and medical diagnosis.

1896

C. Edmund Kells (1856–1928) of New Orleans began the practical application of X rays (or Roentgen rays). He used them as a means of revealing anatomical and pathological conditions of the teeth and jaws, and he developed stereoscopic radiography. Dr. Kells died of overexposure to X rays. Dr. Kells is also credited with having used the first "lady assistant."

1897

Dr. B. F. Philbrook presented a paper before his fellow dentists in Denison, Iowa, in which he described the use of a disappearing wax pattern in casting inlays. This incident prevented Dr. William H. Taggart of Chicago from patenting the process in 1907. Dr. Taggart developed the process and has been given credit for developing inlay casting as we know it today, but he was denied his bid to charge $150 for every inlay placed by another dentist.

1899

Edward Hartley Angle systematized the practice of orthodontics. He developed Angle's Classification of orthodontic cases, used as the standard throughout orthodontia. He founded the first postgraduate school of orthodontics, the first society of orthodontics, and the first journal of orthodontics. Norman W. Kingsley (1829–1913) was one of the earlier pioneers in the field of orthodontics, although Angle is perhaps more widely known.

The Twentieth Century

Dentistry became a profession with stature. Progress continued in many areas.

The Profession

Educational requirements for dentistry were established and are continuously upgraded. By 1917 dentistry required four years of college education. This requirement was raised in 1927 and again in 1942.

In 1924 William Gies performed valuable studies on saliva and its relationship to dental caries for the Carnegie Foundation. The report was publicized in 1926. Nearly all dental schools were incorporated into

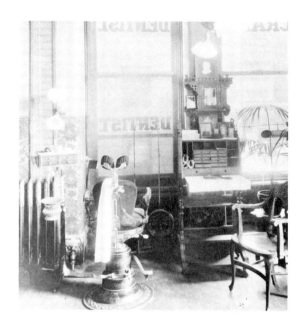

Figure 2.4
A typical dental office at the turn of the century.

the universities after that Carnegie report, which elevated the stature of the profession. In 1928 the National Board of Dental Examiners was established, creating some cohesive national standards. Today dental specialties require graduate degrees beyond the dental degree.

A Connecticut dentist, Dr. A. Fones, began training oral hygienists in his office in 1913. Dental hygienists had been originally visualized by C. Wright in 1877. In 1917 the coursework for hygiene was incorporated into college programs, and Dr. Fones discontinued his training programs. Today hygienists are not only educated, but required to be licensed.

Dr. Edmund Kells, noted for his work with radiography, claimed to be the first dentist to utilize a lady assistant in the southern part of the United States. The photographic proof of his dental team is dated around 1900. By 1924 there were enough dental assistants to organize nationally, and the American Dental Assistants Association was formed. The organization has grown, and it continues to elevate the standards of the profession. Certain functions assistants perform today may be performed only by registered assistants.

Growth of Preventive Dentistry

After World War II, a greater social consciousness of public and individual health care needs developed. During that war, young men and women in the armed services were exposed to health care as many of them had never experienced it before, and they developed an appreciation for it.

At the same time within the health professions, the idea of total health care delivery resulted in the development of the team concept with emphasis on prevention of disease. Within the specialized health area of dentistry the result has been education of the patients and advocacy of certain measures that affect the well-being of the entire population. For example, fluoridation of public water supplies has progressed, resulting in a well-documented decrease in the incidence of caries. Many states have laws that require fluoridation of all communal water supplies. The research on fluoridation of public water supplies, conducted for ten years beginning in 1944 in the communities of Newburgh and Kingston, New York, was responsible for the widespread adoption of fluoridation.

The commonly used fluoride treatments for children's teeth are a direct result of the documented research indicating the lessening incidence of caries in treated teeth.

To assist the patient in his Personal Oral Hygiene (POH) today, dentists and their oral health care delivery teams are teaching home care and utilizing such recent developments as oral irrigating devices, disclosing tablets, dental flossing aids, anticariogenic toothpastes, and improved brushes which supplement the improved brushing techniques taught to patients.

Advances in clinical dentistry, especially endodontics and periodontics, have greatly reduced the number of teeth extracted and the number of prosthetic appliances prescribed.

Oral cytology programs for early detection of cancer have been established. Advanced techniques for treatment of temporomandibular joint dysfunction (TMJ) have been established.

Time and motion studies, pioneered by H. C. Kilpatrick, produced work simplification procedures. Kilpatrick's text first appeared in 1964.

Professional Advances

The total health care concept changed the concept of dental practice. Consequently, dental practices have been reorganized to utilize auxiliary personnel, and the practices have often developed into group practices. The trend is toward more group practices and an incorporation of group and individual practices.

From 1955 to 1967 more effective utilization of auxiliaries developed. Dental schools taught students to work with assistants. Statistics indicate that in 1967, 90,000 dentists utilized the services of 136,000 auxiliaries.

In 1956 the DAU (dental auxiliary team) program was begun in certain select schools. (The DAU program is federally supported.) New techniques of dental health team performance were developed.

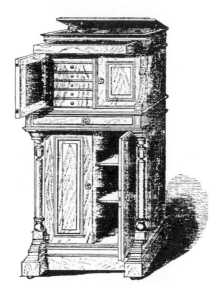

Figure 2.5
Early S. S. White dental cabinet.

Extended duties personnel free the dentist from certain routine operations that auxiliaries can be trained to perform. Today the dentist is likely to be a supervisor of several team members as well as an operator contributing his or her skill and knowledge to the overall production of the oral health care delivery team.

The Council on Dental Health of the ADA was established in 1958. Important advances in public education about dentistry and dental health can be traced to the Council.

Development of dental third-party payment plans began in 1955, and this development continued with Medicare coverage for dentistry in 1965, the ADA dental program for children in 1966, and dental programs that stand alone, such as Delta Dental Plan, initiated in 1969. It is interesting to note that in 1970 Delta Dental paid $414 in claims but paid over $52 million in claims in 1988, covering more than 550,000 persons.[5] Obviously, fee payments for dental services are more frequently included in government health programs, insurance programs, and other third-party payment systems as we near the end of the twentieth century.

Materials and Equipment for Dentistry

Anesthesia improved. For example, in 1905 Einhorn synthesized procaine. It was introduced as "novocaine," a product of Novol Chemical Company. Braun and Bieberfeld introduced its use in combination with adrenalin. This product is one of the commonly used forms of local anesthesia today.

Anesthetics and analgesics have been continuously improved. Today the use of topical anesthetics eases the discomfort of an injection; and the anesthetics, such as sodium pentathol, provide better management of procedures and greater patient comfort.

Antibiotics have revolutionized the treatment of infections. In 1929 Alexander Fleming, an English scientist, discovered the bacteriostatic influence of penicillin. Link, a German botanist, had isolated the penicillin mold in 1824, but no one had perceived its value until Fleming's research indicated its usefulness in medicine. In 1935 Domagk demonstrated the action of sulfanilamide. In 1936 Long and Bliss introduced sulfanilamide in the United States. Aureomycin appeared as a product of Lederle Laboratories in 1948. The field of antibiotics advanced rapidly. New derivatives and new applications are being developed continually.

Polymerized acrylic resin (methyl methacrylate) was introduced as a base material for artificial dentures in 1935. Resins of this and other types have replaced vulcanite denture base material. The Germans modified **methyl methacrylate** as a filling material during World War II. By 1956 **composite filling materials** appeared, and they have changed anterior restorations. The research by the 3M Company began this development. **Spherical amalgam alloy** was introduced in 1962.

Experimentation with materials continues, and new products are tried daily. Some are discarded, but the entire field of dental materials is changing as some of the experiments produce improved approaches to restorations.

Disposables have been introduced. Every disposable item that is used for a patient lessens the opportunity for cross infection, because an item that is used for only one patient cannot *contaminate* (infect) another should there be some failure in the complete sterilization process. Today patient covers, bibs, and saliva ejectors are commonly disposable. Perhaps the most important disposable unit is the disposable syringe: needle, carpule, and syringe can all be used once and thrown away.

Tungsten carbide burs, introduced in 1949, replaced the less efficient steel burs.

Dental engines for rotating the drills changed in 1872 from a hand operated device to the foot-engine. In 1910 the electric engine was added as the power source, and it continued to be used without challenge until 1956 when the **air turbine,** which provided increased rotational speeds, was developed. The process of preparation of teeth was revolutionized. The safety of operation increased, there was less stress for both the dentist and patient, greater control of the cutting instrument, and less pulp damage through trauma and the heat of cutting. The air turbine also provides more comfort for the patient because it reduces to a negligible degree the vibrations the patient feels through the bones of the skull.

In 1878 **diamond instruments** were invented to help reduce tooth structure. Rough chunks of diamonds were pounded into the steel blank, which was shaped like a dental bur or cutting disc. In 1932 modern diamond instruments were perfected, resulting in precision diamonds with accurate sizes, shapes, and grits. The fine diamond pieces were evenly plated on the blanks.

Dental chairs have been made more comfortable for the patient and have given the dentist the opportunity to practice sit-down dentistry.

Dental units have all but disappeared as time and motion studies showed better ways to manage the necessary equipment and hand instruments. The cuspidor has also been restyled. Most dentists utilize the evacuator and rarely need to permit the patient to expectorate.

Development of **ultrasonic cleaners** has simplified the process of cleansing instruments in preparation for sterilization, resulting in more efficiency with greater ease for the assistant.

Prophylaxis units that simplify work and increase efficiency have been developed.

Prefabricated and **prewelded orthodontic bands** have increased the efficiency of orthodontic treatment.

Impression materials for restorative dentistry have undergone developments that allow far greater accuracy, such as hydrocolloid, mercaptan rubbers, and silicones.

The danger of exposure to radiation has been greatly reduced by changes in X-ray equipment. Exposure time has been shortened by the use of **high-speed films** and improved **X-ray equipment.** The area of exposure is reduced by filtering and restricting the useful beam.

Articulators began to be used in the nineteenth century, and their development continued in the twentieth century. In 1910 the first modern adaptable articulator appeared. An adjustable articulator with which it is possible to reproduce the movements of the human jaw was developed and refined by several researchers. The articulator is valuable for prostheses and for gnathology.

The use of composite materials has greatly increased the capabilities of dentists to restore the teeth, not only for function, but for **aesthetics.**

Developments in the area of **dental implants** have made it possible to provide a more stable, functional, and comfortable replacement of missing teeth.

Risk management has become extremely important. The recognition of the prevalence and communicability of such diseases as AIDS and hepatitis demand stricter attention to aseptic office procedures.

The evaluation of the accomplishments of dentistry in the twentieth century indicates that the profession has developed stature as a part of the total health team. Continuing research and experimentation creates further improvements, and only the test of time will keep dentistry on the leading edge of service to the public.

Summary

Dentistry is a relatively young profession, although dental treatment was recorded in very early history—7000 years ago.

Skills, processes, and materials necessary in dentistry have been developed by many people throughout the world.

The knowledge explosion in basic science and dental technology in the twentieth century has increased the academic study of dentists to seven or more years.

Significant developments have occurred in the last thirty years in preventive dentistry, equipment design, and organization of practice. Some of these developments are:

1. Fluoridation of water supplies.
2. POH education of patients, including the use of disclosing tablets, flossing, irrigating devices, improved brushes and brushing techniques.
3. Improved techniques in endodontics and periodontics that help patients retain their teeth.
4. Improved instrumentation, including the air turbine, diamond instruments, and tungsten burs.
5. Improved X-ray equipment, with accompanying reduction in exposure of patients and staff.
6. Disposable supplies to avoid cross-contamination.
7. Ultrasonic cleaners and prophylaxis units.
8. Prefabricated and prewelded orthodontic bands.
9. New philosophy of group practice and use of the oral health care delivery team.
10. Third-party payment for dental services.

Study Questions
1. When was the earliest record of dental treatment and where did the treatment occur?
2. What significant factors have changed the type of dental treatment offered in the last twenty-five years?
3. Name five equipment changes which have greatly affected dentistry.
4. What preventive dentistry measures have been developed?

Vocabulary
attrition   wearing down teeth by friction
contaminate   infect
gnathology   method for occlusal treatment

CHAPTER
3

Dental-Medical Terminology (Nomenclature)

Technical Versus Layperson's Language
Aids for Developing a Dental-Medical Vocabulary
Word Elements
Using Your Knowledge
Sound-alike, Look-alike Words
Word Study

Technical Versus Layperson's Language

Whenever technical language is used to discuss the subject matter of a career, those who are related to that career must understand the terminology if they are to understand and be understood. Any member of the oral health care delivery team should acquire the necessary technical vocabulary to converse intelligently with members of the dental profession.

A dental assistant must further be able to understand the patient's use of layperson's language. (Laypersons are those people you and I meet on the street, who may not possess the technical vocabulary.) They use nontechnical terms often referred to as *colloquialisms*. The following are some common examples:

Correct Term	*Colloquialism*
orthodontics	straightening teeth
dentures	plates or false teeth
upper cuspids	eye teeth
lower cuspids	stomach teeth
gingivae	gums
first molars	six-year molars
second molars	twelve-year molars
third molars	wisdom teeth
deciduous teeth	milk teeth or baby teeth
granulation tissue	proud flesh
cleft upper lip	harelip
restricted tongue movement	tongue-tied

Please remember that there is nothing wrong with these terms, but they are colloquial terms and not the proper professional terminology. Often the oral health care delivery team members explain technical terms to patients. Many dentists consider it important to teach the patients the correct terminology rather than use colloquialisms when conversing with patients.

Aids for Developing a Dental-Medical Vocabulary

A large dental-medical vocabulary must be mastered by anyone who wishes to be an effective member of an oral health care delivery team. Some of the terms look frighteningly difficult, but with the proper approach to visualizing them, you will find you can master all the vocabulary you desire to learn.

Occasionally the vocabulary contains a proper name. Usually an anatomical part of the body or some specific disease has been given the name of the person who first described it. For example, Salk vaccine is so named to recognize the physician who developed it. An example in the field of dentistry is Stenson's duct, named for the man who described the parotid duct.

The English language is composed of many words, some of them similar to each other because they belong to the same family. When words belong to the same family, they usually come from the same "root" or "stem" word. The root, stem, or basic part of the word expresses its primary or essential meaning. Prefixes and suffixes may be added. Some words are constructed from combining forms—words that are a combination of two or more word parts.

Prefixes are letters or syllables placed before the root word. A prefix modifies or qualifies the meaning of the root word.

Suffixes are syllables or letters placed at the end of the root word. A suffix also modifies or qualifies the meaning of the word.

Affixes are both prefixes and suffixes. For example, the root word *part* comes from the Latin word *pars* or *partis*. It means "something less than the whole." Add a prefix, *de*, to make the word *depart*, which means "to go away." Add a suffix, *ment*, and we have *department*, meaning, "a separate division." Or if you wish to add just a suffix and drop the prefix *de*, you may use *parting*, which means "taking leave."

Most dental-medical language is scientific, and scientific language is derived from Greek and Latin. About 75 percent of our scientific language is credited to the early Greek and Latin cultures.

When the Greek era declined, many Greek scientific words were used by the Romans and some were slightly altered. Later the words were altered again in a modern language. When a term was borrowed by another modern language, further change might have occurred. An example is our modern word *surgery*.

The Greek word was:
chirugia (cheir + ergon = hand + work).

The Romans used the Greek word:
chirugia for their Latin language.

The French changed it to:
cirurgeria.

The English changed it to:
surgery.

Most scientific words are constructed by using a combination of two or more words or word parts. Understanding the meaning of the basic words or word parts from Greek and Latin assists in building one's dental vocabulary.

Words in dental terminology can also be classified as root words, root words with prefixes, root words with suffixes, and root words with affixes. If you will learn the meaning of certain dental-medical prefixes, stem words, combining forms, and suffixes, your understanding of a dental vocabulary will be acquired much sooner than if you try to memorize each word individually.

One problem is that some words that look as if they have the same root or prefix may be derived from different words. An example is *melalgia* and *melicera*. The medical dictionary will indicate that melalgia is derived from the Greek, *mel + algia* (limbs + pain), while melicera is derived from the Greek, *meli + keros* (honey + wax). It is important to know that the two roots, *mel* and *meli*, are different. It may be difficult to know at first, but practice will improve the educated guesses. When in doubt, consult the medical dictionary.

Word Elements

Memorize the group of word elements in the right-hand column of this page. These elements will help you learn a dental vocabulary more quickly. At the ends of most of the remaining chapters you will find a list of ten word elements to be memorized. They may have nothing to do with the chapter, but they are grouped around a theme to help you memorize them. The first group is about quantities.

In the left-hand column of this list you will find the word element, what kind of word element it is, and its meaning. In the right-hand column is an example of the word element used in a word and the meaning of that word. Learn to make the associations between word elements and to discern the meanings of new words you hear.

These word elements refer to quantities from 1–10. Other common word elements referring to these quantities are *hex, hexa, hexyl,* and *sex,* meaning six; *hept* and *sept,* meaning seven; and *non* and *nona,* meaning nine. There are many word elements that imply quantity. Some of these are listed in the next chapter.

Using Your Knowledge

Use your knowledge of these word parts to understand many dental-medical terms rapidly. For example, the suffix *itis* means "inflammation of." Let us apply this knowledge to words which are commonly used in dentistry.

Pulp becomes *pulpitis,* meaning "inflammation of the pulp."

Larynx becomes *laryngitis,* meaning "inflammation of the larynx."

Word Element	Example
uni prefix meaning: one	**unicuspid** a tooth having only one cusp
mon, mono prefix meaning: one	**monangle** one angle
bi, bis, bin prefix meaning: two	**bimonthly** every second month
di prefix meaning: two, twice	**dicelous** having two cavities
tri prefix meaning: three	**triangle** three-cornered form
quadr combining form meaning: four	**quadrant** any one of four corresponding parts
tetra combining form meaning: four	**tetracycline** an antibiotic substance composed of four elements
pent, penta combining form meaning: five	**pentavaccine** a vaccine comprised of five microorganisms
octa combining form meaning: eight	**octagon** eight-sided figure
dec, deca combining form meaning: ten, ten times the root with which it is combined	**decimal** division of a number by tenths

Cheil (lip) becomes *cheilitis,* meaning "inflammation of the lip."

Gingiva (gums) becomes *gingivitis,* meaning "inflammation of the gums."

Neur (nerve) becomes *neuritis,* meaning "inflammation of the nerves."

Pharynx (area behind the soft palate) becomes *pharyngitis,* meaning "inflammation of the pharynx."

Tonsil becomes *tonsilitis,* meaning "inflammation of the tonsils."

Stomat (mouth) becomes *stomatitis,* meaning "inflammation of the oral mucosa."

Periodontal (surrounding a tooth) becomes *periodontitis,* meaning "inflammation of the tissues surrounding a tooth."

Thus it is possible to learn many words quickly by being alert to the combinations of word parts.

Sound-Alike, Look-Alike Words

Some word parts look alike and sound alike. They may even be exactly alike but have different meanings. For example, *os* means "mouth" or "opening" and also "bone." Other words are spelled differently but sound much the same. Sometimes only one vowel makes the difference in spelling. For example:

> *Hema* refers to blood.
> *Hemi* means half.
>
> *Para* means beyond, near, or beside.
> *Peri* means about or around, enclosing a part.
>
> *Stoma* means mouth.
> *Stomach* means the most dilated part of the alimentary canal in which part of the digestive process occurs.
>
> *Cocci* is the plural form of *coccus,* a bacterium.
> *Coxa* means hip joint or hip.

Make your own list of such similar looking words. Listen carefully to be certain that you understand the terminology used.

Word Study

Knowledge of word parts is only the beginning of building a technical vocabulary. The second step is to study the words used in your profession. Turn to the Glossary and read it. These are the more commonly used words in dentistry.

You will find the Glossary is given in layperson's language. This will help you understand the terms more easily. When you understand the definitions given in the Glossary, you can then read any of the medical dictionaries listed and better understand the technical language used therein. One book that you may wish to study is *Boucher's Current Clinical Dental Terminology,* edited by Zweemer—an excellent work in the field of dentistry.

The chapters that follow contain much technical language. Apply your knowledge of word construction and similarity in building your vocabulary, and then memorize to aid in retaining the new words.

Summary

Understanding the technical language associated with the practice of dentistry is a necessary part of the education of a member of the oral health care delivery team.

Parts of words, prefixes, suffixes, combining forms, and root or stem words are used to form many of the words in a dental vocabulary. Familiarity with some of these word parts is a great aid in developing an understanding of the language of dentistry.

Some words look alike or sound alike but have different meanings. Be alert to this possibility and be sure you understand the intended meaning.

Study Questions

1. Why is it important to study word parts?
2. What do these word elements mean?

stoma	di	gingiva	bin
cheil	uni	perio	octa

3. What difference would it make if someone wrote *hema* instead of *hemi?*
4. What is the technical meaning of these colloquialisms?

straightening teeth	twelve-year molars
plates	proud flesh
stomach teeth	harelip

Vocabulary

colloquialism an expression that is not incorrect but is below the level of the scientific or technical language of a profession

prefix letters or syllables placed before a root word, modifying or qualifying the meaning of the root word

suffix letters or syllables placed after a root word to modify or qualify the meaning

Dental Jurisprudence

Dental Law
Part One: The Dental Practice Acts
The Need for Regulation
American Law
Laws Regulating Dentistry
   Requirements for Licensed Dentists
   Revocation of License
   Requirements for Auxiliary Personnel
Part Two: Legal Relationship of Dentists and Their
        Patients
Creation of a Contract
The Assistant as Agent for the Dentist
Duties to the Patient
Duties of the Patient
Remuneration for the Dentist
Termination of a Contract
The Dentist's Public Duties
Part Three: Liabilities: Professional and Criminal
Personal Injury Claims
Medical Professional Liability (Malpractice Claims)
   Proof of Negligence
   Res Ipsa Loquitur or "Somebody Obviously
      Goofed!"
   Proximate Cause
   Additional Tort Liability
   Admissions
   Breach of Contract
Professional Liability Insurance
Criminal Liabilities
Part Four: Avoiding Dental Professional Liability
        Claims (Minimizing the Danger of
        Unjustified Malpractice Claims)
Three Defenses for Dental Professional Liability
        Actions
   Contributory Negligence
   Assumption of Risk
   Statutes of Limitation
Minimizing the Danger of Unjustified Medical
        Professional Liability Claims

Dental Law

Dental jurisprudence is the science that concerns the principles of law and the legal relations concerning dentistry. Society gives order to our lives by a system of laws. Those that apply in particular to dentistry are not only of interest but of extreme importance for the oral health care team to understand. Subjects of concern for the dental assistant are how the laws affect the practice of dentistry; the legal relationships that exist between a dentist, the staff, and their patients; the dentist's liabilities in the practice of dentistry; and the public duties of the dentist. Just by knowing the dangers that exist, the alert dental assistant can prevent an unjustified legal entanglement through care of certain office responsibilities.

The difference between jurisprudence and ethics is important. Ethics, discussed in chapter 1, concerns the regulations a profession makes for its members. It is usually a higher standard of conduct than that required by law. Laws set the minimum limits of care required. Ethics set the high, visionary ideals of the profession. Legally it is possible to do certain things that would be ethically incorrect. As long as the act is not illegal, the courts will not be involved. The *profession* may take action against a member who is unethical in his or her conduct, but that is professional disciplinary action—not legal action by the courts. It is important to remember that all who work in the profession of dentistry should abide by the high ethical standards set for their profession as outlined in chapter 1. In chapter 4 we will attempt to understand the legal relationship of dentistry to society and to the persons who are patients.

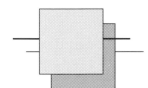

Part One: The Dental Practice Acts

The Need for Regulation

That some people are eager to diagnose the problems of others and prescribe treatment for the "cure" of these problems is a reality that has existed almost as long as civilization. However, sometimes those who are eager to diagnose and prescribe are not educationally qualified to do so. There have been instances of the exposé of unlicensed and uneducated persons who have perpetrated a hoax on innocent laypersons.

A dentist (as well as a physician) is sometimes responsible for the life or death of a patient. The judgment of the professional doctor may determine what happens to that patient. Therefore society has come to be rightfully concerned with the preparation of the health care professionals.

In early history there were some laws aimed at improving medical care, but these were largely repealed until no laws existed by 1850. Because so much quackery developed, all the states passed dental and medical practice acts by 1900. There was much discussion and contention about these laws; some people protested that persons were denied their constitutional rights if they were not allowed to practice medicine. The Supreme Court ruled in 1889 that the states had a right to pass licensing legislation. The state is given power to protect its citizens from harm by persons who are not qualified to perform certain functions such as *diagnose* (determine what is wrong) and *prescribe* (specify the use of a remedy or treatment).

Following this decision, licensing requirements for the health professions have been upheld by the courts in the interests of protecting the general public. Any state may use any requirements that are not "arbitrary, unreasonable, or discriminatory" in issuing licenses for the practice of the health professions. Requirements are not considered "arbitrary, unreasonable, or discriminatory" if they are attainable by reasonable study or application, are appropriate to the profession, and are available to all persons of like age and condition.

Inasmuch as this decision by the Supreme Court set these criteria, any state may reasonably increase educational requirements, raise the licensing fees, and radically revise qualifications by action of the state legislature.

The only federal license for dentists and physicians is a narcotics license. Should a dentist or physician wish to prescribe medications containing narcotics, that dentist or physician must obtain a federal narcotics license.

American Law

There are three general sources of American law: **federal law,** which includes the United States Constitution; **state law,** which includes the state constitutions; and **judicial decisions.** Federal *statutes* are laws that apply to the entire country and regulate everyone who is within the domain of the United States. These are written laws that can be found in the *United States Code.* A **code** is a system of regulations controlling a group. It is a systematic body of law. The *United States Code,* then, is composed of our federal statutes. Unless these laws contradict the United States Constitution, they represent "black letter law," the hard-and-fast rules of the United States.

State laws differ only in that they must also be in accord with the constitution of the state of which they are law. They apply only within the boundaries of that state.

In addition to these two well-known areas of law, there is judge-made law (often called common law). This law is applicable within the jurisdiction of the judge who issues the decree. The only requirement is that it does not conflict with the constitution of the state in which the judge presides and the Constitution of the United States. There are differences in judge-made laws within a state. For example, a local judge in the northwest corner of a state may create a common law that states that all dogs must be kept on a leash, while a judge in the southeast corner of the same state may decree that dogs may run loose so long as they do not attack anyone. Since neither of these common laws is in conflict with the constitution of that state nor the United States Constitution, they both can be part of the body of common law of that state.

The areas for which the federal government can make laws are specifically established by the Constitution of the United States. The Constitution also states that all other areas are to be controlled by the states. Police power (in its broad sense—*regulation*) is one of the areas that the states control. This means that the states control the practice of dentistry.

Common law simply means that the courts must fill in the gaps between the laws that the legislature makes. It is not possible for the legislators to anticipate all the possible problems; therefore, laws are generalized. The judges (courts) then have to interpret and also decree certain regulations. Black's *Law Dictionary* states that these decisions become "common law—those principles and rules of action, relating to the government and security of persons and property, which derive their authority solely from usages and customs of immemorial antiquity, or from the judgments and decrees of the courts recognizing, affirming, and enforcing such usages and customs."

The dentist is controlled by:

1. **Federal law** if he or she prescribes medicines containing narcotics. The dentist must have a federal license to authorize the pharmacist to dispense any narcotics.
2. **State law** in the state in which he or she practices. This state law is the dental practice act. It governs licensing.

3. **Judge-made** or **common law,** in his or her professional relationships with patients.

The legal relationships of dentistry and medicine are intertwined and dependent on each other because judges usually follow **judicial precedents** (earlier decisions by other judges) set in similar cases within their own state.

Common law is difficult to amend. Appeal to a higher court is one way. Another way is to have the legislature of the state enact new legislation that voids the common law.

Common law is the law that usually affects the dentist in his or her relationships with patients. All members of the oral health care delivery team should become aware of the precautions necessary to avoid malpractice claims.

Laws Regulating Dentistry

Dental practice acts are regulatory statutes (laws) that prohibit the practice of dentistry by any person without a license. This means that anyone who indicates he or she is able to perform dentistry—to diagnose, treat, prescribe, or operate for any disease, pain, injury, deficiency, deformity, or physical condition of the teeth, jaws, or adjacent structures—must acquire a license. The individual state dental practice acts may word the definitions differently, but each defines the area of dentistry. Most acts indicate that the use of the title *dentist* (or any of its other forms, such as oral surgeon) or of the letters *D.D.S.* or *D.M.D.* is reserved for those individuals who have been licensed by the state.

Most of the states agree that the applicant for a dental license must meet certain conditions. He or she must:

1. Have graduated from a dental school that has been approved by the State Board of Dental Examiners and/or the Council on Dental Education of the American Dental Association
2. Be twenty-one years of age or older
3. Be a citizen of the United States
4. Be a resident of the state
5. Be of good moral character
6. Not have committed a crime involving moral turpitude
7. Not be addicted to drugs or alcohol
8. Pass an examination both written and oral, both theory and practical, given by the State Board of Dental Examiners

Requirements for Licensed Dentists

Once a dentist has been licensed to practice in a state, and continues to practice, that dentist must renew his or her license annually by payment of the licensing fee as determined by the state. This fee must be paid promptly at the proper time each year. A yearly certificate is issued. The *original license* and the *annual certificate* should be displayed in the office.

A dentist must also have a *narcotics license* in order to dispense drugs that contain narcotics. This license is obtained from the federal government. It is the only medical function that the federal government licenses. The narcotics license is obtained by application to the Bureau of Narcotics, United States Treasury. It is sent to the district branch of the United States Treasury in the district in which the dentist practices. A stamp with the narcotics license number of this particular dentist is then issued. The number must appear on each narcotic prescription blank. The license is renewed annually on June 30, which is the end of the federal fiscal year.

Revocation of License

Since licensing occurs, there are situations where revocation of license becomes necessary. The rules vary from state to state. However, suspension or revocation of a dental license can occur:

1. If the dentist is convicted of a felony (narcotic violations, murder, and rape are specifically included).
2. For unprofessional conduct (such as permitting an unlicensed person to perform dentistry or permitting employees to perform duties not specifically permitted by law, advertising that is unethical or misleading to public morals or safety, giving or receiving rebates, and habitual intemperance in the use of narcotics or alcohol).
3. For personal or professional incapacity. (If a dentist has been judged insane or incompetent, his or her license may be revoked. If a dentist insists on continuing to practice when senile, his or her license might be revoked because he or she is personally or professionally incapable of performing dental service of value to patients. In all probability, every effort would be made to persuade the dentist to retire voluntarily before denying the license renewal.)

The power of revocation or suspension is given the State Board of Dental Examiners by the state legislatures.

Requirements for Auxiliary Personnel

Certain auxiliary personnel in the dental office are either licensed by state boards or registered or certified by the board as competent to perform certain specific operations or duties in the dental office under the supervision of the dentist.

Dental hygienists are licensed after examination. The license must be renewed each year. The license and annual certificate must be displayed prominently in the office where the hygienist works.

Dental assistants who perform expanded duties must be registered or certified as qualified to perform the specific duties. An examination is passed and a certificate is issued.

The degree of delegation of certain skills is the important factor in delineating actions of auxiliaries as either proper or as practicing dentistry illegally. Supervision by the dentist is necessary, and frequently the presence of the dentist is required in the operatory during the performance of tasks by a dental assistant.

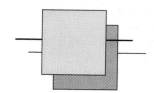

Part Two: *Legal Relationship of Dentists and Their Patients*

A definite legal relationship exists between a patient and a dentist. This relationship can be, and often is, upheld in a court of law. Eleven commonly accepted duties of dentists to their patients are implied by law, while only two such duties of patients to their dentists are implied. Failure to fulfill any of these duties can become the basis for a lawsuit. Thus, it is imperative that all members of the oral health care delivery team become aware of their obligation in order to minimize the possibility of a lawsuit.

As a dental assistant you should be aware that emergency care is being refused by some dentists and physicians. An atmosphere of caution about treating strangers has developed within the health care professions because claims for damages have been filed by some unscrupulous persons who have received such "good Samaritan" treatment.

Creation of a Contract

A dentist is not required to accept everyone who requests service. The legal decisions from the courts have indicated that a dentist may arbitrarily refuse to accept anyone as a patient, even though there is no other dentist available.

The dentist-patient relationship begins when the dentist performs services after a patient has requested such service, either by implication or by direct statement. Administering emergency care does not create the relationship. The dentist must use his or her skill and care when treating an emergency, but this act does not create the dentist-patient relationship. The dentist is also free to limit care to a specific time or place or to one specific treatment. However, after the patient-dentist relationship has been established, there are certain obligations on the part of both patient and dentist.

The first step in any dentist-patient relationship is the creation of a contract. A **contract** is an agreement with an individual patient that indicates the patient is placing herself or himself under the care of this dentist for a specific treatment of a specific condition or placing herself or himself in the dentist's care for whatever services the dentist may deem necessary (as a patient does who engages a family dentist). This agreement may be *verbal;* it may be implied rather than specifically stated.

When a patient is unable to make this arrangement herself or himself, an **agent** makes it for him or her. The agent may be the parent of a child; or in the case of an aged parent, an adult son or daughter. The agent for a mentally incompetent individual is usually a near relative or a court appointed guardian.

A dentist and the staff should know the laws governing **financial responsibility.** These laws vary from state to state. It is important to know the laws governing financial responsibility that apply to the practice of dentistry in your locality. Be certain you are dealing with the correct person when you attempt to collect a fee.

The Assistant as Agent for the Dentist

Whenever an employee is able to act for her or his employer, that employee is considered an agent. The dentist must, of necessity, empower (direct) employees to act for him or her in some circumstances, usually under specific direction. For example, the dentist directs the hygienist to perform prophylaxis for patients. The hygienist, in this case, is acting as the dentist's agent. The dentist who employs an expanded duties certified dental assistant also directs that assistant to perform certain operations. The assistant is the dentist's agent while polishing an amalgam or taking an impression.

Since someone must be responsible for any treatment given a patient, it also follows that the dentist is responsible for the actions of his or her agent. If the hygienist or dental assistant accidentally injures the patient, the patient can sue the dentist for the damage rather than sue the hygienist or dental assistant; or the patient may sue them jointly.

Generally, a dentist is responsible for injury if assistants, apprentices, agents, or employees do not have the proper skill or do not exercise the proper care. However, one employee is not responsible for the negligence of another employee. Thus, if the dentist employs another dentist who in turn gives orders to the dental assistant to perform some treatment that injures the patient, the employed dentist is not held responsible for the negligence of the dental assistant because he or she is an employee, as is the dental assistant.

This area of responsibility for an agent's actions is difficult to define completely because so many factors enter the conditions under which the service is performed.

The dental assistant is the agent of the dentist and acts under the dentist's direction; therefore, the dentist is responsbile for the assistant's conduct and treatment of patients. It is essential that anyone engaged as an oral health care delivery team member be constantly alert to see that *the directions of the dentist are accurately followed and recorded for future reference.*

Duties to the Patient

When a contract has been made (either written or oral), what are the duties of the dentist to a patient? The implied duties are the following:

1. The dentist must be licensed. Anyone who attempts to practice dentistry without being properly licensed to do so is liable for court action.

2. The dentist must use reasonable care and skill in diagnosis and treatment according to the standards of care provided by other dentists in the same type of community.

3. The dentist must use standard drugs, materials, and techniques in treatment and postoperative care.

4. The treatment is to be completed within a reasonable length of time.

5. The patient is to be given instructions for any postoperative care, including instructions to return for postoperative observation when necessary.

6. The dentist may not abandon a patient. Once the contract has been established between a dentist and a patient, it is necessary for the dentist to care for that patient. If the relationship becomes impossible for the dentist, it is his or her duty to give the patient sufficient notice for the patient to be able to find another dentist.

7. The patient is to expect a reasonable charge for services rendered. This fee may be different for different patients, but the dentist is obligated to charge a reasonable fee for services rendered.

8. The dentist is obligated to see that patients have care during his or her absence from the office. If some patient is likely to need care while the dentist is away, it is advisable for the dentist to tell the patient before leaving and to make arrangements with a colleague for this care. (Most dentists make arrangements for the care of emergencies with a nearby colleague prior to being absent from the office.)

9. The patient has a right to a reasonably satisfactory result from his or her dental care.

10. The dentist is to refer a patient to a specialist for proper treatment if such care is necessary.

11. The patient-dentist relationship is a confidential relationship, and any information disclosed to the dentist must be treated confidentially. This rule applies to financial matters as well as health and/or any personal information that is disclosed.

Duties of the Patient

In contrast to this lengthy list of dentist-duties, the patient is required to do only the following:

1. Pay a reasonable fee for the dentistry that has been performed.

2. Follow instructions and cooperate with the dentist in whatever treatment is required.

The contrast of duties only emphasizes the responsibility of all the members of the oral health care delivery team to be aware of the dentist's legal obligations and to be certain that these obligations are met insofar as it is possible for each member of the team.

Remuneration for the Dentist

The dentist may charge the patient directly for services and receive payment from the patient. Frequently, however, **remuneration** (payment) may occur through insurance, prepayment plans, union contracts, employee benefit contracts, and government agencies. This type of payment is called third-party payment. Care must be exercised so that remuneration is actually received when a third party is involved.

The various plans differ in coverage and method of remuneration. It therefore becomes necessary for the dentist's office staff to understand these differences clearly. Inasmuch as the benefits vary from full coverage to deductibles and percentages, accurate understanding of the particular plan is essential, and in some instances the plan must be explained to the patient. In all cases, for complete detailed assistance the patient may be referred to the specific insurance carrier or government agency.

Considering the premium, the patient is remunerated according to some established fees, payable by the insurance company but not necessarily accepted as full payment by the dentist. (The dentist may charge more for the service than the insurance carrier allows.) In the final analysis, the contract is between the dentist and his or her patient rather than a third party. Therefore, the responsibility of the dentist and the patient to each other is of paramount importance.

Payment through a government agency may be handled somewhat differently. If a patient states that the government is responsible for his or her dental bills, the dentist must determine that this patient is eligible for such governmental care and must then file the proper forms and reports. Failure to report the case according to government regulations may mean loss of fee. The various governmental agencies have often refused to pay a claim because it was improperly reported. Workmen's compensation laws in your state should be examined very closely, because some states do not permit patients to choose their dentists if care is to be paid for by their employers under workmen's compensation laws.

The amount a dentist may charge for services is a subject of controversy. Some courts in the United States have refused to permit a dentist to charge fees based on the patient's ability to pay. Other areas do permit just this approach to setting fees. It is important for dentists to know the decisions in their states about setting fees. (Dentists set their own charges.) Fees are based on usual and customary charges made by a dentist for specific services and are more or less in keeping with similar services rendered by others in that community. Fees may become the basis for a lawsuit.

Termination of a Contract

Once a dentist enters into an agreement with a patient, the dentist is under an obligation to continue to care for the patient. The contract continues until it is **terminated** (ended) by either the dentist or the patient. Either one may terminate the contract by indicating that the relationship no longer exists.

For legal protection the dentist needs to complete certain papers when a relationship with a patient is terminated. It is well to have these forms available in the office.

A contract with a patient may be created verbally, but the dentist should terminate it in written form. The patients have a responsibility in the dentist-patient relationship of following the instruction of the dentist and appearing for the requested examinations. Failure of a patient to uphold his or her part of the contract is reason for a dentist to dismiss the patient and terminate the contract. The patient should receive a written statement.

There are certain letters with which a dental assistant should be familiar concerning the dentist who is faced with termination of the patient-dentist relationship. The dentist is under an obligation to care for the patient unless he or she gives notice of his or her intention to withdraw from the case. Thus, one form that a dental assistant must understand is the letter of withdrawal issued by the dentist. The dentist must give the patient reasonable notice if he or she intends to withdraw from the case. This varies with the conditions of the community in which the patient lives (figure 4.1).

JOHN C. RAEYWEN, D.D.S.
104 Any Street
Anytown, Anystate 12345
612-926-1414

July 17, 19—

Mr. John H. Smith
734 Poplar Lane
Anytown, Anystate 12610

Dear Mr. Smith:

I wish to inform you that I will no longer perform dentistry for you because you have failed to follow my dental advice and treatment program concerning your home care.

If you so desire, I shall be available to attend you for thirty days after you have received this letter. This should give you ample time to select a dentist from the many competent practitioners in this city. With your written approval, I will make available to the dentist of your choice your case history and information regarding the diagnosis and treatment which you have received from me.

Very truly yours,

John C. Raeywen, D. D. S.

Figure 4.1
Sample letter of withdrawal from case.

Another way in which services are terminated is at the instigation of the patient. In this case, the dentist's office should issue a letter of confirmation of this discharge (figure 4.2).

Other notifications to the patient or authorizations by the patient are illustrated in figures 4.3–4.5.

These letters should be sent by certified mail. A copy should be kept in the dentist's files, along with the return signature card that the post office will send to you after the patient has signed it. (The returned signature card is your proof that the patient received the letter.) Keep both these papers until the statute of limitations has expired. (The sample letters should be used as guides but are not to be copied verbatim.)

Dentists who use these letters and statements of relationships with patients who leave their care or fail to cooperate place themselves in the position of having established the written facts that (1) the dentist did not abandon the case, or (2) the dentist was discharged by the patient, or (3) the patient refused to follow the dentist's advice.

JENNY C. RAEYWEN, D.D.S.
104 Any Street
Anytown, Anystate 12345
612-926-1414

July 17, 19—

Ms. Mary H. Smith
734 Poplar Lane
Anytown, Anystate 12610

Dear Ms. Smith:

This will confirm our telephone conversation of today in which you discharged me as your dentist.

In my opinion, your condition requires continued treatment by a dentist. If you have not already done so, I suggest that you employ another dentist without delay. You may be assured that, at your written request, I will furnish that dentist with information regarding the diagnosis and treatment which you have received from me.

Very truly yours,

Jenny C. Raeywen, D. D. S.

Figure 4.2
Sample letter of confirmation of discharge of patient.

I have refused to permit Doctor _____ to take X rays (roentgenograms) of my teeth for a diagnosis. The doctor has told me that it is advisable to use X rays for this diagnosis. I waive any claim for damages because roentgenograms (X rays) were not taken.

Date:_____

_____SIGNED:_____
WITNESS   Patient

Figure 4.3
Form for refusal to permit X rays.

I hereby authorize Doctor _____
to disclose complete information to
regarding his or her dental diagnosis and treatment

of the undersigned from   19   until the
date of the conclusion of the treatment.
    Further, I authorize the doctor to testify, without limitation, about all dental findings and treatment of the undersigned, in any legal action, suit, or proceedings to which I am, or may become, a party; and I waive on behalf of myself and any persons who may have an interest in the matter all provisions of law relating to the disclosure of confidential dental information.

_____   _____
WITNESS   Patient

_____   _____
Date   Address

Figure 4.4
Authorization for disclosure of advice.

JOHN C. RAEYWEN, D.D.S.
104 Any Street
Anytown, Anystate 12345
612-926-1414

July 17, 19—

Mr. Albert M. Sorenson
652 Maple Avenue
Anytown, Anystate 12622

Dear Mr. Sorenson:

At the time that you brought your son, William, to me for examination this afternoon, I informed you that I was unable to determine without X-ray pictures whether a fracture existed in his jaw. I strongly urge you to permit me or some other oral surgeon of your choice to make this X-ray examination without further delay.

Your neglect in not permitting a proper X-ray examination to be made of William's jaw may result in serious consequences if in fact a fracture does exist.

Very truly yours,

John C. Raeywen, D. D. S.

Figure 4.5
Sample letter to patient who fails to follow advice.

The Dentist's Public Duties

Dentists have some public duties that they must perform simply because they are dentists. They must have a narcotics license to dispense or prescribe narcotics, and the quantity prescribed is registered by the licensing bureau. It is necessary to keep an inventory of the narcotics in the possession of the dentist. Daily records must be kept of certain drugs dispensed. These drugs are listed by the federal government. Only a qualified person may administer narcotics. The type of records to be kept are discussed in the section on administration of the office. Reports on addicts must be made.

A dentist may be called by the courts to serve as an **expert witness.** An expert gives an opinion on a subject as an authority for the benefit of the jury and the court. This testimony has nothing to do with an individual patient of that dentist. The dentist may not know the defendant or plaintiff in the case. The judgment of the dentist is used for court education.

It is also possible that a dentist may be called to testify in behalf of his or her patient who is involved in a damage suit. The dentist is expected, in this instance, to explain his or her diagnosis, findings, progress of treatment, description of the patient's residual problems, amount of suffering the patient has experienced, and probable permanent impairment.

The statute regarding patient-dentist privilege affects what the dentist may say in court. If the patient does not waive his or her privilege, the dentist may not testify.

If the dentist must appear in court, it is important for the assistant to discover the exact date and time, the courtroom number, and the judge's name. Most attorneys are very cooperative in judging the exact time at which the dentist must appear.

It is important that the dentist take his or her records of the case to court for reference when asked questions about the case. Occasionally, it is necessary for the assistant to testify as to what was said and done in her or his presence.

Sometimes a subpoena is required when a dentist is called to testify. A **subpoena** is an order from the court that requires that the person named in the paper appear in court to testify. A penalty is dealt if the person named does not appear. This subpoena helps waive the confidential patient-dentist relationship.

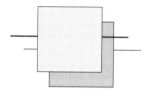

Part Three: Liabilities: Professional and Criminal

There are many ways a dentist may be sued in a court of law. It is important that the assistants of the dentist understand the problems and use care to see that insofar as possible there are no incidents that might give a patient an opportunity to sue.

The matter of patients suing dentists has become a serious problem. Until 1930 the number of cases was insignificant, but from 1930 on, suits for injuries began to increase in many fields. A contractor was sued for injury to children playing in his partially constructed home, even though the children were trespassing. A washing machine manufacturer was sued for injury to a user who had failed to read the directions. The claims against physicians and dentists began to increase, also. Today these claims have become so numerous and large that insurance companies are often unwilling to provide medical professional liability insurance for certain high risk practices. Further, the premiums for liability insurance have been raised to figures that cause some health professionals to be reluctant to continue practicing. Part of the reason that the claims have been so large is that some attorneys charge no fee at all unless they win the lawsuit. The fee, then, is a third of the settlement. This arrangement means the patient suing the dentist (called the plaintiff) pays the attorney nothing unless the patient wins the lawsuit; thus, the risk to the patient is minimal and the patient may receive a large sum of money.

An attorney once stated to all his clients, "Stay out of court if you possibly can!" One of the best ways to stay out of court is to avoid situations in the dental office that invite suits. To do so means that all members of the health team must understand the liabilities that exist in the office—and do everything they can to avoid creating situations that invite suits. Let us examine the liabilities that exist.

Personal Injury Claims

Everyone who has a place of business or a home is responsible for any injury that occurs on its premises. The large department store owner is responsible for any conditions that cause accidents within the premises. If an injury occurs within a building but not within the office space rented by an individual, the owner of the building may be responsible.

Everyone needs protection against this personal injury liability. For the dentist who maintains an office this protection is very important.

Since the dentist can be held responsible for everything that happens in his or her office, it is essential that the staff be alert to common problems and do all they can to eliminate accident-inviting conditions. For example, if there is a screwhead on the doorknob that cuts anyone in opening the door, the dentist is responsible for the injury. If a nylon stocking is caused to snag and run by a rough spot on a chair, the dentist is liable for the cost of the nylons. If a rug causes someone to trip, or a waxed floor causes someone to fall, the dentist is responsible. This is **personal liability,** and a dentist must be protected from such claims by insurance and by extreme care exercised by the staff to eliminate all possible hazards.

Medical Professional Liability (Malpractice Claims)

Personal injury claims are usually not as serious or as frequent as medical professional liability, commonly known as medical **malpractice** (bad practice) claims, for which a dentist may be sued if the patient feels he or she was detrimentally affected by a treatment, was injured by treatment, or that the diagnosis was incorrect.

The term **medical professional liability** is preferred because it best describes the area in which the claims actually arise. Furthermore, malpractice has a special meaning (connotative meaning) that causes people to think in terms of criminal acts or disreputable conduct and can cause prejudgment of the issues in a court case.

Medical professional liability describes all the civil liability that a dentist incurs by any professional act or by failure to properly perform his or her duty to a patient if this failure results in some injury to the patient.

Black's Law Dictionary defines medical professional liability as "bad, wrong, or injudicious treatment resulting in injury, unnecessary suffering, or death to the patient, and proceeding from ignorance, carelessness, want of proper professional skill, disregard of established rules or principles, neglect, or a malicious or criminal intent."

Malpractice claims can be listed under three legal classifications that will help your understanding. There are **malfeasance** claims in which it is said that the dentist has wrongfully treated the patient—for example a dentist extracted the wrong tooth. This is malfeasance—wrong treatment.

The **misfeasance** claims involve lawful action done in the wrong way. If the dentist extracted the correct tooth but did not use necessary care to prevent infection or failed to properly treat the area, a claim could arise out of misfeasance—what the dentist did was lawful, but he or she didn't perform it correctly.

The third group of claims are **nonfeasance** claims—failure to do anything. If a dentist does nothing about a patient's complaints—a wait-and-see policy—or leaves town and does not provide someone to care for the patient's tooth, the dentist can be sued for nonfeasance. If, for example, the dentist looked at the tooth and said, "Let's wait and see if the infection spreads," and the patient went home and soon became seriously ill, the dentist could be liable for nonfeasance.

All medical professional liability claims can be classified under one of these three actions or nonactions by dentists. This complicated area of medical law can be clarified if you are aware of this classification. The dentist may be attacked for not helping, for trying to help in the wrong way, or for trying to help in the right way but performing the procedure incorrectly.

The dentist is expected to use reasonable care, and the tendency is to bring suit for failure to use such care.

The basic standard of reasonable care is one that exists for every citizen in relation to her or his fellow citizens. This means that a dentist is required to possess and use the same knowledge and skill used by other dentists in good standing who have the same general training in the same or similar neighborhoods under similar circumstances. Thus the generalist would be compared with generalists of similar background, but not with specialists, such as oral surgeons. The specialists generally are expected to have a higher degree of skill in the area of their specialty.

Breach of duty is a broad term that covers a number of actions or a lack of action by a dentist for which a patient may sue. The following areas can be involved in a breach of duty:

1. *Diagnosis* requires that a dentist use ordinary skill in acquiring all the data necessary for a complete diagnosis. Should he or she fail to make the necessary tests, take essential X rays, or observe all unusual conditions as colleagues do under similar circumstances, the dentist can be sued for negligent diagnosis.

2. *Standard procedure* refers to treatment as commonly performed by most dentists of similar training.
3. *Prior dentists* need protection. When a patient terminates a contract with one dentist and becomes a patient of a different dentist, the new dentist must not, by inadvertent gestures, looks, or comments, give the patient any idea that the patient might sue the prior dentist. The present dentist cannot know what the circumstances were at the time of treatment, and any indication that the prior dentist was not skillful must be carefully avoided by the dentist and staff.
4. *Instruction of patients.* Patients must be properly instructed about home care of themselves and what symptoms to report to the dentist.
5. *Referral of the patient.* If a dentist feels a specialist is necessary to adequately treat or diagnose the patient's problem, the dentist is expected to make a proper referral.
6. *Exposure of patient.* The exposure of the patient to the public can also bring a lawsuit. The dentist must be very careful that the patient is seen by no one but the necessary office staff without the patient's express permission. This includes being seen by another dentist or being photographed for scientific purposes.
7. *Attention to patient.* The patient must receive the attention his or her symptoms require. Failure of a dentist to give the patient the proper amount of attention has resulted in court actions.

Proof of Negligence

It has been historically true in the courts of the United States that the plaintiff has to prove negligence. Recent court decisions have on occasion cast the burden of proof on the defendant dentist, causing the dentist to prove that he or she was not negligent. Interpretations of laws are changing, and it wise to protect oneself with all the written documents possible.

However, there are some comforting facts to be remembered. An error in diagnosis is not enough evidence by itself that a dentist was negligent. A dentist cannot be held accountable for poor results for dental treatment. Other circumstances, such as contaminated instruments, must be part of the evidence to obtain a verdict of negligence. X ray is one cause of numerous claims.

The **burden of proof** requires that the patient offer more proof that the dentist was negligent. If the jury decides the two groups of evidence are equal, they must decide in favor of the defendant (dentist). The dentist is not considered negligent until proved so by overwhelming evidence. The patient must prove the standard of care dentists in good standing exercise and then prove that this dentist does not exercise that care.

Expert testimony formerly was necessary to prove negligence. However, in recent years there have been two areas of suits in which expert testimony has been judged unnecessary in many courts. They are cases which are tried under *res ipsa loquitur* and the doctrine of common knowledge.

It is said that the jury, from its fund of common knowledge, is able to decide without expert testimony whether or not the defendant is guilty. It is generally felt that some of the court applications abandoning expert testimony are creating unfair situations for the settlement of court claims.

Res Ipsa Loquitur or "Somebody Obviously Goofed!"

Res ipsa loquitur literally means "the thing speaks for itself." The character of the accident and surrounding circumstances determines whether *res ipsa loquitur* applies. If an accident is inexplicable in terms of ordinary and known experience except by negligence, then negligence is either presumed or inferred. Circumstances surrounding the accident must amount to evidence from which the jury can infer negligence. It differs from circumstantial evidence in that the evidence points to no specific fault.

Three conditions necessary for *res ipsa loquitur* are as follows:

1. The accident must be one that ordinarily doesn't occur unless someone is negligent.
2. It must be caused by something within the control of the defendant.
3. It must not have been due to any voluntary action or contribution on the part of the plaintiff.

The difficulty for the dentists with *res ipsa loquitur* is the way in which it shifts the burden of proof to the defendant (dentist), whereas in other court actions the burden of proof is the responsibility of the plaintiff (patient).

An example of *res ipsa loquitur* would be infections caused by contaminated instruments.

The traditional requirement for *res ipsa loquitur* to apply is that the accident that caused the injury must have been under the control of the dentist or his or her employees.

Another doctrine—the **doctrine of common knowledge**—is similar to *res ipsa loquitur*. The chief difference with the doctrine of common knowledge is that no expert opinion is judged necessary for the jury to make its decision.

How do *res ipsa loquitur* and common knowledge apply to the dental assistant? Note that injuries from equipment used in the office—even frayed electrical cords—and diseases and infection contracted from contaminated instruments are common charges in court actions. The office team must be constantly alert to the dangers of injury and accident in the office. "Somebody obviously goofed" becomes a nightmare all too easily today.

Proximate Cause

A **proximate cause** is the direct relationship of an act or factor contributing to a specific result. The negligence of the dentist must be the proximate cause of the injury or death. This negligence must be shown to be such that the injury would not have occurred if the dentist had not acted as he or she did. For example, if the dentist fails to sterilize instruments and the patient develops an infection or dies, the dentist is liable because the proximate cause is obviously the contaminated instruments.

Additional Tort Liability

Tort, a term used in legal discussions, means "conduct that constitutes a civil wrong," making it possible for the injured individual to collect damages from the person who caused the injury. In dentistry the most common liability is the tort of negligence.

Other liabilities are the following:

1. Assault and battery, false imprisonment, and personal restraint
2. Fraud or deceit
3. Defamation, libel, and slander
4. Invasion of privacy and breach of confidential communication
5. Liability for the acts of others

The last item means that the dentist is responsible for the acts of anyone who is employed by him or her. If an employee injures a patient, it is the dentist who is responsible and can be sued. The employee may also be sued, but usually secondarily.

Negligence ordinarily means that the dentist had permission to treat the patient but the treatment did not measure up to the standards imposed by law, or that this particular dentist did not perform dentistry as effectively as members of similar standing in the dental profession in his or her community.

Admissions

No dentist should ever admit error unless directed to do so by his or her attorney and insurance company.

Frequently, the dentist does not know the facts in the situation. Perhaps there were some concealed symptoms at the time of examination. Regardless of what the dentist and office staff think about the case, absolutely no information should be given to anyone but the dentist's attorney and the dentist's insurance company, unless the attorney so instructs the dentist.

Breach of Contract

Another area to consider is breach of contract, in which a dentist promises to correct or promises to perform a service for a patient.

If a dentist agrees to achieve a particular result or effect for a patient and fails to do so, he or she is liable for breach of contract even if the highest degree of professional skill has been used in performing the dentistry.

It is also in this area that one dentist promises another not to compete in the practice of dentistry and then violates this promise. The court case usually concerns two dentists, one of whom had for some reason agreed not to practice dentistry within a certain restricted area (such as within a certain town or within fifty miles of that town) and then reconsiders that promise. Usually one of these dentists has been employed by the other or has purchased the records and space of an older dentist who leaves the community. Eventually the older dentist decides to reopen an office somewhere nearby, and former patients return to the older dentist's practice. Another example might be that the agreement between the two dentists proves unsatisfactory, but the younger dentist likes the area too well to leave, and he or she opens an office nearby. Patients who prefer this dentist leave the older dentist's practice. Both these examples are classified as breach of contract.

Professional Liability Insurance

Obviously, liability insurance is imperative—and in as large an amount as possible. Not only should the dentist be covered by this insurance, but his team members should also be protected.

Criminal Liabilities

Another form of liability which a dentist can experience is criminal liability (the previously discussed liabilities are civil liabilities). In criminal liability cases, the dentist must be guilty of a crime punishable by the court that has jurisdiction over this form of crime.

A **crime** is an act that wrongs the public as a whole instead of injuring one specific individual. Crimes are classified as misdemeanors or felonies. The classification is important to a dentist who is unfortunate enough to be accused of a crime, because state medical practice acts usually revoke the license of a dentist convicted of a felony. Crimes of moral turpitude (such as willfully evading income taxes) can mean suspension of a dentist's license to practice.

Criminal liability is more difficult to prove than civil liability. In civil action the injured party simply has to show more evidence of injury than the dentist shows lack of proof of injury. If the plaintiff can show more evidence, he or she is usually able to collect damages.

In a criminal action the government must prove that the defendant is guilty beyond a reasonable doubt and must convince every juror of it. The defendant is guaranteed the right to a trial by jury and is presumed innocent until proved guilty. The defendant need not even try to defend himself or herself but can remain silent, and the government must prove guilt beyond reasonable doubt. The defendant can then appeal to a higher court.

Narcotic violations, negligence that causes death, and income tax evasion are all areas in which a dental team could be accused of criminal liability. The team members must be exact in recording and dispensing any narcotics to avoid the least suspicion of improper use concerning these drugs. Further, maintaining the sterile conditions required in certain operations is imperative to avoid any suggestion of negligence. Lastly, careless record-keeping could result in income tax evasion charges. Any one of these areas of neglect can bring criminal charges—and loss of license to practice. Be certain that your conduct is not responsible for the initiation of such a charge.

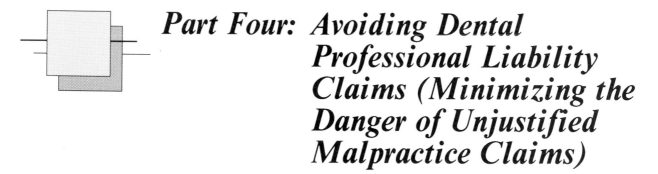

Part Four: Avoiding Dental Professional Liability Claims (Minimizing the Danger of Unjustified Malpractice Claims)

Patients form an opinion of the dental health team as they experience dentistry. If the opinion is favorable, if the patient feels as if he or she is a human being whose health and person are important to the staff, he or she likes the experience. This patient is not likely to institute a suit. Therefore, treat patients as human beings about whom everyone on the staff cares.

Excellent communication with the patient is essential. The discussion of the treatment, the possible results—both good and bad—and the fees charged for the work should occur prior to treatment. Then, in the visits that follow as the work is performed, communication about progress is essential. The patient who feels understood and that she or he understands rarely becomes the plaintiff in a suit.

Should a member of the health team sense that some patient has become antagonistic, the dentist should be notified at once and every effort made to discover why this formerly contented patient is now antagonistic. These observances will aid in materially reducing the attempts at medical professional liability claims.

In addition, the patient should be educated about dentistry. As the work progresses, it is possible for an alert team to express ideas about dentistry that may not be known to the general public. For example, dentistry is a highly skilled profession. All members of the oral health team have been specially trained to perform a service. Then, too, all members of the team must continue to improve their education by attending study groups, meetings, or refresher courses. Scientific research, resulting in better care and improved services, is continually performed; and the members of the team are made aware of these improvements.

To express these ideas casually in conversation with patients over a period of time assists in creating an excellent image of dentistry for the patients who usually are unaware of these factors. It may offset some of the resentments patients often express about the high cost of dentistry.

In addition to creating the right environment in the dental office to make patients enjoy coming (although they may not enjoy the discomfort of some operations), there are ways in which the danger of unjustified malpractice claims can be minimized.

Three Defenses for Dental Professional Liability Actions

Contributory Negligence

If a patient does not cooperate with the dentist by following all reasonable instructions, and this failure on the part of the patient contributes to his or her problem—injury, worsened condition, or death—that patient cannot collect damages because **contributory negligence** causes part of the problem.

Assumption of Risk

Legally, it is assumed that to knowingly pursue a course of action that involves certain risks means that the person cannot recover damages if injury occurs. For example, a skier assumes the normal risks of injury while skiing. In dentistry the **assumption of risk** means that a patient assumes the risks of specific treatment once the patient has been properly informed about them; however, that patient does not assume risk from negligent treatment.

If experimental treatment that, as yet, is not adequately proved safe is to be attempted, the patient must be fully warned and should sign a consent statement to relieve the dentist of liability for possible detrimental effects.

Statutes of Limitation

Time limits are established for the filing of court claims. These time limits vary from state to state. It is important to know the **statute of limitations** for your state. If a claim is not filed within that period of time, it can never be filed.

Minimizing the Danger of Unjustified Medical Professional Liability Claims

Some of the medical professional liability claims that are filed against dentists have legitimate bases; however, many of the cases are unjustified claims. What can the oral health team members do to avoid unjustified medical professional liability claims?

1. All team members can communicate with the patients. A friendly atmosphere discourages lawsuits. At the first awareness that some patient is dissatisfied, the dentist should be informed. All team members should be asked for, and should provide, any data concerning the patient who seems to be developing dissatisfaction. Attempts to reinstate the friendly relationship should be made.
2. Delegation of tasks by the dentist to other staff members must only be those tasks which they can perform legally.
3. Equipment used in the office must be maintained regularly.
4. Avoid making any statements that may invite a lawsuit.

    Suppose, for example, there has been an accident in which the dentist has inadvertently injured a patient in the presence of an assistant. Anything that the assistant says at that time is a part of the action, and the patient can quote the assistant in court.

    A dental assistant should be very careful to avoid making any statement that might imply that the dentist made a mistake or was at fault. No comment should be made about the dentist's work at this time. Even the comment "This never happened before" is an invitation to some patients to sue. The dental assistant should remain silent.
5. Dental assistants must be careful not to prescribe for patients in conversation with them, nor to discuss the relative merits of methods of treatment or medication. To do so would be practicing dentistry without a license.

    If you discuss medication or its effect, without specific instructions from the dentist, you are liable to be charged with practicing dentistry without a license to do so.

    The dental assistant is permitted to take dictation from the patient or a member of the patient's family concerning the effects of the treatment he or she has received. However, the dental assistant may not discuss the probable effects or predict what she or he thinks the dentist may do when the dentist receives the report.

6. Never permit the refill of a prescription without first consulting your dentist.

7. The instructions given to a patient for home care must be specific, detailed, and clear. Some of them should be in writing to avoid misunderstandings. Frequently, a medical professional liability claim is begun by a patient due to the poor results of treatment. Be sure that the poor results are not due to the fact that the patient was not carefully instructed as to his or her obligations in home care.

8. Be optimistic. Optimism, like courtesy, is infectious. Optimism is the inclination to anticipate the best possible outcome and leads to confidence on the part of the patient in the ability of his or her dentist and the anticipated results. It should be instilled into the minds of the staff and, in turn, be infectious to the recipient of the services.

9. Dental records are of extreme importance. A complete, legible, carefully written clinical record is essential. It may make the difference between a verdict in favor of the dentist rather than one against the dentist.

   It is also wise not to correct or write over these records. It is better practice to note the correction as such. Draw a single line through the incorrect statement so that the statement is still readable. Then note the correction and the date on which the correction was made. It is also helpful to initial the correction.

   An example of incorrect care of records occurred in a situation where a dentist was sued. His prescription for the patient was well within the normal limits of the general prescription policies for that drug. However, this patient suffered a severe allergic reaction to it. When the patient's attorney approached the dentist, the dentist became disturbed because the dosage was somewhat more than he usually prescribed. He erased the record of the amount of the drug administered and wrote over it. When the insurance company made a photocopy of the record, the erasure showed clearly. A quick out-of-court settlement was made because the record had been altered, not because there was anything wrong with the original dosage. Be certain that your records are neatly and accurately kept, and be certain all

corrections are visible and noted as having been made on the date that you prepared the record, or close to that time.

Frequently, a professional liability claim is begun by a patient due to poor results of treatment. Actually the poor results are due, at least in part, to the fact that the patient did not follow the dentist's orders, or the specific drug or dosage was inadequate. However, in a jury trial, the aggrieved individual is a far more appealing object to the jury than the dentist. The complete, carefully written record, substantiated by letters to the patients indicating the need to follow the treatment schedule carefully, is one of the best defenders of the dentist in the courtroom. Be certain that your office protects your dentist as completely as possible by keeping such records and by writing any necessary letters that should be sent by certified mail.

10. Be sure to have a written request from a patient who wishes to have records sent or given to a new dentist. Without the written request from the patient, you are liable for releasing confidential information without the consent of the patient.

11. Keep the office scrupulously clean and neat to avoid charges of carelessness and negligence.

12. Be certain that two persons are present when the patient is in the operatory. A reliable witness for examinations is required to avoid lawsuits. The second staff member can verify the report if necessary.

13. Be accurate and complete in preparing insurance records. It is possible to have an insurance report used against a dentist by both the patient and the insurance company. Examine insurance reports carefully. Call the attention of your dentist to any items which might cause trouble. Be certain that you have a copy in your file of every insurance report that leaves the office.

    Some of the items you should think about as you look over an insurance form to be mailed are these:

    a. A medical professional liability suit can start from an indication by the dentist or staff that the problem encountered in the office was not entirely the fault of the patient. In this instance the patient collects from the insurance company and then sues the dentist.

b. Any statement that might be interpreted as placing the responsibility on your office for any accident or unfortunate occurrence should be rephrased so that it does not admit or assume blame.

c. A statement made by the dentist that uses the wrong words to describe the patient—words that can be termed libelous—should be rewritten. For example, the dentist should write, "I was unable to discover any physical conditions that would account for the patient's complaints" instead of writing the patient is a "malingerer."

d. Be certain the insurance form is completed properly. An insurance firm can sue a dentist for incomplete reports.

If you have any misgivings about these reports, it is far wiser to consult your dentist and gain permission to present the papers to his or her attorney than to mail in a report that might create a legal problem.

14. Refrain from criticizing another dentist. Only the dentist in attendance knew the conditions existing at the start of the treatment. Careless derogatory remarks about the treatment prescribed by another dentist or physician have started unjustified lawsuits. The reputation of the health profession suffers every time there is a lawsuit. The public certainly deserves to keep its faith in the health professions. You can help by not destroying that faith by careless remarks.

15. The general standard of care dispensed by a dentist should be the equivalent of like dentists practicing under similar conditions.

16. Experimental treatment should be performed only with the full knowledge and consent of the patient. A law exists that a dentist shall use only such methods as are generally approved by other dentists in the community. Thus, for any experimental treatment it is wise to have the written permission from the patient because the dentist is violating a law if he or she experiments on a patient without this permission. If the patient requests this care, the patient has released the dentist from the violation.

17. Diagnostic tests that are usually used for specific symptoms must be performed if the dentist is to escape the accusation of inadequate diagnosis.

18. Specialists and consultations should be used whenever the dentist deems them necessary and proper. Failure to request the care of a specialist for a condition that is not normally treated by the dentist could lead to a charge of negligence.

19. Consent of the patient is necessary to perform treatment or surgery. A dentist who proceeds without the written consent of the patient is inviting claims of assault and battery. It is necessary for the dentist to inform the patient of the course of treatment and its probable outcome, and to permit the patient to decide whether to undergo the particular treatment. The same is true for oral surgery. Any surgical procedure must be preceded by a specific consent for the particular surgery to be performed.

20. A substitute dentist is sometimes necessary. Patients are to be informed that the dentist plans to be away. They should also be told whom to see in the dentist's absence. To some patients the discovery that their dentist is not present to care for them is very upsetting. Soothing, tactful reassurance is a strong deterrent to possible court actions.

21. Prescriptions have been the cause of some court problems. A written prescription by the dentist is the best insurance against being charged for an error in prescription for which the dentist is not responsible. Sometimes there is misunderstanding when a prescription is given verbally over the telephone, and an error is made in filling a prescription. The problem can be avoided by insisting that the written prescription be presented to the pharmacist.

22. Guard against carelessness or negligence by scrupulous care in the office. The alert assistant will maintain a constant vigilance against dirt, lack of order, and outworn materials. Records will be accurately maintained. The assistant should frequently look at the office through the eyes of a patient to see wherein some detail needs attention. The office should look immaculately clean and neat. The appearance of a tidy office is a deterrent to accusations of carelessness and negligence.

Attention to patients' needs, and consideration of each patient as worthwhile are important in establishing this office as one in which negligence does not occur because the staff is too interested in the welfare of the patient.

23. Fees should be discussed with candor and understood before treatment is begun. It prevents serious misunderstandings and is fair to the patient. The patient will appreciate this kind of consideration.

24. Withdrawal from a case is sometimes necessary or wise. As discussed earlier in this chapter, there are certain precautions that are necessary when a dentist wishes to withdraw from a case. Send the patient a certified letter stating that the dentist is withdrawing and suggest how the patient can find another dentist.

25. Attitude of the staff toward patients is extremely important in maintaining the desired atmosphere of thoughtful consideration of each patient. The tactful care of the patients by the entire staff can be a preventive measure when considering medical protective liability suits. If a patient seems to change his or her outlook (grumble, be somewhat antagonistic or withdrawn), it is time to communicate. A review of the case history in consultation with the patient may tell the dentist why the patient appears dissatisfied. In turn, this may prevent a medical professional lawsuit.

    Consideration of each patient as an individual human being with a life to lead and interests beyond your office will be one of the best deterrents to medical professional lawsuits any dentist can have. A patient who feels kindly toward the entire staff is not going to start a suit. That patient thinks of the dentist and staff as friends.

26. Avoid discussing cases. A patient must reveal information that he or she may not wish known to anyone else, including family. The law protects each human being by stating that he or she has a right to privacy. The dentist cannot reveal any information to anyone without the express permission of the patient. This also means that the dentist's staff is unable to divulge any information regarding any patient. Special circumstances, such as insurance examinations, require the listing of information. The patient must be made aware of this procedure before the information is released.

    Never reveal information about a patient to an unauthorized person. It may surprise you to know that to be legally correct in giving information to an authorized person, it is necessary to have the request for information in writing. Never give information about a patient over the telephone. Ask the caller to write the request and mail it to you. Be sure to ask the caller to furnish the authorization by the patient or a responsible member of the family. Be certain that the written authorization is actually a document executed by the patient or responsible member of his family. It pays to double-check the authenticity of this request.

    If a dentist is requested to give information to an attorney, a release must be signed by the patient. The release includes the name and address of the person to whom the report is to be sent. It should be dated and signed by the patient whose signature should be witnessed by someone other than the dentist or staff members.

    It is interesting to know that in addition to the right to privacy, the patient-dentist relationship is one of **privileged communication;** that is, it is the privilege of the patient to request the dentist to keep the information private or to reveal it in a court of law. The statute regarding privileged communication does not apply to the dentist's staff. No staff member can reveal any information at any time. They are all required to keep the records confidential.

    One exception to the right to privacy and privileged communication is that of the dentist who is employed by an insurance company. The dentist examines a patient with no thought of treatment, and reports the findings to the insurance company. The information from this examination is not privileged. The dentist may testify in a court of law about the findings without the permission of the patient.

27. Sometimes a lawsuit occurs in reaction to a fee. The patient has decided the bill is too high, or for some reason doesn't want to pay when payment is due. The charge, of course, should be correctly just and owing

before the initial billing. In the event of a patient's dissatisfaction with the fee charged, the patient is urged to discuss his or her dissatisfaction with the dentist. Should this discussion fail to produce any satisfactory arrangement for the patient to complete his financial obligation, verify the time limits on medical professional lawsuits in your state because medical professional lawsuits are outlawed after a certain period of time. Perhaps by careful consideration of just when you should apply pressure to collect an account, a suit may be avoided.

28. Legal advice concerning lawsuits should be accepted from the attorney whom the dentist employs. A simple list of rules about such matters ought to be posted where the staff can be reminded of their duties, such as refraining from discussing any case and avoiding the temptation to inadvertently prescribe for the patient.

29. Settlement of lawsuits is a matter to be handled by the insurance company with whom medical professional insurance is carried and/or the dentist's attorney. Be very certain that no comment about any matter pertaining to a lawsuit is ever made by any staff member except as required by the attorney of the dentist or the court of law.

Summary

The dental practice acts: The eagerness of people to diagnose and prescribe for others has made it necessary to establish controls over who is entitled to practice in the health sciences.

There are three general sources of American law: federal, state, and judicial decisions. Federal statutes are found in the *United States Code*. Federal statutes must not contradict the United States Constitution; state statutes must not contradict the constitution of that particular state. Judicial or judge-made law is often called common law. It applies within the jurisdiction of the judge who issues the decree.

Police power (in its broad sense of regulation) is the privilege of the states; therefore, states control the practice of dentistry by licensure.

The dentist is controlled by (1) federal law, to prescribe narcotics, (2) state laws in the state in which he or she practices, and (3) judge-made or common law in relationships with patients.

The dental practice acts are regulatory statutes that prohibit anyone from practicing dentistry without a license.

Licensing is by state, by the National Board of Dental Examiners, and by reciprocity.

The annual certificate and original license must be displayed in the dental office.

Narcotics may not be prescribed without a narcotics license.

Licenses can be revoked for specified actions. The power of revocation belongs to the State Board of Dental Examiners of each state.

Legal relationship of the dentist and the patient: A definite relationship exists between a dentist and a patient and is upheld in a court of law. A contract is created when a dentist agrees to perform services for a patient who requests such care. The dentist may limit care specifically or agree to provide continual care. This agreement may be verbal, but a wise dentist terminates such an agreement with a written document. An agent may complete the agreement if a patient is unable to do so for himself or herself.

Financial responsibility laws should be understood by the dentist and staff. The dental assistant is an agent for the dentist. The dentist is responsible for the conduct and treatment performed by his or her employees.

It is important that the dentist and his or her staff make proper arrangement for payment for services if an agent requests dental care for anyone.

Insurance programs, prepayment benefits, and government agencies present specific problems in collections. The staff should be acquainted with the regulations pertaining to such plans in their locale.

A contract must be properly terminated if a dentist is not to be held liable for neglect. Forms for such terminations are available through medical professional insurance companies. These termination letters should be sent by certified mail.

Termination can occur if the dentist gives notice of intent to withdraw or if the patient indicates he or she no longer desires the services.

Public duties that a dentist must perform include reporting narcotic addicts and recording the use of narcotics in the office.

Professional and criminal liabilities: It would be unwise for an assistant to look with suspicion on all persons who enter the office—they are not all intending to sue your office for personal liability or medical professional liability. It is wise, however, for the assistant to be alert to conditions that encourage such suits, because in the course of seeing hundreds of people it is only logical that some of them may become claimants.

We cannot urge you too strongly to be alert to the dangers that exist in your office. Be constantly vigilant. Watch for safety features: furniture, fixtures, rugs, waxed floors, sharp edges, frayed electric cords, furniture which tips easily, step stools that are weak or do not have a wide base. Never leave a patient alone in a room in which there is equipment that could be inadvertently activated, such as X ray if the controls are in the room.

To avoid malpractice claims, see that your records are accurately and clearly kept and that all assistants observe the regulations that are so necessary in preventing these claims.

Criminal liability means an act has been committed that wrongs the public as a whole rather than one individual. Such crimes usually result in loss of license to practice dentistry. Among the crimes in this classification are narcotics violations, negligence, and evasion of taxes. Careful records must be kept to prevent the slightest doubt of accuracy with either narcotics records or income statements.

Avoiding liability claims: Defenses to medical professional liability actions are as follows:

1. Contributory negligence. (Proving the patient contributed by not taking proper home care of himself or herself.)
2. Assumption of risk. (Proving the patient was informed of the risks involved.)
3. Statute of limitations. (Allowing the collection of the case to wait until the statute of limitations becomes effective and makes it impossible for the patient to start a suit.)

Twenty-nine ways to minimize the dangers of unjustified medical professional liability claims are stated.

Study Questions

1. Why should a dental assistant understand the basic laws relating to dentistry?
2. Why are there laws regulating the practice of dentistry?
3. What are the sources of American law?
4. Who licenses dentists?
5. What body of law regulates the relationships with patients?
6. What are causes of revocation of license?
7. Why must dental assistants understand the rights, privileges, and laws concerning the care of patients?
8. What is a contract with a patient?
9. Discuss laws governing financial responsibility.
10. What is meant when it is stated that the dental assistant is the agent of the dentist?
11. What knowledge must a dental assistant have about insurance programs?
12. Why should a dentist terminate a patient contract in writing?
13. What public duties must a dentist perform?
14. For what two reasons might a dentist be called to appear in court?
15. Why is the use of narcotics recorded so accurately in the dentist's office?
16. Why is it so necessary today to be alert to dangers in the office which may bring lawsuits?
17. What kind of claims are filed?
18. Discuss malpractice claims.
19. What are breach of duty claims?
20. Discuss burden of proof.
21. What is *res ipsa loquitur*?
22. What is proximate cause?
23. What are the tort liabilities for a dentist?
24. Discuss breach of contract.
25. What protection does professional liability insurance provide?
26. Why is a criminal liability accusation more serious for a dentist?
27. List the defenses to malpractice actions.
28. Write an explanation of the dental assistant's role in maintaining equipment in excellent condition as an aid to prevent lawsuits.
29. Discuss complete clinical records and their importance to the dentist.

Vocabulary

agent   a person who legally represents another person. Examples include a parent acting for a minor child, an adult child acting for an incompetent parent, or a dental assistant acting for the dentist who has directed the assistant to perform certain tasks

assumption of risk   patient assumes risk when properly informed of the risks involved, and patient consents to treatment

breach of duty   a broad term covering many actions or nonactions by a dentist, for which a patient may sue

code   a system of regulations controlling a group

contract   an agreement with an individual patient that indicates the patient is placing herself or himself under the care of this dentist for a specific treatment of a specific condition, or placing herself or himself in the dentist's care for whatever services the dentist may deem necessary

contributory negligence   failure of patient to cooperate with the dentist by following reasonable instructions

crime   an act that wrongs the public as a whole

diagnose   determine what is wrong

expert witness   an authority gives an opinion on a subject for the benefit of the jury and the court

malfeasance   wrong treatment

malpractice   detrimentally affecting a patient (including injury and misdiagnosis); also called medical professional liability

misfeasance   lawful action done in the wrong way

nonfeasance   no treatment; failure to do anything

prescribe   specify the use of a remedy or treatment

remuneration   payment

res ipsa loquitur   the thing speaks for itself; a type of suit

statute of limitations   time limit established for the filing of court claims; if claim is not filed within that period of time, it can never be filed

statutes   laws

subpoena   an order from the court that requires that the person named appear to testify in court

terminated   ended

tort   conduct that constitutes a civil wrong, making it possible for the injured individual to collect damages

Word Elements	
Word Element	*Example*
amphi prefix meaning: both, doubly	**amphicarcinogenic** tending to both increase or to decrease carcinogenic activity
centi combining form meaning: one one-hundredth (indicates fraction in the metric system)	**centimeter** one-hundredth part of a meter
chron combining form meaning: relationship to time	**chronometry** measurement of time or intervals of time
diplo prefix meaning: double	**diplogram** a double X ray
hect combining form meaning: 100 times the unit of measurement (indicates multiple in the metric system)	**hectogram** 100 grams
hemi prefix meaning: half	**hemisection** the complete sectioning through the crown of a tooth (endodontics), or the removal of one or two roots (periodontics)
kilo combining form meaning: 1000 times the unit of measure (indicates multiple in the metric system)	**kilocycle** 1000 cycles per second
milli prefix or combining form meaning: one one-thousandth (indicates fraction in the metric system)	**milliampere** one one-thousandth of an ampere
poly combining form meaning: much, many	**polymerization** formation of a compound from several single molecules of the same substance (prosthetics)
semi prefix meaning: half, partly	**semicoma** mild coma from which a patient may be aroused (anesthesia)

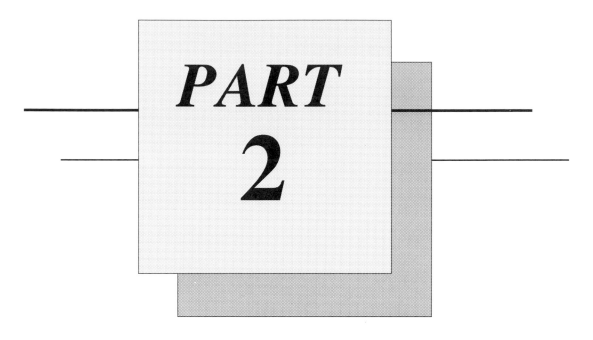

PART 2

People and Personnel: The Human Element

A dental office is centered around relationships among people and is a place where people meet to give and receive service.

Some patients are apprehensive, some are relaxed, some are joyous, and some are withdrawn, fearful, or belligerent. The gamut of emotions is expressed by patients.

The attitudes of the personnel who dispense service for these patients can and do affect the attitudes of patients, and vice versa. Those who provide the service ought to remain pleasant and cheerful even when attitudes encountered in patients cause frustrations. The dental office personnel should be able to accept the problems as part of a day's work.

The chapters in Part Two are written to help the dental assistant gain perspective for work as a member of the oral health care delivery team. These chapters provide information about techniques in the areas of communication and human relations, essential for work as a member of the oral health care delivery team.

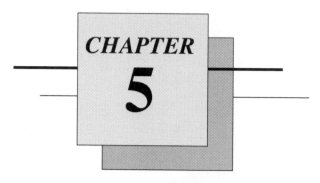

Fundamental Principles of Human Relations

Working with People
Fundamental Human Needs
Tools for Patient Motivation
Favorable Empathic Response Creates Cooperation
Psychology in the Dental Office: A Developmental
     Perspective
Behavior Characteristics of Children
   Characteristics of Specific Age Groups
Behavior Characteristics of Adolescents
Behavior of Adults
   Indirect Approach to People
Public Relations
   Create a Friendly Atmosphere in the Office
Factors Establishing Good Public Relations
   Listen to Patients
   Treat the Patient as a VIP
   Allay the Patient's Fear
   Give the Patient Immediate Attention
   Use the Patient's Name
   Explain a Delay to a Waiting Patient
   Some Individuals Need Special Care

Working with People

After the dentist has received a license to practice and has opened an office, the dentist must have patients to treat. What brings patients to the office? Why do they continue to come to this dentist instead of finding another dentist?

Obviously, something brings the patient to the dentist. It may be pain, poor appearance, or knowledge that regular dental care is desirable, although perhaps not always enjoyable. Patients frequently enter the office apprehensive of the treatment they are about to receive.

What causes a patient to return for a second office call? Aside from the area of the country where there is only one dentist for miles around, a patient returns to the dentist because the patient has confidence in the dentist and likes the way he or she has been treated in the office. Let's say that again: *The patient likes the way he or she has been treated in the office.*

The dental health team can help create an atmosphere in which the patient feels comfortable and appreciated. How? By understanding how patients are motivated and using this knowledge to create rapport.

Fundamental Human Needs

All people experience basic needs or wants that motivate them to take certain actions. This fact can be utilized effectively in working with people. An explanation about basic needs has been given by Maslow. His theory helps us understand why people behave as they do. Some needs are more important to an individual than other needs; and until those highly important needs are satisfied, that individual will not experience other needs. Maslow arranged these basic needs in order of importance: physiological, security, belonging, and esteem. Howell further adapted Maslow's work by developing the ladder of deficit motives (figure 5.1). If we arrange the needs as the rungs of a ladder, it suggests that the needs described as the first rung of the ladder must be satisfied before one can step up to the second rung of the ladder and so on. In other words, until a person's physiological needs are satisfied, that person will not experience security needs. Physiological needs include food, air, protection from physical harm, sleep, and activity.

Next, everyone is concerned with security needs. If they feel safe and secure, then they can experience social needs, such as developing relationships with others. When they have enough social satisfaction, then they become concerned with esteem and prestige needs—with being important.

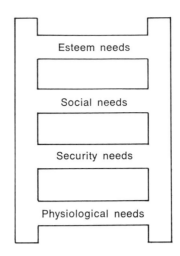

Figure 5.1
Ladder of deficit motives developed by William S. Howell.

If we look at these needs in relationship to the patients in the dental office, we can readily see that there may be a patient who has such pain that he or she is struggling with the physiological need of relief from pain.

Most patients may have problems with security needs; that is, there is a strong desire for a predictable, organized environment—an environment in which a person is not worried about disruptive changes. If the future is uncertain, then the person is more likely to feel insecure, and therefore needs a sense of security.

These four classifications of needs are referred to as *sequential* because a person who is hungry is going to think only about getting food until he has satisfied that desire for hunger. Then, and only then, will he or she be able to think about something else. As long as he or she is hungry, he or she will be thinking about satisfying the hunger. Therefore, the deficit needs are referred to as *motivators*. If a person is hungry, his or her motivation is to acquire food so that he or she is no longer hungry. Motivation is something inside an individual that drives that individual to do something special. How hard it drives him or her depends on how important that particular goal is to the person at that particular time. If we are mildly hungry we may be motivated to eat a little food. If we haven't had any food in three days we are going to be very strongly motivated to find food. The source of energy to find food within the person who is very hungry is much stronger than this same source in the person who is only mildly hungry. Once that hunger has been satisfied, the energy to find food decelerates so that a person may look to security needs—to finding a better job, for example. When he or she has a job and feels safe and secure, then he or she may be motivated to care for social needs—those of belonging and being loved by someone. When the person has a satisfying relationship with other people, he or she will begin to feel motivated to satisfy esteem needs—those of being important.

Now, how does this apply to the dental office? Staff in the office should be aware of the fact that this motivation ladder does exist, that many persons who enter the office have physiological needs—not necessarily hunger. Pain of dental origin may affect their basic physiological state. Others are going to have security needs because they do not feel safe and secure. For example, a patient who has a cyst in his or her jaw may feel very insecure while the possible cancer diagnosis is being determined.

If a patient is in the office for preventive dentistry, he or she may be a very well adjusted individual with all four levels of needs satisfied. Staff members should be able to recognize the motivations affecting the patients. It is also important to recognize that a person can be on one level one time and another level another time. Example, the patient has a biopsy performed and is insecure until learning that the results are negative. The patient suddenly returns to seeking esteem satisfaction rather than remaining on the second rung of the ladder.

Unsatisfied needs prevent action; therefore we refer to them as **deficit motivators.** If a patient is struggling with a basic physiological need, he or she is prevented from being concerned about security, social, or esteem relationships. Therefore, his or her motivation is directed toward physiological needs. No other action can occur. Once a need is satisfied, it will not motivate behavior because satisfied needs do not motivate behavior. It is the anxiety, the lack of something, that causes a person to take action.

Let's look at these needs now in relationship to the dental office. The patient with basic physiological needs of self-preservation is concerned about:

1. Keeping alive.
2. Avoiding or retarding the aging process.
3. Avoiding injury.

That patient may have a need for sleep, for activity, or for sexual experience. This drive runs the gamut from just protecting oneself from the automobile that is careening around the corner and may kill you, to being concerned with little acts that preserve one's health and youth.

The security needs include:

1. Feeling secure and safe.
2. Being protected from whatever imagined or real foes exist.
3. Having a safe, predictable, organized environment.

Patients may be interested in security in the sense that they want to feel that their dentist is competent and that they are safe in trusting her or his judgment. The dental staff must also inspire the patient's confidence.

Social needs, the third-level, concern belongingness and giving and receiving affection. Often a patient wants to "belong" to the doctor and/or staff.

The esteem or prestige needs are the highest level of the ladder. People want to be thought of as worthwhile by other people; they want to have a feeling of personal worth. This is a very important drive. It is easy in the busy rush of the dental office to ignore patients' needs to feel worthwhile. Too often, patients complain that they aren't a "person"—but just a "body." Careful attention to patients as worthwhile individuals is of utmost importance.

The oral health care delivery team that can help a patient recognize the dental service as an asset—better appearance, health, or success—has succeeded in eliminating the stage of negation (often expressed as "How large a filling, Doctor?").

Tools for Patient Motivation

These drives, then, are tools with which to work in the office. Learn something about the background of your patients so that you may better understand their moral and socioeconomic problems (their background—their income level and the type of society in which they live). This will help to individualize the patient and perhaps explain his or her drives.

Psychologists have stated that to some degree, all people are driven by imaginary or real fears. All fears are real to the individual experiencing them, but sometimes someone is unnecessarily afraid. Some fears—or most fears—stem from experiences in childhood that we no longer remember but the emotional memory lingers on below the level of the conscious mind and affects our behavior.

It really doesn't matter what causes the fear. *The important idea for you to remember is that people have fears and need to be treated with kindness and reassurance.*

Your understanding of motivation is important. Actually the motivation of these basic needs in people may be negatively expressed as fear that they will not be able to preserve themselves; that they will not be loved; that they will not have the security of a good job, social position, and so forth; and that they will not be recognized as important by other humans. These feelings are very basic to every human being. They are brought into your office, and you must cope with them. Most patients who come to your office will be unaware that they are being controlled by one or all of these basic feelings.

Patient Motives

The motives of these patients for seeking the service your office offers are:

self-preservation
People fear the aging of their bodies, wish to protect themselves, wish to keep on living.

love
People want love from other humans—love between parents and children, between siblings (brothers and sisters), between other family members, between friends.

security
People need to feel secure and safe, need protection from any real or imagined foes, need a safe, predictable, organized environment.

recognition (esteem)
People wish to be recognized and feel important with other human beings.

It is possible to use these drives to help the patient develop his or her appreciation of the services that your office offers. The indirect presentation of an idea (often referred to as "suggestion") is one of the better approaches in helping patients. It simply means that you express an idea in such a manner that the listener begins to accept it as his or her own idea, or as a very desirable idea because it relates him or her positively to people he or she wishes to emulate: a TV star, a successful business person, a socially recognized woman. Once the patient has recognized the service you are providing as an asset to him or her—as better appearance, health, or success—the patient's fears will decrease.

Favorable Empathic Response Creates Cooperation

From a patient's first contact with the office, whether by telephone or office call, that patient should be made to feel as much at ease as possible—to form an emotional response of contentment or satisfaction with your office—if he or she is to remain a long-term patient. The attitude of the entire staff helps set an emotional tone in the office that makes a patient feel comfortable or uncomfortable, depending upon what attitudes the staff holds. The feeling aroused in the patient in your office is known as **empathic response**. In the dental office it is most important to arouse favorable empathic response.

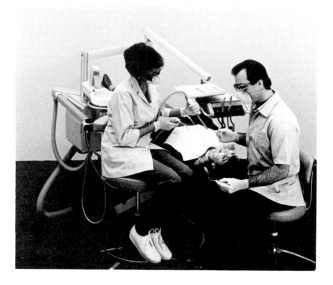

Figure 5.2
Providing every comfort for the patient creates confidence in the dental health team.

You know that a patient's cooperation is necessary to practice dentistry. It is necessary for the patient to open his or her mouth, sit still, and offer some degree of cooperation if the dentist is to prepare a tooth for an amalgam restoration. Learning how to make the patient like to cooperate is important to the long-range success of the office.

Income in the office is increased or decreased by the time consumed in producing a given unit of dental service. The income in your office usually affects the salary of the dental assistant. The time consumed by each patient is important. It is unwise to allow any patient to feel "rushed"; neither can you afford to allow a patient to dillydally and consume your dentist's precious time with long conversations. It is therefore necessary for you to learn how to work with people in such a manner that the patient will look forward with a sense of satisfaction to a visit to your office, yet you do not allow any patient to use more of the dentist's time than is necessary.

You should be able to read the behavior of others, to understand why they act as they do, to offer motivation for the kind of behavior you wish from the patients, and to lead them in the office routines that you must maintain if the oral health care delivery team is to perform successfully.

Everyone possesses a desire to be of value. You can utilize this drive effectively in the dental office to fulfill the patient's need for a sense of personal worth. If you are able to satisfy the patient's need—to make him or her feel that in your office he or she is a very important person whose feelings are considered, whose physical well-being is uppermost in your mind, whose fear you understand, sympathize with, and allay—you will have achieved the objective of making him or her a long-term patient.

In order to be successful in this task, you must watch for cues about the patient's emotional state. Sometimes the same patient will need to be approached in different ways on different days because his or her emotional tone may vary from day to day—even hour to hour.

It is also necessary to recognize that different ages make differences in the way people react. A person's sense of values varies with changing age. The three-year-old offers a different reaction to the dental office from that which the six-year-old exhibits. This difference holds true throughout life. Each age group varies. Each individual in the age group may be different from the others in that age group. That is why you must be alert in observing the behavior of every person who enters your office, realizing that his or her reaction today may differ from his or her behavior six months ago—or last week.

We will discuss some psychological principles to be applied in working with patients and try to illustrate them with reference to situations in the dental office.

Psychology in the Dental Office: A Developmental Perspective

Psychology has been called the science of the mind. Psychologists do not agree on any one definition. Modern psychology is a science that studies all the interactions between living organisms and their environment. The ideas (concepts) of emotions, consciousness, instincts, and intelligence are described in relationship to the individual as a whole. The individual is exceedingly complex. Furthermore, the individual changes constantly in some areas of behavior and remains the same in other areas. No two individuals change or behave in the same manner or at the same time.

Human beings are referred to as a "bundle of traits" with varying amounts of abilities for each trait. People and conditions surrounding a person influence that individual, who reacts according to the way he or she feels about these people and conditions.

For example, a five-year-old child who, because of small stature, is usually called a three-year-old by strangers will react to social situations very differently from the five-year-old who, inches taller than his or her playmates, is thought to be older than five.

It is necessary to understand the development of the individual from birth if you are to understand and work with adults. Development does not stop with the end of childhood. The processes we go through of discovering what we can do as individuals and of trying new skills and ideas continues throughout life.

We will consider some generalizations about behavior of all ages, recognizing that no one person is a specific age. Most people, whether they are five or fifty, show characteristics of several ages. However, one is more likely to see three- to eight-year-old behavior exhibited by a five-year-old. Thus, we have isolated behaviors according to the age at which they are generally exhibited.

Behavior Characteristics of Children

Generalizations about behavior from early childhood through adolescence are listed here because we believe they have application in working with youngsters in the dental office. These generalizations will help you understand the conduct of children and will indicate what subjects you can discuss with them or how to help them conform to office routine.

Because children are developing their large muscles they may be engaged in constant activity. They may be "wigglers" in the dental chair until they are almost eleven. However, with a good friendly relationship with the dentist, some three year olds will sit still and be more cooperative patients than some adults.

Before six, most children do not have good eye-hand coordination. If you distract the child by asking her or him to help in some fashion, be sure that it is something easy for her or him to do.

Between ages nine and eleven, control of the small muscles develops, and more physical control is possible.

In early childhood, the only interest children have in health is when they are ill. Therefore, you cannot expect them to care for their teeth without parental assistance.

Children suffer a serious handicap in their ability to get along in society because their speech development is exceedingly limited. It is years before children have enough ability to think and express themselves so others can understand what they really want. This ability is called *language facility*.

Language and social development grow together. As children gain language facility, they get along better socially.

The child's home life affects speech development. Some parents unintentionally prevent a child from developing speech ability because they anticipate the child's desires or needs and provide the materials before the child can express the need, thus sharply cutting the need for language development. (Why try to express an idea with difficult words when someone will give you what you want if you just look and wait?)

Lack of language facility is one of the causes of negativism in the two- to four-year-old. In this negativistic period, children usually respond to any suggestion with a "No, no!" Usually some discipline is needed.

Give it pleasantly and firmly to show that this negative attitude is not going to be accepted; that in the dental office cooperation is in order. (Negativism, if not properly treated, may continue into adult life in an otherwise normal individual.)

Three-year-olds usually can speak in simple sentences and answer simple questions; however, they cannot tell whether the event happened yesterday or during the morning of the very day you ask the question. They may not remember, they may not be able to frame a sentence, or the sense of time may be too great for them. (Any past event may be said to have happened yesterday—even though it was really six months ago.)

For the three- to six-year-old, laughter is a way of conversing.

Relationships with adults vary with age. In early years (three to six), adult smiles mean friendliness to the child who is more interested in relationships with adults than with peers. The young child wants to be friends with adults and seeks their approval.

Your friendliness is important in making the child like your office. Smile for the young child.

Young children like to have you put your arm around them, they enjoy the sense of protection it gives. By the time children are eight or nine, however, they may not want you to put your arm around them because now they feel that adults are less necessary in life. (They are able to do so much for themselves.) They still desire adult approval, so be sure to compliment eight-year-olds on the things that they do well. However, if a child shows any signs of desiring physical affection, be sure to give it.

Characteristics of Specific Age Groups

The following observations, based on research studies, are useful if you remember that the divisions are not precise according to ages. There is overlapping in either direction in some individuals. At age three, some children will show characteristics of the five-year-old—and perhaps some of the characteristics of the two-year-old, also. The classifications are a guide, however, for your recognition of the type of behavior to expect until you know the child personally.

The Twenty-Two Month to Twenty-Six Month Old Youngsters

1. Are frightened about being separated from mother at first and may cry.
2. Are curious about surroundings and will usually become interested and stop crying just as soon as the dentist starts doing something for them at the dental chair.

Therefore, be gentle, slow, ignore the crying, and carry on a process in which they can develop an interest just as soon as possible. Never make fast movements around youngsters of this age.

The Two-Year-Olds

1. Are negativistic.
2. Can be made interested in the surroundings, but must be handled firmly to prevent so negativistic an attitude that it is impossible to work with them.
3. Have just succeeded in learning how to manipulate people (including parents) and will manipulate you as well unless you are alert.

Therefore, be firm, gentle, slow, and carry on a process in which the two-year-old can become interested.

The Three-Year-Olds

1. Enjoy simple imaginative play. (Join in, in all seriousness, if you want a real thrill. If they feel that you really want to play and understand, you will have little friends who include you in secrets otherwise not divulged.)
2. Understand what others do in relationship to their own desires. Their language, activities, and life revolve around their own needs and ideas.
3. Do not want to share their possessions. Anything they hold in their hands is theirs—anything they want is theirs. (Watch your choice of language regarding toys and supplies they are using that belong to the dental office.)
4. Know the differences between one, two, and "a lot of."
5. Are angry when you interfere with their bodily activity.

The Four-Year-Olds

1. Wish to make their own decisions.
2. Wish to understand each problem facing them.
3. Have keen imaginations.
4. Like animals and small children.
5. Respond to comparisons of their physical size with others. Be careful! Too many people may have commented on how little a certain four year old is.
6. Are angry with whoever or whatever upsets them and may attempt to inflict physical punishment on the person or object.

The Five-Year-Olds

1. Show off for attention.
2. Sometimes are very shy.
3. Sulk or become destructive when you prevent them from doing what they want.
4. Begin to show interest in everything around them. This interest continues through the seven-year-old period.
5. May embarrass you with the direct way in which they ask you personal questions. Treat the questions casually.
6. May panic with real fear, or just put on a display in order to stop procedures. (Learn to tell the difference.)

The Six-Year-Olds

1. Begin to be afraid of doctors, blood, a fainting person, dark, and being alone. These five items should be remembered in connection with any six year old's visit to your office. Other fears that may appear at this age are fear of ghosts, death, and dead animals. These fears persist through age ten and sometimes last throughout life.
2. Are interested in simple factual explanations of everyday life.
3. Are angry when you interfere with their plans or possessions, or when you ridicule them or call them names.
4. Begin to question who, what, and why (with more language facility). They are curious about the environment and eager to experiment by asking questions for more information. You can answer the questions simply, in brief sentences, reducing the language to their level.

The Seven- to Eight-Year-Olds

1. Compare themselves with others their age. They feel superior if they are physically larger or more skillful in any phase of work or play and inferior if they are smaller or less skillful. (Therefore, praise them for their skills.)
2. Must dress like their classmates, play as they do, and live by the same code of conduct.
3. Are upset by ridicule, loss of prestige, or failure.

The Eight-Year-Olds

1. Begin to be interested in past cultures. (Good conversation material for your interaction with eight-year-olds.)

2. Enjoy imaginative play as pioneers, Indians, and pilgrims.

The Eight- to Nine-Year-Olds

1. Have their closest friends among members of their own sex. They are less interested in the opposite sex.

The Nine- to Eleven-Year-Olds

1. Gain more satisfaction as they see their personal improvement in skills.
2. Are interested in factual, historical information, but not in political history.

Behavior Characteristics of Adolescents

The eleven- to thirteen-year-olds may be entering adolescence. Many adolescent characteristics begin to show as early as ten. The adolescents:

1. May be embarrassed by poor posture, awkwardness, pimples (acne), and excessive perspiration.
2. Are interested in gang approval rather than adult approval.
3. Are learning social graces and trying to be pleasant in their relations, especially with adults.
4. Wish to be treated as adults when privileges are being considered (driving the car, hour established for bedtime, etc.).
5. Wish to remain children when responsibilities are involved (helping with housework, yard maintenance).
6. Want their adolescent friends to think of them as adults.
7. Are especially anxious to do as their contemporaries do about dating, dressing, and spending money.
8. Have huge appetites.
9. Often have physical coordination and finger dexterity far superior to adults.
10. Now feel that being well-groomed and physically attractive is important.
11. Behave in a cocky manner sometimes because they have grown suddenly and are proud of their new height.
12. Grow up mentally, becoming more interested in present environment, ecology, and space programs, and in social, political, and economic life.
13. Are interested in good health, in why and how smoking, drinking, and drugs affect health. The wise adult can do much with older adolescents on these subjects.

14. May be upset emotionally if their parents have failed in marriage or business—family awareness has developed.
15. May be more interested in one or two hobbies than in any school subject.
16. May steal due to the pressures for items that the family or part-time job cannot provide.
17. Often wish to discuss their personal problems and may ask an adult whom they admire for advice. They are curious about human relationships.
18. May be distressed by a growth spurt that makes them suddenly much bigger than they were a short time ago.
19. In late adolescence want to be a success in adult terms. They recognize that they are changing and even want to give protection instead of being protected.

An adult other than the parent is in a position to help an adolescent to a more responsible use of freedom, since some adolescents revolt against parents who refuse to allow them to make certain decisions. You may find that you are in a position to help a number of adolescents realize their responsibilities as well as their freedoms.

Behavior of Adults

Adults, too, can be encouraged to exhibit desired behavior in the office if you remember the fundamental human needs and how the satisfaction of those needs affects behavior.

Let us look at some methods of accomplishing your work each day while making the patients feel safe, important, and having them like you, your dentist, and your office. These are certain basic ways of approaching people that are more pleasing than other ways.

Indirect Approach to People

Presenting ideas indirectly is usually a better way of working with people than presenting your ideas directly. Some people have developed very negativistically and will not respond to being told directly what to do. They "blocked" at the two-year-old level.

If your attitude is dictatorial or "bossy," patients may feel that you see them as puppets or some subhuman species to be pushed around. A patient who feels this way will surely oppose your suggestions and will dislike you intensely. It is wise to avoid the direct approach. The patients will either refuse to do as you

command, do so when your back is turned, or walk out on you—except for a few who are very easily influenced or tractable.

Tractable persons will do what you ask without hesitation. Many persons, however, are either passively negativistic (refusing to do what you tell them to do) or actively negativistic (doing the opposite of what you tell them to do).

The indirect presentation of ideas keeps patients from feeling less important than you, makes them feel their independence, gives them credit for having a good idea, or makes them afraid that unless they follow through with their good idea they will lose prestige.

Here are seven indirect approaches to people:

1. **Assume that the patient will do as you wish him or her to do. (Suggest the behavior if necessary.)**

    When you act as if a person knows the correct thing to do and will do so without being told, you are complimenting her or him most skillfully. You are really saying (without saying it) that this patient is in a very special class. Not all people know the correct thing, and fewer people do the correct thing even when they know how they should behave. Because this is true, this patient holds a very high place in your esteem—and in the patient's mind it makes her or him even more important in your office than other patients who do not know and do not do the correct thing.

    Assume that the child will do what is expected without a fuss:

    "It's your turn now, Jane," to the seven-year-old when you are ready to lead her to the chair.

    "Hop up in the chair now, Bobby. You're so big I can't lift you," to the four-year-old.

    "There are some new books on the reading table, Jimmy," to the nine-year-old who must wait a few minutes in the waiting room. You may keep him from undesirable behavior.

    Before the adult patient lays his coat on the chair, you say, "You will find the coat rack in the corner, Mr. Jones."

2. **Praise correct behavior when you see it.**

    When anyone does what you want him or her to do, it is a good idea to offer praise. That person will feel like doing it again.

"I like the way you remembered to put the books back on the shelf, Jimmy."

"Isn't Mrs. Jones a wonderful patient, Dr. Smith?"

3. **Credit the patient with already knowing what you are about to say.**

It is sometimes necessary to remind patients of office procedures because the long time-lapse between visits can cause them to forget routines. It is wise to use great care in approaching the patient, since people often resent being told something they already know—even when they would have forgotten it anyway.

Before you make the statement of what you wish the patient to do, use such expressions as "There is no need to remind you that. . . ." or "You probably remember . . . ." or "As you already know. . . ."

4. **Show a patient that a certain way of behaving is very desirable.**

Imply that most people do what you are about to suggest to this patient. This is appealing to the desire for social approval.

"The boys and girls who come to see Dr. Smith like to sit on this chair made especially for children" (to keep small children from occupying big chairs needed for adult patients).

"Since the usual Coke or soda snack is so unhealthful, a number of high school students are switching to a snack of fruit after school. Maybe you can convince your crowd to do the same." (Since adolescents feel that they must do as the gang does, you are suggesting that this adolescent is a leader.)

"It is a good idea to have your teeth checked regularly. Most young adults come for a checkup every six months, but some people find that they need to come every four months."

"Some people have immediate dentures, and their friends hardly know that they have had dentures made."

5. **Disagree tactfully with a patient.**

There are times when it is necessary to disagree with a patient. Be pleasant. Be careful to oppose ideas gently. Listen to the patient carefully and courteously and disagree courteously and quietly—and indirectly, if possible.

A patient may say, "I don't want my teeth cleaned this time. It injures the enamel."

You respond with a question: "Many people feel that way, Mrs. Jones. I wonder whether you know how hard the enamel is on your teeth?"

"No-o-o, I really don't."

"Enamel actually is about the same hardness as steel. The cleaning agent used for a prophylaxis is only as cleansing as necessary to remove the soft deposits on the surface of that enamel. It is almost always possible to demonstrate the presence of a bacterial plaque—even with the most careful brushing. This plaque is what the dentist removes in cleaning your teeth." (See chap. 27 for a discussion of this topic.)

Or you may answer: "Although the cleaning agent is very slightly more abrasive than toothpaste, if your teeth were cleaned only twice a year from birth to age eighty, it would only be 160 cleanings—not enough to injure the enamel. Brushing even once a day would be 365 times each year!"

6. **Give the negativistic adult an opportunity to express himself or herself.**

The haughty or domineering person may only be very negative. Sometimes the negation developed between two and four years of age continues throughout life. Sometimes emotional factors in the lives of adults cause them to be very negativistic toward people. You must learn to work well with these persons. Sometimes you can induce these patients to do what is necessary in your office in spite of their negative attitude. Sometimes you find that you must work around the negativism.

A negativistic adult may be approached with any of these wordings before stating the idea you wish to have accepted favorably:

"You may not like this . . ." or "I may have made a mistake, but . . ." or "You don't think that . . . , do you?"

Any of these approaches gives the patient a chance to disagree and yet agree with you. Negativistic people usually say no just out of habit. They can't bring themselves to say yes, so you provide the opportunity to allow them to at least partially disagree with you.

If a patient disagrees with the suggestion you made, drop the idea. If it is a good suggestion, the patient may bring it up later as his or her idea. If this happens, let the patient continue to think so.

Comment on the excellence of the *patient's* idea. Be happy that he or she does as you wish rather than attempting to take credit for the idea.

7. **Be pleased with every person who enters the dental office.**

   Think in terms of being gracious and kind to everyone—of being pleased with every person who enters the reception room. No matter what a person does to earn a living, be sure that you express approval of that job. Occasionally, a question about some phase of his or her work may be used as your lead question when the patient enters the office. You may learn much from such an approach.

   Many patients make the comment, "I can't understand how anyone can be a dentist!"

   This is an example of a comment that you must never make about anyone's way of earning a living. Never even imply dislike of any patient's occupation. A comment of interest in the patient's work, such as "Being a baker must be fascinating," is helpful.

   People must find some satisfaction in their work, or they are not happy. This applies to you in your work too.

Public Relations

Public relations in the dental office is one of the most important phases of assisting. Remember that the patient is constantly appraising you as a person. Are you gentle? Are you cooperative in explaining things? Are you gruff? These intangible, elusive factors make good or bad public relations.

Public relations, as we know it, came into use as a term about 1900. Since that time, much effort has been placed in the promotion of good public relations in every field of human interaction. Briefly, the development of good public relations means the cultivation of goodwill. It is devoted to improving the relations of an organization or individual with the public.

We do not develop good public relations by accident. It is necessary to be constantly aware of the importance of everything we say and do—how it is said, how it is done—in relationship to the individual with whom we are dealing.

The success any one person may have in maintaining good public relations might well be considered on a percentage basis. There will be, under the best circumstances, a small percentage of persons with whom there will be unpleasant relationships. As long as this percentage remains very small, we should feel that our efforts are successful. If the percentage shows a tendency to rise, the time has come for a close examination of our own personality, our own outlook toward people in general.

In order to work well with people, we must communicate with them. However, most people are preoccupied. Most of what you say is not even heard. What can you do? Let us try to understand preoccupation first, then perhaps we can do something about it.

Preoccupation usually begins in infancy, or is the result of problems from infancy. Powerful emotions that control our lives usually cause preoccupation. The most powerful of these emotions seems to be fear, and most people do not even realize that they live with fear.

Children are often treated in ways that produce fear that they must hide. Parents usually do not consciously set out to make their children afraid. However, just the enormity of the size of an adult in the eyes of a child can be fear-inspiring.

One of the authors remembers being towered over by an immense first-grade teacher. When the author was age twenty-two, she had occasion to see this teacher again. She towered over the teacher who was five feet tall. Even a five-foot-tall adult can seem like a giant to a six-year-old.

A young man, as a high school senior, commented upon seeing the playground of the elementary school where he had been enrolled, "Why, I used to think it was immense. It's small!" He laughed. "You know, I used to wonder how those teachers could bat the ball the whole length of the playground! They were tremendous. Why, it's no trick at all. The playground is so little."

We must remember that the adult world viewed through the eyes of a little child is decidedly different from the view of an adult.

If, in addition to seeming like a giant, the adult happens to be stern or angry, the child can be terribly afraid. Timmy is helpless and cannot protect himself effectively from the anger or punishment heaped on him. If his parent is insecure and takes out his hostilities against society on those he can dominate, the child is helpless. He cannot fight effectively, he cannot run away, he cannot even say, "Look, Dad, I'm not to blame that you didn't get that promotion."

The human has one more problem. In addition to protecting himself physically, Timmy also must protect his ego—his opinion of himself. The child has to build an image of himself with which he can live the rest of his life. If he is encouraged as a child, he builds a confident image. If he is belittled or not allowed to try certain activities, he soon acquires the idea that he is not very effective. The emotional memory carries into adult life on an unconscious level.

The treatment begins at birth. Children who feel important to their families develop a better picture of themselves than the youngsters who are constantly belittled. If Mary is afraid of one of her parents, she usually is afraid to let her parents know she is afraid. She becomes anxious. Anxiety keeps her from doing well on tests at school, or anything else that measures her achievement—even making her bed. Anxiety in adult life tends to produce preoccupation. The world is full of adults who were ruled by fear when they were children. Emotionally they are confused, ending as anxiety-ridden adults unable to admit or even know that they are afraid. They are preoccupied.

The sooner you, the assistant, can recognize a person's problems, the sooner you have conquered the problem of fitting the individual into a smoothly-run office routine. We must remember that problem persons are problems to themselves as well as problems to others. They see situations as their minds allow them to visualize. Their perspective of situations is different from that of other persons. Problem persons act on what is reality for them: on how they interpret what they see. No person can do more than that. If you are color-blind and cannot see that the stop light is red, you will not stop for it. It is your inability to *see* that prevents you from behaving as society thinks you ought to behave. Problem persons use a self-centered approach in every situation. They are preoccupied with their own problems.

Persons who continually blunder and create tension are persons who are never free enough from problems within themselves to be interested in the world around them. They are controlled by fear and hostility and create problems for others because they have no relief from being problems to themselves. An example in the dental office is the patient who otherwise may not be a problem person at all. Mr. Jones has an upsetting fear of any dental treatment. He tenses, squirms, grabs the dentist's arm just as the dentist is about to insert the needle, moans, and shoots hostile glances at the assistant; in short, he creates a problem by succumbing to his fear. He is so preoccupied with his fear that he can concentrate on nothing else.

When a person feels that he or she doesn't amount to much, that he or she is a cog in a huge factory, an underling, a nobody, that person has a hard time living with himself or herself. Sometimes home life can make a person feel this way; sometimes a visit to a dental office can make a person feel unimportant. Giving patients emotional acceptance and approval can raise their opinions of themselves.

You can accept people as they are and give them what they deserve: your interest and courtesy. You can give them polite attention even if they are rude. Simply remember that they are being rude to a memory of past treatment by someone else. They are not intentionally being rude to you. Your attitude of the importance of everyone who enters the office will pay off in time. Even the grouches will be less grouchy. This attitude of accepting people as they are, liking them as they are, will help them like themselves, and they will be more pleasant.

For example, in a dental office, a querulous old man came in shouting for the bookkeeper. He waved a letter he had from the dentist. He kept shouting at the receptionist that he wanted the bookkeeper. The waiting room was full of people. Most patients would expect to wait their turn. Not he. He continued shouting. The bookkeeper appeared and said calmly, "I am Mrs. Simpson, the bookkeeper."

He began to wave the letter at her. She nodded and invited him to sit by her desk. She disposed of his problem and sent him off in quiet satisfaction.

Many people would have reacted to his antagonism and anger with a hostility that matched his. In some offices he would have been told to sit down and be silent—eventually they would get to him, but the receptionist and bookkeeper were soothing, giving recognition to the seeming urgency of his complaint, commanding his goodwill by providing the environment for him to give goodwill—that which they were giving him. They did not stop and demand his goodwill and courtesy first. The bookkeeper extended the basic courtesy to human nature as she found it in a human being, difficult as it might be. You can help people live with their mistakes and shortcomings without being overwhelmed by them. In the final analysis, you must realize that people must be treated as whole beings and you must recognize the socioeconomic and moral problems they may have, in addition to their dental problems.

By remembering that patients are people and people are preoccupied and fearful, although they don't always know it, you can do some specific things in order to have a smoothly-run office. The section of this chapter "Factors Establishing Good Public Relations" is an attempt to give you some actions to take as you remember some specific things to do as you bear in mind that people are preoccupied and fearful. You can overcome these two problems with the right approaches in the office.

Create a Friendly Atmosphere in the Office

It is true that the attitudes that you possess are often reflected in those with whom you come into contact. A friendly approach will usually bring a friendly response. A cynical approach will usually bring a response of distrust and dislike. Just what should your attitudes be toward the people you meet in the dental office? Since it is important for you to help patients like your office, you must be friendly, sympathetic, and courteous, no matter what attitude the patients have. It is up to you to make them feel your friendliness. How good are your self-control and self-discipline?

It is possible to run a very businesslike dental office and yet miss the little touches that build good public relations. Cultivating the habit of letting people know that you appreciate something that they have done for you builds better public relations. It is good practice to close telephone conversations by saying, "Thank you, Mrs. Blank," if you place the call, or "Thank you for calling, Mrs. Blank," if Mrs. Blank telephoned you.

Factors Establishing Good Public Relations

Some of the factors involved in establishing good public relations are discussed in the rest of this chapter. Perhaps you will think of other ways to accomplish good public relations in the office in which you work.

Establishing a friendly atmosphere in the office does not mean that one forgets why the dental office exists. Cultivate the habit of thinking in terms of what is to be accomplished in the office. Act accordingly. Guide the patients. Direct conversations into the correct channels to accomplish what you desire to achieve in office administration. The ideal situation in the dental office is one in which friendly relationships with patients are maintained while dentistry is accomplished on schedule.

Listen to Patients

Listen carefully and plan your reply carefully. It is helpful to think through the explanations which you must give. They should be phrased so that they are understood correctly and completely. Consider the feelings of others. Try to place yourself in the other person's position in order to consider what that person may be feeling. In short, treat people as they want to be treated, and you build good public relations.

Treat the Patient as a VIP

Dentistry is the performance of a personal service for an individual personality. The dental health team will share the responsibility of making the individual feel that he or she is the most important person in your office. All efforts are made with one point in mind: to serve that patient to the best of your ability. The patient will feel your pride in "your" dentist, your office, and your work. The impression the patient forms of your dental office is one to which you contribute by your appearance, efficiency, and tact.

Since each individual is human, he or she will have failings or shortcomings. We must accept the fact that each patient will have peculiarities and weaknesses. Do we practice looking for the good, the interesting, in each patient—even when obvious defects are visible? Someone phrased it this way: "There is so much good in the worst of us, and so much bad in the best of us, that it little behooves any of us to speak ill of the rest of us." Or, as Will Rogers put it, "I never met a man I didn't like." He did not mean to say that he had never disliked anyone; rather, that when he learned to know a person, the pleasant, interesting, and good part of his or her character always outweighed the unpleasant characteristics.

The peculiarities and idiosyncrasies of patients should be learned and remembered. The large majority of patients exhibit good common sense and rational behavior with perfectly normal desires to know what is being done for them, how it is to be done, why it is to be done, and for what cost. Maintaining a pleasant professional relationship with this majority is a source of considerable satisfaction to the person who likes people.

By learning to adjust quickly to the individual personality of the patient and by exhibiting courtesy and consideration for that patient's interests, you place good public relations in action in the dental office.

Allay the Patient's Fear

Fear has been cited as the most important cause of dental neglect. When assisting, remember that the patient may consider dental work an ordeal. Be sympathetic and reassuring in your comments if the patient expresses such a thought to you. Use these reactions in a constructive manner by indicating the ease of regular care at regular intervals. Do not ridicule or laugh about any indication of discomfort or fear.

One of the best ways to allay fears of the patient with whom you haven't had an opportunity to develop personal ties is to show him or her an office that runs as smoothly as the proverbial well-oiled machine—one in which each member moves with sureness and certainty to perform an obviously perfected task.

Give the Patient Immediate Attention

Patients who enter the reception room should receive immediate attention. They are being treated most discourteously if they are forced to wait while a personal conversation is carried on either among the office staff or by a staff member over the telephone. Smile when you first see anyone enter the office! Patients should be made to feel important, to feel that their needs are your first interest no matter where they may be—in the reception room, operatory, recovery room, or in any other room in your office.

Use the Patient's Name

Learn the patient's name and the names of family members. Use them at every opportunity.

The primary interest of patients centers in themselves. They like to hear their names. They like consideration and attention centered completely on their needs and care. Due to this normal human characteristic, it is wise to listen carefully to the conversation between the patient and the dentist whenever possible. If something is said about the patient's immediate family—a trip to be made, a graduating student, etc.— unobtrusively make a note of the item on the patient's record card in pencil, or clip a note to it so that either you or the dentist will be reminded to ask or comment about that personal item at the next visit of that patient.

New parents, or about-to-be-parents, are almost always very proud of the fact. Show an interest in their new child, or the expected child, whenever the opportunity is presented. A final reminder to the expectant mother to be sure to send the office an announcement will be received with pleasure.

When the announcement comes, immediately send a congratulatory card or a set of miniature dentures (usually available from dental supply houses). In either case, the dentist's personal signature on the card is important. On the outside jacket of both parents' records list the name and date of birth of the new baby. The fact that this is noted allows the dentist an opportunity to say to the patient at the proper time: "I see that Kay will be eighteen months in June, Mrs. Jones. It would be wise to bring her for a training prophylaxis and examination before she is two years of age. Started at this age and recalled every four months, Kay will learn to look forward to dental care instead of fearing it, as you and I do."

In the patient's mind this shows evidence of interest in the dental care of the family. To ignore the youngster until one of the parents suggests a dental visit can seem like lack of interest in the family's dental health.

When you do have occasion to make a remark about a patient in the chair, always do so by naming the patient: "Mrs. Jones certainly is a good patient, Doctor."

Do not use the third person pronouns he or she.

Explain a Delay to a Waiting Patient

Should an appointment exceed the time reserved, promptly notify the next waiting patient of the delay and the approximate time involved. Specify the approximate time, rather than a "few minutes."

Let your voice show a sincere respect for the fact that Mrs. Jones is one of the two very important people in your office at that moment—the other being the patient still in the operatory. Patients will not develop respect for their appointments with your office unless your office has respect for their time also.

Some Individuals Need Special Care

The occasional unpleasant person, either in the office or on the telephone, is most diplomatically handled with an affirmative reply. It is not possible to argue with a *yes*. The person whose voice has risen to an intensity indicating emotional strain is not in a logical frame of mind. That person is not ready to hear a reasonable explanation of the problem. It is not, usually, the time to try to give him or her one. The use of yes should include a short sentence suitable to the situation: "Yes, Mrs. Jones, it does look that way" or "Yes, Mr. Jones, I can understand your viewpoint" or "Yes, Mr. Jones, I will check that again."

This reply should be given seriously, not with a smile. You really are concerned about how to get this individual back to a calm discussion of the situation. It may be possible to do this immediately; but frequently it is preferable to defer further discussion until Mr. Jones's emotions have had time to return to a normal level. Either later the same day (soon after a mealtime is good) or the following day will be a better time. At that time, be certain that you understand the situation completely, from his viewpoint as well as yours, before discussing it again with the individual concerned. You may discover that the patient has a valid complaint!

Occasionally, you will work with a patient whose manner irritates you severely. In such cases, do not allow your feelings to become obvious by the slightest expression of dislike, either facial or verbal. Remain friendly in any and all contacts with those very important people—patients. Again, no matter what occurs in your contacts with patients, remain calm, friendly, poised, and in complete control of your emotions and verbal responses. It is your job to do so.

Another type of person, only rarely encountered, can be quite rude and difficult in routine contacts with the assistant, but becomes most courteous and polite to the dentist. Circumstances such as this are more likely to occur during telephone conversations.

Assume that such a situation arises concerning arrangement for an appointment. If it is your job to make all appointments, then see to it that you do handle the situation diplomatically. If the difficulty concerns some phase of dental practice that is not under your control, do the very best you can to avoid asking the dentist to help you. If you cannot keep the situation under your control, then inform the patient that you will have Dr. Smith call as soon as possible. Should the patient be present in the office while the dentist is with another patient at the chair, ask if Dr. Smith can telephone at a specified time. Very often these situations are only an attempt to see the dentist personally without an appointment to do so.

Summary

Patients are people who like to be treated as worthwhile human beings, as welcome guests in the office, and as VIPs whose problems are important to the staff.

Motives that lead people to seek dental care include self-preservation, love, security, fear, and recognition. The indirect presentation of ideas, or the power of suggestion, may be used to help patients recognize the value of dental services. It is important for the dental assistant to understand the approaches and purposes of her or his dentist in working with patients.

The feeling aroused in the patient when he or she is in your office is known as an empathic response. It is desirable to arouse a favorable empathic response in patients—that is, to make them like you and the office. It is wise to learn to read the behavior of others and to offer the kind of motivation that results in the conduct and attitudes necessary to a successful dental practice.

Everyone desires to be of value—to feel worthwhile. To make patients feel that they are very important persons in your dental office is to make them continuing patients.

Principles of psychology are helpful in working with patients. Generalizations regarding behavior of all humans—children, adolescents, and adults—are an aid in successful dental assisting. Indirect approaches that work well in the dental office include the following:

1. Assume that the patient will do as you wish.
2. Praise the correct behavior when you see it.
3. Credit the patient with already knowing what you are about to say.
4. Show a patient that a certain way of behaving is very desirable.
5. Be tactful when objecting to or disagreeing with a statement.
6. Give the negativistic adult an opportunity to express himself or herself.
7. Be pleased with every person who enters the dental office.

The development of good public relations means the cultivation of goodwill.

Factors that contribute to development of good public relations include:

1. Establishing a friendly atmosphere in your office
2. Thinking in terms of office accomplishment
3. Cultivating the art of listening to patients
4. Treating patients as if they were very important persons—they are!

Remember that patients are human beings, and allay their fears; give them immediate attention; use their names and not a third-person pronoun when speaking to them or about them; notify them of a delay if one occurs; and remain calm when working with upset individuals.

The patient is a very important person. Remember to keep him or her pleased with your office!

Study Questions
1. List four motives that cause patients to seek dental care.
2. What indirect approaches work well in the dental office?
3. Discuss good public relations.
4. List four factors that contribute to attainment of good public relations.
5. What philosophy should you have about patients?

Vocabulary
deficit motivators   unsatisfied needs
empathic response   feeling aroused within a person by an environment (the patient has an empathic response to your dental office)
motive   something inside an individual that drives him or her to do something special
sequential   one follows another in order

Word Elements	
Word Element	*Example*
bi prefix meaning: two (see chapter 3)	*bicuspid* premolar; usually has two cusps
di prefix meaning: two (see chapter 4)	*diaphragm* a partition that separates (in the body, the diaphragm separates the thorax from the abdomen)
bi combining form meaning: life	*aerobic* living only where oxygen is present
bio combining form meaning: relationship to life	*biopsy* removal of living tissue for microscopic examination
dia, di prefix meaning: through or apart	*diastema* a spacing between the teeth
dis, di prefix meaning: apart, away from	*disinfectant* an agent that destroys or inhibits microorganisms that cause disease
gram suffix meaning: tracing, picture	*roentgenogram* a photograph made with roentgen rays
gram root word meaning: a unit of weight in the metric system	*kilogram* 1000 grams
iso prefix or combining form meaning: equal, alike, same	*isometric* characterized by equal measures
meso, mes combining form meaning: middle	*mesial* situated in the middle: toward the center line of the dental arch

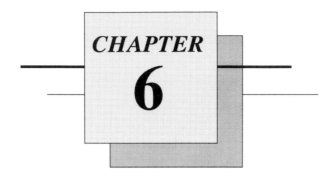

CHAPTER
6

Communicating and Interacting with People

Communication IS Public Relations in the Dental
        Office
Basis for Understanding
Ways We Communicate
The Process of Communication: An Overview
Transferring a Message
Feedback
Practical Applications
Interacting with People
Observation, a Necessary Tool
Office Conversation Technique
Co-workers and Communication

Communication IS Public Relations in the Dental Office

Each year students of a certain learned professor hear him say, "Your success will depend about 15 percent on your technical skill and 85 percent on your ability to communicate."

He may be right. A research study by Evans on insurance sales showed that when the insurance salesperson and the client liked each other, a sale was made. If they did not like each other, no insurance was purchased. The principle is reflected in other areas of life. If two people like each other, they work well together—cooperation is apt to occur.

The personnel in the dental office may make a better team if they like each other. If the personnel build warm personal relationships with the patients, there can be more cooperation from the patients. Communication in the one-to-one relationship is one of the most important skills a dental assistant can develop.

Basis for Understanding

How many times this week have you said, "They don't understand" or "I don't understand"or "No, that's not what I meant at all?"

Understanding and being understood are common problems all of us face. Communicating ideas is important because we must work with other people, and to do so necessarily means being able to communicate with them. It would be difficult, indeed, to attempt to perform dentistry if we could not understand and communicate in some form with the patients and our co-workers.

Communication is transmitting an idea or feeling to another person. The *accurate* transmittal of an idea from one human to another is an ideal not often achieved. *The accurate transmittal means that the receiver understands the idea as the sender intended it to be understood.* How a person feels while making a request may affect the inflection that he or she uses. In turn, the listener may assume that the speaker meant something else because the listener *interpreted* the inflection according to the way the listener was feeling. The alert, sensitive person will attempt to evaluate the message received and will verify the message with the sender after receiving it. This individual will also ask himself or herself, "How can I phrase my request (or statement) to be best understood by my listener?"

The process of transmitting an idea from one person to another (or several others) becomes complicated. Even the way one says "Good morning" differs with circumstances. Consider these instances:

1. The first patient arrives fifteen minutes early. She is an enthusiastic, talkative individual. You are still dusting and have yet to prepare the setups for the operatories. No one else is in the office, the telephone is ringing, and the behavior of this patient in the past indicates that you should give her your undivided attention. Knowing all this, how do you say "Good morning?"
2. An aggressive, overbearing salesperson bursts into the office every Tuesday morning at nine, right in the middle of your busy schedule. Your dentist has left instructions that he or she does not want to see this salesperson—ever. Yet your dentist has also instructed you to be courteous to all salespeople but to prevent them from disturbing him or her. Say "Good morning" to this salesperson.
3. An attractive single patient of the opposite sex enters. Your dentist has been clear about professional attitudes toward all patients. Smile and say "Good morning."

If making or interpreting this simple greeting is complicated, consider, then, the problem in transmitting the idea that the X rays have been ruined by some problem with chemicals or that the laboratory has been unable to return the appliance for a difficult patient who is in the office expecting to receive it.

Ways We Communicate

Words are the smallest part of communication. Mehrabian measured communication and demonstrated it to be 7 percent verbal, 38 percent vocal, and 55 percent nonverbal (facial and bodily movement) (figure 6.1). Thus, according to Mehrabian, 7 percent of our communication is accomplished with words; 38 percent depends on our tone, inflection, and the sounds we make that are not words (the "uh's," "er's," and so on); and 55 percent depends on our nonverbals—what others see us do as we try to communicate.

1. The **words**—those tiny, but very important parts of our communication—seem simple enough. They have meaning—but what meaning? Most of our commonly used words have several meanings, depending on their use and the interpretation that the users give the word. The word *post* is an example of a word with many different meanings, depending on the person who is using it. A dental office bookkeeper may think of transferring charges for services rendered to the patient's account record; a farmer may think of building a fence; and

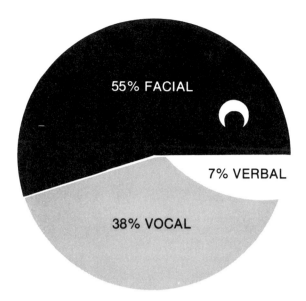

Figure 6.1
The component parts of communication as measured by Mehrabian.

a dentist may think of construction of a prosthetic device. The dictionary gives nineteen meanings for the word *post*. Clearly, we must be aware of the exact meaning we intend when we use a word and whether the listener may have the same meaning in mind.

Words have connotative and denotative meanings. Some words are more likely to have connotative meanings than others. *Denotative* words have meanings from the dictionary. The word *table* is denotative. For a test of whether a word has a denotative meaning, see if you can point to an object and have people understand what you mean.

Connotative meanings are a little different. They exist because you have an emotional feeling about the words, such as "The clouds reminded me of the gray dust rolls under my bed."

One difficulty in communicating is due to the fact that words that are normally thought of as having only denotative meanings really do have connotative meanings. For example, if someone says *chair,* what do you visualize first? the chair you sit on at work? an overstuffed armchair? a ruby red tapestry seat on an Early American cherrywood rocker? Your personal vision of *chair* is present because you have had experiences which cause your mind to select a specific

chair to remember. The person sitting next to you has another vision colored by his experience. The symbol *chair* can have as many meanings as there are people present to hear the word.

We must remember that even words that we think of as factual, reportive words have different meanings for different people. If words have an emotional meaning, this, too, colors the individual's reaction. For example, what does *watermelon* mean to you? Does it mean a delightful treat enjoyed especially on the Fourth of July? Does it bring back memories of wonderful family picnics? Most people think of watermelon as a happy memory. Let us consider the case of eleven-year-old Suzy. She had developed this wonderful feeling about watermelon. It was a treat reserved for such special occasions as Fourth of July. One Saturday, shortly before the Fourth, her father called Suzy and her brother and sister to the kitchen "for a treat." It was watermelon. Suzy could scarcely contain her joy and excitement. She popped a huge piece of the heart into her mouth and let the juice run all around until she could scarcely keep it from trickling down her throat and choking her. While Suzy was enjoying the sweetness and texture, her father said, "Children, your mother and I are going to get a divorce. You will have to decide which of us you wish to live with."

Suzy began to cry, and soon the salt tears, the thick saliva, and the watermelon sweetness mingled until she could hardly swallow. Years later when Suzy was grown, the mention of watermelon reminded her unconsciously of her parents' divorce. Her reaction to watermelon was unpleasant. Its meaning for her was different from its meaning for others whose emotional memories were not so unpleasant. She didn't even know why she disliked watermelon!

This is a risk you take with every person you engage in conversation. They may have had life experiences that make their emotional responses to a word different from your emotional response.

There is no "one word, one meaning." All words are surrounded by a cloud of experiences and emotions inside each individual, namely the connotative meanings the words have acquired for that individual. It is necessary for each individual to sort out from this cloud of meanings the one he or she thinks is the meaning intended by the speaker. How many times does the listener guess correctly?

A third problem is that some words create emotional responses of hate or love reactions. They are often called "snarl" and "purr" words. Some words create negative prejudice, such as "Jack is a *rotter*" or "Jack is *yellow*." Other words create affirmative prejudice, such as "Mr. Smith is a *noble, kindly* person." And still other words are inclined to shock you— *nigger, wop, hick, Red,* and others.

These problems are all concerned with the meaning found in words:

  a. Which dictionary meaning is being used?

  b. Which connotative meaning is being used?

  c. Which meaning does the listener perceive?

  d. What effect emotionally does the word produce in the listener?

2. **Tone, inflection,** and **vocalizations** add to the meaning. "It's about time," can mean that the impression should be removed from the water bath, or that someone is late and ought to have appeared much sooner. The latter meaning would require a sarcastic tone and some inflections that would be quite different from the gentle way the same words would be said if one were indicating it was time to remove something from the water bath. Often the "uh's," "er's," and other vocalizations we use are attempts to control people—to indicate to them, for example, that we wish to continue speaking and are just gathering our thoughts. In addition to this use, the nonword vocalizations all have meaning. They may indicate nervousness, a necessary time lapse, and so on. They relay a message about the speaker (the actual emotions and meanings the speaker is experiencing that he or she may only partially express verbally).

3. **Nonverbal communication** (*facial expression and bodily movements*—the 55 percent of our communication) concerns *body language.* Most of us are not conscious of what we do in this area of communication. Our bodies often communicate messages of which we are unaware.

For example, the way an individual holds his arms often indicates tension, withdrawal, or openness. Consider Mrs. Doe. She stands before you, arms crossed, body tense, lips set in a firm line, and she says, primly, "I am open to suggestions."

Do you feel certain that she would accept a suggestion? Her body tells you that it would be difficult to find her "open" to anything yet her words tell you that she is.

A second area of nonverbal communication concerns the individual's personal and cultural space needs. Each person requires a certain amount of space around him or her—referred to as *personal space.* The space needs of persons vary according to the culture in which they have been raised. Some cultures, such as the South American cultures and the Arab cultures, encourage closeness. The majority of North American cultures require more distance between persons. Research indicates that in the United States we need about eighteen to twenty-four inches of space around us to feel comfortable. The invasion of this space can be an irritant to some people.

Consider Jenny, the co-worker in your office, who takes your arm and says, "I wouldn't dream of intruding." Yet, she is standing so close to you that she is touching your shoe with hers, and you find it necessary to draw back to keep her hair from tickling your nose. She has actually invaded your personal space. You have just received a *double message.* Her body and actions tell you one thing, her words tell you another. Quite probably Jenny is unaware that she has given you the message you received from her body language.

Another important aspect of nonverbal communication is *territory.* We humans have need of space that belongs to us. Notice how some patient will always sit in the same chair in the reception room. That chair becomes (unconsciously of course) the "territory" of that particular patient. If he or she enters the reception room and the chair is occupied, quite likely the patient will feel uncomfortable. Often,

Table 6.1
Misinterpreted Silences

Person B has just made a statement or asked a question and is waiting for Person A to respond. However, Person A doesn't respond. There is silence. During the silence Person A is thinking what you read in column A, and Person B is thinking what you read in Column B.

A is thinking	while	B is thinking
"I will cry if I try to talk."		"She won't share anything with me."
"I will laugh at you if I say anything."		"You must think I'm good!"
"I'm tired, and I don't feel like talking."		"What a bore—just won't respond."
"My throat is so sore it hurts when I talk."		"Sure is silent and uncooperative."

siblings in a family will say, "Get out of that chair, it's mine!" Co-workers may unconsciously assume that certain areas of the office are theirs.

We communicate by touching: the gentle touch, the directional push, or the caress. We also communicate by fidget behavior which is what we do with our hands, our stance, etc. All these mannerisms affect our relationships with others, who unconsciously interpret these behaviors.

4. **Silence** communicates—often something the individual doesn't intend. For example, your dentist may make a statement about a dental office policy or situation. You remain silent, thinking, "I don't want to disagree with my boss so I won't say anything." The dentist notes your silence and thinks, "Good, she or he agrees with me."

Look at table 6.1 for a few examples of misinterpreted silence.

Remember that what you don't say can be interpreted differently from what you intended. Next time you fail to answer someone, be aware that a message of some kind is being given. Are you sure it is the message you wanted to give?

5. **Timing** is another aspect of communication. The longer the pause between the question and the answer,
   a. the greater the degree of discomfort the listener feels.
   b. the more negatively the response to the message is interpreted.
   c. the less important the listener feels.
   The statement "Of course you can do it!" said quickly with positive inflection makes the person waiting for the answer feel

encouraged and capable. The timing used creates a message—perhaps subtle, but often thoroughly comprehended.

Involuntary communication is often unintentional and usually the communicator is unaware of his or her communication. The involuntary physical reactions convey messages. Tests have shown that when a person becomes excited or overjoyed, the pupils of the eyes dilate involuntarily. An inner emotion of elation can be seen if the observer is alert because there seems to be no way an individual can control the involuntary physical reaction of dilated pupils.

6. **You always communicate something!** Actually, when two people contact each other, there is interaction and communication whether or not the individuals want to communicate or are aware of their communication. There are two kinds of communication that are important to understand. They may be referred to as open communication and blind communication:
   a. Open communication is information that Jan is willing to share with Marge. (Jan states the information and is aware that she is giving Marge the information.)
   b. Blind communication concerns information Marge discovers about Jan by observation. (Jan doesn't realize that Marge has discovered this information.)

Here is an example:

Dr. Raeywen: "Mrs. Jones, your second molar needs to be crowned."
Mrs. Jones frowns, is silent at first, and then says: "I see. Maybe I should have it pulled."

Dr. Raeywen is immediately aware that Mrs. Jones is uncomfortable. She is unaware that she has given an indirect message of concern. It could be concern over expense or discomfort. Some personal problem that has nothing to do with dentistry could also be the cause of her expression. Since Dr. Raeywen is sensitive to this unspoken communication message, he explains the problems and costs of the two treatments, and the need for a bridge should the tooth be removed. He also explains the minimal discomfort with good dental crown preparation. Mrs. Jones better understands the dental problem she faces.

A sensitive individual utilizes the impressions obtained in conversation to help interpret the entire message being received. That is what Dr. Raeywen did.

A person who is skilled in techniques of communicating will learn as much as possible about his or her own message-sending and will attempt to control his or her nonverbal communication and make it agree with verbal communication. (The person who listens and observes carefully while another is speaking has a more complete idea of the message given. That individual has acquired much data to use in his or her interpretation of the spoken message.)

7. **Listening** is another important part of the complicated communication process. The person who is speaking wants to reach the listener and get a response. The listener hears what the speaker says, interprets it, and responds according to his or her interpretation of the speaker's comments. The listener may or may not remember what the speaker said.

Listening is a complicated process. Hearing and listening are not the same thing. First we have the hearing of a sound, then we have the interpretation of the sound followed by a response of some kind. If the interpretation has been important enough *to the listener,* he or she remembers what the speaker said. Thus, listening really has three parts: the hearing of the sound, the interpretation of the sound, and the remembering of those interpretations that are important to the individual.

In addition, listening really starts even before the person begins to speak. The instant the listener sees the speaker, the listener begins to assimilate (absorb) impressions about the speaker and continues to formulate impressions during and following the speaker's presentation. This applies whether the situation is a formal speech or a conversation between two people. If the speaker is depressed, that depression will affect his or her entire appearance and speech. If the speaker happens to be resentful of his or her niche in life, the resentment will show in the speaker's bearing and tone of voice. The listener responds involuntarily to this emotional communication even before responding to the verbal message of the speaker.

The Process of Communication: An Overview

Communication is achieved by the use of words, sounds, tone, inflection, facial expression, body language, silence, timing, and listening. Sometimes our communication is involuntary and unintentional because we always communicate something whether we want to or not.

If we put it all together, the communication process can be illustrated as in figure 6.2. The speaker, Mary Smith, feels a need to communicate. She forms a message. She then gives that message (arrow 1) to listener Joe Jones who receives it, including the impressions he has received as well as the words. (This is called

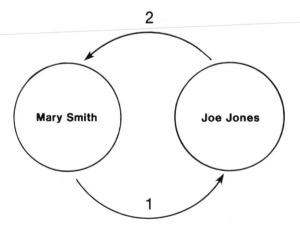

Figure 6.2
The process of communication as visualized by W. S. Howell.

getting the data.) He then *processes* it. (He analyzes it—What does it mean?) Then it is treated creatively. (What will I do about it?) The listener, Joe Jones, packages and organizes a response. This becomes his data. He asks himself, "How can I best respond to this message?" He forms the message on the basis of all this data, his emotional responses, and his normal way of responding to others. Then he sends the message back to speaker, Mary Smith, who now becomes the listener (arrow 2).

Most of the communication process occurs inside the individuals involved. The messages given reflect each individual.

Let's apply this formula to the dental office.

Transferring a Message

You are about to try to transfer a message, to try to communicate effectively. Suppose you are a receptionist in a dental office. Your next task is to see that seven-year-old Janie is seated in an operatory and that her mother remains in the reception room.

Step number one is to transfer the idea to Janie that it is now time to go to the operatory. Janie is a somewhat fearful and negative child, rather strongly attached to her mother.

You decide on the sentence that you think will accomplish your goal. The message is "Janie, it's your turn now."

Step number two is to state the message. How you say this message will determine, at least in part, her response. If you are nervous and you look imploringly at her mother or at the ceiling, hoping that Janie will respond nicely, Janie may refuse to go, and may cling to her mother, or scream.

You are showing Janie security if you assume a cheerful, positive attitude and demonstrate warmth and love for her. Look directly into her eyes as you smile at her sincerely.

If you express genuine love for a little child and show Janie by your attitude that she is to receive only kindness and love from you, she is more likely to respond to the security that you offer and come with you.

Notice that you attract Janie's attention before you tell her what she is to do. The full impact of your message will be received only when you have her full attention. Further, if you will walk across the reception room and stand near Janie, smile, and hold out your hand, you will be inviting her participation. It would be very hard for her to refuse an offer of such loving attention.

Another approach might be to look through the reception window and say, "Come on, Janie. Doctor's waiting for you," perhaps a little gruffly because you feel distracted. (The other assistant is asking about Mrs. Jones' appointment, and the telephone is ringing.) Under these circumstances, Janie is quite likely to cling to Mother, scream, and refuse to go into the operatory.

If you say "Do you want to come now?", it is easy for her to say "No!" and then you have a problem in forcing her to come anyway.

Whatever method you use, the message is received by Janie (step number three). She translates into personal meaning all the communication that she receives: your words, your bodily messages, your facial expression, your attitudes, and the atmosphere of the office. She interprets these things in relationship to her past experiences with her parents, her teachers, other "nurses" and "doctors," and whether her previous dental visits have been pleasant. She is also affected by her present emotional state. If she has been fighting with siblings for parental attention and love that morning, or if she has been belittled, she will react differently from the way she may react on a day when she has been praised and loved. If she has been taught to be afraid of life or the assistant or adults, it may show in her reaction. All her emotional pressures will affect her answer.

If the sense of love, gentleness, and security she receives from your manner and tone is strong, it will offset negation on her part, and she will respond to your held-out hand by putting her hand in yours and walking with you—perhaps slowly, but nevertheless trusting you to care for her. The more kindness and interest in Janie as a person you can show on (what seems to her) that long walk to the chair, the more secure she will feel.

Briefly, the process of transferring a message from one person to another is this:

1. The need for a message is recognized
2. The message is formed
3. The message is given
4. The message is received
5. The message is translated or interpreted by the receiver
6. The response is given (which becomes a form of feedback)

Note that the message may not be interpreted as the giver intended, but some kind of meaning is received.

Feedback

How can you be sure the message you intended is the one received? Asking for feedback is helpful. Feedback is a way of judging whether or not the message was received as intended. Some feedback can be obtained by observing the persons to whom you addressed your comments. However, asking for their interpretation of what you just said may be more helpful. The speaker must observe the listener's responses carefully to be reasonably sure the message has been received correctly.

Practical Applications

Communication is complicated. When it is important to be accurate, remember:

1. Sometimes the interpretation that an individual makes when receiving a message may change the meaning of the message the sender thought he or she was transmitting. Sometimes what the sender fails to say or do affects the receiver as much or more than what the sender says. So get feedback if you wish to be certain the patient or co-worker understands your message as you intended it.

2. Meanings are in people, not in words. Unless the receiver understands the sender as the sender intended, there is a communication breakdown.

3. How an individual is treated when communicating often determines his or her willingness to communicate later. For example, if a boss, Mr. Sartell, becomes angry when told some unpleasant facts about his business, his employees are more likely to avoid communicating unpleasant news thereafter. People tend to respond well to kindness. Should it be necessary to be the bearer or recipient of unpleasant news, treat the person involved with kindness—not anger. Your most important responsibility is to keep the channels of communication open. With a gentle, kindly approach, it is possible to do so.

4. Misunderstandings are bound to occur, but corrections can be made if the persons involved use feedback and openly say, "I'm not sure I understood" or "I'm not sure you understood me, let me state it another way."

5. A wise response to trouble is, "How can we correct this problem?" not "Whose fault is it?" or "It's not my fault, it's hers!"

Concentrating on correction of the difficulty rather than placing blame results in accomplishment of goals instead of ego crushing.

Interacting with People

We have discussed these two ideas:

1. Establishing a friendly one-to-one relationship with each patient is important.
2. You can improve your ability to communicate more effectively.

The friendly relationship is established through effective communication.

Now let us add another important concept: *People do things for their reasons—not yours.*

So how can you communicate with people to help them agreeably fit into the necessary office routines? Your approach must include several factors.

Build on the basis of your understanding of that individual, but be aware that patients may be affected by factors of which you are unaware. Meet each encounter by asking yourself why the patient feels as he does rather than by agreeing or disagreeing with that patient. It is important to respond calmly to all emotion-charged words. You may or may not agree with the patient. You must try to understand why the patient makes the statement.

It doesn't matter whether the patient thinks the president of the United States is the best president we ever had, or the worst. What is important is that the negative emotions be allowed to exhaust themselves harmlessly and that you continue to remain calm and friendly.

It is important in the dental office that you control your emotional reaction to people and give them all a warm, attentive reception, regardless of the messages they may be sending your way by their actions.

Research studies in listening have indicated strongly that the most important single attribute in a manager is *listening to the individual employee.* The principle behind this discovery is just as applicable in the office situation. Listen attentively. Concentrate on what the patient is saying. Try to evaluate (1) why the patient is saying what he or she is saying, and (2) what the patient's emotional state is at the moment. If you try to see the situation from the patient's perspective, your response will be more successful because you will have more empathy for that patient's particular problems.

Observation, a Necessary Tool

It is necessary to observe carefully the people you meet. The keen observer can recognize little movements (a twitch of a muscle, the blink of an eye) and be more aware of what the person being observed is actually thinking. It is wise for a dental assistant to develop this ability. It is rather easy to do if you can discipline yourself to keep your mind on the subject you wish to consider. If you can concentrate on listening attentively to the patient who is speaking to you and at the same time be observant of that patient's expression, posture, and ease or lack of ease, you are much more aware of what he or she is trying to tell you. You are also discovering much about that patient that you would otherwise miss entirely.

To train your powers of observation, examine some little object for a minute and then try to list everything you can remember about it. Then look at the object again and see how accurate you were. It can be a leaf from a tree, or any object with which you are familiar. When you have done this exercise to your satisfaction, try concentrating on a person—a classmate, a co-worker, or someone you see on the bus. Make a mental note of everything you can about that person in a specific length of time—as for example, in one minute.

Gradually, you will sharpen your powers of observation. If you listen carefully to a patient and observe his or her physical movements and expressions, you will eventually be able to guess with fair accuracy what that patient's next comment will be.

One of the greatest satisfactions in life is found in the interaction of human personalities. Your day will be far more satisfying if you are able to be an observant, sympathetic, and attentive listener.

Office Conversation Technique

Conversation occurs when two or more people exchange ideas of interest to themselves. In normal conversation, the emphasis is on the word exchange. In the dental office, your job is to keep the conversation centered on the patient's interests and to make dentistry one of those interests. Continue to make remarks and ask questions that encourage the patient to speak. You must be careful, however, to see that conversation does not interfere with dental work. Use it wisely—just enough to make the patient feel appreciated—and sparingly enough so that you do not interfere with the proper functioning of the dental office. Greet the patient with a personal comment and, after his or her answer, change the interest to dentistry—the purpose of this office visit.

To attain this mature status as an expert conversationalist under the specific conditions of the dental office, you must be a good listener, be alert to the interests of the patient, and be able to make the patient the center of interest. Your comments should be made in a sincere and straightforward manner.

Since your patients are apt to be interested in a wide range of topics of conversation, try to be informed about as many currently interesting subjects as possible: sports, national events, movies, plays, books, international affairs, business conditions, styles, TV programs—to mention several. The object is to know enough to make a personal contact with the patient on this patient's favorite subject. It is not intended that you expound on it. Actually, to be informed requires little effort beyond reading the newspaper, noting TV programs, and glancing at a magazine or two. This will also make a delightful difference in your social life.

As mentioned earlier, a note clipped to the patient's record of an important family event gives the office staff something personal to mention at the next visit of the patient. A note listing a patient's favorite subjects of conversation that is clipped to the record is also a great aid to the dental assistant when the patient comes in for a recall. For example, some people love to talk about plants, and a simple note of one word, *plants,* clipped to the record reminds the dental assistant to ask a question casually about some houseplant, to the delight of the patient.

After you have asked a patient a question, be interested in the answer. Attention at this moment is the basis of being a good listener. It also gives you an opportunity to learn to read the behavior of the patient. Only by learning what to expect can you anticipate situations that could be problems unless they are properly met.

Most of us go through life without observing other people's reactions to what we do and say. The first step in learning to know what the patient is thinking is to listen to that patient and watch him or her closely.

When you talk with a patient who reacts unfavorably, remember what you said that brought about this reaction from the patient. Later, analyze your remarks. Try to recall the particular phrase you used that caused the trouble. Find a substitute phrase. The next time you have a similar situation, try the new phrase that you have worked out. Keep experimenting until you know that what you say to patients is pleasing.

Co-workers and Communication

Understanding and communicating with office personnel are also areas of importance. For patients, one ordinarily plans and follows through with planned communications, but co-workers are another matter. One is inclined to feel that planning communication with them or working to express a message in the most diplomatic terms is unnecessary, but remember that barriers to communication exist in all phases of life.

Communicating with co-workers may be even more difficult than with patients because a close working relationship exists in a dental office, and the exposure to co-workers is usually for eight hours a day. Any personal frictions can create attitudes that form barriers to understanding.

The person who attempts to do an effective job of communicating with people remains alert for these three barriers to communication:

1. *Misunderstanding.* Never assume meaning. Always ask for clarification. Ask "What do you mean?" and listen to the response. Ask for explanations of expressions that could be interpreted in several ways. When something is described as satisfactory or unsatisfactory, try to discover how it is satisfactory or unsatisfactory. Under what circumstances? In what way? Try saying, "Let's see if I understand you." Repeat in your own words the message you have just received. The speaker then has an opportunity to correct your interpretation of the message. The difference in meaning may surprise both of you.

   It may help you to understand the problem if you remember that of the words most frequently used by Americans, 500 of them have 14,000 dictionary definitions! There is possibility for misunderstanding simply because a word has two different meanings to the persons trying to communicate.

2. *Disagreement* may also build barriers to communication. Occasionally, some of the office personnel have purposes they wish to accomplish that they may never share with the rest of the staff. For example, if Mary wishes to keep the spatulas in drawer *A* and Susie wishes to keep them in drawer *C,* this can become a barrier to communication. Disagreement may be about something as simple and as small as spatulas. It may also be a fundamental disagreement about the philosophy of working in a dental office. Unless the disagreement can be aired and resolved, problems may arise in communicating.

3. *Misinformation* can cause barriers to communication, also. If Sally thinks Doctor said he was dissatisfied with the arrangement of the recall file, whereas what he really said was that it would have to do until something better was discovered, Sally may not be able to communicate effectively about the file until she learns that what she has done with the file is acceptable for now.

Listening—actually listening—can probably do more for staff accord than almost anything else. We simply do not listen well to others. Usually we are planning what we are going to say while the other person is talking. To be able to listen, think, and then answer takes self-discipline. But without having heard what the other person had to say, how can one understand and respond effectively?

Try to give the same attentiveness to your co-workers as we have suggested you give to your patients.

Summary

Communication in the one-to-one relationship is one of the most important skills a dental assistant can develop.

Communication is the transmitting of an idea or feeling to another person. The accurate transmittal of an idea is the desired ideal.

Two of the most common problems in the communication of ideas are understanding others and being understood.

We communicate in many ways other than words. Actually, words are only 7 percent of our communication. Often an individual is unaware of some of his or her communication. What you fail to say and do is as important as what you say and do. You always communicate something. Thus, it is reasonable to attempt to communicate the message you really wish to express.

A message is transferred from one person to another by a process that includes the need for recognition of the message, formation of the message, giving the message, receiving the message, translating or interpreting the message, and giving the response (which becomes a form of feedback). Feedback is a way of judging whether the message has been received as intended.

Complexities of person-to-person communication include these problems: variations occur in interpretation of the message; meanings are in people, not words; treatment of persons during communication varies; and misunderstandings are to be expected.

People do things for their reasons, not yours. Thus, the dental assistant should attempt to phrase the necessary communications about dentistry in ways which appeal to the patients' motivations. Skillful observation assists staff to be aware of the needs of patients.

Office conversation requires that staff members keep the conversation on the subjects of interest to the patient and on dentistry.

Communication with co-workers is often neglected, but it is very important. Ask "What do you mean?" rather than permit a misunderstanding to occur. Try to repeat the message for clarification.

Listening is vitally important for staff accord.

Study Questions

1. Discuss the importance of a dental assistant's ability to communicate.
2. What steps are necessary for one person to effectively transfer a message to another person? Illustrate these steps with the skills used to encourage Janie to leave her mother and go with the assistant to the operatory.
3. What problems can be avoided by giving thought to the complexities of communications?
4. What three factors build barriers between staff members?
5. How can barriers to effective communication be avoided?

Vocabulary

connotative   meaning suggested by a word or thing

denotative   specific and recognized meaning (readily found in the dictonary) of a word or thing

double message   one from words, another from actions (usually conflicting)

dyad   one-to-one relationship in communication

feedback   receipt of information from listener that indicates to the speaker whether he or she was understood as intended.

haptics   communication by touching

kinesics   communication by body position

nervantics   fidget behavior

personal space   space people need between themselves and others to feel comfortable

proxemics   use of space and physical relationships of people to implement communication

Word Elements	
Word Element	*Example*
brachy combining form meaning: short	*brachygnathia* marked underdevelopment of the mandible
graph suffix meaning: to write, record, describe	*radiograph* an X-ray record of a tooth or other body part as recorded by the X ray
macro prefix or combining form meaning: long, large	*macrogingivae* abnormally large gingivae due to heredity, disease or hormonal stimulation
megalo, mega combining form meaning: large, of great size	*megadontismus* abnormally large teeth
megaly suffix meaning: enlargement	*acromegaly* enlargement of bones, soft parts of hands and feet, tongue, mandible, and separation of the teeth
meter suffix meaning: measure, especially an instrument used in measurement	*dosimetry* accurate and systematic determination of the amount of radiation to which a patient has been exposed during a particular period of time
micro combining form meaning: small size	*microglossia* abnormally small tongue
multi combining form meaning: many, much	*multicell* many cells
oligo, olig combining form meaning: few, less than normal	*oligodontin* having only a few teeth
sub prefix meaning: under, below, deficient	*submarginal* a deficiency of contour at the margin of a pattern or a restoration

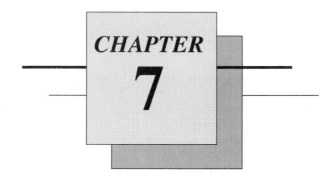

CHAPTER

7

Reception Procedures

Creation of a Cordial Reception
Reception Room Procedures
   Receiving Previous Patients
   Receiving Strangers
     The New Patient
     Receiving Salespersons or Detail Persons
     The Professional Colleague
     The Unidentified Caller
   Dismissing Patients
Telephone Procedures
   Telephone Technique in the Professional Office
   The Professional Telephone Call
   Recording Telephone Calls
   Taking the Message
   Specific Suggestions for the Dental
       Office Telephone Problems
   Assisting New Patients Who Call by Telephone
   Appointments for Children
   Difficult Calls
   Outgoing Calls
   Telephone Answering Service

Creation of a Cordial Reception

The warmth, cordiality, and friendliness of the staff are necessary attributes in the reception procedures for all who contact the office. One never knows who strangers entering the office are, what their businesses are, and what they will say about their reception in that office once they are outside again. Word-of-mouth advertising by persons who contact the office either personally or by telephone is extremely important. Cordial treatment of all persons is one of the best ways to establish good empathy with the public. In addition, patients appreciate a cheerful, pleasant attitude from the assistant and feel wonderful if the assistant also treats them as persons. Learn to work well with patients so they like you and your office. Some of the treatment that has been accorded waiting patients is shocking. We who serve the public in the health fields should view these instances of rudeness with concern.

A garage mechanic was heard to say in a vicious tone, "Let him wait! It'll make up for some of the time my wife has spent sitting in doctors' waiting rooms." He was referring to a doctor who was waiting for his car. The mechanic didn't know the doctor in question. Perhaps this doctor did not keep patients waiting, but as long as some do, the profession as a whole is condemned.

In a milder form this same resentment is expressed by housewives. Contrary to the opinion of most people who receive a paycheck for their working hours, a housewife's time is just as valuable to her and to her family as the office worker's is to himself or herself and his or her employer. It is important to take patients on time insofar as it is humanly possible. If delays are encountered, it is exceedingly important to be fair to all patients—housewives and children as well as office workers . . . or your best friend.

The garage mechanic was generalizing that since some doctors have no respect for patients, all doctors have no respect for patients, and therefore doctors should be treated with disrespect. This is not true, and it is necessary for all the personnel in dental and medical offices to help change this idea that is prevalent among lay people today.

Actually observed in a waiting room was this example of disrespect for people. The waiting room was full; patients were standing. The receptionist looked at the group impassively. Names were called indifferently. The waiting period beyond an appointment was close to an hour. She glanced coldly over the group and said, "You, there in the green chair by the lamp, come here."

There was no trace of common courtesy in her tone. There was no consideration of the people there as

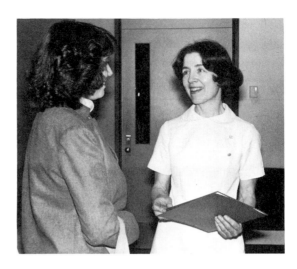

Figure 7.1
Be respectful and courteous when greeting patients.

individual human beings with obligations and appointments beyond this office. She was totally disinterested in anything except that she had to call the next patient.

You may feel that this is an extreme example, and certainly in our better-administered offices this treatment does not occur, but it does exist in enough offices to create a negative impression for some of the public.

We have also heard assistants complain of the treatment they have received from patients who have been rude. We are not suggesting that only the office personnel are inconsiderate. We know that some patients can be very inconsiderate and rude. However, there is one extenuating circumstance in connection with patients. Remember that most of them are apprehensive. They may also be dreading the treatment they are about to receive. Their ability to be pleasant is directly limited by their physical and mental conditions.

It is your job to make such a person as comfortable as possible and to refrain from responding to rudeness with rudeness. One can be firm and remain courteous regardless of the attitude of the patient. The most important attitude to develop with patients is to make them feel that each one is a VIP whose health and welfare receive top priority in your office.

It is the objective of this chapter to help the dental assistant become aware of and develop the skills that permit her or him to treat patients to this well-deserved care.

The dental assistant who is aware of the importance of personal attention to patients will avoid treating people as impersonally as if they were chairs. She or he will also remember that the patients have obligations beyond the office and will appreciate a well-planned schedule of appointments. Only rarely will a patient object to waiting due to some unforeseen emergency—provided every day is not an emergency. It is the business of treating every day as an overload that upsets patients.

Reception Room Procedures

A reception room for receiving guests—rather than a waiting room where nonpersons are allowed to sit until they are called—is the important differentiation to be made in your work with patients. Try to maintain the concept that you are receiving VIPs. Think and speak of the *reception* room.

Everyone should be greeted warmly with a smile, just as you would receive people who call on you at your home. They should be greeted promptly upon arrival. When the doorbell rings, indicating someone has entered your reception room, respond as quickly as you possibly can. Be a very gracious hostess or host to all who enter the office. Remember that patients who return do so because they like the way they were treated on previous visits.

What you do after the initial greeting depends on the nature of the caller's business.

Receiving Previous Patients

1. Know the name of the patient you are expecting and use it when you greet him or her.
2. One of the finer touches in hostessing or hosting that you can use, if time permits and your dentist agrees, is to greet patients with a coat hanger in your hand and hang their coats for them. This moment, if available, gives opportunity for that personal contact you wish to make with patients and makes them feel cared about.

    In cold climates, the really heavy work of dressing children for travel to the dental office, removing their outer clothing for the appointment, then dressing them again for the trip home is tiring for the parent. Assistance with children under these conditions is appreciated. It also gives you the opportunity to remove overshoes or boots that otherwise might be left on to track snow or mud into the operatory.
3. If for any reason the dentist will be late in beginning work for the patient who has already arrived at the office, inform the patient of the fact. Include the probable time of waiting involved—do not say "Just a few minutes" when you are actually

twenty minutes behind. You say, "I'm sorry, Mr. Jones, we have been delayed. We will be ready for you in twenty minutes."

4. See that the patient is seated and that reading material is available. If children are present, see that they are entertained. A few coloring books and a supply of soap crayons (which will wash off almost anything) can do much to keep most children occupied for short periods.
5. Do not permit a patient who comes to the office without an appointment to receive dental care unless it is a true emergency (pain or hemorrhaging). Give the drop-in patient an appointment in the future. Once patients learn that they can drop in and have dental treatment immediately, they will continue to do so repeatedly. Therefore, it is wiser to avoid this behavior by insisting on appointments made in advance for everyone except the true emergency. Even if your dentist is idle from a cancellation, do not take an unappointed patient. Use your call list to fill any cancelled appointments.

Receiving Strangers

Greet the stranger with a smile and say, "May I help you?" The first thing to discover is the purpose of this stranger's visit to your office.

The New Patient

If the stranger is a potential patient and is having pain of dental origin at the moment, give him or her the Acquaintance Form on its clipboard, and say "Will you please fill this out? I will ask Doctor Smith how soon he can see you."

Immediately notify your dentist, by note if the dentist is operating. The dentist will suggest your next step. It is helpful if the assistant can inform the dentist of the patient schedule at the moment. For example, the dentist may be finishing the present patient and the next appointment may not have arrived.

If the stranger is a potential patient but is having no pain or discomfort, give him or her the Acquaintance Form on its clipboard, and say, "Will you please fill this out for Doctor Smith?"

Have possible appointments in mind. When you have received the completed form, check it rapidly. Note which day of the week is preferred. Then say "Doctor Smith would like to see you for examination on (day), at (hour) or (hour). Which time will be more convenient for you?"

Write the patient's name in the appointment book at the proper time, then write on an appointment card the date and time of the appointment. Double check to be certain the information on the appointment card agrees with your appointment book entry. Give the patient the card when you say goodbye.

Receiving Salespersons or Detail Persons

Salespersons should rarely see the dentist except by prearranged appointments. Almost all purchases can be handled by the dental assistant. If it is desirable for the dentist to talk with a salesperson, make an appointment. Time is valuable for both the dentist and the salesperson, and an appointment with a specified length of time respects that value. The time of this appointment must be limited. Make certain that the salesperson understands the time limit. According to the day's schedule, you say, "Doctor can see you at 1:50 for ten minutes" or "Doctor Smith is free from 1:50 until 2:00." Make the appointment between patients—not at the beginning of the lunch hour or at the close of the day. It is advantageous to be able to interrupt the conference at the end of the allotted time. When that moment arrives, you say, "Doctor Smith, your patient is in the chair."

During office hours the dentist sees only salespersons who sell dental products and equipment. The dentist can see other salespersons away from the office.

Salespersons frequently bring detail persons with them. A detail person is a new products expert who skillfully presents the product to the dentist. Often the dentist does not wish to spend time with the detail person. Protect your dentist from anyone whom he or she does not wish to see. Remember that if you continue to politely refuse to allow the individual to see the dentist, that person will stop coming. Several refusals should convince even the most obtuse individual.

Perhaps your dentist prefers to see dental salespersons as soon as it is convenient. In this case, the suggested handling of the stranger who is a salesperson will be altered. The salesperson who has entered the office should be informed of the time-wait involved or of a more opportune time to call.

Whatever methods are used for controlling interruptions in your dentist's schedule, all salespersons should be treated courteously. They earn their living by selling and very often they can be helpful.

The Professional Colleague

If the stranger who enters your reception room introduces himself or herself as "Doctor Jones," immediately ask him or her to be seated and excuse yourself. In a clear, distinct voice tell your dentist immediately that Doctor Jones is in the reception room. Your dentist will tell you what he or she wishes you to do. Unless your dentist specifically indicates otherwise, always remember that the privacy of the patient in the chair should be respected. Ordinarily, any other professional person, or any person not a member of the office staff, is never brought to the chairside without the express permission of the patient beforehand.

The Unidentified Caller

Occasionally there will be individuals who merely indicate that they would like to speak to Doctor Smith, without giving you either their name or business. Usually, this would indicate in itself that if the dentist knew the reason for the visit, he or she would refuse to see the caller. Some judgment is required in these situations, but if you do feel doubtful due to the appearance of the individual and his or her reluctance to tell you his or her name and business, inform that person firmly and courteously that you must have his or her name and the subject of the visit, indicating that you will then be able to ask Doctor Smith if he or she will see the visitor. Should he or she refuse again, say, "I'm sorry, but in that case you will have to reach Doctor Smith at home after office hours." Then leave that individual.

This same technique is used with telephone callers who insist on speaking to the dentist but refuse to give their name or business after you have gone through the regular routine.

Once in awhile, an individual will ask a question (in response to your greeting) such as, "Are you the only employee in this office?" or, "How long have you worked for Doctor Smith?" Such an approach, a rapidly given personal question, is often a device used to gain the initiative in the conversation and is widely used by door-to-door salespeople. Keep in mind that personal questions are not the privilege of a stranger. Do not follow the impulse to answer.

Reply with a question of your own, such as "What is it you are selling?" Or simply say, "What is it you wish, please?" Do not waste your time or your employer's time unnecessarily.

Dismissing Patients

Helping a patient to leave the office feeling worthwhile and valued is also important. Frequently the dismissal begins at the dental chair.

The receptionist's duties usually include escorting the patient from the operatory back to the reception room. All possible assistance should be given with coats, boots, and gathering of personal belongings. If the patient is elderly, helping him or her put on his or her coat is often appreciated. If a parent has small children, that parent can be very grateful for assistance at the time of departure.

These courtesies to patients can only be performed when time permits and the dentist approves. One of the advantages of this type of reception and dismissal of patients is that it permits the receptionist to protect the dentist from a problem situation that might develop. The dentist cannot afford to spend more than the allotted time with patients, salespersons, or anyone else. During the patient's appointment, the dentist and staff must make certain that the patient is made to feel valuable, appreciated, and important as a person. When the allotted time has elapsed, the dentist must be ready to devote his or her undivided attention to the next patient. At this point, the receptionist or other staff member can give the departing patient attention so that the patient leaves the office feeling appreciated.

Telephone Procedures

A patient enters a dental office by one of two methods: either by appearing in person or by calling on the telephone. The usual procedure is to telephone prior to coming to the office; thus, the telephone becomes an important means of entry. The dental assistant whose assignment includes answering the telephone must possess skillful techniques in telephone usage. She or he must be aware of the factors that encourage patients to take the next step—appearing in person at an appointed time.

The success of a telephone contact is dependent on how well the two persons involved understand each other. All the physical factors that are present to help that understanding in a person-to-person contact are missing in a telephone conversation. It is possible to have a satisfying interaction over the telephone, provided the message content is carefully selected and effectively presented. The individual who is gracious, sincere, and courteous while interacting on the telephone usually creates a favorable impression.

Telephone Technique In the Professional Office

The telephone is such a common part of our everyday life that some of us are apt to use it carelessly. In a professional office, care must be taken to use this instrument properly. The fact that the physical management of the telephone can be stated simply does not lessen the importance of following the instructions for its effective use.

The telephone should be held so that the transmitter is one-half to one inch from the lips. Since the telephone transmitter is as sensitive as a microphone, the voice must be directed into it. A person must be especially careful not

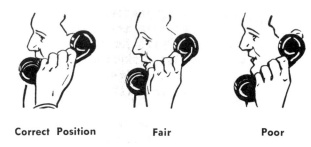

Correct Position   Fair   Poor

Figure 7.2
Hold the telephone correctly.

to let it slip under the chin, or to cover the transmitter with the hand.

A well-modulated conversational tone of voice carries best over the telephone. Of course, it goes without saying that impediments—like a pencil or gum—should not be placed in the mouth when talking. This could lead to annoyance or misunderstanding and create unfavorable impressions.

Care should be taken to hang up gently, since banging the receiver is unpleasant to the ear and is like slamming the door in someone's face.[1]

Following the rules set forth in the foregoing quoted paragraphs will care for the mechanics of telephone usage. In addition, when speaking on the telephone, always speak as you would if the person were standing before you—the same courtesy, the same warmth of expression, and the same friendliness of manner. Try smiling while speaking. Only your voice contacts the person with whom you are speaking. You must make it so cordial that the person on the telephone feels the warmth of your personality just as though you were speaking to each other in the same room. *Remember that how you say what you say affects the person on the telephone more than in a person-to-person conversation.*

The Professional Telephone Call

A professional telephone call may be divided into four parts:

1. Identification of caller and person called
2. Purpose of call, including any specific arrangements to be made
3. Conclusion of business, including verification of information or specific arrangements
4. Termination of call, including courteous closing remarks, such as "Thank you for calling"

Additional suggestions to render effective telephone service include the following:

1. Answer the telephone promptly, thus making the caller feel that he or she is important, that this is an efficient dental office, and that you value the patient's time as well as your own.

2. When you make calls, allow time for the person to answer. A minute is a very short time for a person to reach the telephone. In one minute the telephone will ring about ten times.

3. Try to avoid calling a wrong number by having the correct number at hand and then dialing carefully after you have heard the dial tone. If you do receive a wrong number, apologize and hang up gently.

4. Give information regarding an appointment slowly.

5. If it is necessary to leave the telephone to get information, remember these three items:

   a. Be sure to excuse yourself and indicate that you will return in a specific length of time, such as a few seconds, one minute, or two minutes.

   b. Return to the telephone to assure the caller that you haven't forgotten him or her if it takes longer than you said it would to find the information.

   c. Attract the caller's attention on your return by saying his name or "Thank you for waiting, Mr. Jones." Then give the desired information.

6. Always close any telephone conversation with a pleasant, "Thank you, Mrs. Jones," or "Thank you for calling Mrs. Jones." The first phrase applies if you called Mrs. Jones; the latter phrase applies if Mrs. Jones called your office.

7. Upon completion of a call that a patient made to your office, the caller should be the first to hang up the receiver. It is courteous to let the other party be the first to hang up.

Recording Telephone Calls

Often it is necessary to take messages from telephone callers. The telephone notebook is the ideal record of telephone calls. A bound notebook used for this purpose means that every call that is written in the book remains there to be seen later. It is impossible to lose a telephone message if it is bound into a telephone notebook that is much like a receipt book. A carbon

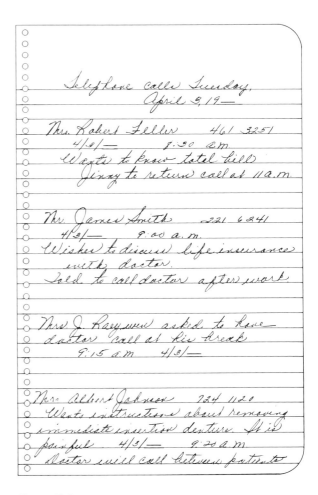

Figure 7.3
Sample page from a telephone notebook.

copy of the written message remains bound in the book for future reference; the original copy is removable. This means the message can be kept for future reference and, at the same time, be given to the person who is to receive the message. A notebook containing a list of the telephone calls received should be kept whether or not the dentist for whom you work wishes to use the telephone book with carbon copy. A sample page from a telephone notebook is shown in figure 7.3. Notice that specific information is given for each call.

Taking the Message

Be helpful if you are taking a message. Be certain that you have the name, the telephone number of the caller, the date (with year), and the time of the call—written legibly. Agree on an approximate time to report back to the caller. Be certain that this information is recorded on your note of the call:

1. Name of caller
2. Telephone number (can you read it?)
3. Date and time of call

4. Desired information
5. Time at which the call will be returned
6. The name of the person who is to return the call

Specific Suggestions for the Dental Office Telephone Problems

1. *Answering routine.* In answering the telephone, say "Doctor Smith's office." Your dentist may like you to add, "Mr. (or Ms.) Jones speaking." Use an agreed-upon wording and do not alter it.

2. *Expressing competence.* You must give the telephone caller the positive assurance of your ability. You do not say so, but you give this assurance by using a tone with no rising inflections at the ends of sentences. A calm, low voice is good, providing it is cheerful.

3. *Visualizing the caller.* Try to put yourself in the caller's place. Think what the caller is thinking—and treat the caller as you would want to be treated. Be pleasant!

   Individuals who telephone the office will occasionally abuse this form of entry and become discourteous. Never give anything but courtesy in return, even under the most trying circumstances.

4. *Two jobs at once.* If the telephone rings while you are caring for a patient— welcoming, dismissing, or accepting payment, for example—answer the telephone after excusing yourself, ascertain the name of the caller, then courteously ask the telephone caller to wait until you have finished with the patient in the office.

   You say, "Mr. Jones, will you please wait while I complete an appointment?" If he indicates he is too busy, then you may say, "May I call you in a few moments?" and take his number and call him immediately after you finish the business with the patient who is standing in front of you.

   However, most callers will be willing to wait, understanding that you are working with another patient. In this case, finish your business with the patient in the office as quickly and as courteously as possible, then return to the telephone and say, "Thank you for waiting, Mr. Jones. Now may I help you?" It is extremely irritating to·a patient to find his or her business with you interrupted by a

telephone call and to have you give the telephone call precedence in your attention. It is discourteous to the patient who is present in person.

   If a patient enters the reception room when you are telephoning, smile at that person and bring your business conversation to a close as quickly as possible to care for the needs of the patient in the reception room. If your conversation is personal (a rare occasion), immediately terminate it and finish your personal business later.

5. *Screening telephone calls.* Should the caller ask to speak with the dentist, your reply usually is, "Doctor is with a patient. May I help you?"

   Avoid the phrase, "Doctor is busy just now." Be more specific: "Doctor is with a patient," or "not in," or "in conference," or "I cannot interrupt Doctor just now."

   Ascertain the reason for the call.

   Always secure the name of the caller.

   If you cannot take care of the problem this particular caller presents, ask for and write down his or her telephone number and name. Ask if you may have Doctor return the call.

   Telephone calls from colleagues, hospitals, and pharmacies, as well as long distance calls, are usually extended to the dentist immediately. Of course, if your employer gives other instructions, it is your responsibility to follow those instructions.

   All calls not given to the dentist immediately should be written in the telephone notebook. The name of the caller and his or her business and telephone number are to be legibly written. If the person expects to have the call returned by any specific time, it should be stated. Any remark by the receptionist to the effect that the person will be called requires a report back to that person, even if the dentist is unable for some reason to return the call. It is desirable not to interrupt the dentist when he or she is with a patient. If an emergency does occur, it may be necessary to interrupt the dentist-patient relationship, but every effort should be made to refrain from such interruption.

6. *Know to whom you are speaking.* It is important that you know to whom you are speaking before you give any information or answer any questions. It is customary to identify the office and state your name,

then ask for identification of your caller unless the person has already given it. Refer to the proper professional call procedures. (Pages 83–84)

7. *What NOT to say.* Do not inadvertently give information to a caller if that information is not necessary. It is very easy to do. If the dentist, for example, is taking two days away from the office, it is not necessary to tell a patient that the doctor won't be in on the twenty-second or twenty-third, but he can see the patient on the twenty-fourth at three. Say, rather, "The first appointment we have available for you, Mrs. Jones, is Wednesday, the twenty-fourth, at three o'clock in the afternoon."

There is one exception to this procedure, however. If your dentist is attending a convention, a study course, a postgraduate course at a school, or a dental committee meeting, always be sure to state the cause of his absence: "Doctor Smith will be attending a postgraduate course at the University that week, Mrs. Jones. The first appointment available is the following Wednesday, the twenty-fourth, at nine o'clock in the morning." This information indicates to the patient that Doctor Smith is refreshing his or her education and therefore must be a good dentist.

8. *Fees.* A disagreement about a fee should not be discussed in a telephone conversation. Should a patient telephone to argue, invite a patient to come to the office to see you. Make a definite appointment with the patient for this visit—an appointment with you, not the dentist. Inform the dentist of the call when convenient and get the details of the account or charges for use during the appointment.

9. *Confidentiality.* When you telephone a patient about an overdue account or payment or any other strictly personal matter, never give this information to anyone but the patient personally. Other members of the patient's family may be insistently curious about the subject of your call. For example, if the patient is a young adult who still lives with parents, brothers, or sisters, it may be difficult for him or her to maintain privacy. Your only statement in these circumstances is, "This is Mary at Doctor Smith's office. Will you please ask John to call me as soon as possible?"

10. *Shoppers.* Individuals who call various dental offices to ask what it costs to have a tooth filled, a tooth pulled, or plates made are called shoppers. Should someone call and ask such a question, respond with the question, "May I ask who is calling please?" Usually a caller will not give his or her name. If the caller does comply, he or she will also repeat the question. Your answer is, "I'm sorry, Mr. Jones, but Doctor Smith would have to examine your mouth before he could give you an estimate. Would you like an appointment for an examination?"

11. *SOS for dentist.* At times there may be a telephone call that you cannot personally care for or delay until your dentist is free. Note legibly the name of the caller and the subject of this emergency. Show it to the dentist, preferably so that the patient on whom he or she is operating is unaware of the process. Your dentist will tell you what to do or will give you an answering note.

12. *Cancellations.* Should a patient call to cancel an appointment, ask if you may make another appointment. The purpose of this approach is to avoid having the patient say that he or she will call you. Memories can be short—and then you have lost contact with a patient. If the time involved is a matter of weeks or even months before the patient expects to be available for another appointment, ask if you may call at that time. The patient will usually agree to this arrangement. Immediately make a note of the call to be made—in the appointment book, in pencil, on the proper date, or on another calendar of the note type used for this purpose. See that these calls are made promptly.

13. *Expectations.* In order to preserve the value of any set routine in handling telephone calls as well as in-person calls at the office, it is necessary that your dentist keep you informed of anticipated personal calls or visits and indicate willingness to accept these contacts immediately. If this routine is followed, you will be aware of calls that some individuals may imply are personal but are really commercial in nature, for which your dentist does not wish to be disturbed.

14. *Keeping the dentist away from the telephone.* The dentist should not come to the telephone except to speak with another

professional person regarding professional work.

A patient rarely needs to talk on the telephone with the dentist. You can relay most messages, even in an emergency.

In an emergency, ask specific questions:

a. The name of the caller
b. The address and telephone number
c. The location of the trouble in the mouth, and the severity of the problem

With the information obtained, write a note for your dentist stating the problem. Your dentist will instruct you in what measures to relay to the patient for relief (hot or cold packs, etc.) and will also indicate whether the patient should be seen either immediately or at the emergency appointment time. You can then return to the telephone with the information for the patient while your dentist continues to provide dentistry for the patient in the chair.

15. *When to be uninformed.* Often, the patient who has had an examination and is called after X rays have been read may immediately say, "How many cavities do I have?"

To the patient, this means "How much work do I need?", and patients use this as a basis for estimating probable costs.

To the dentist, the number of cavities does not indicate the amount of work. A cavity may require a one-surface restoration or it may require a full crown.

One example of effectively meeting the problem is illustrated in this conversation:

Dental Assistant: Doctor has studied your films. You need to have some work done. Would you like to come in the morning or afternoon?
Patient: How many cavities do I have?
Dental Assistant: About an hour's time will be required, Mrs. Jones.
Patient: But how many *cavities* are there?
Dental Assistant: Mrs. Jones, I'm not qualified to read these films, but Doctor asked for an hour's time for your work.

There are times when it is wise to be uninformed, and this is one instance.

16. *Keeping your promise.* If you tell a patient that you will perform some service (call him or her back, etc.), write yourself a note immediately! Don't trust your memory. There are too many things to remember. Write notes!

17. *Mind your job.* None of the conversations that you hold with people can be "stiff" if you are to be successful in leading them or in keeping them as patients. All this has to be automatic. You must be on your toes and a jump or two ahead of everyone. Your mind must be on your work in the office.

18. *A habit to avoid.* Remember that the telephone forms one of the main entrances for new patients into your office and should be kept as free as possible for this purpose. Using the telephone for personal calls, while occasionally necessary, is a habit to be avoided.

19. *Space outgoing calls.* When you use the telephone to make a series of outgoing calls, space them out well. Make one or two calls, then wait ten minutes or so before making the next one or two calls. This procedure allows time for incoming calls to be received. If your office has two or more incoming telephone lines, this precaution is not necessary.

20. *Answer the telephone promptly.* Answer the telephone as promptly as possible. Because it is the way most patients contact the office, it should be answered quickly.

21. *Retain the initiative.* The ideal in patient control is to retain the initiative, whether on the telephone or in person, without hurting the patient's ego or being discourteous in any way. The easiest way to achieve this end when you are inexperienced is to have a set routine that is used without variation to resist the usual pressures some patients will exert for special consideration. As you gain poise in your office, you may vary the routine to suit the occasion.

Either you manage the patients or the patients will all too willingly manage your office.

If you lead, the patient will follow. It must be done lightly. Inject humor occasionally, yet let the patient know that you mean what you say.

For example, a dental assistant was confronted with a longtime patient who always insisted on personally talking with the dentist to make an appointment. In previous conversations, the dental assistant had mentioned that she was making all appointments now, so this particular day she avoided mentioning it again.

The dentist happened to be at his dentist's office having some necessary work done from noon to one o'clock.

Dental Assistant: No. Dr. Smith is not in. Who is calling, please?

Patient: Do you expect him back today? (*Refusal of patient to give his name*)

Dental Assistant: Yes, I expect him back. May I help you?

Patient: I'll call later. (*Still wants the dentist*)

Dental Assistant: It would be better if he were to call you—otherwise you may call when he is unable to come to the telephone. (*Said with a smile*)

Patient: This is Mr. Appleby. (*Capitulation*)

Dental Assistant: Oh, yes! May I help you? (*Recognition*)

Patient: Well, I want to see the doctor at five tonight.

Dental Assistant: What seems to be the difficulty? (*What do you want to see him about?*)

Patient: Well, . . . I have a sore spot. (*Reluctant capitulation*)

Dental Assistant: Doctor Smith could see you for your emergency at a quarter of two, Mr. Appleby. That will be so much better than you having to wait around all that time after work. Doctor has a five o'clock patient so he would not be able to see you today after that hour.

Patient: All right, I'll be in at a quarter of two.

Dental Assistant: Goodbye, Mr. Appleby and thank you for calling.

The purpose of the dental assistant's approach was to keep the patient from doing what she did not want done—to overcrowd an already overloaded late afternoon—and to prevent the patient from speaking with the dentist. (The dentist might have felt it necessary to say, "Come when you want to.") She saw the opportunity to work in this emergency at a better moment and proceeded to set it up her way instead of allowing the patient to set it up his way. She did it with cordiality in her voice—helping a regular patient find satisfaction through accepted office procedure without loss of the assistant's authority.

Had the dentist been in the office, she would still have proceeded as she did— preventing the patient from contacting the dentist directly. What the patient desired— an appointment—is the business of the assistant, not the dentist.

In reviewing this conversation, we see the attempts of the patient to achieve his desire to talk with the dentist, and the assistant's deft sidestepping to avoid an open clash as she frustrates his intent—and satisfies him sufficiently to keep him as a patient.

Assisting New Patients Who Call by Telephone

The assistant should start an Acquaintance Form for the new patient who calls by telephone. Ask the caller's name, home address, home telephone, and the name of the person who referred this individual to your office. Then you ask, "Do you wish an appointment for an examination, Mrs. Jones?"

If the caller is having pain, she will so inform you at that time. If such is the case, make whatever arrangements are customary in your office for emergency care, and at the appointment complete the arrangements for an examination appointment. If you should ask Mrs. Jones if she is having any pain, this very frequently serves as a suggestion to that individual to claim discomfort as a means of securing an earlier appointment with your office. If you suggest an appointment for examination and do not mention pain, you will experience less pressure of this sort.

Should Mrs. Jones indicate that an appointment for examination is the purpose of her call, ask what day of the week is usually most convenient. Check for a possible appointment time in the appointment book, then say, "Doctor Smith will see you for an examination on (day), at (hour) or (hour). Which time will be more convenient for you?"

Appointments for Children

Should you receive a telephone call from a parent desiring an appointment for a child, the responsible person's name should be asked, and that person's first name, middle initial, and last name should be placed on the Acquaintance Form. The name of the child, date of birth, the child's nickname, and whether or not the child has been to the dentist previously should be ascertained and noted. If the answer to the last question is yes, ask if the child objected to seeing the dentist. Note the reply.

Ask for the name of the person responsible for the child. Sometimes if you ask for the name of the child's father, you may receive some objection. Estrangements or divorces are common. Should you note any resentment at the question, merely indicate that your office wishes to know the name of the person responsible for the child. This is a reasonable request.

Keep the age of the child in mind as you check your appointment book. In accordance with the suggestions given under "New Patients Who Call by Telephone," offer a choice of two appointments. One of the parents should accompany the young child for the examination visit.

Difficult Calls

Callers sometimes present difficulties for the assistant. A patient may request information that you are not at liberty to give, a patient may be upset about a bill, someone may call to inquire about a patient, or a shopper may call to quiz you about fees.

It is a good idea to think of as many of these difficult calls as possible and try to have some answers ready in your mind or in a file by the telephone. After you have worked awhile, these calls become much less difficult.

The patient who is easily upset by changes in routine may call and be disturbed because you are not the assistant he or she talked with before. Listen for the name carefully, use it soothingly in speaking with him or her, and assure the patient that you will see that he or she has careful attention. The patient should soon become accustomed to your presence.

A patient may call to change an appointment. Be sure you make it clear that your dentist sees patients by appointment and give the caller a specific appointment at a time that is open. The patient should not be allowed to crowd into an already filled day simply because he or she is unable to keep the appointment. Find another appointment for the patient.

A patient may call to complain about a bill. Courteously ask the patient to wait. Pull the patient's financial card and clinical record from the file. Return to the telephone and be courteous about the matter.

Sometimes you will receive a call asking about the dentistry performed for one of your patients. Never give information to anyone about a patient. Tell the caller that you will have your dentist return the call.

Outgoing Calls

It is frequently necessary for the assistant to call patients or other dentists. Before you make one of these calls, have at hand all the materials necessary for completing the business of the call. Be certain that you have the correct telephone number. Try to place the call at a time when you anticipate the least amount of interruption within the office. (If you know the dentist is within a minute of needing you, it is not a time to place a call.)

If you are calling a patient, a dentist, or a physician with whom your dentist wishes to speak, be sure that your dentist is available before you place the call. If you are calling a patient about an appointment, have the appointment book in front of you. If it is necessary for you to change the appointment, give the patient all the consideration possible. A parent may have already engaged a babysitter, or an employed person may have already asked for the time off. An explanation of the reason for the change is courteous.

It may be necessary for you to call a patient with instructions. Be certain that your information is accurate before you make the call.

Telephone Answering Service

Today dental offices may have some type of telephone answering service that cares for calls during the periods when no one is in the office. The answering service is notified when the receptionist leaves the office. The information to be given to callers is stated at that time. It may be the telephone number where the dentist can be reached, or the answering service may be requested to take the name and telephone number of the callers for the receptionist until she or he can return the calls.

Summary

Friendliness, warmth, and cordiality are necessary attributes in the reception procedures for all who contact the office—whether by telephone or through the reception room door.

Be prepared for previous patients as they enter the reception room. Greet them as old friends. Strangers must be identified and given attention on the basis of the purpose of their visit. The new patient is given an Acquaintance Form and eventually an appointment. Salespeople receive an appointment. Professional colleagues are either ushered into the dentist's business office or given immediate care in the reception room. Unknown callers are identified or are not permitted to see your dentist.

A reception room for receiving guests rather than a waiting room where nonpersons are allowed to sit until they are called is the important differentiation in your work with patients. Try to maintain the concept that you are receiving VIPs. Think and speak of the reception room.

Patients who do not enter the dental office through the reception room door, enter by means of the telephone. The success of the telephone conversation depends on how well the two persons understand each other. Since the only contact is by voice, there is room for misunderstanding that doesn't exist when two people can see each other as they speak.

General technique of telephoning demands the same courtesy and warmth as one would express in a personal contact. Speak directly into the telephone with a normal voice and good diction.

A business call can be divided into four parts: (1) identification of caller and person called, (2) purpose of call, (3) conclusion of business, and (4) termination of call.

Prompt answering, care in writing messages received, ascertaining name and telephone number of the caller are all important points to remember in using the telephone.

It is important that there be an agreed-upon method of answering the telephone in the dental office. Special care should be exercised when the telephone rings while you are working with a patient in the reception room. Other important ideas to be remembered in working with the telephone are the following:

1. When the dentist is with a patient, refrain from calling him or her to the telephone.
2. Give only the information necessary to the business of the moment.
3. Answer the telephone as promptly as possible.
4. Close every call with a "thank you" in one form or another.
5. Confer with your dentist by note about telephone matters that cannot be delayed.
6. Allow time between outgoing calls.

Lead the patients rather than allow them to lead you in matters of appointments and office routines. Emergencies can be handled by relayed messages rather than by interrupting the contact your dentist has with the patient in the chair—a very important person who is paying for that undivided attention from your dentist.

Study Questions

1. Why are reception procedures so very important?
2. Discuss the fundamentals of reception room techniques for the dental assistant.
3. Discuss the variations in reception for (1) previous patients, (2) strangers, (3) unidentified callers, (4) salespeople or detail persons, (5) professional colleagues.
4. Discuss the best form for a professional telephone call.
5. Discuss telephone courtesies and routines.
6. What information must you secure in case of an emergency?
7. What routine do you follow when a new patient calls on the telephone?
8. What information do you need when a parent calls for an appointment for a child who is new to your practice?

Word Elements	
Word Element	**Example**
a, an prefix meaning: without	**anesthesia** without sensation, loss of sensation
e, ec combining form meaning: without	**edentulous** without teeth
en, em prefix meaning: in	**encyst** enclose in a cyst
endo, end prefix meaning: inward situation, within	**endodontics** specialty in dentistry concerned with infection within the tooth
ento prefix meaning: within, inner	**entocyte** within the cell
im prefix meaning: in, within	**impression** imprint or negative form within which is found the likeness of the object
in prefix meaning: in, within	**injection** forcing liquid in
intra, intr prefix meaning: situated or formed within	**intrapulpal** within the pulp
intro prefix meaning: into or within	**introvert** to turn inward on itself
in prefix meaning: not	**indirect** not direct (as in indirect inlay impression)

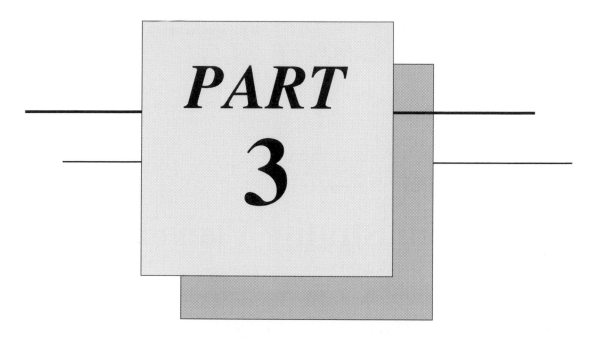

PART 3

Administration of the Business Office

The administration of the dental office, with all its minute details, is the job of the dental assistant, office receptionist, or someone designated as manager, depending upon the size of the staff. The dentist should be occupied with the practice of dentistry. Since no one else is so qualified, it is the responsibility of the staff to see that the dentist only performs services that no one else in the office can do—namely, diagnosing and treating patients—using the skill that only he or she possesses. Clinical team members should also spend their time practicing the skills for which they are trained. All the work that can be done by someone else should be done by someone else.

The achievement of this goal means that the responsibilities of the office administrator are:

1. Organization of time in the office: dentist's, patients', and staff members'
2. Maintenance of open channels of communication with all other health-related services, organizations, and practitioners, as well as with the patients
3. Maintenance of proper records so that the dentist is protected professionally and financially and that the staff is paid accurately
4. Organization of all details of office operation so the office functions smoothly

Part Three presents the organization of the business office services, including appointing patients.

Administrative Planning

A Dental Office Administrator
Coordinating the Office Staff
Procedure Manual
The Staff Conference
Sources of Information
Commercial Communication Services
The Dentist's Personal Reminder Service
Understanding Patient Recall Philosophy
Succeeding as an Office Administrator
    Solving a Problem
    Discovering Which Problem
    Examining the Problem
    Selling Your Dentist
Orderly Office Routines
    Work Schedules: Their Successful Operation
    Advance Record Preparation
    Laboratory Schedule
    Verification of Information
    Thank-you Notes
    Current Invoices
    Come-up Card Files
    Patient Recall Control File
    Office Task Control
    Birthday Card Control

A Dental Office Administrator

Whenever two or more people work together, some form of cooperation and communication is necessary. If these two or more people are working together to provide a service to others, the cooperation must be organized and administered to avoid confusion and to encourage efficiency.

The dentist may hire an office coordinator (administrator or manager), or the dentist may assign the office administrative details to one staff member. The delegation of these tasks to one person should result in certain advantages:

1. More efficient dental service to patients
2. Less mental, emotional, and physical strain for all members of the oral health care delivery team
3. Lowered operating costs

The administration of the dental office with all its minute details should be the responsibility of one person: dental office assistant, receptionist, office manager, or office administrator, depending on the size of the staff. The reasons for employing an administrator are to see that:

1. The dentist produces dentistry—utilizing the skills and training that no one else has.
2. All members of the oral health care delivery team perform the skills for which they have been trained.
3. The details of the dental practice are controlled, which includes maintaining

adequate, accurate, professional and financial records, and organizing all details of operation so that the result is order—not chaos.

The administrator will attempt to gain an overview perspective of this particular dental practice as outlined by the dentist-employer. The duty of the administrator is to appraise continually the office routines in an effort to maintain the highest quality service to patients.

Visualization of the office organization through the use of the diagram in figure 8.1 may be helpful. The relationships between staff members can be understood. This diagram does not necessarily apply to all dental offices. It is important that the dentist give careful thought to his or her needs and develop an individual plan of organization.

Coordinating the Office Staff

Perhaps one of the most difficult problems in a large office—or even in an office with only two employees— is to coordinate the work of the staff members in order to avoid overlapping of duties. Dentists should be given the assistance they need when they need it by the one person appointed to give this specific assistance. Two employees should never be standing around, each waiting for the other to give the necessary assistance. It is important that all employees know what is expected of them and when that service is to be rendered.

The ideal is to have the coordination of the staff explicitly stated in a procedure manual. However, even when the duties are carefully written in a procedure

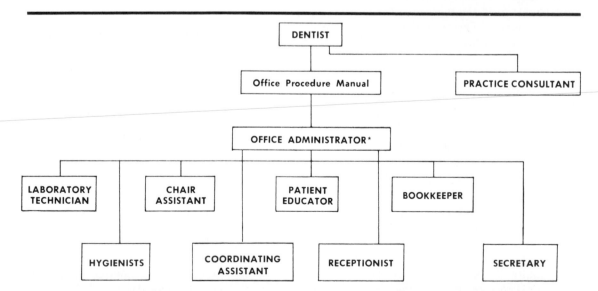

*However the dentist wishes to designate this function. The employee may perform only administrative tasks or may have another responsibility, such as reception or bookkeeping. The concept is that some form of administration must occur if the dentist is to spend his time practicing his profession.

Figure 8.1

Functions in the dental organization.

manual, a certain amount of attention must be given to the staff to see that the directions as set forth in the manual are kept in operation in the office. Writing something on paper doesn't necessarily make it happen in working relationships between people.

The employee who is assigned to coordinate the efforts of the oral health care delivery team must have a sense of timing and the ability to manage intuitively to keep the traffic flowing. This type of intuition is developed with practice, alert observation, and notation of details such as the amount of time:

1. the dentist uses for specific preparations;
2. the chair assistant takes to prepare the operatory;
3. the hygienist spends with patients of different ages, and
4. the laboratory technician needs to complete certain operations.

A knowledge of traffic-flow studies is helpful. In such studies, the observer uses a floor plan of the area and draws the walking pattern of the individual(s) involved. A study of this pattern may lead to improved ways of performing specific tasks. Perhaps steps can be eliminated by rearranging materials or equipment.

The goal of the well-coordinated office is to keep the dentist occupied in providing care for patients that no one else can provide. Some of the employees may perform specific services that no one else on the staff can provide. The employee may be certified in a specific area of oral health care. No matter what the job differences are, the central idea is that all team members perform the tasks for which they are trained and any other tasks that are assigned them in the overall plan as visualized by the dentist. The duty of the coordinator or administrator is to utilize this previously-agreed-upon plan.

Procedure Manual

A manual of office procedures is important regardless of the size of the office staff. It is most helpful in acquainting a new employee with the office routines. In addition, all staff members know what is expected of them because the information is carefully written in the procedure manual. Each duty of every assistant should be listed, and detailed instructions should be given about the dentist's preference in the way certain routines are performed.

The manual is usually divided into sections: the first presenting the general considerations that the dentist deems important for his or her individual office, followed by specific information about certain areas of

work in the office. Such a manual might contain brief summaries of the following areas:

I. The philosophy of dentistry as practiced in this office
   A. Ethics for the staff
   B. Philosophy of dental practice
II. Employer-employee relationships
   A. Salary
      1. Beginning salary
      2. Schedule of raises
      3. Amount of raises
      4. Reasons for raises
   B. Working hours
      1. Specific hours for each employee (Usually one employee remains in the office as long as the dentist is treating a patient. A statement should indicate which staff member is responsible for this extra time.)
      2. Remuneration for the responsibility of extra hours (either time off or increased salary)
   C. Vacation policy
      1. Schedule of amount of time allowed per year of employment
      2. Vacation restrictions (Times when vacation may be taken are specified in some offices.)
      3. Accrual of vacation days
   D. Holidays: annual holidays on which the office is closed, for example New Year's Day, Memorial Day, Fourth of July, and so on
   E. Sick leave
      1. Amount of time with pay allowed
      2. Unused sick leave privileges (added vacation or extra pay)
   F. Uniforms
      1. Types permitted (slacks or dresses)
      2. Requirements of style, color, hose, shoes, cap, slip
      3. Purchase policy (who purchases?)
      4. Laundry policy (who launders?)
      5. Special considerations for short-term employees
      6. Requirements for clean uniforms
   G. Dentistry for employees
      1. Conditions under which dentistry is performed
      2. Discounts for employee and family (family defined)
   H. Coffee breaks: when, how long, and where permitted
   I. Smoking: if permitted, where and when

J. Activity in professional organizations
   1. Financing of annual dues and dinner meetings
   2. Attendance requirements
K. Dental meetings
   1. Meeting attendance requirements
   2. Financing of meetings
L. Personal appearance: grooming requirements—hair, jewelry, perfume, nails
M. Personal hygiene
   1. Daily bath requirements
   2. Other personal requirements
N. Probation period of employment
O. Use of telephone for personal calls: calls may be limited to before and after office hours, or there may be a specific statement that no personal calls are to be made or accepted except in case of an extreme emergency. It is possible to make your personal telephone calls on coffee break at a nearby public telephone so that the office telephone is available for the office business, including emergencies that, of necessity, form a part of every day in a dental practice.

III. Staff meetings
   A. How often
   B. Responsibilities of staff for meeting
IV. Responsibilities and duties of the dental personnel
   A. The dentist
   B. The office administrator
   C. The dental chair assistants
   D. The dental clinical assistants including coordinating assistants and those performing expanded duties
   E. The dental secretarial assistants
   F. The dental receptionist
   G. The dental hygienists
   H. The dental laboratory technicians
V. Office policies concerning:
   A. Financial arrangements for patients (The specific items in this section state exactly how to complete arrangements and follow through on collections.)
   B. Assignment of appointment control (ideally, one person uses the book)
   C. Care of telephone calls: suggested phrases for best telephone communication with patients
   D. Recall control
   E. Birthday card control, if used

VI. The forms that are used in the office (All the forms that are used in the production and administration of dentistry should be included with notations about any special instructions for their usage.)
VII. The patient education program (complete description)
VIII. Inventory control
   A. System explained
   B. Regulations for ordering supplies carefully outlined
IX. Housekeeping and maintenance routines and responsibilities outlined
   A. Dusting and tidying the office, assigned by area. The receptionist in a large office may have the responsibility for the care of the reception rooms; a chair assistant may have the responsibility for the operatories; the laboratory technicians may be responsible for the laboratory and so on.
   B. Laundry records, sorting and verification of laundry
   C. Autoclaving and related duties
   D. Cleaning and management of supply cupboards
X. Patient reception routines clarified

With this kind of detailed description of the working routines of the office, all staff members can verify their individual responsibilities from time to time. Should someone fail to abide by the regulations, it is possible to refer the individual to the regulation in the manual.

The Staff Conference

Plans of operation are just that—plans. The successful administration of a plan necessitates action. In the dental office, cooperative action is necessary. One of the most efficient methods of assuring the success of an action plan by a group is to set aside a time when the team members can confer about the problems that arise—about irritations as well as pleasant experiences. A regularly scheduled meeting of the staff can become one of discussing mutual problems and of making suggestions to improve the efficiency of the entire staff.

The decision to conduct staff conferences is the responsibility of the dentist, who should be given every opportunity to discover that working conditions are more satisfying for everyone when the team can meet to coordinate their efforts successfully.

The meeting should be scheduled at a regular time each week. It is not to be treated casually nor held when some patient cancels an appointment. This meeting can become the key to successful team cooperation and should be treated as one of the most important occurrences during each week.

All staff members should make notes during the week of the subjects they wish to discuss. In a normal office relationship, frictions often occur. The team members are better prepared to handle their irritations in a mature way if they know there is a time when this closely interdependent team can sit down and discuss how they can work together more effectively.

The dentist should also be prepared to make comments. Comments should not make one staff member uncomfortable and "at fault" for a problem. Comments might be, "The cooperation of the entire staff was excellent on Wednesday when we inserted Mr. Jones' immediate denture. Everyone was alert and did an excellent job"; or "The schedule was really fouled up Wednesday. What happened? Can we avoid it another time?"

This allows for an evaluation of the activities on Wednesday without making a particular person the brunt of the criticism even though it was caused by careless appointing on that person's part. That staff member will perceive the problem.

In addition to a time to air one's feelings and improve working relations, the staff conference is a time for the dentist to teach the staff whatever they need to know. It may be a talk of five to ten minutes on the dentist's philosophy of preventive dentistry. It may be that a new product has been introduced that the dentist believes the staff should understand. The information can be presented by the dentist or a detail person. Other subjects the dentist might wish to present to the staff include information from a dental consulting firm; psychology of working with patients; or information to prepare the staff to meet the emotional problems staff face when working with the public.

To use some staff conference time to further this kind of understanding is a wise investment for any dentist or oral health care delivery team.

Sources of Information

One of the marks of an educated person is to know where to find information. In any career it is impossible to know everything; thus it becomes important to know where to find missing information.

Books that will prove invaluable in finding required information will be found in your dentist's library. Two journals that ought to be delivered to your office are the *Journal of the American Dental Association* and *The Dental Assistant,* the journal of the American Dental Assistants Association. In addition, many of the pharmaceutical houses send out bulletins and pamphlets that are helpful. "Throw away" magazines about dentistry will be delivered free in the mail, and your dentist may subscribe to others.

A dictionary is one of the most valuable aids. The ability of an individual to define a term usually means the individual has insight into the full meaning of that term.

Specialized dictionaries and terminology books are valuable and ought to be found in your office library. Use them frequently. One that is most pertinent to dentistry is *Boucher's Clinical Dental Terminology,* edited by Zweemer. Blakiston's *New Gould Medical Dictionary* and Dorland's *Medical Dictionary* are also helpful.

If you are uncertain whether some piece of information is available, consult the local county dental society or their library.

Commercial Communication Services

Communication to distant places is now as common as calling your neighbor. Often, telegraph or long distance telephone services are used in the dental office. Should it be necessary for the assistant to work with any of these services, special instruction is available from the services, such as Western Union or telephone companies.

The telephone is probably the most common and most dangerous means of communication in the dental office. The promptness with which it is answered, the manner of the person who answers it, the comments made by the answerer all affect whether or not the caller feels pleasant about this contact and desires to remain a patient of this dentist.

The size of the telephone unit will depend on the size of the office. The greater number of telephone lines installed, the more complicated the equipment, but training in the use of the equipment is provided by the telephone company. It is conceivable that some dental offices will utilize automatic answering systems or telephone answering services. Either of these services provide an answer when the telephone rings, regardless of whether someone is in the office.

The Dentist's Personal Reminder Service

Most dentists have numerous details to remember in connection with their professional and personal lives. Their social and professional engagements must be kept. The little courtesies that mark them as considerate individuals should be accomplished. The dentists want to remember to perform these little acts and attend the meetings, but usually their minds are so busy with diagnosis and treatment plans that it is difficult for them to remember. A wise and well-organized assistant will keep notations of these necessary activities. They can be recorded on cards kept in the comeup file; they can be noted on the appointment book; or they can be kept in a separate calendar or booklet. The assistant should be efficient in reminding the dentist about these matters. A note can be placed on the dentist's desk suggesting that the dentist call a colleague to offer congratulations on some attainment or that plans should be made for the celebration next week of his or her spouse's birthday. The dentist will be grateful for these reminder notes.

Any meetings or social events should be written on the calendar, with the appropriate hours marked off. Reminder notes of these meetings should also be placed on the dentist's desk and perhaps a verbal reminder should be given during the day.

The assistant and the spouse of the dentist can confer regularly to see that the social events are recorded at the office and the professional meetings are recorded at home.

Understanding Patient Recall Philosophy

One philosophy of preventive dentistry is regularly scheduled examinations and prophylaxis of each patient. To achieve this goal patients are "recalled"; that is, the dentist determines how frequently the particular patient needs to be examined. (Four- and six-month recalls are common, and some patients who have exceptionally clean mouths may be placed on nine-month recall.)

On or before a patient's last appointment for work he or she needed as a new patient, the dentist or the assistant will explain the desirability of regular examination and prophylaxis visits. At this time the good intentions of patients are highest. They are determined never again to neglect their dental health. They look forward to recalls that do not include any serious amount of dental work. Therefore, now is the time to obtain a definite commitment, phrasing your question exactly: "Mr. Jones, if you wish we will be happy to place you on our recall list and send you an appointment in six months. Would you like us to do that for you?" The patient who will answer negatively at that particular time is very unusual.

If Mr. Jones gives his consent to the recall arrangements, check with him immediately to discover, if you do not already know, the day of the week and time of day that are usually most convenient for him to come to your office, and the address at which he

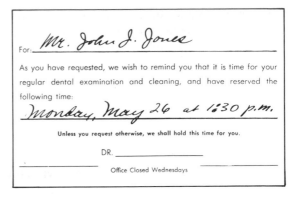

Figure 8.2
The recall card as sent to the patient.

wishes to receive the notice. A recall control card is prepared. The recall control card will be discussed later in this chapter.

When time for the recall appointment arrives, the patient receives a card worded as in figure 8.2, if he was asked about participating in a recall system.

Mr. Jones will remember, as he reads the recall notice, that he did ask for it voluntarily. The sense of pressure from the dental office is eliminated, while the tendency to keep the appointment, since it is by his request, is increased. The patient may call to change the time or date of the appointment, but very few will not be in your office for a recall. The average patient will require little or no dental work at this time. A comparison should be made between the amount of work necessary on his first contact with the office and the amount necessary now. The case of maintaining oral health by regular recall will please the patient, and the patient's acceptance of regular dental care will be established.

The dental office that employs a dental hygienist can maintain a separate recall control file under the care of the hygienist.

The profession of dentistry performs a service to the patient in restoring the mouth to good health and in teaching good oral habits and care. Most dentists should assume a moral responsibility for the regular care of their patients by making it possible for them to have recall appointments promptly and as frequently as necessary.

Succeeding as an Office Administrator

An office administrator maintains a perspective of the entire office operation, attempts to provide an equitable division of labor, and facilitates the team operation. How? The personnel functions diagram (figure 8.1), the procedure manual, and the staff conference are three tools to which can be added certain organizational procedures for the business office, which are discussed in the succeeding chapters of this section of the text. Careful organization and supervision of these details will permit the office administrator to concentrate her or his attention on people and problem situations.

Solving a Problem

The operation of a well-organized, pleasant office cannot be left to chance. It must have constant attention. An open-minded attitude, a willingness to challenge the present system, and an attempt to try out new ideas to develop better ways of doing the "dailies" are very important to successful administration.

Keep a list of your problems. Keep it current. Add to it. Keep it in your desk drawer, but take it out frequently and look at it. Then rank the problems in order of importance. Try to do first things first.

Discovering Which Problem

First, ask yourself which problem causes the greatest difficulty to you, to your dentist, or to the patients who come to your office. This is the problem to attack first.

Second, ask yourself, "How severe is this problem? Is it worthy of the time it will take to solve it?" To answer your question, you might try to count the number of times this irritating situation recurs in a day, a week, or a month. Walk through the routine if necessary. (Suppose it is the interference of two assistants when one is trying to remove materials from the file and the other must pass through that space to another part of the office.) List the number of times the problem occurs in a specified length of time.

Third, ask yourself how soon the problem must be solved. If it is a serious matter that requires immediate attention, it must receive priority in the thinking process that occurs in problem-solving.

Fourth, if some problems can be solved, which problem, if eliminated, will give the greatest benefits to the dentist, the patient, and the staff? This is the process we can call investigation of the problem; that is, selection, or recognition of which problem to attempt to solve. Now that you have decided on one problem to solve first, examine this problem.

Examining the Problem

Keep a record about this activity that is causing problems. A chart that lists the activity in question and has columns for listing the time, the distance involved, and any other notes needed will help clarify the situation. A diagram showing the floor area and the traffic pattern is also helpful. Make the diagram after watching the interference for a period of time.

Next, ask questions to try to discover an alternative method of accomplishing the task. Ask what,

why, where, when, who, and how. If a file is the object of interference because the assistant who is filing is in the way of those who must pass back and forth to assist the dentist, or if patients must pass by the file to get to the operatory, a listing of the number of interruptions of the assistant's work per hour—of the number of times she or he must push in the file drawer, straighten up, and lean against the file—should be made. The office should be reexamined critically and creatively. There may be another location for the file that would eliminate the crowding of the passageway. Lacking this, perhaps the filing could be done prior to the patients' arrivals and after their departures.

Through the creative process, the members of the office staff can take the problem as outlined on paper and find some better methods of meeting the situation. One of the most important things to remember in any administrative work is to keep asking questions about the present routines. Usually, there is room for improvement no matter how effective the past thinking has been.

Selling Your Dentist

Suppose you have now arrived at a solution to the problem. The next step is to sell your idea to your dentist, who must be agreeable to the change.

Some methods of approach work better than others. Timing is exceedingly important. When your dentist is tired, hungry, or frustrated is no time to ask for a change. If he or she is having difficulty with the problem you are concerned about, perhaps this is the moment to suggest a change. If the dentist must wait by the file until the file clerk has placed a handful of papers in the drawer in order to avoid spilling them on the floor before closing the drawer, this is a good time to suggest that perhaps a new place could be found for the file. Stress those ideas that will interest and appeal to the dentist. Be enthusiastic, but don't push. Use a question approach—ask the dentist, don't tell him or her. When the dentist accepts the idea, you can establish a timetable to get the approval of others for your idea if the matter is one that involves approval from the rest of the staff.

Improvement cannot be left to chance. Constant attention must be given to the office problems. There must be open-minded attitudes to challenge the status quo if new ideas are to be developed. Remember that the greatest strides have come from creative thinking about a problem. New ideas can be developed and used if people are open-minded and willing to experiment.

Staff conference is an ideal time to develop new ideas. It is far easier to discuss the problem and solutions at a staff meeting. Education of the staff to the need for change can occur at this conference. It is also possible for staff to create changes. Creative thinking engaged in by several people may be many times as effective as creative thinking by one person. Discussion of problems at a staff meeting is usually more effective and easier than discussion on an individual basis when the problems concern more than one member.

Orderly Office Routines

There are routines that, when regularly performed in a dental office, allow the office staff the pleasure of working without the frustration caused when certain duties are overlooked. The patients and the oral health care delivery team are directly, as well as indirectly, benefited when these details are performed as an orderly routine.

Work Schedules: Their Successful Operation

Working by appointment means that work is scheduled. Maintaining the schedule can be facilitated by a routine concerning the schedule.

The day's work schedule is a list of patients who are coming to the office, the time of their appointments, and the service for which you must be prepared for each patient. It is a reminder of all that must be accomplished during the day. Thus, the day's work schedule is posted where every member of the oral health team can see it frequently and be prepared to stay on schedule.

After all appointments are verified and any canceled appointment time is filled, it is time to prepare the day's schedule for the next working day. An easy way to prepare the schedule is to type the time of the appointment, patient's name, and work planned on a 4-by-6 inch paper with carbons for the required number of copies. Commercially prepared forms are available if your dentist wishes to use them instead (figure 8.3).

After necessary copies are typed, place a copy in each operatory where it is not visible to patients. Place a copy in the dentist's private office and one in the laboratory. If there are any other areas where staff may work or relax, it is desirable to post a copy there also.

If the office is a clinic, each dentist will have his or her own patients listed on a daily work schedule. Any hygiene appointments that interlace with the dentist's schedule are written as illustrated in figure 8.3. However, dentist number one has no need to be aware of the patients of dentist number two, so individual work schedules should be made for each dentist.

Here is a day's work schedule based on the appointment book example in figure 9.3 in chapter 9, Time

Control: The Appointment Book. Our four-inch by six-inch paper would include the following information:

SCHEDULE, Thursday, March 18

8:00	Drake, Mr. W. S., operative
9:00	Hoover, Randy, operative
9:30	Emergency break
9:45	Coffee break
9:55	Carlson, S. J., salesperson
11:00	Fischer, Mrs. S., operative
12:00	Lunch
1:00	Wagoner, Mr. J. R., impressions
2:00	Jones, Mrs. T., operative
4:15	Berg, Mrs. Andy, case presentation
4:30	Smith, Ms. Mary, impressions
5:30	(District Dental Meeting at 6 P.M.)

Advance Record Preparation

With the daily work schedules prepared, it is time to collect the folders for those patients who are to be seen the next day. Blank record cards and folders clipped to the Acquaintance Forms for new patients are also prepared. These Acquaintance Forms were either filled out by the patients when they came to the office to arrange their first appointments or were begun by the assistant who received their calls on the telephone.

Usually these collected folders are placed together in a locked file overnight. In the morning the folders are placed in the proper operatories. The office administrator assigns some staff member the responsibility of placing these records in the proper operatories.

Laboratory Schedule

The work performed in the laboratory can be roughly divided into two general classifications: (1) cases that are carried to completion entirely within the dental office, and (2) those that are forwarded to a professional dental laboratory for all or part of the processing. Depending upon the individual dental office, varying degrees of preparation will be involved in cases that are forwarded to the professional dental laboratory. Some dental offices may perform very few of the laboratory procedures for any cases; others may perform all procedures for their requirements.

A laboratory schedule for all cases, whether accomplished in the dental office laboratory or the professional dental laboratory, should be maintained properly and should be posted in the laboratory. This schedule should include the name of the patient, the type of case to be completed for that patient, and the date the case

DAYS PLAN		DATE _Thursday, March 18_
	Dr.'s Patient	Procedure	Hygienist's Patient
8	Drake, Mr. W.S.	operative	Murphy, Mr. John
9	Hoover, Randy	operative	Murphy, Mrs. John
	Emergencies		
	coffee break (9:55 Carlson – salesman)		
10	Fischer, Mrs. S.	operative	coffee break / Danover, John
11			McIntosh, Mr. R.
1	Wagoner, Mr. J.R.	imps	Tarchow, Randy
			Tarchow, Rudy
2	Jones, Mrs. T.	operative	Tarchow, Mrs. Peter
3		(coffee break with / Mrs. Jones)	coffee break / Olson, Mary
4			Peterson, Mr. Rolf
	Berg, Mr. Andy	case pres.	
	Smith, Ms. Mary	imps	
5			
	District Dental Mtg. at 6 P.M.		

DAYS PLAN – STYLE "A"
SPILLANE'S, INC. – MINNEAPOLIS, MINN.

Figure 8.3
A commercially available form for posting the day's work schedule.

must be finished. If more than one professional laboratory is used, the name of the one that has each particular case should be indicated. As cases are completed, they are removed from the laboratory schedule. As new cases are started, they are added to the schedule (figure 8.4).

Verification of Information

Form the habit of casually verifying the home address, work address, and telephone numbers when the patient comes in for regular recalls. If there have been changes, the corrections on the record card and envelope should be made immediately. A recommended procedure is to keep a record of the old address on note paper placed

DATE ENTERED	NAME OF PATIENT	PROSTHESIS	NAME OF LAB	DATE SENT	DATE REQ.	CASE COMPLETED	INITIALS OF PERSON WHO SENT
5/5	Zambolini, George	upper partial	Erickson's	5/5	5/12	5/12	LS
5/6	Terreno, Sylvia	upper anterior bridge	Kraus'	5/6	5/13		SP
5/6	Smith, Don	#3 crown	ours	5/6	5/10	5/10	LS
5/10	Maxwell, John	anterior crown	Kraus'	5/10	5/17		SP
5/12	Franklin, Mary	lower denture	Erickson's	5/12	5/19		LS

Figure 8.4
A laboratory case schedule.

in the record envelope. When this procedure is followed, it is wise to date each note completely so that the chronology of addresses is not lost. Any note or information made on a separate piece of paper should be dated with the month, day, and year. Once the habit is acquired, you will find it most convenient to have dated notes.

It is very reassuring to be able to look at your own writing and know that Mrs. Brown moved on January 10, 1985, to 124 South Elm Street or that it was on Tuesday, February 9, 1990, that the laboratory called to ask about a particular bridge and told you it would be delivered on Friday, the 12th. You won't have to guess about the day of the call or the date of delivery.

Thank-you Notes

A thank-you note sent to all individuals who have referred patients to your dentist is a gracious gesture. Preferably, these notes should be written by hand if the job is delegated to you; however, many dentists prefer to write these notes themselves. The assistant should not sign the dentist's name to such a note whether a printed form or a hand-written note is used.

Current Invoices

It is a convenience to have a file folder labeled "Current Invoices" in your subject file. All invoices received may be kept in this folder until the monthly statements arrive. This procedure will prevent the misplacement or loss of any invoices before the arrival of the monthly statements.

Come-up Card Files

A come-up card file, or reminder file, is an easy method of controlling duties that would otherwise be overlooked or would require more cumbersome reminder methods. This method of control can be applied to equipment maintenance, general office tasks, recall control, and birthday card lists. It can serve as a reminder method for any detail that is to receive future attention. For its successful operation there is but one requirement: the file must be checked each day. Variations in the manner of setting up the reminder cards are numerous, but the cards used for any one type of reminder—for example, the recall control—should be of the same color and same layout form.

The come-up card file is best used in a file drawer at the desk or in a drawer converted to operate as a file drawer in the desk. For general use in the dental office, four-by-six-inch cards are perhaps the best size to use for all purposes, although three-by-five-inch cards are satisfactory. The size must be the same for the entire file. A different color is used for each classification of detail: one color indicates equipment maintenance and general office tasks; another color indicates recall control cards; a third, birthday card reminders; and other colors are used for other classifications.

Patient Recall Control File

The patient who volunteers to be placed on recall requires a patient recall control card. A four-by-six-inch card is prepared similar to figure 8.5. The patient's name and birth date are typed or written in ink; other information is written in pencil to facilitate change.

Jones, Mr. John J.	645 Elm Street	926-1414
Name	Home address	Home phone
May 23, 1955	204 Main St.	333-0000
Birthdate	Office address	Business phone

Recall due: 6 months

Preferred time: Mondays, early afternoon

Due for recall: May 1991 ✓ 27

    Nov 1991

Figure 8.5
A recall control card.

When patients consent to recall, they are asked to state the most convenient time to come and the address at which they wish to receive the notice. The assistant records these two pieces of information on the patients' records.

On the recall control card, note in pencil the length of time between recalls. (Your dentist has indicated this period on the patient's service record.) Also note the patient's preferred time for recall, and write in the first month that patient will be due for recall (in figure 8.5 it is May, 1990). Place a check mark by the address to which you are to send the recall notice.

When all information is complete on the card, file it in the come-up file behind the appropriate monthly index tab. Recall control cards should be filed in the come-up card file behind the monthly card index one month before the month noted for the recall. This is done to allow for the lapse of time necessary to place an appointment in the appointment book and for mailing the recall notice to the patient two weeks before the appointment date. Therefore, in the sample shown, the recall control card would be filed behind the *April* index tab.

When April 1 arrives, all cards behind the *April* index tab are removed. Our sample recall control card will be in this group. This patient is then dated in the appointment book for his or her recall during the month of May, accommodating his or her preference for day of the week and time of the day as nearly as possible. Since you will be arranging all the May recalls at this time, it is possible to balance the work load by spreading the appointments throughout the month.

At this time, write (in pencil) the date of the appointment after the month and year, which has already been recorded on the card. The recall notice, which is to be sent to the patient two weeks before the appointment, is prepared at the same time and checked twice against the appointment book entry for accuracy. The recall notice may be a postcard or a card to be placed in an envelope. Either one is addressed as indicated on the recall control card, and the date of mailing is written in pencil in the upper right hand corner of the envelope, where it will be covered by the stamp when the card is mailed two weeks before the actual appointment date.

The recall control card for this patient is then filed behind the *May* index tab, and when May 1 arrives, the card is placed behind the correct date tab. When the patient records are pulled for the day on which this recall comes, the recall control card is clipped to the patient's record and, after the examination and prophylaxis are completed, the dentist will indicate the month and year when the patient should again be recalled. The month and year are written in pencil below the former entry. Since our sample patient was recalled in May, 1990, and is to be in at six-month intervals, the next penciled date is November, 1990. The recall card is then filed behind the *October* index tab in the come-up file.

Should the patient fail to keep his or her appointment, the recall control card in the come-up file is a reminder to reschedule the patient so that he or she is not neglected. If the recall control card was filed with his or her patient service record, this opportunity to contact the patient would be lost.

Office Task Control

This classification of cards to be used in the come-up file should be a different color from those used for the patient recall control cards. The average dental office will require but one color for one copy of this classification. In the large office or clinic practice that has an employee in charge of general office duties, it is more convenient to have each card of this classification in duplicate, preferably in two colors (neither color the same as used in any other classification, however). These cards list the regular recurring duties of maintenance of equipment and periodic work such as changing X-ray solutions, cleaning sterilizers, cleaning and waxing equipment, and cleaning surgical cabinets and instruments, laboratory cabinets, and storage shelves. The cards used in the multiple office should be numbered to facilitate handling and matching the original with the duplicate card. The supervisor can give the original card to the assistant delegated to take care of the particular task and can leave the duplicate out of the file and on her or his desk as a reminder that this task has been assigned for accomplishment. When the task has been completed, the assistant gives the original card to the supervisor, who returns original and duplicate cards to the come-up file under the proper index card for the next date on which the task will be performed (figure 8.6).

```
┌─────────────────────────────────────────────────┐
│  QUARTERLY    First Friday of March,   DENTAL UNIT │
│               June, September and                  │
│               December.                            │
│                                                    │
│                                                    │
│                                                    │
│                                                    │
│  Remove and clean water supply screen.             │
│                                                    │
│                                                    │
└─────────────────────────────────────────────────┘
```

Figure 8.6

An office task control card.

The office task control cards may be typed or printed in the following form: at the extreme top left, place the frequency of the task, such as daily, weekly, semimonthly, monthly, six weeks, bimonthly, quarterly, semiannually, or annually; at the extreme top right, place the name of the item to be serviced, such as dental unit, X-ray tank, or laboratory; and at the top center, place the day for which the job is scheduled. Working out the proper arrangement to balance the workload throughout the year is a very important feature—and not too difficult to accomplish.

In any dental office there are so many duties to be performed that it is imperative to arrange recurring office tasks so they may be accomplished as required without overloading any one period of time. Incompetent work schedules cause some dental offices to neglect the majority of these tasks. Performance of these tasks increases the efficiency of operation and creates more pleasant working relationships.

All daily tasks should be typed on four- by six-inch cards and kept behind the *Daily* tab in the come-up file. This procedure relieves the assistant of memorizing daily routine jobs.

When all cards for the "office task" classification are made out, sort them according to the upper-left hand notation, the frequency of the operation.

Daily Tasks: Cards for these duties are filed under the *Daily* guide card for daily checking. An alternate method of handling daily tasks, which may be preferred in the smaller dental office, is discussed later in this chapter.

Weekly and Biweekly Tasks: These cards are filed according to the date the work is to be performed. Assume that a job is scheduled for Tuesday of each week. The calendar is referred to for the date of the next Tuesday. This card is then filed behind the guide card of that particular date, in the 1 to 31 section of the come-up file. When the work has been completed, the card is filed under the date of the next Tuesday. If the first Tuesday was the 7th, the job is completed on that date and the card is refiled under 14, the date of the next Tuesday.

Monthly, Bimonthly, Quarterly, Semiannual, and Annual Tasks: These cards are filed behind the monthly guide cards on the particular month in which the work is to be done. On the twenty-seventh day of each month, the cards filed under the following month are removed from the monthly section and refiled behind the 1 to 31 guide cards; they are filed under the particular date (shown by the calendar) for the day given in the upper center of the card. When the job specified on the card has been completed, the card is filed behind the next appropriate monthly guide card. Thus, the sample card shown in figure 8.6 would be filed under March. On February 27, it is removed, along with the other March cards, and this particular card is placed in the 1 to 31 file behind the date of the first Friday in March. If that should be March 3, you file it behind 3. On March 3, the card will be removed and the job accomplished. The card will then be filed in the monthly file behind June, the next month this task is to be performed.

Alternate Methods for Daily Tasks: Tasks to be performed on a daily basis may be listed on a stiff-backed paper and either posted in the laboratory or kept in the desk for ready reference. If the list is posted in the laboratory, it may be protected with a transparent plastic cover.

The following are lists of daily tasks described in this textbook. The dental assistant may use these lists as guides to make up a copy that will apply to the office in which she or he is employed. Add items necessary in your office and delete those not applicable.

Daily Tasks Upon Opening the Office

1. Thoroughly air the office.
2. Turn on all necessary switches to place equipment in readiness.
3. Run sterilizer if necessary.
4. Have instruments replaced correctly or have trays ready for use.
5. Dust office thoroughly.
6. Check reception room and its magazines.
7. Check entire office for proper lighting.
8. Patient's records should be placed in the proper operating rooms.
9. Day's work schedule should be in operating rooms, private office, and laboratory.
10. See that dental chairs are clean.
11. Wipe with a damp cheesecloth pad all enameled surfaces of equipment. Do not forget X-ray arm.

12. Check medicine bottles in cabinets for a workable daily supply in each bottle.
13. Check the come-up file for today. Lay out office task cards.
14. Clean all surfaces, equipment, and work areas of both the dentist and chairside assistant.

Daily Tasks to Be Performed During the Day

1. Polish outside of sterilizers with soft cloth or chamois. Wash with soap and water or use a nonabrasive cleanser, when necessary.
2. Check operation of sterilizers, including liquid levels.
3. Weigh and load silver-filing capsules whenever necessary, if used.
4. Take care of the jobs for the day as indicated by the come-up file. This includes recall notices, birthday cards to be sent, and office tasks to be accomplished.
5. Call patients scheduled for the next workday to remind them of their appointments. Space outgoing calls so that the office telephone line is not monopolized.
6. Keep the required bookkeeping entries as current as possible.

Daily Tasks Upon Completion of Appointments for the Day

1. Call any patients not already reached to verify the next workday's appointments.
2. After all appointments for the next workday have been verified, type the required number of copies of the next day's work schedule.
3. If necessary, sterilize any instruments needed for the first patient in the morning. Set up required trays of instruments.
4. Flush a glass of slightly soapy water through the evacuation hoses.
5. Relieve tightness of belt on dental engine arm if one is still used.
6. Clean up after last patient.
7. Run motor-driven chairs all the way up.
8. Turn off all switches.
9. Close windows.
10. Leave radiators turned on during cold weather.
11. Put all records out of sight, filing in the proper section of the files those not needed for the next workday—after all bookkeeping is completed for which they may be required.

12. Refile the come-up cards under their proper dates.
13. Double-check to see that all sterilizers, units, lights, and water valves are off, and that no X rays are left in the washing tank.
14. Be certain that all files are locked.
15. Take all outgoing mail.
16. Be certain that the office door is locked when you have closed it.

Birthday Card Control

In any office that cares for children, the benefits derived from sending birthday cards to children through the age of ten are often surprising. Children have such little personal mail that the birthday card from someone outside the immediate family carries a tremendous psychological impact. Children have been known to take their dentist's birthday card on a tour of their neighborhood. Young families have been most grateful for the personal touch of a card for a youngster who happened to be ill on his or her birthday. When cards are purchased by the box, sending them is not an expensive item for the promotion of goodwill. The type of birthday card that displays the age is preferred because it adds another personal recognition of this individual child, who can identify himself or herself with the card even more completely.

The birthday card control file should have a different color from any other used in the come-up file. Whenever a new child under the age of nine years is registered with the office—that is, through the age of eight so that he or she will receive at least two cards from the office—a birthday control card is made up for him or her. The letter *B* is placed in the lower-left-hand corner of the child's personal record envelope to indicate that a birthday control card has been made out. The form followed for this classification is shown in figure 8.7.

When the birthday card is prepared for mailing, the year and age are written on the control card as an indication that the card has been prepared for mailing.

As with the recall control cards, it is preferable to file these control cards under the month previous to the birthday to insure mailing the cards in time to arrive before or on the birthday—never late. The birthday control card can be ignored each month until about the 20th if the dental assistant will keep a reminder card under the date *20* in the 1 to 31 guides. This card should state that the birthday cards for the next month should be prepared at that time for mailing. The dentist can then sign the entire month's birthday cards in one group. The assistant places them in their envelopes and marks

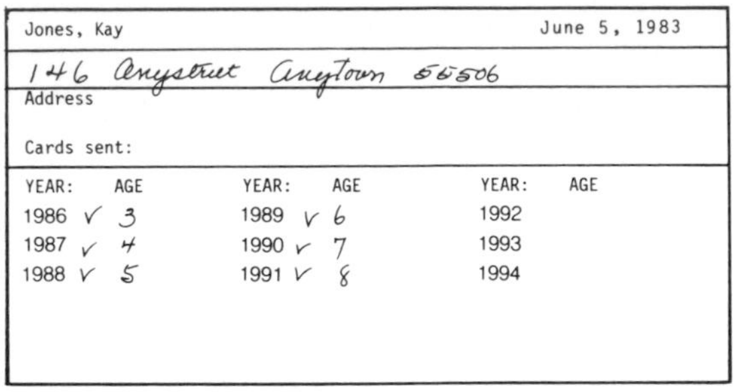

```
Jones, Kay                         June 5, 1983

146 Anystreet Anytown 55506
Address

Cards sent:

YEAR:    AGE        YEAR:    AGE        YEAR:    AGE
1986  √  3         1989  √  6         1992
1987  √  4         1990  √  7         1993
1988  √  5         1991  √  8         1994
```

Figure 8.7
A birthday control card.

the mailing date for each card in pencil in the upper-right-hand corner of the envelope, where the postage stamp will cover it.

Recall notices and birthday cards prepared in advance for mailing may either be placed behind the proper date in the 1 to 31 guides or, if too bulky, may be arranged in mailing sequence and kept in a separate desk drawer. In this event the assistant must be certain that the cards are mailed on the proper dates.

Summary

The coordination of the efforts of the oral health care delivery team is extremely important and can be accomplished best by the appointment of an office administrator.

The first goal of the well-coordinated office is to keep the dentist occupied in using the unique professional skills that only the dentist can perform. The second goal is to delegate duties so that the other members of the oral health care delivery team provide services for which they have been uniquely trained. All team members ought to be enabled to accomplish their responsibilities in dental care, and to relate to each other in the total office production schedule.

The delegation of tasks should result in three advantages:

1. More efficient dental service to patients.
2. Less mental, emotional, and physical strain for members of the oral health care delivery team.
3. Lower operating costs.

The office administrator is charged with the responsibility of administering a plan that will accomplish these goals. An office procedure manual that acquaints new staff members with office routines is one useful tool. The manual should list each duty of every staff member and certain statements about working conditions, fringe benefits, and salary.

A regularly scheduled staff conference allows the office team to become an efficient, harmonious unit and permits instruction of the staff about new materials or team operations.

Every dental assistant should be aware of sources of information such as clinical dental terminologies, periodicals, reference manuals, medical dictionaries, and texts.

A dental office administrator can succeed by being constantly alert for problems. Such problems can be listed and considered for solution. There are four questions that the administrator can ask in determining which problem to attempt to solve. Timing is important in presenting the suggested solution to the dentist.

Maintenance of certain written schedules and come-up files assists in the performance of office routines.

Study Questions

1. Describe a procedure manual and tell why it is valuable.
2. Explain the office administrator's role on the oral health care delivery team.
3. Describe a good staff conference.
4. What are sources of information and why are they valuable?
5. Describe a come-up file system.
6. What are a number of orderly office routines that assist in administering a dental office?
7. What information is included on a day's work schedule?
8. What are the two general classifications of work performed in the laboratory?
9. What information is included on the laboratory schedule?

Word Elements

Word Element	Example
cata prefix meaning: down, lower, under	*catalyst* provides a pathway that requires less energy for a chemical reaction to occur
de prefix meaning: down or from	*decalcification* removal of calcium from the tooth surface by acid
infra prefix meaning: below or beneath the stem word	*infraorbital* below the eye
ex, exo prefix meaning: beyond, out of, without, from	*exodontics* the art and science of the removal of teeth
para prefix meaning: beyond, beside	*paradental* beside the teeth
ultra prefix meaning: beyond, excess	*ultraviolet* beyond the violet end of the spectrum
opistho combining form meaning: backward	*opisthognathism* receding jaws
post prefix meaning: behind, after	*posterior* situated in the back part of a body or structure
re prefix meaning: back, again	*rehabilitation* restoring a person to useful activity
retro prefix meaning: backward, back of	*retromolar* behind the molars

CHAPTER 9

Time Control: The Appointment Book

The Importance of Time Management
Preparation of the Appointment Book
Managing the Appointment Book
Judging Time Allotment
Planning Appointments
Scheduling Appointments
   The New Patient
   The Recall Patient
   Patients Not on Recall
   The Emergency Patient
   Courtesy Service (for a Patient of
      Another Dentist)
   Salespersons
   School Children
The Appointment Book Entries
A Practical Example
Patient Awareness of the Importance of
      Appointment Time
The Appointment Card
Reducing Appointment Failures

The Importance of Time Management

Time is a critical factor in dentistry. Appointments with patients must be skillfully controlled. Should the appointments be scheduled too closely, the schedule will be impossible to maintain, resulting in pressure on the staff. The staff can become irritated. Perhaps the dentistry performed will not be as well done. The patients may become angry because they are forced to wait. However, if too much time is left between appointments, the staff will be idle, and office income may not meet expenses. Efficiency of operation is of prime importance. Expenses in the dental office go on whether or not the staff is working. Thus, if the appointments are so spaced that the team is idle five, ten, or fifteen minutes between patients, the necessary income to meet the payroll may be lacking. The assistant responsible for controlling the appointments must know how much time is required for each operation performed.

The **appointment book** may be bound, spiral bound, or loose-leaf. Each working day is divided into time intervals—usually a line appears for each fifteen minute interval. Some books list each entire week on the opened double page, enabling one to see the entire week at a glance. Appointment books may be purchased from the American Dental Association, practice management companies, and dental supply houses. Dated books for the next year can be obtained in the autumn. This supply should be ordered as early as possible. Some supply houses carry undated loose-leaf appointment sheets. The assistant writes in the dates as she or he prepares the pages. This type of sheet can be ordered any time it is necessary. Appointment books will have space for one dentist, a dentist and hygienist, or will have several columns for use in an office with multiple dentists and hygienists.

Often, when more than one dentist is practicing in the same office, each dentist has his or her own appointment book. Sometimes one book is used for several hygienists—particularly if they work for all the dentists in the practice. Thus, the assistant who manages the appointment book may be controlling one book, one book with two persons' appointments (dentist and hygienist), two, or several books.

Preparation of the Appointment Book

When the appointment book has been purchased, go through the book and draw a red *x* through the times your dentist is not available. In addition, write in the necessary information or draw the required lines as stated in these points:

1. Mark off the days your office is regularly closed. For example, your dentist is not in the office Wednesday afternoons and Saturdays. Draw a red *x* through each Wednesday afternoon and each Saturday.

2. Mark off all holidays observed by your office. Your office is closed on New Year's Day, Memorial Day, Independence Day (July 4th), Labor Day, Thanksgiving, and Christmas—legal holidays. Each of these is marked with a red *x*. Your dentist also closes the office for Christmas Eve Day. Mark this day.

3. Check with the school superintendent's office in your area or the local dental society office to discover when school holidays occur. Write "School Holiday" just above the appropriate days in the appointment book. These days should be used to accommodate as many school children as possible—particularly those in junior and senior high school.

4. Check your dentist's scheduled meetings. The regular monthly district dental meetings, the state convention, and other specialized society meetings are advertised well in advance. The days of those meetings should be marked to indicate the hours your dentist will be away from the office. (Some of these meetings are evening meetings, which may mean stopping early. Others may be day-long meetings, which mean the office will be closed all day. The book should reflect the time the dentist will be away.) Regularly scheduled meetings that occur once a month or once a week should be indicated. For example, your dentist attends the Business Executive's Luncheon Club Meeting on the second Tuesday of the month from noon to 2 P.M. The appointment book should be marked with red so that work will be finished by 11:30 and will resume at 2:30 (or whatever other time allotment your dentist needs to reach the meeting on time and return). Mark a red line at 11:30 and another at 2:30 and note the meeting name, time, and place between these lines.

Your dentist attends the District Dental Meeting, which occurs on the third Thursday of each month at 6 P.M. Draw a red line at 5:30 P.M., which is the time your dentist must be completely finished. Below that line write "No more. District Dental Meeting 6 P.M." Be certain that the last patient scheduled will be *finished* by 5:30.

5. If the appointment book is loose-leaf, at the end of the month remove the used appointment sheets and add the same number of new ones.

Some dentists who use a loose-leaf appointment book keep appointment sheets for three or six months in the current book. When the end of the month arrives, the used sheets are removed and new ones added. For example, on January 31 the January sheets are removed and the April or the July sheets added, thus keeping three or six months of appointment book sheets in the book at all times.

Managing the Appointment Book

Managing the appointment book requires a plan. Two plans are commonly used. The less commonly used method is that of restriction of appointments to a specified period of time. The dentist states that he or she wants appointments restricted to a specific period, such as one month or three months. All patients who cannot be appointed within the time limit are placed on a call list and called as appointments become available.

The more commonly used method allows for appointing patients as far in the future as necessary to accommodate them. If this method is used, the dentist must plan his vacations and attendance at meetings well in advance. Without such farsighted planning it may be impossible to attend the meeting or to take the vacation. Blocks of unappointed time need to be left because unexpected emergencies occur. For example, the dentist may become ill. These time blocks can be used to reschedule patients whose appointments are affected by the emergency.

Another method of appointing patients who need a series of appointments over several weeks is to schedule the patients in the appointment book, but only inform the patient of his or her next appointment. At each subsequent visit, the patient is informed about the next appointment. In this way, the appointments can be changed if necessary without calling all the patients to rearrange their appointment time.

The responsibility for management of the appointment book is best left entirely to one individual in the office. The greater the number of individuals allowed to make appointments, the greater will be the inefficiency in management of the appointment book.

Judging Time Allotment

The dentist and the assistant who make appointments must know the amount of time necessary for each operation performed in the dental office. A specific amount of time is designated as a *unit*. It may be ten minutes, fifteen minutes, or twenty minutes. The unit figure is utilized in planning dental work for each patient.

The dentist decides how many units it will take to complete the necessary dentistry for the specific patient. The dentist is aware that certain patients may require more time than others for the same preparation. Therefore, the dentist usually writes the number of necessary units on the record for the assistant to use in planning appointments. Should a bridge be involved that requires laboratory time between the necessary appointments for preparation and completion, that amount of time lapse is stated. Perhaps in some situations, the assistant becomes familiar enough with the dentist's time utilization to know without being told how many units are necessary; but, at least in the beginning, the dentist will specify the necessary units.

A list of the usual unit requirements for most dental operations kept with the appointment book is helpful for the new dental assistant. With such a guide, the dentist only notes the times for the unusual preparations and for the patient who requires additional time for the usual operation.

Another advantage of the unit system is that the number of units can be mentioned in the presence of patients. The association between time to perform dentistry and cost of services does not exist if one speaks of two units rather than half an hour. The hourly rate for dentistry performed includes not only expenditures for salaries, materials, and space, but for time spent in preparation when the patient is not in the chair. Patients usually are unaware of these additional costs and are likely to think, "Half an hour, I only earn _____ per hour. Why does dentistry cost five times that?" Thus, it is important to avoid the association of time spent in the chair with the charge for services rendered. This can be accomplished if the dental health team members speak of units, not minutes.

Planning Appointments

Dentists who carefully plan the work of each patient assist themselves and the patients. Research studies indicate that less time is wasted when longer appointments are utilized. Planning the scheduled work for a patient into the largest blocks of time possible for that particular patient is desirable.

Patients who come for a larger block of time require fewer trips to the dental office—a fact that most people appreciate. The dentist's time is used more efficiently because chair-time is lost whenever a patient-change occurs in the operatory (three to ten minutes are lost for each chair-change).

If the dentist has only one operatory, it is possible to have as much as ten minutes of unproductive time between two patients' appointments—time that is necessary to excuse one patient and seat another. Changing patients every half hour can mean as much as two hours and thirty minutes lost chair-time. (Six half-hour appointments mean fifteen patient-changes.)

If there are multiple operatories (two or three for each dentist), the time loss can be negligible, providing the assistant seats the second patient before the dentist finishes the first one.

Sometimes a patient comes a little early. Seat him or her at once! If the dentist finishes with the current patient early, the dentist can begin immediately with the next patient without loss of time.

Accuracy in judging the necessary length of time for each operation is important. Be certain the appointment selected is long enough to actually complete the planned work. Should there be a forty-five minute break in one day but an hour is required for the patient, find another appointment during which the dentist can actually complete the patient's dentistry.

Scheduling Appointments

If you are going to do the finest kind of time organization for your dentist, appointments should be scheduled when you are alone and have a number of appointments to make and are not pressed for time. It is only under such circumstances that you can really see how to organize the time to the best advantage. It takes careful planning to arrange appointments so that there are no unused units of time in your book.

Some appointments must be made when a patient is present, but you can keep them to a minimum if you will follow these suggestions about making appointments.

If your office is open on Saturdays, either all or part of the day, there will be considerable pressure to make appointments available on this day. A good policy is to apportion Saturday appointments equally among the different groups in your practice—employed persons, school children, and so on.

In some offices hygienists schedule their own appointments. However, the assistant in charge of appointing the dentist's patients may also arrange the hygienist's appointments. The hygienist's patients must be examined by the dentist after the prophylaxis. Time for these interruptions must be allowed. Some dentists allow for the interruptions in indicating the number of units for operative dentistry. There must, somehow, be an allowance in the dentist's schedule to accommodate the interruptions experienced while completing the hygienist's patients' examinations, whether the assistant

or the hygienist makes the appointments. Normally, the interruption is approximately five minutes. This time can be allowed in the unit scheduling.

The New Patient

The new patient is first given an appointment for an examination. In this example, the appointment is for one hour, or four units. Indicate by a red pencil that this is a new-patient appointment. ("NP" or "new" written in red by the patient's name in the appointment book is easily seen.) At the close of this appointment, the patient is given an appointment for a conference (case presentation), at which time the dentist will explain the necessary work, sometimes suggesting two or more ways to accomplish the required dentistry. The patient then selects the desired service.

The length of the conference will be determined by the dentist. A fifteen-minute period spent in the dentist's private office is usual. At the close of the dentist-patient conference, the dentist is able to inform the assistant of the number of units required for the patient's work. With the unit figure in the dental assistant's possession, it is possible for the assistant to make the necessary number of appointments to complete the patient's work. If at all possible, schedule all the work during one appointment.

If it is necessary for this patient to have a series of appointments, give the patient just one while he or she is waiting for you. Be sure that you know the most convenient day and time of day for the patient. Plan the rest of the appointments when you are alone and not under pressure.

Not all offices use a patient conference. Necessary dentistry is scheduled as soon as the X rays are read. The assistant is informed of the number of units of time needed for the patient. The assistant then appoints the patient while the patient is present or informs the patient by telephone later.

The Recall Patient

A recall patient is a regular patient who has indicated a desire to be recalled on a regular schedule that is determined by the dentist. The purpose of the recall appointment is to give a prophylaxis and to examine the teeth and mouth for any conditions requiring treatment. Some patients are on four-month recall, although the most common recall period is six months. Recall appointments are usually scheduled from the information on a recall come-up file card (see "Come-Up Card Files" in chapter 8).

On the first of the month all the recall control cards are removed from the come-up file, appointments are scheduled, and the recall appointment cards are mailed to the patients two weeks prior to the appointment. The recall control card is placed in the patient's service record envelope until the recall appointment has been completed.

The dentist studies the findings of the oral examination and X rays and indicates the necessary amount of time to complete the patient's work. The assistant telephones the patient to give the necessary information about additional appointments.

Some offices call patients whether or not additional work is needed. It affords a person a wonderful sense of satisfaction to be told, "I thought you would like to know that there is no further dental work necessary at this time. You will hear from us in six months." Patients so treated usually respond with a "Thank you for calling!"

Your relationship with patients determines whether this type of call should be made. Time-pressed patients can be told, "Unless you hear from me next week, we won't be seeing you for six months."

Patients Not on Recall

Some offices do not run a recall system. They allow their patients to take care of making their own appointments for checkups instead of placing all patients on recall. When these patients call in, appoint them for an examination as you would a recall patient.

The Emergency Patient

When a patient calls and is in pain, that patient is to be seen as soon as possible. If your office has an emergency period reserved each day, the patient is asked to come at that time only. If your office operates without such a break, look over the schedule and select the most likely looking break in time. If it is a true emergency, the patient will come at that time. If it is not, there is no need to crowd your schedule.

When you offer this emergency patient an appointment, you specifically say, "Doctor will see you at _____ to take care of the pain (or to care for the emergency)." No patient should be permitted to crowd into the day for work other than a real emergency. If further work is required following the relief from pain (and there usually is), the patient should be appointed for an examination, and the procedure for regular patient care should be followed.

Courtesy Service (for a Patient of Another Dentist)

Occasionally, a dentist asks your office to care for his or her patients during his or her absence. These appointments are almost always emergencies. When the patient calls, you explain that your dentist works by appointments, that the patient can see the dentist at _____ (time) to care for the emergency. Give the patient an appointment as you would for an emergency among your own patients. After the appointment that gives relief from pain or irritation, no further appointment is given. It is your dentist's responsibility, ethically, to see that patients return to their regular dentist as soon as the dentist returns. Usually, this emergency service is given without charging a fee.

Salespersons

Appoint salespersons according to the instructions given in chapter 7, "Reception Procedures," or see them on available emergency time.

School Children

Many school systems have some arrangement for the release of children to keep dental appointments when necessary. When the arrangement has been worked out, it is usually between the local dental society and the school superintendent. The requirements of these arrangements should be scrupulously kept by your dental office.

The time of day selected for children's dental appointment is extremely important. Preschool children should generally be given only early morning appointments, the time during which they are most able to adapt themselves to cooperation in the dental office. The average child under ten is preferably seen before noon. The early school years demand much energy from children in relation to stamina. Appointments after school for children will usually be difficult from the standpoint of cooperation because children have expended so much energy during the course of the school day that they have little ability left to cope with the tensions to be experienced in the dental office. After these children are thoroughly adjusted to the dental procedures, recall appointments can be made during after-school hours. However, performance of operative procedures is usually more successful in the morning.

Discuss dental appointments for children with your dentist and learn his or her wishes. Try to use this information, then, as a set routine in arranging such appointments.

The Appointment Book Entries

Let us assume that you have arrived at the time when you can sit down with the appointment book and make appointments for several patients. It is March 1 and you have just pulled from the recall control file the recalls to be appointed between March 15 and 31. You also have the records on several patients who have had conferences or case studies with your dentist. What must you remember as you schedule these appointments?

1. Schedule appointments for as long a sitting as possible. There is an exception to this rule, however. Some patients are exceedingly sensitive and dread dentistry so much that they are emotionally unable to endure long sittings. It is then necessary to schedule their work in shorter units of time until you have overcome their fears. Your dentist will recognize any such serious emotional disturbance and will note the information on the patient's record. (Premedication is frequently used for such tension.)

2. Be sure that you know the length of time needed for the dentistry to be completed and give your dentist that much time, but no more!

3. Include, insofar as possible, a variety of types of dentistry in the day. Work is more interesting then.

    As a general rule in arranging appointments, each day should follow, as closely as possible, a regular sequence: work that requires most concentration and effort should be scheduled for morning hours, with a gradual trend toward work requiring less tension and concentration. Thus, appointments for operative work, bridgework, denture impressions, and preschool children should be scheduled for the morning hours. The first two types of work mentioned are usually given long appointments.

    The early afternoon hours can best be devoted to the shorter operative appointments: new patient appointments (except for children); denture work necessary between impression and final insertion appointments; appointments with new patients for discussion of necessary work (appointments for case presentation); and recall appointments for prophylaxis and examination, if your dentist does the prophylaxes.

    It is not always possible to adhere strictly to such an arrangement of dental appointments, but the general thought in giving appointments should be to take the greatest advantage of those hours during which the dentist is best able to concentrate on difficult work.

4. Write only in pencil in the appointment book. (It is easier to correct or change, should this be necessary.)

5. If a patient has a complete mouth reconstruction or some operative work, bridgework, and perhaps a partial denture to be prepared, the patient will require appointments over a considerable period of time. No one likes to continue going to the dentist for three months. Try to organize these appointments into a four- to six-week period. Use the longest sittings possible considering the nature of the work to be accomplished.

6. If a series of appointments is to be given, it is preferable to give the patient an appointment on the same day of the week at the same time of day until the series is complete. It helps the patient remember the appointment more easily.

7. Your dentist may want a "break" period in the morning and/or afternoon. A period so maintained is very useful for emergency work when required or for a relaxation period. There are times when an unforeseen difficulty prolongs an appointment beyond the original plan, and the "break" period will be of help in maintaining the balance of the schedule. However, some dentists prefer to work without such a break, risking their lunch hour if necessary. Be sure that you set up the appointment book on the basis that pleases your dentist.

8. In arranging appointments try to organize the time so that the unused time is easy to fill. For example, if your patient requires a one-hour appointment on a morning that is open from 8:30–11:30, give that patient either 8:30–9:30 or 10:30–11:30, rather than giving him or her an appointment in the middle of the open time. If the patient is given 9:30–10:30, the remaining time is cut up into periods that are difficult to fill. It is more efficient to leave the remaining time in a larger single period.

    Some dentists insist that the appointments be made beginning at noon and working back toward the early morning, and beginning at lunch and working toward the evening. Such a practice means that if there are not enough patients to fill the morning, the day might start at 10 or 9 A.M. It eliminates the possibility that one patient would be

```
NAME                    AGE      WORK                    BEST TIME

Andrews, Mr. K.B.       30    Bridge impression       Thursday, mid-mornings
                                --10 units

Drake, Mr. W.S.         40    Operative               Thursday, early mornings
                                --4 units

Berg, Mr. Andy          28    Case presentation       after 4:00
                                --1 unit

Hoover, Randy            5    Operative               Thursday A.M.
                                --2 units

Jones, Mrs. Timothy     45    Operative               Monday and Thursday P.M.
                                --8 units

   (Conference revealed she needs 48 units of work, five separate appointments allowing
   one week between each of the last three for laboratory work to be completed.  First
   appointment for operative work prior to impressions should be for 8 units.)

Price, Mr. J.E.         38    Operative               Thursday, early mornings
                                --2 units

Smith, Ms. Mary         55    Denture impressions     Thursday, at or after 4 P.M.
                                --4 units

Zambolini, Mr. I.F.     21    Operative               Thursday, late P.M.
                                --4 units
```

Figure 9.1

Entries for completing sample appointment book page.

scheduled at 8 A.M. with an unproductive wait till the next scheduled patient at 10 A.M. Such a request by the dentist precludes appointing the business executive who desires an 8 o'clock appointment—or arranging most appointments at the time of patient preference.

9. Remember to schedule children according to their age and physical ability.

10. Certain information must be entered in the appointment book. This information is essential for efficient office management. Check the following list as you fill in the appointment book. Until you are more familiar with the list, perhaps you could copy it and put it on the appointment book cover as a reminder to be sure you have all the necessary information.

   a. The patient's full name (in order not to confuse him or her with some other patient whose name may be very similar). Include the person's title: Mr., Mrs., Ms, Miss, or Dr.

   b. Telephone number (so that you may reach the patient in case of emergency or necessity to change the appointment)

   c. Time of appointment

   d. Length of appointment

   e. The nature of the work to be done

   f. Who is to do the work (dentist or hygienist)

A Practical Example

Now you are ready to write the names and times in the appointment book. Although you will work with a much larger group of patients and many more days in such a planning session under ordinary office conditions, we will limit our list for this example to eight patients, all desiring Thursday appointments. For the purpose of this example, a unit will be fifteen minutes. The information you would normally know about each patient appears in figure 9.1.

You also have a note stating that S. J. Carlson, the supply house salesperson, makes a regular call on Thursday (5 minutes). Your dentist likes to see this particular salesperson.

Before arranging appointments for this group of patients, the page of your appointment book will look something like the one in figure 9.2. There probably will be three single columns (each from 8:00 to 5:45) on a page, a double page making up the total week in order that you can see the week's schedule at a glance, but we are working only with Thursday.

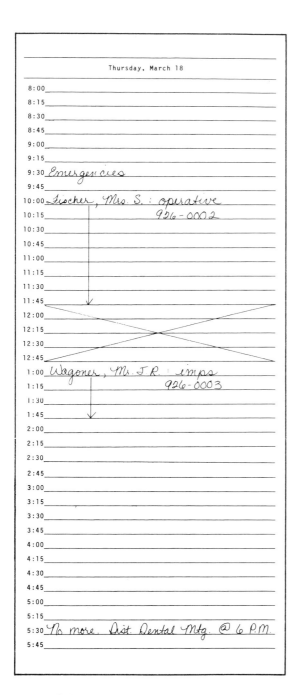

Thursday, March 18

8:00	
8:15	
8:30	
8:45	
9:00	
9:15	
9:30	*Emergencies*
9:45	
10:00	*Fischer, Mrs. S. : operative*
10:15	*926-0002*
10:30	
10:45	
11:00	
11:15	
11:30	
11:45	
12:00	
12:15	
12:30	
12:45	
1:00	*Wagoner, Mr. J R. : imps*
1:15	*926-0003*
1:30	
1:45	
2:00	
2:15	
2:30	
2:45	
3:00	
3:15	
3:30	
3:45	
4:00	
4:15	
4:30	
4:45	
5:00	
5:15	
5:30	*No more. Dist. Dental Mtg. @ 6 P.M.*
5:45	

Figure 9.2

Appointment book page prior to organization of appointments.

Fit the patients who are to come on Thursday into the schedule on the basis of the most efficient work plan that you can visualize. If it is impossible to schedule all the Thursday patients on this one day, some may have to be postponed to the next week. With the entire appointment book before you, that is possible.

Already filled in from previous appointment-making sessions are 10:00–12:00 and 1:00–2:00. Notice that lines are drawn from the patient's name downward through the hours consumed by his or her appointment, with an arrow indicating the last unit.

This is the third Thursday of the month, and the District Dental meeting is held at 6 P.M., which means that Doctor must leave the office by 5:30. Draw a red line across the page just below 5:15 and write, "No more. Dist. Dentl. Mtg. @ 6 P.M."

Now look at the list of people to be scheduled for Thursday. Mr. K. B. Andrews needs a ten-unit period in mid-morning. Since that time is already filled, leave his work for the following Thursday. Randy Hoover, age five, needs a morning appointment. Schedule him for 9:00. This leaves one hour between 8:00 and 9:00.

Both J. F. Price and W. S. Drake need early Thursday morning appointments. However, Mr. Drake needs four units while Mr. Price needs only two units. The space available is a four-unit space; so Mr. Drake is given the appointment and Mr. Price will be appointed the following Thursday. Write in Mr. Drake's name and information.

Look again at the morning. There is a fifteen minute break after the emergency period. No coffee time has been set aside, so use the 9:45 time for a ten minute coffee break, and schedule Mr. S. J. Carlson, salesperson, at 9:55—to permit him his five minutes with Doctor prior to the 10:00 patient. Mark the coffee break and insert the time of Mr. Carlson's appointment and his name. The morning is now complete.

The afternoon begins with Mr. Wagoner, already appointed. Since everyone enjoys a break in the afternoon, schedule Mrs. Jones, who needs eight units of operative work, at 2:00 for two hours and fifteen minutes, utilizing the fifteen minutes as a coffee break in the middle of her appointment, including Mrs. Jones in the coffee break. The rest of Mrs. Jones's appointments would be scheduled on successive Mondays and Fridays if you were working with the complete book. Mrs. Jones would know of her next appointment. Her folder would contain the complete list of future appointments, and at each appointment she would be given the card for the next appointment.

Mr. Berg is to have a case presentation—a one unit appointment. It is desirable to start new patients as soon as possible. Thus, he should be scheduled at 4:15, a time he will appreciate because he can come right after work.

Denture patients must have additional appointments. It is, therefore, important to start such a patient. To choose between the denture impression and the operative work means that Ms. Smith will be chosen and Mr. Zambolini will be given an appointment the following Thursday. Thus, Ms. Smith comes at 4:30. This appointment will finish the day with no time to spare, since Doctor must leave at 5:30.

Note that the complete name, telephone number, and type of work to be performed are all written in the appointment book.

Be sure you write the times of the appointments in pencil on the patient's record or on a special paper or card used for this information and kept in the patient's file. Whatever method is used is unimportant. *It is important, however, to keep a record of future appointments in the patient's file.* Should anyone fail to remember appointment times, the patient's record allows the information to be found and verified in the appointment book quickly. If your office only tells patients of the next appointment, it is imperative to keep this list of future appointments with the patient's record.

Avoid, if at all possible, leaving a single unused unit. It is better to find another appointment and a different patient whose requirements fit the space allotment.

Check to be sure the proper time for laboratory work has been allowed in situations where laboratory work must be done between appointments. Your appointment book page will look like figure 9.3 when you have finished writing in the names. Note that the complete name and telephone number are given for each patient appointed (figures 9.4 and 9.5).

Should you be responsible for the appointments for the hygienist also, try filling in the examples of appointments for the hygienist.

The Murphys both require morning appointments. Mr. Murphy needs an early morning appointment. He can be appointed for the 8:00 time, with Mrs. Murphy following at 9:00. At 10:15 it would be possible to see the seven-year-old (for three units), allowing the hygienist a break of fifteen minutes.

The rest of the day can be completed. Be sure to schedule Mr. Rolf Peterson at 4:00 as the last patient of the day.

Appointments for hygienists are either four, three, or two units. The critical factor is that your dentist is to examine each recall patient. This interruption of the dentist's work should coincide with a break in the dentist's schedule.

Patient Awareness of the Importance of Appointment Time

Writing the appointments in the appointment book is important. Still more important is to see that the patients keep these appointments—on time. What can you do?

You can help patients become aware of the importance of the appointment time.

When the patient is verbally informed of an appointment, you can say something like this, "Doctor Raeywen has reserved 9 o'clock on Tuesday morning,

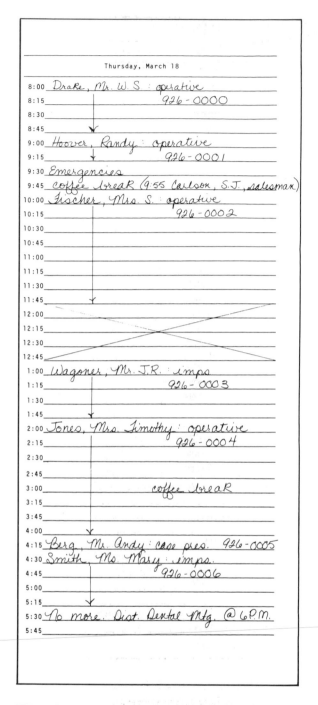

Figure 9.3

Appointment book page after organization of appointments.

September 9 for your dentistry. Should you be unable to keep this appointment, please notify us immediately so we can schedule another patient. It would also help if you arrive a few minutes early. That way your dentistry can be started promptly, assuring its completion before Dr. Raeywen must begin work for another patient."

NAME	AGE	WORK	BEST TIME
Danover, John	7	Recall -- 3 units	Thursdays
Murphy, Mr. John	38	Recall -- 4 units	Thursday, early mornings
McIntosh, Mr. Kenneth	25	Recall -- 4 units	Thursday mornings
Murphy, Mrs. John	36	Recall -- 4 units	Thursday mornings
Franklin, Mr. Andy	21	Recall -- 4 units	Thursday mornings
Jarchow, Mrs. Peter	35	Recall -- 4 units	Thursday afternoons
Jarchow, Randy	5	Recall -- 2 units	Thursday afternoons
Jarchow, Rudy	5	Recall -- 2 units	Thursday afternoons
Olson, Mary	9	Recall -- 3 units	Thursday afternoons
Peterson, Mr. Rolf	60	Recall -- 4 units	Thursday, at or after 4 P.M.

Figure 9.4
Entries for completing a sample hygienist's appointment book page.

The Appointment Card

An appointment card reminds the patient of his or her appointment in writing. It may be as small as a calling card or it may be somewhat larger. Some offices use appointment slips made out in duplicate, with a carbon copy kept at the office for verification in case of confusion about an appointment. Some offices may have the patient write in his or her name and time of appointment so that the carbon copy shows the patient's handwriting.

The appointment card has spaces for the patient's name, the date, and the time of appointment. The dentist's name, telephone number, and address are printed on the card, and some cards state that twenty-four-hour notice must be given if the appointment must be cancelled. Sample cards are shown in figure 9.6.

When the patient is present in the office, the dental assistant copies the appointment date and time from the appointment book onto the appointment card. The card is then given to the patient. Some offices mail the cards to patients whose appointments have been made by telephone.

Reducing Appointment Failures

After making the appointments, it is also necessary to see that appointments are kept, or your dentist will be resting when he or she should be operating. As you have

time during the day, call the patients who have appointments for the following day. (Their telephone numbers should be in the appointment book by their names.) Post cards should be mailed as a reminder to patients living beyond the local telephone exchange; the cards should be mailed early enough to reach patients a day or two before the appointment.

If a patient scheduled for a recall appointment has previously telephoned to verify his or her appointment (after receiving the recall notice specifying a definite day and time), that patient's recall appointment in the appointment book is marked with a red *x*. This patient is not reminded by telephone the day prior to his or her appointment. You know the patient is aware of the appointment.

The telephone call confirming the appointment for the next day requires only a simple statement: "This is Dr. Smith's office calling to confirm your appointment at 10:00 tomorrow morning, Mr. Jones."

Mr. Jones will usually respond with an indication that he will be there as scheduled.

"Thank you, Mr. Jones," is a correct response. Wait for Mr. Jones to hang up his telephone first.

In the event that Mr. Jones is ill or for some reason cannot keep his appointment, the office will have sufficient time to arrange to use Mr. Jones's appointment time either for a patient from the call list or to extend the work, when possible, that is scheduled for the patient preceding Mr. Jones's appointment.

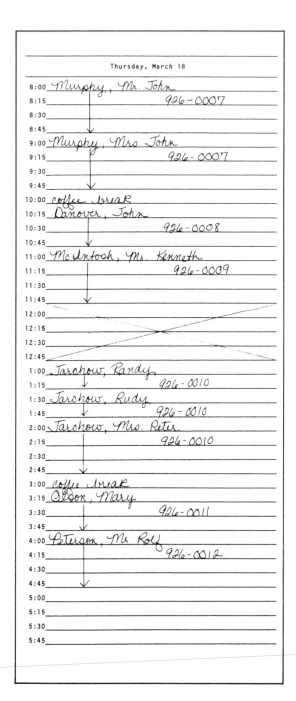

Figure 9.5

Hygienist's appointment book after organization of appointments.

Summary

Proper management of the appointment book is one of the factors that contribute to the success or failure of the dental practice. It keeps your dentist busy or allows

has a reservation with

DR._____

_____

For _____

at _____ o'clock

This time is reserved for you. If, for any reason, the appointment cannot be kept, notification should be made 24 hours in advance, please.

PHONE: _____

HAS TIME RESERVED WITH

John C. Raeywen, D.D.S. 926-1414

Day	Date	Time
1.		at _____ o'clock
2.		at _____ o'clock
3.		at _____ o'clock
4.		at _____ o'clock
5.		at _____ o'clock
6.		at _____ o'clock

THIS TIME HAS BEEN RESERVED FOR YOU
Twenty-four hour notice required for change

This is a sticker. Moisten back and attach to your calendar or other prominent place.

Figure 9.6

Appointment cards.

him or her to be idle. It should be managed by one person rather than by several people.

Good management includes using a unit system of measuring time for dental operations, knowing the amount of time needed for each operation, appointing a sizable group of patients at one time in the quiet and privacy of an inner office where it is possible to pay attention to time organization, and seeing that general rules for the use of time are followed. Appointments should be as long as possible for the benefit of both the patient and the dentist. If possible, include a variety of work in each day. Include a break period each day in order to allow for emergencies, unless your dentist specifically dislikes this procedure.

The following information is to be included in the appointment book: the patient's full name, the patient's telephone number, the time of appointment, the length of appointment, the nature of the work to be done, and who is to do the work. Adults' names are preceded by Mr., Mrs., Ms., Miss, or Dr. "New" patients are so indicated for statistical use.

As soon as a new appointment book is received, the holidays, vacation days, professional meeting days, and any other days on which the office will be closed should be marked off with a red-penciled *x*. School holidays should be so indicated at the top of the page.

An appointment card offers patients a reminder of their appointments.

Reducing appointment failures is an important part of dental assisting. Patients should be called one day in advance of their appointment to be reminded of the appointment. Recall patients need not be called if they have telephoned their acceptance of the date.

Proper management of the appointment book is an art and a skill. A well-managed appointment book allows a dentist to produce more dentistry and serve more people.

Study Questions

1. Discuss the importance of time management in the dental office.
2. What is important to remember in making appointments for (a) the new patient? (b) the recall patient? (c) the emergency patient?
3. What are your responsibilities in rendering courtesy service to a patient of another dentist?
4. Discuss appointments for school children.
5. Explain the ten steps to be remembered in making appointment book entries.
6. What is an appointment card?
7. How can you help patients become aware of the importance of being present on time for their appointment?
8. How can you help reduce appointment failures?

Word Elements	
Word Element	*Example*
agogue, agig root word meaning: lead, drive, make	*sialagogue* an agent that promotes the flow of saliva
anti, ant prefix meaning: against or over against	*antidote* medicine given to counteract a poison
contra prefix meaning: against, counter	*contraindication* any symptom or circumstance suggesting that a form of treatment is inadvisable, although otherwise the treatment would be used
ec prefix meaning: out of	*eccentric* out of center or away from center
extra prefix meaning: outside of, beyond	*extracoronal* outside the body of the coronal portion of the tooth
levo combining form meaning: to the left	*levorotation* turning to the left
morph combining form meaning: form	*morphology* the science that deals with the structure and form of organic beings
neo combining form meaning: new, strange	*neoplasm* any abnormal new growth, such as a tumor
per prefix meaning: throughout space or time	*perforate* to puncture, bore, or pierce through
zoo combining form meaning: relationship to animal	*zoology* branch of biology concerned with the animal kingdom

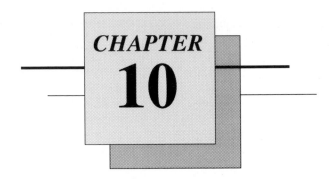

Mail Service and Care

Classes of Mail
Incoming Mail
    Working with the Mail
    Payments on Account
    Dental Office Purchases
Outgoing Mail
Care of Mail During Dentist's Absence
    When the Office Is Closed

Just keeping up with the mail in a dental office can be a time-consuming job. Today the quantity of advertising by mail is enormous. Some of this material is valuable to the dentist and/or the office staff. Some of it is best deposited in the wastebasket. However, judgment is necessary to determine which advertising is important for your dentist to examine. Until such time as the dental assistant has developed this judgment, the dentist should see all advertising.

Classes of Mail

Mail is divided into several classes. The post office has determined rates based on type of material and speed with which delivery is executed.

First-class mail is personal, private communication. The rule is that first-class mail cannot be opened by postal workers. Such mail also receives attention before the second-, third-, and fourth-class mail. It supposedly travels faster.

Regulations state that handwritten communications and typed communications are first class and must bear first-class postage. Usually first-class mail is sealed and will be forwarded if the individual has left a forwarding address.

Second-class mail is newspapers and magazines that have been registered at the post office as such.

Third-class mail and fourth-class mail include packages and mail that have not been classified as first-class mail or second-class mail.

Books may be sent by any class by paying the proper postage. However, there is a book rate for packages plainly marked as "books" or "library rate." This rate is considerably cheaper, and the delivery is slow. Books marked with "bulk rate" receive attention only after first- through fourth-class mail has been delivered.

Weight and size limitations exist for post office packages. Consult your local post office for the latest information concerning the largest and heaviest package you may send.

Second-, third-, and fourth-class mail can be opened and inspected. The rates for sending these classes is cheaper.

The post office offers special services.

1. *Airmail* is still used outside the United States. Inasmuch as mail is now sent by plane anywhere in the United States, the airmail classification formerly used within the country has been abolished. It is stated that all first-class mail moves as fast as the former airmail. However, this is not true outside the United States. If you are sending a letter to any foreign country,

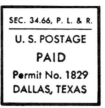

Figure 10.1
A "permit" postage mark often used on circulars and other advertising mail.

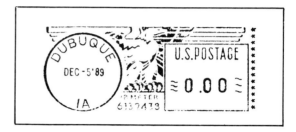

Figure 10.2
Pitney-Bowes metered postage used on first-class mail quite frequently, as well as on some advertising.

airmail is useful. The time differential to Europe is about five days versus six weeks—airmail versus boat.

The airmail rate to foreign countries varies with the country so one must call the post office to discover the correct postage, which is stated by the half ounce or fourteen grams.

Packages can be sent by *priority mail*. Priority mail is sent by airplane along with the first-class mail and it receives the same treatment as first-class mail. Insurance is available for priority mail.

2. Services within the United States for which one pays an additional fee include the following:

Express mail is a service that guarantees next day delivery. The post office furnishes a special large envelope. Your packet can weigh up to 2 pounds.

Registered mail is mail that is protected because it is personally registered as having been delivered. The mail carrier must have the recipient sign a card which states that the mail was received at the address given. For an additional fee it is possible to ask that the card be signed by the person to whom the mail is addressed. This card is then returned to the sender.

It is also possible to *insure* mail that you send. The fee for insurance depends on the value of the package.

Cash on delivery (COD) is a way you can send an item for which you have not been paid, and the receiver will pay for it upon its delivery. The money for its purchase is then returned to you by postal money order.

Certificates of mailing furnish evidence of mailing only. A receipt is not obtained upon delivery of the mail.

Special delivery is a service that means the mail is delivered immediately upon receipt at the post office. A special car takes it to its destination.

Special handling is a service available for fourth-class mail. It speeds the service somewhat but does not mean the package is delivered by special delivery.

Certified mail provides for a receipt to the sender and a record of delivery at the office of address. It is handled in the ordinary mails and no insurance coverage is provided.

Money orders, by which it is possible to send money to someone else, may be purchased at the post office.

3. There are services for misaddressed mail. Sometimes mail cannot be delivered. (The person may have moved and left no forwarding address.) Therefore, it is important to use a *return address,* which is the address of the sender written, preferably, in the upper left-hand corner of the envelope. If no return address is provided, the letter is sent to the dead letter office, where every attempt is made to find either the sender or the addressee, but much mail is auctioned or destroyed each year because it is impossible to discover either the sender or receiver.

4. Mail that fails to reach its destination within a reasonable time can usually be traced. Should you discover that mail you sent has not been delivered, consult your post office for the proper forms to complete. The post office will then make every effort to find the lost mail.

Receipts from the post office for money orders, insured mail, certified, and registered mail should be kept until you have received notification that the mail was received in good condition by the person to whom the mail was sent.

5. *Zip code directories* containing the zip codes for local areas are available. Such a directory should be used. For codes of distant cities, call the post office zip code number listed in the telephone directory.

6. Postal regulations change frequently. Consult your local post office for any *bulletins* they furnish.

Incoming Mail

Processing *incoming mail* is important. Most of the money paid for dentistry is sent by mail. Some patients even send currency through the mail, in spite of all admonitions our society expresses concerning the dangers of this practice. Payments, whether by check or cash, must be accurately recorded. In addition, professional meeting notices of utmost importance to your oral health team are sent through mail, as well as most of the paperwork concerning the practice of dentistry. The assistant charged with receiving and distributing the mail must be aware of the types of mail and what to do with each.

Incoming mail can be divided into three groups:

1. Mail that should be placed on the dentist's desk:
   a. personal mail,
   b. letters from professional colleagues, and
   c. announcements of meetings for the dentist.
2. Mail that is the responsibility of other staff members:
   a. letters from patients other than questions of accounts (Such mail may request information or action that some staff member is authorized to perform. That staff member should answer the letter unless the dentist gives other instructions);
   b. letters concerning statements or accounts other than payments; a patient might question a charge or need information for an insurance policy;
   c. payments on account;
   d. insurance forms;
   e. invoices for dental supplies or business supplies;
   f. monthly statements for the office supplies;
   g. magazines;
   h. laboratory cases (if mailed); and
   i. letters soliciting contributions.
3. Advertising matter, to be handled with discretion by the assistant.

Working with the Mail

The mail arrives. The assistant carefully examines each piece. The letters that are personal communications for the dentist are placed together.

The rest of the envelopes are to be opened. Minutes can be saved each day if you will use a letter opener to slit all the envelopes first, without removing the contents until all envelopes are cut. Tap the envelopes against the desk to be certain that the enclosures are away from the edge before you use the letter opener.

When all the envelopes are opened, lay down the letter opener and carefully remove the contents of each envelope. Be certain that nothing is lost. Clip the contents and the envelope together. Verify the address inside the envelope with the return address on the envelope. Also verify your records. A patient or correspondent may have moved, and this letter indicates the new address.

Ascertain which staff member is best qualified to handle each letter. Place the letter with the mail for that staff member.

The dentist's mail is placed on his or her desk immediately (group one).

Distribute the mail classified in group two. Each staff member should attend to the mail to be answered as quickly as possible.

Some letters require information that the dental assistant can ethically and legally furnish. Such a request should be answered the day it is received. The dental assistant signs her or his name—not the dentist's!

Letters from a patient, especially when they concern any complaint, and a copy of your reply should be placed in the patient's record envelope. Should you have any question about such letters from a patient, ask your dentist for his or her recommendation.

If any mail refers to previous correspondence, this correspondence should be removed from the files and placed with the current letter. Read the letter carefully. Know whether you have removed all the necessary records. Your dentist may have to examine an X ray or reread an examination record to answer the mail intelligently.

Payments on Account

A large part of the mail will be payments from patients. Examine checks and money orders carefully. Ascertain that they are correctly prepared. A bank will not accept a check for deposit unless:

1. It is dated no later than the date of deposit (that is, a check for deposit on October 1 must be dated October 1 or earlier, not October 10).
2. The amounts of money, numerical and written, agree.
3. The check is properly signed.
4. The check is properly made out to your dentist.

Verify these items and then immediately turn the check over and endorse it "For deposit to the account of Dr. _____." Most banks today furnish a bank stamp that states the number of the dentist's checking account and endorses the check so that no handwritten endorsement is necessary. The important fact is to endorse every check on receipt. Should the check be lost or stolen it cannot be cashed with the endorsement on its reverse side.

Dental Office Purchases

Invoices for dental office purchases will arrive either in the package of supplies or separately in a first-class envelope. The invoice is an important paper and must be kept. The merchandise must be verified with the invoice to be certain that the invoice is correct and that you are not charged for something you have not received. Invoices are filed in a file folder labeled "Current Invoices" until the end of the month. (See chap. 17 for complete details.)

Statements for dental office purchases are received near the end of the month. The invoices from the firm which have accumulated during the month are to be verified with the statement. When the statement arrives, remove the invoices for that firm from the current invoices file and attach them to the statement. These papers are then given to the staff member who is responsible for bookkeeping.

Laboratory cases received in the mail should be opened and the invoice located. Many dentists like to have the laboratory charge indicated on the patient's record card. This charge should be entered on the patient's record as soon as the invoice is received for each case, before the invoice is placed in the current invoices file. Laboratory cases that consist either partially or wholly of processed acrylic, such as jacket crowns, full crowns with acrylic veneer, facings on bridges, or denture bases, should be removed from their protective wrappers and placed in water in the laboratory as soon as unpacked. A slip of paper identifying the patient for whom the case is constructed should be placed in such a manner that it cannot be separated from the proper laboratory case. Items that do not require immersion in water are placed in small plastic, metal, or cardboard boxes in the laboratory, with the identifying slip of paper containing the patient's name attached to the box. Large plastic boxes may have the name written directly on the box with a china pencil. The marking can be wiped off when the box is to be reused.

Supplies received should be opened carefully. Locate the invoice. Verify the contents. Store as indicated in chapter 11, "Supplies and Their Control." File invoices in the current invoices file.

Insurance forms received in the mail must be given to the staff member responsible for completing such forms.

Advertising, the third group of mail, is examined only after group two has been completed. Some advertising material is definitely desirable in the dental office because it may acquaint the dentist with a new product. On the other hand, some advertising material is not related to the practice of dentistry, is of no interest to the dentist, and is devised to look like personal or first-class mail. If one of the end flaps of the envelope is merely tucked in for closure and carries a statement in fine print that it may be opened for postal inspection if necessary, it is advertising. In addition, such mail will usually have a permit postage mark (fig. 10.1) rather than an attached postage stamp or a metered postage mark (fig. 10.2), due to the large number of pieces the originating office will place in the mail at one time. Open this mail and place it on the bottom of the pile for your dentist.

Your dentist should brief you on the types of samples he or she wishes to see, the advertising literature he or she wishes to read, and what you should do with the rest of such mail. Samples not used in your office can be given to a charitable organization.

Outgoing Mail

Mail to be sent from the office must also receive care. When letters have been dictated, typed, proofread, and signed, they should be properly folded and prepared for mailing. Weigh letters to be certain that enough postage is used on any mailing. The last person to leave the office should mail the letters. Sometimes a report is finished late, or the dentist signs a letter just before leaving.

Care of Mail During Dentist's Absence

When the dentist is attending a meeting or on vacation, it is important that there is a complete understanding about mail. Personal mail may need special care. The dentist will decide whether or not it should be opened. Perhaps instructions will be that the assistant is to call the dentist concerning certain pieces of mail. Sometimes it is necessary to forward mail, but the decision will be made by the dentist.

If a delay in answering mail will occur, the secretary can write a brief note of explanation to the correspondent indicating the probable time the dentist will return.

If the information sought is something the secretary can supply within legal and ethical restrictions, she or he can answer the letter and explain that she or he is caring for the matter in the dentist's absence.

Some mail may demand an immediate decision by the dentist. Perhaps your dentist will arrange with you before leaving to call him or her at the meeting. In the absence of such an arrangement, use your best judgment about any action you think necessary.

If you are to send any mail to your employer while he or she is away, make a copy of it to send. If it is lost in transit, you will still have the original.

If your dentist does not want you to open letters marked "Personal," send a note to the return address on the envelope, explaining the dentist is away and will receive the mail on his or her return. Also, indicate that if there is anything you can do to help, the writer should contact you personally. Sign your name.

When the Office Is Closed

Notify the post office or mail carrier if your office is to be closed for any length of time. The mail can be held at the post office until your return. It will eliminate lost mail and possible loss of income through theft of the letters that contain payments. In addition, any accumulation of mail at the door of the office is indication to a would-be thief that now is the time to break into the office.

Summary

There are several classes of mail that the dental assistant should recognize and understand both for classifying the importance of mail received and for understanding which type of service to use for mail to be sent. These classes include first-, second-, third-, and fourth-class mail, air-mail, express mail, priority mail, registered mail, COD, special delivery, special handling, certified mail, and money orders. Zip code is necessary on all mail sent.

A postal manual which will contain the correct regulations may be purchased.

Incoming mail must be sorted and processed according to its urgency. Mail that must be seen by the dentist should be opened and placed on his or her desk, with the most important pieces on top.

Outgoing mail is to be proofread by the secretary before it is mailed. It should be mailed just as soon as possible after the dentist has signed the letters.

Special care must be taken of personal mail for the dentist during his or her absence from the office. Mail that can be answered by the secretary should be answered. Mail that the dentist wishes to remain unopened should be placed on his or her desk or in a special file. The secretary should send a note to the return address on each envelope, explaining the absence of the dentist and indicating that if the matter is urgent, the addressee can write the secretary directly.

If the office is to be closed for any period of time, such as a week, the mail carrier should be notified so that the mail can be held at the post office for reopening of the dental office.

Study Questions

1. Why is it desirable for the assistant to recognize the classes of mail?
2. Describe the proper sorting of mail.
3. Why should outgoing mail be proofread by the secretary?
4. Describe the special care of mail during the dentist's absence while he or she is attending a convention.
5. Why should you notify the mail carrier if the office is to be closed for a two-week period?

Vocabulary

invoice an itemized list of merchandise shipped, specifying the price and terms of sale, and usually accompanying the merchandise

statement a summary of a financial account showing the balance due, and usually listing by number the invoices included in the balance due

Word Elements	
Word Element	*Example*
ante prefix meaning: before, preceding in time	*anterior* front or forward part (The anterior teeth are the six front teeth in both arches.)
antero prefix meaning: front	*anteroclusion* malocclusion of teeth in which mandibular teeth are in front of their normal position
pre prefix meaning: before	*prescription* written directions for giving or using a remedy
pro prefix meaning: forward, forth, before, for, in front of	*prognosis* forecast as to possible result of a disease or condition
hyper prefix meaning: excessive	*hypercementosis* excessive formation of cementum usually at the apical portion of the tooth
hypo prefix meaning: deficient	*hypoplasia* incomplete or defective development of any tissue (Enamel hypoplasia is defective development of enamel-forming cells leaving pits or ringlike grooves.)
trans prefix meaning: through, across	*transverse* placed crosswise, at right angles to the long axis
ana prefix meaning: upward, backward, excessive	*anaphylaxis* a violent allergic reaction characterized by sudden collapse following injection
super prefix meaning: above, or implying excess	*superior* situated above
supra prefix meaning: above or over	*supraclusion* abnormally deep overlap of a dental arch or group of teeth

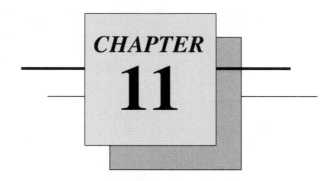

CHAPTER
11

Supplies and Their Control

Selecting the Suppliers
Control of Expendable Supplies
Methods for Control of Supplies
Care of Supplies on Delivery
Damaged Merchandise
Proper Storage
Care of Laundry

Few businesses can be run effectively without control of the supplies that are used. It is necessary to know the quantity of each supply on hand and how to reorder before the supply is exhausted.

Supplies used in a dental office are varied. **Professional supplies** used in the actual practice of dentistry depend on the type of practice. For example, the supplies for an orthodontist will be quite different from those for an oral surgeon.

Business supplies used for keeping the records and controlling the income and outgo vary with the method of bookkeeping and dental record-keeping system preferred by the dentist.

Some supplies are used once and thrown away (the **disposables**), some are used for a short period of time, and some instruments and pieces of equipment will be used for many years.

We speak of expendable and nonexpendable materials. For tax accounting purposes the materials used in a profession or business must be categorized. Thus, materials whose cost is over fifty dollars and whose life is three years or more are labeled **nonexpendable.** Materials that cost less than fifty dollars and that are replaced in less than three years are **expendable.** See chapter 18, "Records for Taxes . . ." for further explanation of this terminology. In this chapter we are considering the expendable supplies—those items that are used and must be replaced frequently.

Selecting the Suppliers

Whatever the life expectancy of a material, the time comes when it must be replaced. For most supplies in daily use this may be frequent.

Where one purchases a supply depends on what that supply is. Dental materials—those supplies used in the actual performance of dentistry—are ordered from a dental supply house. (Materials such as alloy or impression materials are *dental* supplies.) Drugs are usually ordered from a pharmacy. The necessary supplies for the dental business office are usually ordered from a printer of dental office supplies, or a dental practice management firm, or sometimes from the dental supply house. These supplies are business supplies—record-keeping materials. Cleaning supplies and coffee can probably be purchased most cheaply at a nearby grocery or department store.

Control of Expendable Supplies

The amount of each supply purchased at a given time is governed by four factors: (1) the dentist's preference in quantity purchasing; (2) the space available for storage of the supplies; (3) the rapidity of use; and (4) the shelf life of each particular supply.

Quantity purchasing can mean a considerable savings over a period of time. The degree of such purchasing must be governed by the practical aspects of space availability and shelf life of the particular article. Quantity purchasing must be considered carefully and utilized only when it provides an economic advantage.

Supplies should be ordered in quantities that will be used within a year. The rapidity with which changes in dentistry occur means that it is possible for supplies to become obsolete.

The *space available* for storage determines the quantity of all items. Some items are very small and require little storage space, but some items are bulky and require large space.

The *rapidity* with which the item is used will affect the quantity required. An item that is used at the rate of three dozen a week requires more duplicates on the shelf than an item that is used at the rate of three dozen a month.

The *shelf life* of an item is an important factor in considering the quantity to purchase. Never purchase more than the amount the office uses within the limits of the shelf life period. If the shelf life is three months, and in three months the office uses nine of this particular supply, then the purchase should never be more than nine—even if a special rate is offered for the purchase of a dozen. Manufacturers mark the expiration date on each product and it appears as either an actual date or a code. If a code is used, the manufacturer will supply the explanation of the code on request. Usually, the dental product supplier will have this information for you.

Methods for Control of Supplies

Several different approaches to controlling supplies are utilized. In some dental offices an order is placed when a staff member notices an item is missing or the last box has been taken. Some dentists use partial control, such as a running inventory. Still other dentists utilize a highly accurate and complete supply control system.

Briefly, the **running inventory** method, often used in small offices, consists of two items: (1) the running inventory list and (2) the supply control cards, kept in a special file.

The running inventory is a list of supplies on hand that is kept inside the supply cupboard door or on the wall near the supply cupboard. It bears the name of each expendable supply, its location, quantity on hand, and reorder point. Each time an item is removed from storage, the quantity on hand is corrected.

ITEM	AMOUNT ON HAND	REORDER POINT
Alginate	~~10~~ ~~9~~ ~~8~~ ~~7~~ 6	2
Alloy	~~12~~ ~~11~~ ~~10~~ ~~9~~ ~~8~~ ~~7~~ ~~6~~ 5	5
Bibs	~~30~~ ~~35~~ ~~34~~ ~~35~~ ~~32~~ ~~31~~ 30	3

Figure 11.1

A running inventory.

Bibs				
Date	Quantity (Cases)	Firm	Brand	Total Price
6/5/87	1	G. Marcus	KP	$28.50
7/5/87	3	"	KP 3 Case price	85.50
10/8/87	3	"	KP "	85.50
1/10/88	3	"	KP "	85.50
4/10/88	6	"	KP 6 Case price	156.00
10/10/88	6	"	KP "	156.00

Figure 11.2

A supply control card.

If the staff is accurate in recording each removal from the supply cupboard, the assistant charged with ordering supplies has only to check the running inventory each day and order those supplies that have been reduced to the reorder point. (Figure 11.1 is a running inventory.)

When the reorder point is reached, the supply control card becomes important. The supply control file contains, in alphabetical order, a card for each supply used. This card gives all the information necessary for purchasing the supply (fig. 11.2). The record on the control card of the date and quantity purchased indicates the time lapse between purchases, and thus the rate of consumption can be calculated. A decision can be made about the quantity to order. If the item has not been satisfactory, the supply control card can be marked to prevent reorder. Each time you place an order, verify the most desirable quantity rate for the storage conditions in your office. A change in quantity purchase rates may have occurred since you last placed an order.

When the new package of supplies arrives, the assistant adds them to the remainder in the supply cupboard and changes the running inventory to correspond with the actual quantity on hand. Thus, if three cartons of bibs were ordered (twelve packages to a carton), and when they arrived there were two packages left in the supply cupboard, the assistant would write a new line for bibs and indicate the quantity on hand as thirty-eight (thirty-six new ones plus the two in the cupboard).

The disadvantage of this method is that it is very easy for a staff member to be in such a hurry that the running inventory is not marked on removal of the supply. Since no one person is solely responsible for the removal of the supplies, the failure to mark the running inventory may go unnoticed until the moment when no supply is on hand.

Dr. Leo Hoffman's inventory control system eliminates this possibility. He recommends the following requirements for inventory control:

1. A *code number* for each supply used in the office. The code number is used on each item of the supply and on the indices of that supply.

2. A *supply control file card* for each supply, arranged alphabetically in a special file. Each card has, in addition to the record of orders of the supply, the code number of that supply.

3. A *cardex tray file* or a *visirecord tray*. This file consists of flat one-inch high trays. Each tray holds about fifty cards flat, with the bottom quarter-inch exposed. When looking at this tray, one sees the bottom quarter-inch of all the cards at once. The code number and the subject of each card is written on the bottom quarter-inch for reference. The top of each card is attached to the tray by a clip or wire so that the card may be raised without removing it from the file. Thus, if you glance at the series of fifty cards in the tray and see a card you wish to study about a third of the way up the tray, you simply lift up the card above the one you want to see. All the cards will move up, and the card you wish to study will be clearly exposed.

In the inventory control system, this four-by-six-inch card (fig. 11.3) has the name of the supply, the code number of the supply, the description of its stability, the maximum amount to be kept on hand, and the reorder point or minimum number. These items are all at the bottom of the card. The upper three-fourths of the card is devoted to an accounting of the use of the supply: date, amount of supply in, amount of supply out, and the balance. When the balance reaches the minimum order point, the supply is to be reordered.

DATE	AMT. IN	AMT. OUT	BAL.	DATE	AMT. IN	AMT. OUT	BAL.
8/1	36	—	36				
8/5	—	2	34				
8/15	—	2	32				

CODE	ITEM	STABLE	PERISH.	MAX.	MIN.
107	Bibs	✓		39 pkg.	3 pkg.

Figure 11.3

An inventory control card.

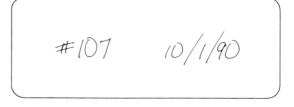

Figure 11.4

A code label.

The cards in the cardex file are filed in numerical order by the code number for that supply.

4. A *container for code labels* removed from supplies. This may be a box or jar placed on a laboratory bench or by the supply cupboard. Perhaps several containers can be utilized in various places around the office.

5. *Code labels* prepared for each supply. Each label bears the code number of that supply and the date it was received. Self-adhering labels are used. One label is attached to each individual packet of the supply. When a packet or individual item is removed from the supply cupboard, the label is dropped in the container kept for this purpose.

6. An assistant who *gathers the labels* from the containers and enters the label information on the cardex file cards.

7. *Crimped color signals* to indicate various stages in the process of ordering supplies. Any set of colors is acceptable. For our example, we will use red markers to indicate that the supply must be ordered. When the balance on the cardex card shows the same number as the minimum, a red color signal is placed on that card.

The order is placed, and at that time a green color signal is attached to the cardex card next to the red one. When the supply arrives and has been checked in and recorded, these signals are removed.

If an item is back-ordered, an orange signal is placed on the card and the red and green signals removed. If an item is

returned to the dealer for credit, a blue signal is placed on the cardex card until the credit slip has been received and verified.

How the assistant works the system: Mary, the assistant who records the used supplies, has just entered the balance on the cardex card number 107, which is the card for bibs (figure 11.3). She notes that it is the same as the reorder point—three. She places a red signal on the bib card.

Later in the day Mary uses the alphabetical supply control file and discovers that the supply is ordered in quantities of three cartons (twelve packages in each carton). She calls the supplier, orders the bibs, and verifies the price for three cartons. She still receives the quantity price for three cartons, but the price has been raised. She notes on the control card the order and its price increase. She places a green signal next to the red signal on cardex card # 107. Three days later she receives the three cartons of bibs. She verifies the invoice against the bibs, removes the red and green color signals from the cardex card # 107, records the amount in, and the balance, which now shows thirty-eight since another package has been taken from the supply cupboard since she placed the order. She then prepares thirty-six labels with # 107, and puts one on each of the thirty-six packages of bibs. At the supply cupboard, she removes the two packages and stacks the new supplies in back, replacing the two old packages in front so they will be used first.

Care of Supplies on Delivery

Anyone responsible for receiving supplies must exercise care in examining the supplies as they arrive.

1. Open the package carefully and find the invoice. Check each item against the invoice to be certain you have received the quantity you ordered and that the price is correct. If no invoice is found in the package, hold the supplies until the invoice arrives in the mail. Sometimes the mailed invoice precedes the package. Under these circumstances remove the invoice from

John Marcus Dental Supply Company
3037 LYNDALE AVE. SO • MINNEAPOLIS, MINNESOTA 55408 • PHONE 827-6125   Salesman **Dick**

TO
John C. Raeywen, D.D.S.   Customer
104 Any Street
Anytown, Anystate 12345   Date April 8, 19—

MANUFACTURER	BACK ORDERED	QUAN. ORDERED	QUAN. SHIPPED	DESCRIPTION	UNIT PRICE	AMOUNT
K.P.		3	3	Bibs (Rate for 3 or more cases)	$28.50	$85.50
Eastman	3	6	3	Kodak D.F. 58	$23.93	$71.79
					SUB TOTAL	$157.29
					SHIPPING	--------
					TAX	$9.44
					TOTAL	$166.73

ITEMS APPEARING IN BACK ORDER COLUMN WILL FOLLOW SHORTLY

Figure 11.5
A dental supply invoice. Notice the back-order marking.

your current invoice file and verify the contents of the package. This *verification is to determine that you have received everything for which you have been charged.*

2. Carefully examine each item in the package to determine that it is not damaged. Be certain that merchandise is not damaged before it is stored.
3. If the item has a shelf life limitation, examine the expiration date or code to be sure the material is fresh. (If the shelf life is three months and the expiration date is one month away, the merchandise should be returned for credit.)
4. Label each acceptable piece with its code number and date (to be sure old stock is used first).
5. Make entries in the inventory control cardex system or the running inventory.
6. Store these items. To do so, remove the old stock; place the new merchandise in the cupboard, then place the old stock in front.

Damaged Merchandise

Damaged or old merchandise must be returned to the supplier. If your dental supply house delivers its merchandise, call them for pickup. If your office is beyond delivery zone, mail or send the merchandise back with a letter of explanation. This letter may be placed inside the package. In some areas a delivery service will be used instead of the mail service.

You must receive a **credit slip** for this damaged merchandise. It is easy to forget unless you remind yourself. If an inventory control system is used, indicate the fact that you are waiting for a credit slip by attaching the correct crimped signal to the correct cardex card. If an inventory control system is not used in the office in which you work, make a card for your come-up file to remind yourself to watch for this credit slip. Place it behind the daily index and keep it there for a week. If no credit slip has been received by that time, call the firm and begin tracing it. Keep using your credit slip reminder in the come-up file until you do receive the credit slip.

Back-ordered means that merchandise was not in stock at the supplier's and will be sent automatically as soon as the supplier receives it. Should an invoice be sent with this notation on it, you must decide whether to order the item from another supplier or wait for the back-ordered item. If you call another supplier and receive the merchandise, be sure to call the original supplier and cancel the back order—or you will have more supplies on hand than you wish. Sometimes the supplier will send you part of an order and back-order the rest (fig. 11.5). If the quantity received will supply your needs for a long enough period, perhaps you can wait for the rest of the shipment. Handling back orders requires judgment concerning the length of time you can wait for the supply.

Proper Storage

Some supplies must receive special storage care. For example, X-ray film must be stored in a lead-lined box unless it is stored in a cool, dry place, well away from the area in which the X-ray machine is used; X-ray developer and fixer must be stored in a dark, cool area; and gypsum materials (artificial stones and plaster) must be kept dry.

Learn the arrangements for special storage that your dentist prefers.

Care of Laundry

Disposables have reduced the amount of laundry required in a dental office today. However, some offices still use towels that must be commercially laundered. Some dentists employ a commercial laundry to launder all uniforms. Some laundries furnish the uniforms and towels.

If your office uses a commercial laundry, it is important to know how to manage this service. The driver usually stops at regular intervals, such as every other day or once a week. Before the driver's scheduled arrival:

1. Count all the soiled linens
2. Record the number of each kind for your future reference
3. Count the number and type of uniforms if you are sending them with the linens
4. Record the number of each kind

When the driver returns the clean laundry,

1. Count the linens (the figures should agree with your note of the number of pieces sent)
2. Check the charge to see that it is correct
3. File the invoice in the come-up file
4. Store the linens

Summary

Supplies, without which dentistry could not be performed, require control so the necessary supplies are always on hand. Supplies are varied depending on the type of practice, but all dental offices use both professional supplies and business supplies. For tax records, supplies are considered either expendable or nonexpendable, depending on their life-expectancy and cost.

Quantity purchasing can be valuable, but it must be controlled by factors of amount used during one year and storage space available. Shelf life also determines quantity purchases.

Supplies can be controlled by use of a running inventory or an inventory control system that requires labels and a visible tray record of supplies.

Supplies must be examined on delivery and verified versus records to ascertain supplies received are those ordered, that the quantity is correct, and that merchandise is not damaged.

If a supplier indicates an item is back-ordered, the dental office staff must decide whether to wait for that supplier or to try another supplier.

Proper storage of supplies includes arranging the merchandise so the oldest supply is used first. Care must be given to certain supplies such as X-ray film.

Laundry must be counted and recorded before being sent and then counted, recorded, and examined on return to be sure that the laundry received is the laundry sent, and that the number of pieces received is the same as the number of pieces sent.

Study Questions

1. Why do you carefully store and plainly label dental supplies?
2. What supplies are expendable?
3. Differentiate between business and professional supplies.
4. Why is a control system for supplies desirable?
5. Describe a control system.
6. How do you make a running inventory and what is its use?
7. Describe an inventory control system.
8. Describe the assistant's duties when a package of supplies is received.
9. What is a back order?
10. Describe your care of the laundry from the time you gather the soiled items until you place the clean ones in their proper storage places.

Vocabulary

back-ordered   merchandise that was not in stock at the suppliers but that the supplier has ordered and will deliver as soon as it arrives.

business supplies   those used for business records

credit slip   acknowledgment from suppliers that some specific item has been returned and is to be credited to the account of the purchaser

expendable supplies   those consumed in less than three years and costing less than fifty dollars

inventory   the record indicating the amount of supplies on hand

professional supplies   those used in the actual practice of dentistry

running inventory   a list of supplies with quantity on hand, which is altered each time a supply is removed from storage

shelf life   length of time a supply can be stored before it deteriorates

Word Elements	
Word Element	**Example**
ab, abs prefix meaning: away, away from	**abrasion** grinding or wearing away of teeth
al suffix meaning: of, like, pertaining to	**palatal** referring to the palate—the roof of the mouth
circum combining form meaning: around	**circulation** orderly movement through a circuit, as blood moving through the vessels
peri prefix meaning: around	**periodontal** around the tooth
ad prefix meaning: to, toward	**adaptation** modification to fit the conditions of the environment
co, com, con combining form, meaning: together with	**congenital** any condition present at birth ("together with birth")
epi prefix meaning: on, upon, over	**epidermis** skin (on the outside of the body)
inter prefix meaning: between	**interdental** space between two teeth
juxta prefix meaning: near	**juxtaposition** placed side by side
stasis suffix meaning: standing still	**hemostasis** arrest of blood circulation

CHAPTER 12

Preservation of Written Records: Filing

Files in General
Dental Office Filing
The Filing Process
    Steps in Filing
Removal of Filed Materials
    Charge-Out Methods
Accuracy in Recording
Record Search
Shelf Filing with Numeric System
Grouping of Patient Records
Retention of Records
Files for Patient Account Records
Filing Color Slides
Dental Office Files: Recapitulation

Files in General

Files are indispensable in conducting a business—including the business of dentistry. Filed papers are the memory of the business. Files are containers in which papers are stored, usually vertically, to aid in ease of handling the materials. (It is easier to find papers placed on end than stacked horizontally on a spindle.)

The basic function of filing is the storing of records in a safe place in a way that permits finding them quickly when needed. It means to file only papers that ought to be kept and file them so they can be found. The filing equipment should conserve time and space and should provide adequate protection of records. Cabinets are available for storing every standard-size record including X rays. Filing cabinets can be obtained with or without locks; shelf filing cabinets are also obtainable with slide-out covers with or without locks.

Filed materials consist of:

1. Records or papers that come into the office and must be kept
2. Copies of materials that leave the office
3. Records made in the office for use within the office

The employee to whom the task of filing is delegated:
- must understand how to organize the filing system,
- must use good judgment in what is filed, and
- must decide when to dispose of material that has been filed.

Usually the employer sets policies for preservation and disposition of the records.

Dental Office Filing

Filing records in the dental office presents some considerations not found in a business. All patient records must be retained until the statute of limitations has expired for that particular patient. Each patient has a clinical record and an account record. These confidential records are the core of the dental practice. The **account record** is the history of the financial transactions with the one patient or family. The **clinical record** is necessary for any dental work performed and becomes the patient's dental history. Complete records about a patient, dating from the first visit to the latest, can be of invaluable assistance to the dentist in planning a course of treatment and in observing gradually changing physical conditions. Thus, patient records must be preserved until the dentist is positive that they are of no further use.

These two files must be kept separately from other office records. Thus, the dental office may have three or more separate filing systems.

1. **Clinical records** are filed either in an alphabetical or numerical file.
2. **Account records** are filed the same way as the clinical records, but usually in a separate file.
3. All other important papers are filed in a **subject file,** which usually is an alphabetical file.

The subject file contains records of taxes, salaries, dental office charge accounts, professional correspondence with organizations such as ADA, colleagues, and any other materials kept in the office except for patient records—both clinical and financial.

Good judgment is necessary in selection of materials to be retained in the subject matter file as well as selection of materials to be destroyed later. The dentist should set up criteria to be used in the selection process.

The Filing Process

Filed materials are placed in folders. Each folder contains similar material—material relating to one subject. The file folder has a raised tab on the top back edge on which the file clerk writes the name, subject, or number of the material contained in that folder. The name, subject, or number written on the tab is called the **caption.** Each file folder will have a caption.

The manilla folders are inserted in a file drawer or on a file shelf in some sort of order—either alphabetical or numerical. (We will assume the subject matter file is alphabetical and discuss numerical filing later.)

File drawers may contain a rack for *hanging folders* or they may contain heavy cardboard dividers on which are printed letters of the alphabet and sometimes a specific subject. The specific subject dividers are used when several file folders are needed to contain different segments of the file for that particular subject. For example, the subject "TAXES" could require several manilla folders—one for each of these topics: Federal Income Compensation Assistance (FICA), Federal Withholding Tax, State Withholding Tax, Federal Unemployment Compensation Tax, State Unemployment Compensation Tax, Income Tax, Property Tax. If a hanging file is used, several manilla folders can be placed in one hanging envelope. If a subject requires too many manilla folders to fit in one hanging

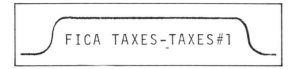

Figure 12.1
A caption for a file folder.

envelope, the captions on the consecutive hanging envelopes can be labeled "TAXES # 1," "TAXES # 2," and "TAXES # 3." The manilla folders would bear the caption location on the tab as well as the caption, thus: "FICA TAXES–TAXES # 1" (figure 12.1).

Steps in Filing

The process of filing papers in the subject material file requires judgment and accuracy. The steps to be taken include these:

1. **Caption classification guide:** The employee responsible for filing needs a written list of classifications used in the subject matter file. This list will include such subjects as taxes, dental supplies, office supplies, bank records, ADA correspondence, and any organization with whom the office personnel correspond. Many other subjects will be used. A typed list of file subjects, with notations concerning the material to be filed under each subject, is necessary to prevent misfiling of materials.

2. **Inspection:** Not all material that is received in an office is worth saving. Therefore, the person responsible for the filing must decide whether this particular letter or paper is to be filed. If the answer to any one of the following questions is *yes,* the paper should be filed.
   a. Will the information in this letter be needed later?
   b. Is this record required by some government service?
   c. Is there a legal necessity for keeping the record?

3. **Indexing:** Decide which caption is best for this particular item so that the paper can be retrieved easily. Anticipating the caption most likely to be used by someone requesting the item later is helpful. That caption should then be used for this item.

4. **Coding:** Code the paper by underlining the words used to determine the caption. It will be returned to the proper file folder if it has been identified by code.

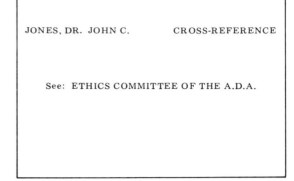

Figure 12.2
A cross-reference index card.

Write the caption used in the upper right-hand corner with colored pencil. No mistake can then be made.

5. **Cross-reference:** Often a paper has more than one possible caption. The secondary possibilities can be utilized by cross reference. The Cross-Reference Card is made (figure 12.2) and filed under the secondary caption. For example, your dentist may be chairman of a committee on ethics for the American Dental Association. He or she corresponds with a number of dentists who are on this committee, and this correspondence is filed under "Ethics Committee of the ADA." One day your dentist wishes to see a letter from Dr. John C. Jones about the Ethics Committee, but may not be specific enough to add the last phrase. You look under "Jones, Dr. John C.," but you do not find the letter since it is filed under "Ethics Committee." However, you do find a cross-reference index card in the file. The caption is headed "Jones, Dr. John C." On the card is written "See: Ethics Committee of the ADA." This card has been placed in the file with the caption "Jones, Dr. John C." at its top. When you look for "Jones, Dr. John C.," you are directed to the "Ethics Committee" by **cross-referencing.**

6. **Sorting:** Sorting is the next process. The file folders ready for filing are sorted alphabetically by the captions on the tabs. Sometimes, several folders on the same subject will be grouped under a special topic in the file. If the file is alphabetically arranged, the folders within the special topic will be arranged alphabetically. For example, a dentist who is involved with

ADA work may have a special section of the file labeled "ADA" and have a dozen or more folders relating to this organization, which are filed as a group behind the ADA cardboard divider, or within a folder.

7. **Storing:** The folders are now filed in the proper place in the files. All records or papers that require filing in the dental office should be filed accurately and immediately on completion of any service that required their use. In other words, all records should be filed promptly when your work with them is completed. There should be no stack of records on your desk for days awaiting action—posting of charges, for example. The records may be needed in the operatory, and another staff member may search for many minutes for a record that has not been returned to its proper place in the files.

Removal of Filed Materials

As important as proper storage of filed materials is the appropriate way to remove the filed materials for work. Proper safeguards prevent the loss of materials by the misfiling of an item.

The bookmark method of removing a file from its normal position is a time-saver. The folder is raised until the left end can rest on the edge of the file drawer. The right bottom edge is now at the bottom of the drawer, or slightly higher. The folder is somewhat diagonally exposed. It is easy to extract or insert a paper and replace the folder without having to relocate that folder.

In another filing system in which folders must be removed for use, colored cardboards are placed in the file at the place the folder is removed. When the folder is to be replaced, it is easier to find its exact location. At this time the cardboard is removed from the file.

Charge-Out Methods

An **out-guide** (or out-folder) is a colored cardboard the size of the manilla folders. When a folder is removed from the file, an out-guide should be inserted to replace the missing folder. When a single paper is removed from a file folder, and the file folder is left in the file, a substitution card should be placed in the folder exactly where the paper was removed.

A charge-out form with space for date, item, and name of user should be attached to the out-guide or substitution form. The person who takes the filed material signs it out.

The advantages of this charge-out system are:

1. It shows the records are being used, and are not lost.
2. It tells the file clerk whom to contact for return of records.
3. It makes refiling easy by marking the place from which the material was removed.

Accuracy in Recording

Accuracy is an absolute necessity in any filing. Misfiled papers are essentially lost. Care must be exercised to be certain that papers are filed correctly.

Filing by names of individuals requires particular care. *Accurate spelling* of the name is essential. The importance of obtaining the correct spelling of a new patient's name can hardly be overemphasized. Once it has been obtained, it should be carefully printed or typed to avoid errors in transcription. Although original mistakes may be discovered later, it is difficult to rectify errors that have been recorded in a number of different places—recall files, birthday files, radiograph files, patient service and account records, and even visible index files that are used in some offices. Meticulous care at the first visit is essential.

Equal care with respect to the spelling of the name on return visits will save much lost time in searching for previous records.

Adopt a **standardized method** of filing names. Many names could be filed in more than one way. These basics may prove helpful.[1]

1. As alphabetical files of names are traditionally arranged according to the surname, it is important to determine which is the surname, and which are the first and middle names, and to record and file them in that order. Many names offer no problem.
   Example: John J. Brown
   Filed as: BROWN, John J.
2. It is customary to file a married woman's record by her own name and add her husband's name as a cross-reference.
   Example: Mary Williams Brown
   Filed as: BROWN, Mary Williams (Mrs. John J.)
3. In some names—including many of foreign derivation—the surname is not always obvious.
   When it can be determined, it is filed according to rule 1.

Example: C. D. Abd El Naur
Filed as: ABD EL Naur, C. D.
(Initials indicate abbreviations)
Otherwise, it is recorded as written.
Example: Ah Hap Akee
Filed as: AH HAP AKEE
(Note: no initials are found in this name.)

4. Hyphenated names are filed as one name, disregarding hyphen and second capital.
Example: Richard Baron-Opits
Filed as: BARON-OPITS, Richard

5. Prefixes of one or more syllables, with or without capitals and apostrophes, are considered part of the surname.
Example: Charles M. DeLacy
Filed as: DeLACY, Charles M.
Example: Joseph P. D'Agostino
Filed as: D'AGOSTINO, Joseph P.
Example: Alfred de la Durantye
Filed as: de la DURANTYE, Alfred
Example: James R. McKenzie
Filed as: McKENZIE, James R.

6. The alphabetical filing of names means that alphabetical order is used throughout the entire group of names, such as Abbott through Zenith. It also means that the same order is used from the first to the last letter of the name when filing names beginning with the same letter.
Example: John M. Anderson and George L. Abbott
Filed in this order:
      ABBOTT, George L.
      ANDERSON, John M.
b in A*b*bot precedes *n* in A*n*derson.
Example: Jane Anderson and Mary Andersen
Filed in this order: ANDERSEN, Mary
      ANDERSON, Jane
e in Anders*e*n comes before *o* in Anders*o*n.
    If there are several identical last names, the given name is used, and if necessary, the middle initial.
Example: Paul K. Anderson and Paul J. Anderson
Filed in this order: ANDERSON, Paul J.
      ANDERSON, Paul K.
    If the middle initials are the same, the middle name is used if available.
Example: Paul John Anderson and Paul James Anderson.
Filed in this order:
      ANDERSON, Paul James
      ANDERSON, Paul John

    If there is no middle initial, the rule that nothing comes before something is followed.
Example: Mary Brown and Mary A. Brown
Filed in this order: BROWN, Mary
             BROWN, Mary A.
    Initials precede a full name.
Example: J. Phillip Sorenson and James Bruce Sorenson
Filed in this order:
      SORENSON, J. Phillip
      SORENSON, James Bruce

7. If two persons have identical names, other verification must be used, such as birth dates and addresses.

8. Titles are disregarded in filing but are included in parentheses at the end of the name.
Example: Dr. J. Phillip Sorenson
Filed as: Sorenson, J. Phillip (Dr.)

Record Search

In order to find names, it is necessary for the searcher to know the rules by which they have been filed. There are inevitably a certain number of occasions when records filed alphabetically cannot be found, either because the name was originally misspelled and hence misfiled or because the name given at return visits was different. In searching for these records, time can be saved if you understand and keep in mind the likely sources of error and search in a logical manner. The majority of errors in names are caused (1) by failure to ascertain the correct spelling of names pronounced; (2) by errors in transcribing from handwriting; and (3) by transposition of first name and surname. A few typical situations follow:

1. Incorrect spelling.
  a. Names pronounced alike, or almost alike, but spelled differently.
    Examples: Jeffrey / Geoffrey
          Catherine / Katherine
          Kohn / Cohn
          Acheson / Atchison
          Kennedy / Canady
          Miller / Mueller
          Caine / Kane
          Bach / Bock
          Atkins / Adkins
          Carroll / Carrol
          Schwarzrock / Schwartzrock
          Reed / Reid

2. Errors in transcribing from handwriting.
   a. Initial letters that may look alike.
      Examples: C/G; K/R; A/O; U/V; G/Y
   b. Internal letters or combinations of letters that may look alike.
      Examples: *u/ei/ie/n; a/o; i/e; m/ni*
   c. Transposition of letters in typing.
      Examples: A*dl*er / A*ld*er
                   D*ei*gert / D*ie*gert
3. Wrong designation of surname.
   Examples:
   Henry James / HENRY, James
   Craig Douglas / CRAIG, Douglas

Occasionally problems arise that are not due to errors in recording or filing the name. One source of trouble is a change of name since the previous visit. A patient of foreign birth may have anglicized his or her name. A woman may have married or resumed her maiden name. A child's name may have been changed by adoption. A patient may have begun to use a middle name rather than the first name. When a record cannot be found for a patient who claims previous examination, tactful questioning may be necessary.

Shelf Filing with Numeric System

Often dental offices use a numeric filing system for patient service records. A **numeric file** is one in which a number is assigned to each patient record, and the records are filed by number. This file has a numeric guide file of names arranged in alphabetical order, which lists the patients by name, their birthdate or other identifying fact, and their file number. Usually this numeric guide file is a visible file. It may be a series of one-inch flat trays mounted vertically on a post so the trays rotate. Each tray has a tab on which its section of the alphabet is indicated for ease in locating the desired tray. The tray contains strips on which are typed the patient's complete name, birthdate, and file number. The assistant refers to the patient's name, reads the file number, and finds the patient record in the numeric shelf file.

The numerically filed records are usually in an open shelf file. This filing cabinet consists of a vertical series of open shelves (fig. 12.3). The records are filed edgewise on these shelves, with a patient's number or name on a visible outer end of the patient folder. A sliding door that locks in place over the records when desired can be part of the file purchased from some manufacturers.

Terminal digit numeric filing consists of three pairs of numbers for each folder, such as 71–18–01. The last two digits (01) indicate the shelf compartment in which

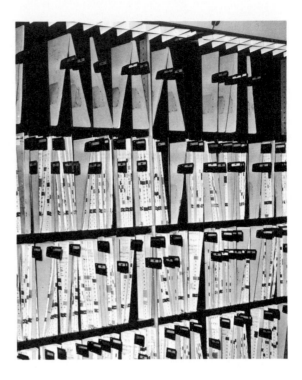

Figure 12.3
Open shelf files.

the record is filed; the middle two numbers refer to the tabs sticking out on the compartment (18); and the last two numbers on the left are the patient's folder number. Thus for the patient whose number is 71–18–01, the assistant would find his or her folder was the seventy-first folder behind the eighteenth tab in the first shelf compartment.

Patient account records will usually be filed separately but similarly. If alphabetic filing is used for patient service records, then patient account records will also be filed alphabetically.

Grouping of Patient Records

Patient records are usually filed in two or three groupings. The separation of patient records into these groupings is to place together the records of patients currently being treated. Records of patients who have not been in for treatment for a period of time are filed separately.

Thus, there may be an active file and an inactive file of patient service records. There will be a file of accounts receivable in the patient account records.

In an office where patient service and account records are a combined form, there will be an **active file** of records of patients being treated, an **accounts receivable file** of records of patients whose treatment is finished but who are still paying for their dentistry, and an **inactive file** of records of patients who are not having dental work performed at present and owe no money for past work.

The separation of patient records allows the staff to work with a smaller number of folders. With hundreds of patients receiving treatment during a year, the numbers of file folders can be voluminous. Therefore patient records are likely to be divided into active, inactive, and accounts receivable.

A fourth classification is the **dead file,** which contains records of patients who have not had dental work performed for several years. All patient records must be retained. (See the next section, "Retention of Records" for reasons.) The dentist determines the length of time during which a patient has not had any dental work performed before the record is removed from the inactive file. This period may be two years or five years—or whatever time lapse the dentist decides. At that time the record is placed in the dead file.

The use of a dead file clears the inactive file of an overwhelming number of folders that otherwise would have to be handled each time the folder of a patient seeking care is removed for use.

When it has been determined that a patient's record is to be placed in the dead file, the patient account record, X rays, recall control card (if the patient had one), and any other records concerning the patient are all placed in the patient service record file.

The patient's name, address, date of transfer, and reason for transfer are typed on a four-by-six-inch transfer card which is then filed in the **transfer file.** The patient records are sent to the dead storage file, which may be located in a storage room somewhere in the office building. Transfer card records are filed alphabetically in a separate file so labeled. Transfer of records to the dead storage area should occur on a planned schedule, such as quarterly.

Transfer cabinets of inexpensive materials are available for storing old records that must be kept. Some of these cabinets are corrugated fiberboard. The records so filed are kept in these transfer boxes in the same alphabetical or numerical order they had in the office.

Retention of Records

Why keep patients' records when the patients have presumably left the practice? One reason is that patients sometimes return to a practice that they left as long as ten years before. It is helpful to have a record of the last contact with these patients. Sometimes patients move out of town but eventually return to the community, and they return to the same dentist.

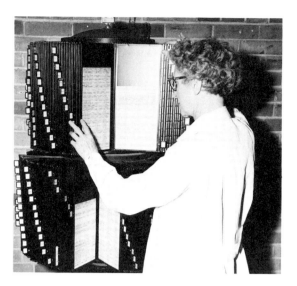

Figure 12.4
Master (cross-index) file of patients and their terminal digit numbers.

The legal reason for keeping a patient's records in a dead file is that a patient can sue the dentist for malpractice any time before the statute of limitations expires. This limitation is regulated by the state governments, and it is wise to know the length of time specified in your state.

The records of a deceased person should be retained, as well as the records of patients who no longer come for dental care, until the statute of limitations has expired. After minors reach their majority, they are privileged to sue for a period of time equal to the statute of limitations. Records of minors must therefore be kept until they are no longer considered minors, and then for the number of years specified in your state statute of limitations law. Consult an attorney who is familiar with this law.

If space is not a problem, it is wise to keep all the records of all patients, except perhaps those of a deceased person, for as long as it is possible to store them.

Files for Patient Account Records

Some patient account records are filed on cards for posting. They are vertical files or visible files (cards standing upright or cards laid in a drawer with the front edge of each card showing) (fig. 12.5).

Both visible and vertical files are used to refer to existing information and to record new information. These files are frequently used for patient account records because new entries can be added easily, payment habits of the patient can be readily ascertained, and the amount owed by any patient is easily seen.

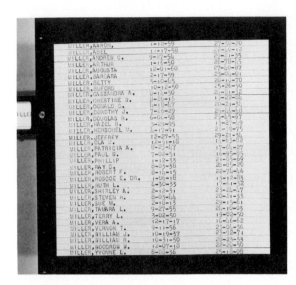

Figure 12.5
One portion of the master file shown in figure 12.4.

In some very large clinics, a motorized rotary file may be used in which the drawers are brought into position by motor. (They rotate inside a huge metal compartment.)

Filing Color Slides

The enthusiasm for photography with dentistry indicates a need for well-filed slides. The number of slides collected usually grows rapidly. To have them properly filed is useful.

Slides are used to show patients "before" and "after" shots of their mouths and to help them see the need for improvement in dental health or appearance. Slides are also used to help educate patients about dental conditions. Sometimes your dentist talks to a high school science class or other meeting, and these slides are helpful for such a presentation.

The slides may be filed by subject matter, or patient name, or whatever method of organization the dentist prefers. Sometimes, slides are mounted in a book under plastic protectors. The notation about the slide is written on the mounting page so that the slides may be replaced easily after use. Whether the slides are kept in a book or in a file, they should be filed accurately and protected from dust and moisture.

Dental Office Files: Recapitulation

The files found in a dental office may include these separate files:

1. A subject matter file
2. A patient service record active file
3. A patient service record inactive file
4. A patient account record accounts receivable file
5. A patient account record inactive file
6. A transfer file
7. A dead file (maintained outside the office)
8. A color slide file
9. A come-up file for office maintenance and routines
10. A patient recall control file
11. A birthday card control file

(The last three items are discussed in chapter 8.)

Summary

Filed papers, including records or papers that come into the office, copies of papers that leave the office, and records made for use within the office, are the memory of the office.

Dental office files include patient clinical and patient account records in addition to a subject matter file. The patient records must be kept separately from other files.

The caption on a file folder is the subject of the material stored in the folder.

A caption classification guide is maintained to assure proper filing of materials.

There are seven steps in preparing papers for filing.

There are three reasons for using a *charge-out system* for removing records from the file: to show the records are being used, to tell who has the records, and to make refiling easy by marking the place in the file from which the material was removed.

Care must be taken to spell accurately names to be put in the file. Rules for filing sequence in your office should be established and followed.

Shelf filing is a vertical series of open shelves that allow easier access to the materials.

A *numeric system of filing* known as terminal digit filing is commonly used in large offices. A *rotating visible file* may be used with this system.

Patient records are filed in four groupings: *active file, accounts receivable, inactive file,* and *dead file.*

Patient records must be kept as long as the statute of limitations indicates in the state in which the dentist is practicing. *Dead storage filing* is used to hold records of patients not currently in the practice until the statute of limitations expires, at which time the dentist may decide whether to destroy the file.

There are three questions that you can ask yourself to determine whether or not to retain a record.

Transfer of the records to dead storage should occur on a planned schedule, such as quarterly. A card indicating the transfer should be made out and kept in a file in the office.

Vertical or visible files frequently are used for patient account records.

Color slides may be filed or stored in book form.

Study Questions

1. List the three types of filing that may be used in the dental office.
2. Explain indexing.
3. Define cross-referencing and explain when it is used.
4. What steps are necessary to prepare a paper for filing?
5. State three reasons for using a charge-out system.
6. Describe a terminal digit file.
7. Describe a visible file.
8. How long must patient records be kept?
9. How do you determine which material is to be placed in dead storage?

Vocabulary

account record   record of financial transactions with one patient or family

accounts receivable file   accounts of patients still paying for services rendered, but not presently receiving treatment

active file   patient records of patients receiving treatment presently

caption   name, subject, or number written on tab of file folder

clinical record   record of dentistry performed

corrugated   shaped in alternate ridges and grooves

cross-reference   an indication in a file that the subject is filed under a different heading

dead file   file of records of patients no longer receiving care

inactive file   patient records of patients not being treated at present time

standardized   following an already established model

subject matter file   records of materials filed by subject, not including any patient records

Word Elements	
Word Element	*Example*
erythro combining form meaning: red	*erythema* abnormal redness of the skin
leuk prefix meaning: white	*leukocyte* white blood cell
melano combining form meaning: black	*melanoglossia* black tongue
xantho prefix meaning: yellow	*xanthoma* small yellow nodules generally in subcutaneous tissue
genous suffix meaning: arising or resulting from	*homogenous* similarity of structure
gen suffix meaning: to produce	*pathogen* disease producing
ics suffix meaning: practice, skill	*prosthodontics* branch of dentistry concerned with making replacements for missing teeth
ism suffix meaning: state of being, process, result of action	*bruxism* an involuntary clenching of the teeth
ize suffix meaning: subjection to action of the root word to which it is attached	*cauterize* to destroy tissue by application of an agent
logy suffix meaning: the study of	*pathology* study of nature of disease

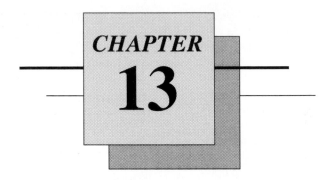

CHAPTER 13

Written Communications

The Right Impression
The Preparation Center and Equipment
Assisting the Dentist with Dictation
Note-taking Shortcuts
Business Letter Form
Signatures
Written Communications Created by the
   Dental Assistant
      The Beginning
      The Middle
      The Ending
Typing Reports
Other Writing

The Right Impression

Earlier in the text we discussed the importance of greeting new arrivals in your reception room with warmth and cordiality. We spoke of creating the right impression with the public and of considering everyone as a very important person in whom you are interested.

The same philosophy in working with people is necessary in written communications. The letters, reports, and statements that leave your office tell a tale about you, your dentist, and the way your office operates. What sort of impression is being created?

What is the receiver going to think about the office if a letter is received that is written on the cheapest typing paper available without a printed letterhead? In addition, the typist has struck over some errors and erased others, leaving smudges. No planning was used in creating the format of the letter. Some words are misspelled and grammatical construction is incorrect, to say nothing of inadequate punctuation.

Obviously, the recipient will wonder and may feel sorry for the dentist who is unable to hire a better employee, but may also wonder whether the chairside dental assisting in the office is of the same poor quality—whether instruments are sterile when they need to be and whether this dentist is capable of providing patients with adequate care.

Reports from a dental office ought to be on bond paper of fine quality. It should use the same grade of bond paper for letterhead stationery on which the dentist's name, address (plus zip code), and telephone number, including area code, have been printed or engraved. The stationery should be businesslike in appearance. This does not necessarily eliminate an artistic, beautiful design, or even the use of sophisticated color: off-white, pastel, or bright. Effective letterhead designs that distinguish the stationery are often used. The minimum requirement is a printed letterhead giving the name of the dentist with his or her degrees after the name, the street address under the name, including city, state, and zip code under the street address.

Envelopes to match the stationery should be available, with a printed return address on them. Envelopes for other purposes should be available, too. Window envelopes are often used for billing purposes. The dentist's name and address should be printed in the upper left corner.

The administrative dental assistant who is assigned to secretarial duties should keep the same kind of inventory of stationery supplies as the chair assistant keeps of dental supplies. Prior to running out of stationery, an order should be placed in ample time to receive the new supply before it is needed.

A satisfactory grade of paper should be kept for carbon copies. Plenty of high-quality carbon should also be available. Correction sheets and fluids are excellent aids in making neat, almost unnoticeable corrections. Erasers are also helpful. Some typewriters now have mechanisms that hold correction ribbon. By pressing the x key, the correction ribbon is activated.

It is possible to purchase copy paper for which no carbon is necessary. Simply place the sheet behind the original letterhead you are to type on, and the copy appears on the second sheet. This paper is somewhat more expensive but is, perhaps, worth it when you consider the cost and bother of carbon paper.

Some offices use a duplicating machine to make copies of all letters and reports, eliminating the necessity for carbon paper.

The Preparation Center and Equipment

The typing area within the office should be equipped with a well-built desk of proper height for typing, drawer or cabinet space for all the supplies that are needed at the typewriter, a rack on which to rest copy (whether the copy be a report or a secretary's notebook), adequate light, a good typewriter, and a chair that encourages the best posture for typing.

Should any of these items be missing, consult your dentist and try to acquire the necessary equipment to make it possible for you to do an excellent job of public relations via the written communications from your office.

The typewriter should receive your best care. It should be covered at night, and cleaned and dusted each morning before it is used. How you care for the machine will be determined by the kind of typewriter you are using. Whatever the type of machine, a professional inspection and cleaning by a typewriter service is most desirable. It can be arranged on a contract basis. If this type of service is used, a representative will call regularly—monthly, quarterly, semiannually, or even weekly if desired. Some of these services also include the privilege of calling the service department for any problems encountered between the regularly scheduled visits of the service personnel.

Many typewriters use film ribbon—ribbon that is used only once. Other typewriters are supplied with ribbon that is used until the ink is faint. Should this type of ribbon be supplied for the machine you use, change the ribbon frequently enough to produce legible communications. In addition, clean the keys frequently with a brush to avoid filled-in letters.

If the typewriter is a standard machine, letters may at times be out of alignment. Keep a record of any keys that strike a little higher or lower than the rest so that when the serviceman arrives, you can give him a list of the keys that need realignment. If the machine is a "Selectric" typewriter, key alignment will not be a problem since the mechanism for typing is somewhat different from the standard typewriter, and the letters cannot be out of alignment.

Some offices will have a computer or word processor with a printer instead of, or in addition to, a typewriter. The use and care of such equipment requires special training that will be provided. In today's dental office, not only is the typewriter or computer a necessity, its effective operation is essential.

If you are skilled in using shorthand, you know the appropriate supplies that you need to keep available. If you work in an office in which a dictaphone or tape recorder is used instead of shorthand, the typing center must also contain the necessary equipment for playing tapes of records and listening to them without the patients in the reception room or any of the rest of the staff being able to hear. Headphones or an earpiece similar to a hearing aid are usually provided.

There are some aids for working with a dictating machine that can be helpful. For example, if the dictator has not keyed his or her letters or commented at the end of each letter about the enclosures for that letter, it is a good idea to keep a notebook handy and list the enclosures as he or she comments on them during the dictation of the letter. It is also desirable to listen once to the tape before beginning to type the letter. In this way, you will pick up the corrections and have a good idea of the length of the letter before you make that excellent copy that is to leave the office.

Assisting the Dentist with Dictation

Although letter writing may be infrequent in the dental office, it does occur in some offices.

A planned time for dictation is a part of good office organization.

You can help your dentist most if you will adopt the attitude that you are not expected to assume anything. Ask about anything you do not understand. Ask immediately, or if he or she objects to being interrupted, ask at the close of the dictation.

Be certain that you understand names: full names, spelling, titles, and addresses. After you become acquainted with your dentist, most of these names will be familiar to you and will not present the problem they do the first time you hear them.

When your dentist gives you instructions about the correspondence, put a number by the part of the letter to which the instructions apply and write your instructions as an additional note to your work with the same number by it. In this way each instruction will be numbered, and there can be no mistake about which instruction fits which piece of dictation.

Be sure your dentist dictates slowly enough for you to be accurate in your work. It is inconceivable that anyone would attempt to take dictation from a dentist without first having mastered the most frequent dental terms used by this particular dentist.

When you are certain you know just what is expected of you and that your dentist has finished the dictation for this period, take with you the material to be answered and your notebook and pencils, being certain to leave the chair in which you sat in its proper position. (Be a good housekeeper. Keep looking for straightening-up jobs as you work around the office.)

Prompt transcription of shorthand notes, dictaphone records, or tapes is most desirable. If the dentist has not indicated which material is most important, it is necessary for the secretary to use her or his best judgment in deciding the order in which to type the notes.

Make at least one copy of every paper that leaves the office. Sometimes a dentist prefers to have two copies. This is usually true in an office that uses a follow-up file.

Occasionally it is necessary for a secretary to correct a statement found in the dictation. If the statement is unclear, if the grammar is incorrect, or if for some reason it is necessary to reevaluate the statement, it is important that the dentist be consulted before any change is made in the dictated notes. It is absolutely necessary to correct any errors before the transcript leaves the office, even if an extra consultation with the dentist is required.

Note-taking Shortcuts

Sometimes it is necessary for an employee who has not had shorthand to take dictation or notes from an employer. The trick is to work out a system of abbreviation which may be unique to you, but which you can understand.

You can learn a system like Gregg Notehand or you can make your own from longhand abbreviations. The longhand abbreviations are not as fast, but if you haven't already learned a system, longhand abbreviations will help you until you can learn one. The only caution is to be sure to write legibly.

For example, drop all unnecessary letters.

learn = lrn	can = cn
abbreviations = abrvns	communications = cmcns
true = tru	may = ma
be = b	become = bcum
you = u	our = r
for = 4	are = r

JOHN C. RAEYWEN, D.D.S.
104 Any Street
Anytown, Anystate 12345
612-926-1414

December 15, 19___

Mrs. Alfred Swenson
234 Norwegian Street
Anytown, Anystate 12615

Dear Mrs. Swenson:

The lefse which you gave me yesterday was delicious. My family and I enjoyed it last evening, and the "ohs" and "ahs" over its delicacy would have pleased you. My wife and children join me in expressing our appreciation to you. We know that making lefse is a difficult task which only an expert can accomplish with the results which you brought me.

I have read your X rays and am delighted to report that you have no work to be done at this time. We will look forward to seeing you in six months at the time of your regular recall in June.

Thank you for your generous gift to us.

Cordially,

John C. Raeywen, D.D.S.

Figure 13.1
A well-planned letter with even margins.

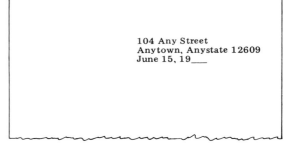

Figure 13.2
A letterhead typed on plain typing paper.

104 Any Street
Anytown, Anystate 12609
June 15, 19___

JOHN C. RAEYWEN, D.D.S.
104 Any Street
Anytown, Anystate 12345
612-926-1414

June 15, 19___

Mr. James R. Jones
251 South Magnolia Avenue
Anytown, Anystate 12610

Figure 13.3
Letterhead stationery properly dated and addressed.

This system can be used for dental terminology, which is long and hard to write. Be sure you have a medical dictionary for unscrambling the abbreviations at the time of deciphering.

Business Letter Form

Design the letter that is to leave the office so that it is an excellent representative of you and your dentist. From one point of view a letter is an ambassador—it *represents* the office. Sometimes it is the only criteria by which the receiver can judge the quality of dentistry and professionalism of the office.

Here are some helpful suggestions.

1. A letter should be a beautiful work of art—even margins at both right and left sides and preferably the same margin on the top, with a slightly larger one at the bottom whenever possible. Consider the letterhead as part of the letter when planning composition of the page to look like a picture (fig. 13.1).

2. All business letters have the writer's address and the date at the top. If your dentist's stationery has a printed letterhead, type the date below the address. If your letters are written on plain typing paper, the address and the date are typed on the right-hand side of the paper, at the top (fig. 13.2).

3. The name of the person to whom the letter is written and his or her address are placed on the left-hand side. This information is often referred to as the "inside address" (fig. 13.1 and 13.3).

4. In formal business letters the salutation is still "Dear Mr. Blank," or "My dear Mr. Milquetoast".

5. The body of the letter is then typed.

6. A complimentary closing follows, but instead of the formal "Yours truly," more and more business people are substituting "Sincerely."

7. Leave space for the dentist's signature. Type the dentist's name and degree letters below the space. Correspondence dictated by the dentist should be signed by the dentist. In the rare instance that this procedure is impossible, sign the dentist's name, initial the signature, and write a note explaining why the dentist was unable to sign the letter (left town abruptly, for example). Of course, any letters composed by the assistant should be signed by the assistant.

8. Be certain to consult your dictionary if you are in doubt about the spelling of any words. See that the letter is correctly punctuated, also.

9. Avoid typographical errors. Correct any errors neatly with fluid or tape. Such corrections should be unnoticeable.

10. Single-space letters of normal length. Double-space between the paragraphs. If a letter is very short, double-space it.

11. Decide on the form of the letter. If you prefer to use block form, there will be no indentation. The division between paragraphs is recognized by the double-spacing. If you wish to use an indentation at the beginning of a paragraph, this is acceptable form. The first sentence of the paragraph is usually indented five spaces from the left margin. Double-spacing between the paragraphs then becomes a matter of choice rather than necessity.

12. The length of a letter determines the margins and placement of the letter on the page. If there is any speculation that a letter is too long for one page, widen the margins and make it a two-page letter rather than crowd it all on one page.

Normally, the second page of a letter is written on plain paper of the same quality as the stationery with the dentist's name imprinted on it. It is numbered -2- at the top and frequently bears a line of type giving the names of the addressee, sender, and the date (fig. 13.4).

13. It is sometimes necessary to type up a rough draft for the dentist to read prior to final typing.

Signatures

After you type a letter, *proofread* it. If it is perfect, clip the enclosures and envelope to it. Place all letters on the dentist's desk. The dentist should always sign his or her own letters.

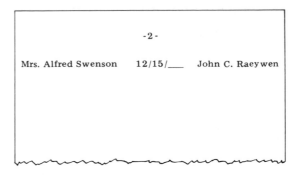

Figure 13.4
Sample top for second page of letter.

After the letters have been signed by the dentist, fold them and put them in the envelopes with the proper enclosures. File the carbon copies and the letters that prompted the dentist to write.

Be sure to weigh any letters that are more than two sheets of paper to be certain you have the correct postage on them.

Written Communications Created by the Dental Assistant

During your career as a dental assistant, you may be required to write some original memoranda and perhaps some original letters of your own. The composition of such letters is important.

Most letters are written with the purpose of getting someone to do something willingly. The advantage and desirability of the action suggested must be "sold." The letter should be planned to bring about willing cooperation; in the letter use persuasion rather than force, inducement rather than threats. The grammar and punctuation must be correct, and the sentences must be complete.

Business correspondence today aims for simplicity and conciseness. Letters are supposed to tell a story in the fewest number of words. Expression is direct and to the point. At the same time, business letters play an important part in developing good public relations; therefore, the qualities of friendliness, courtesy, and thoughtfulness are necessary.

The business letter can be divided into three parts: the opening—to prepare the reader for a favorable reception; the middle—to give the reasons why the reader should do as you wish; and the closing—to stimulate the desired action.

Business letters must create a receptive attitude in the reader before any action is suggested. Because every person is interested primarily in himself or herself, the beginning of the letter should be about the reader.

The Beginning

A good opening gains the attention of the reader. It is an opportunity to make a good impression. Don't waste the opening on trivialities. Capture its full value.

How? By thinking—and writing—of the reader's interest. Put the reader in the center of the stage. Search for the point in the particular letter you are writing that will please the listener.

Just as the salesperson relies on a friendly smile and a cordial handshake to win the prospect before making a sales presentation, so also should letter writers use the letter opening to help to establish a cordial relationship.

Letters written from the *We, Me, Us, Our, I, My* viewpoint are less likely to bring results than those that begin with the readers' interests. Examples of such letter openings include: "I feel sure that you overlooked this statement," "I am afraid that you have overlooked us in the matter of payment," and "We need money in order to pay our own bills."

Imagine the jolt to the reader receiving a letter that begins:

We have made many requests for payment of your delinquent account, and your failure to respond is very disappointing. You have not kept your word. We must take strong action to force payment.

Admittedly, this paragraph might be contained in a letter sent to a person whose account is in poor condition. However, if that person were to come into the office personally to discuss the account, do you suppose the conversation would begin so abruptly? Surely some pleasantries would precede the business discussion.

Yet many collection letters swing into offensive action with the first sentence. The thunderbolts are shot without any preliminaries. The usual result is that the reader is upset and angered, and chances of securing favorable action are much lessened.

Here, for example, are two openings selected from letters dealing with the partial-payment problem.

1. We regret that we have been unable to secure your cooperation in maintaining your account according to our established terms.
2. Your partial payments on your account show a splendid spirit of cooperation. For that we thank you.

Which one do you suppose would make the patient more inclined to improve his payment pattern? Actually, there is not too much difference in words, but there is a great difference in the approach and attitude of the writer.

The Middle

The message—why the reader should do as you wish—should be stated clearly; however, few business letters should be more than four paragraphs in length. Just looking at a full sheet of solid type discourages attention. Cluttering a letter with unnecessary explanations or arguments lessens its effectiveness. Ask yourself, What does this mean? Can I say the same thing more simply? Remove all unnecessary wording, but do write what you feel must be communicated. Use a separate paragraph for each main subject or argument.

Preserve the patient's dignity and self-respect. It is easy to make strong statements in your letters, but nothing is gained by such actions. Keep your own temper; the reader will more likely keep his or hers. Write only what you would be willing to say in person. Use restraint. Remember you are not going to be present to reassure with a smile or give the inflection that clarifies the meaning you intend.

The Ending

The ending of the letter is the climax. The ending idea should be a fairly short paragraph by itself.

Select the best possible action you wish the reader to take. Together with the positive ending, the appeal to immediate and definite action, try for some statement that builds goodwill. Those two direct words, *thank you,* can be used much more often than they are.

The effective letter, then, begins on the *you* note. It attracts the favorable attention of the reader. Something is said to create a favorable atmosphere for the message. In the middle, the reasons why the reader should follow a course of action are stated. The last paragraph is the ending and the *we* angle. It is here that the reader is told what the writer wants done.

The formula is: you-why-we, or interest-explanation-action. Writing a letter using this formula is more likely to produce the desired results in action and in relationships.

The sample letters that follow are not meant to be copied. They are examples of the form that might receive good results. You may use them as a guide, but make your letter to your patient a personal letter in your own style of writing.

Figure 13.5 is a sample of a mild letter to be used after an impersonal series of stickers or stamps has brought no results and it is felt a letter would be more effective.

The same principles of writing business letters can be applied in a letter that is not about collections. Figure 13.6 is a fine example of a letter in which you-why-we and interest-explanation-action are effectively expressed. Here the dentist has opened with a pleasant

JOHN C. RAEYWEN, D.D.S.
104 Any Street
Anytown, Anystate 12345
612-926-1414

Mr. John C. Patient
560 Any Street
Anytown, Anystate 12345

Dear Mr. Patient:

Just a note to tell you that if we can be helpful in the matter of your account, we would welcome the opportunity.

The usual reminders have been sent to you, but we have had no word from you. Perhaps you have been waiting until you could pay the whole bill at one time.

Sometimes, in every family, unexpected circumstances arise that upset well-laid plans. We certainly would be willing to make special arrangements with you should that be the case.

In any event, it is important that you come in or write us as soon as possible. You will find us most cooperative.

Cordially yours,

John C. Raeywen, D.D.S.

Figure 13.5
A collection letter.

February 22, _____

Mr. Fred J. Schwaemmle
Delta Air Lines
Atlanta Airport
Atlanta, Georgia

Dear Mr. Schwaemmle:

It's a beautiful day in Chicago this morning and a perfect day for Delta to be flying.

Our American Academy of Dental Practice Administration is looking forward to your Delta-ing to Chicago to speak before us at 9:00 A.M., Friday, February 2, 1968, at the Conrad Hilton Hotel.

I have personally admired the advances of Delta through the years and felt they had a story to tell about the philosophy of Communication and Motivation in developing the wonderful personnel presentation they offer to the public.

You are probably aware that dentistry is one of the greatest needs of modern man. All we in dentistry have to do is to make people want that need. In other words, it is our challenge to make them aware of their problem and create a want of their needs. This requires the type of mental attitude that I have witnessed in Delta personnel nationally.

It is hoped that the foregoing two paragraphs give you an understanding of the objectives I have in mind. Would you please correspond with me and give me the title of your presentation. Also, would you require one or one and a half hours to present your story? Please do not hesitate to telephone me if you have any personal concern that we could better handle by direct communication.

With kindest regards,

Herbert Gustavson, D.D.S.

Figure 13.6
An excellent example of letter writing.

reference to the firm of the man to whom the letter is addressed. This is the *you* approach. The writer capitalized on the recipient's interest in himself and his business, then the writer tied the reader's interest to the writer's interest—and finally asked for the action he desired, even suggesting a long-distance telephone call for more direct communication. The last paragraph, the closing, asks for action and attempts to make it as easy as possible for the reader to comply. This letter illustrates the three steps in a business letter: interest, explanation, and action.

Typing Reports

Some dentists use a tape recorder to record their initial examination of a patient. A dentist will often have this recording typed as a case study and included in the patient's record envelope. Whether it is typed on a special report form or on plain typing paper, be sure to proofread the record for accuracy before you file it.

Reports to other dentists, to physicians, or to hospitals require careful typing on appropriate paper. The finished report should be typed with neat margins, no errors, and no smudges. Each page of the report should bear the title and page number. (The title may be a patient's name if the report is a case study.)

You may also type reports on special forms. Use the skills you have learned in adjusting the typewriter platen so that you can type on the lines provided on the form.

Lengthy reports of committee meetings should be carefully prepared, single-spaced, and properly indented. The object of indentations is to provide ease in reading.

Form letters, prepared individually as a personal letter, are often sent from the dental office. The dentist may have composed several special letters to use when responding to specific requests. When the dentist asks you to use one of these form letters, type it as carefully as you type a letter he or she dictates. An example of such a form letter might be a thank-you note for referral of a patient.

```
                                SUBJECT:  HISTORY

      Prinz, Herman. Dental Chronology. Philadelphia:
        Lea & Febiger, 1945. p. 96.

      At a meeting of the American Society of Dental
      Surgery, Chapin Harris motioned, "The use of
      amalgam was declared to be malpractice "—a mo-
      tion which was rescinded in 1850, ending the
      Amalgam War. (original motion in 1843)
```

Figure 13.7
Example of notes for research.

I WANT TO TALK TODAY ABOUT INTEGRITY.

I HOPE THAT AFTER I AM THROUGH

WITH MY REMARKS SOMETHING OF

THE SHINING AND WONDERFUL QUALITY

OF THIS VIRTUE WILL REMAIN WITH US.

Figure 13.8
A readable sample manuscript with enlarged type.

Insurance reports must often be completed. It is important to keep a carbon copy of each report for future reference.

Other Writing

There are other types of original writing to be accomplished in the dentist's office. The dentist may be conducting some research and thus needs help in gathering data and bibliographical material. You may be asked to help in this work. It will require good note-taking on the books and sources you read in the dental library. Be sure you prepare the bibliography correctly: copy the author, title, publisher, date of publication, place of publication, and any page numbers to which you refer in your notes. Copy the page numbers of the material you read so that your dentist can refer to the quotation (fig. 13.7).

When it is necessary to type the final manuscript, follow the rules in whatever procedure manual your dentist uses. There are several, and different universities require different manuals.

When you have completed the typing, proofread with care to be absolutely certain your copy is correct.

Sometimes your dentist may be asked to read a paper before a society or study club. Special typing preparation will be needed for this presentation. If you have a Selectric typewriter, you can purchase an Orator ball of type, which is enlarged print. Or you can rent a special typewriter with convention type, which prints the large letters used to make name tags at conventions. The use of this size type, triple-spaced, makes a very readable manuscript. However, the capital letters of your own typewriter and proper spacing of the sentences will also facilitate the reading of a paper. Adequate space around the sentences allows the reader to see them in units and lessens the possibility of losing one's place in the manuscript (fig. 13.8 and 13.9).

```
I WANT TO TALK TODAY ABOUT INTEGRITY.

I HOPE THAT AFTER I AM THROUGH WITH MY REMARKS

SOMETHING OF THE SHINING AND WONDERFUL QUALITY

OF THIS VIRTUE WILL REMAIN WITH US.


        INTEGRITY IS A LATIN WORD

            WHICH MEANS UNFLAWED,

                UNCORRUPTED, UNTAMPERED WITH.
```

Figure 13.9
A readable sample manuscript using capital letters on a standard typewriter.

Summary

A proper impression should be created by the written materials that leave the dental office. Adequate and proper supplies are necessary. Shortcuts should be visualized and used for accomplishing the tasks necessary to project this impression.

When taking dictation you can assist your dentist by asking questions about anything you do not *completely understand.*

A business letter must conform to specifications. Thirteen suggestions are given.

Typing reports will be a necessary part of the work of the dental assistant and should conform to the preference of the dentist. All typed materials must be proofread for accuracy.

After the dentist's signature has been written, promptly fold, insert, seal, and mail the material.

Shortcuts in note-taking are desirable. Omit all unnecessary words such as *the, a,* and *an.* Work out a system of abbreviation that you understand.

The dental assistant who composes letters signed by herself or himself should use care in the preparation of these letters.

A dentist who is doing research may have his or her assistant gather data and bibliographical material. Careful note-taking and references are important. The use of a manuscript manual in typing these reports is desirable.

Study Questions

1. Why should you ask your dentist about anything that you do not understand during dictation?
2. Why is prompt transcription essential?
3. Describe a well-written business letter.
4. Describe a system of shortcut note-taking.
5. Describe a well-written letter composed by an assistant.
6. What must you include in your notes when you are gathering data and bibliographical material for your dentist?

Word Elements	
Word Element	*Example*
aer combining form meaning: air	*aerobic* living only where oxygen is present
ambi prefix meaning: on both sides	*ambidextrous* a person who can perform manual skills with either hand equally well is ambidextrous, whereas other persons are either left-handed or right-handed
aniso prefix meaning: unequal, dissimilar	*anisocytosis* inequality in size of cells, especially RBC's
homo, homeo combining form meaning: same, similar	*homogenous* same kind, similar in makeup throughout
ortho prefix meaning: normal, straight, right	*orthodontia* dental specialty in which malocclusions of teeth and jaws are corrected
para prefix meaning: beside, beyond	*paralgesia* any condition marked by abnormal pain
steno combining form meaning: contracted, narrow	*stenosis* narrowing or stricture of a duct, canal, or vessel
hydro, hyd combining form meaning: relationship to water, hydrogen	*hydrated* combined with water, forming a hydrate or hydroxide
phono combining form meaning: sound	*phonetics* study of production and classification of speech sounds
oid suffix meaning: resemblance, form of the thing specified	*celluloid* a thermoplastic composed, in part, of cellulose

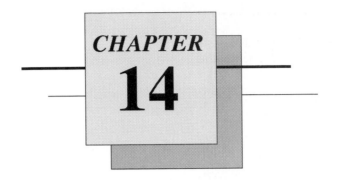

CHAPTER 14

Arrangements for the Meeting-minded Dentist

Reservations
    Travel and Convention Reservations
    Hotel Reservations
Travel Necessities
Preparation for Return
    Homecoming
Arrangements for Meetings and Conferences

Reservations

Special preparation may be needed by your dentist for a meeting of a dental society. A notice of the meeting is usually received through the mail, together with a request for notification of attendance. Sometimes a reservation for luncheon or dinner is necessary.

If your dentist is to attend the meeting, the necessary time must be blocked off in the appointment book and the proper notifications returned to the secretary of the society. If your dentist is an officer of the organization, there may be additional activities for you—secretarial notes to be typed (and even duplicated), treasurer's reports to be prepared, dues to collect, and programs to prepare. Should your dentist be responsible for a program, it is sometimes necessary for you to contact the speakers and arrange for their accommodations. Your dentist, if president, is responsible for the **agenda** (plan of what is to be discussed at the meeting). This agenda should be typed in advance.

Travel and Convention Reservations

Your dentist may attend conventions, study courses, and association meetings held in some other city. Considerable planning is required to complete the necessary reservations for travel, hotel, and attendance at the meetings. This is detail work that you can do. You may be asked to take care of such details for other travel as well.

Let us assume that one day your dentist lays a folder on your desk and says, "I plan to go to this convention. Please make the necessary reservations."

Look over the convention material. Write the following information on a sheet of paper.

1. The date and hour the convention begins
2. The date and hour the convention closes
3. The location of convention headquarters (both building and city)
4. Any special events that require reservations and/or extra fees
5. Where the convention fees are to be sent— if it is wise to register in advance—and what those fees are

The brochure describing the convention usually lists the reservations that are made with the convention personnel. Often this includes hotel. (The persons responsible for the convention usually order a block of rooms held for the convention attendees. By using the order form enclosed with the brochure, you can obtain accommodations for your dentist.) In addition, the convention brochure will offer information about luncheons, dinners, and special meetings for which there may be an added fee.

Ask your dentist the following questions and write down the answers:

1. Do you wish to arrive by the opening hour of the convention?
2. Do you plan to stay until the conclusion of the last meeting?
3. Do you have any preference for hotels? Any instructions about cost?
4. Are you an associate member of the organization holding the meeting? (Associate members have some special privileges and often pay lower fees. Some dentists belong to out-of-state organizations as associate members.)
5. Do you wish to attend any of the special events? (Ask this question only if there are any courses or luncheons requiring advance registrations.)
6. How do you wish to travel?
   a. If by air, ask whether limousine service to the airport is desired.
   b. If the limousine is to be used, where is it to pick him or her up?
   c. Ask what class of air travel is to be used.
   d. Ask whether you should reserve a rental car for arrival.
   e. If your dentist is to travel by car, ask whether you should have a travel agency plan a routing.
7. Do you plan to travel alone, or for how many shall I make reservations?

With the written answers before you, you can complete the entire convention registration, disturbing your dentist only for check-signing.

Write to the address in the convention brochure to make the reservations your dentist has requested, including the hotel reservation if it is to be made through the convention headquarters. If hotel accommodations are not reserved through the convention bureau, you will need to make them or have a travel agency make them.

The transportation reservations must also be made either by you or an agency. Should your dentist have a travel agency preference, call them. If not, use the agency that is most helpful in answering your questions.

1. Ask for the most economical air fare available in the class of travel your dentist prefers.
2. Now is the time to request a rental car for arrival.

3. Get a firm commitment on the price of the hotel or motel before making a reservation.

4. When the reservations are made, ask about ticket delivery. Are the tickets delivered to you or must you pick them up? If you are expected to pick up the tickets, ask when they will be ready and where you are to pick them up.

Hotel Reservations

However the hotel reservations are made, you will need to include this information:

1. Name of your dentist
2. Number of persons in your dentist's party
3. Type of room and beds desired (accommodations)
4. Date of arrival
5. Time of arrival
6. Number of nights room is needed

If you are making the reservations personally, indicate whether the confirmation of the reservation should be made by mail, telegram, or a long distance telephone call, depending upon the time at your disposal in finding your dentist a room. Some hotels require a deposit to hold a reserved room. It is therefore wise to include a sentence that states that a deposit will be sent if it is desired.

You will receive a reply. If there are no rooms available at your dentist's first-choice hotel, try the second-choice hotel, and so on until you locate a room.

If the convention is the national convention, blanks for hotel reservations will be found in the *Journal of the American Dental Association,* in the issue published approximately six months prior to the convention.

Travel Necessities

Itinerary: Now you are ready to write an itinerary for your dentist. It tells your dentist in outline form just what to do from the time the transportation leaves.

Attach all tickets, necessary papers, and a convention pamphlet.

It is important for you to keep a copy of your dentist's itinerary and know how to contact him or her in an emergency. Perhaps your dentist will set up specified times for telephone calls. The sample itinerary (fig. 14.1) is a very simple one.

It is possible that your dentist may travel to several places on the same trip. Then an itinerary might look something like figure 14.2.

Funds for travel: Your dentist should have traveler's checks, credit cards, or money orders available for his or her use.

Dr. Raeywen:

Your plane leaves from the International Airport at 3:30 p.m., VA Flight 762, Sunday, November 19.

You arrive in Convention City at 4:30 p.m. (3-hour trip, cross 2 time zones).

You have a room at Convention Hotel. A $50.00 deposit has been made on it. Your registration for the special course is attached.

You leave Convention City on Thursday, November 23, at 4 p.m., on VA Flight 681 and arrive at International Airport at 9 p.m. (lost 2 hours).

Figure 14.1
A short itinerary.

Ordinarily the convention hotel will cash checks for small amounts for a registered guest, but should some emergency arise, added funds may be needed. Credit cards offer considerable help in providing the extra funds.

Preparation for Return

While your dentist is away is an excellent time to do some of the thorough housecleaning tasks that are difficult to accomplish when patients are constantly present. In the one-dentist office, any accumulated tasks can be accomplished. If you have more than one dentist in your office, there probably isn't a less busy time.

Be sure you have cared for the dentist's mail and have it ready—grouped according to importance.

Homecoming

When dentists return from trips, they are usually somewhat fatigued from travel. The patients who have been unable to see them are anxious and sometimes aggressive about seeing the dentist now. You will do your dentist and the entire office staff a favor if you will see that the schedule is light the first two or three days after the dentist has returned to the office. There will be more emergencies those days that will help absorb any free time caused by scheduling lightly. Your dentist will appreciate the opportunity to ease back into a tough schedule, rather than feeling two days' work has been scheduled for each day.

The same is true of the last two days before the dentist leaves. A little time to prepare for the meeting or vacation prevents the dentist from starting on the trip exhausted.

A leisurely send-off and a cordial, but easy, welcome back is desirable. Hold the unpleasant things out of the way, if you can, until the routine is under control.

"Doctor, the autoclave broke while you were away and the water pipe upstairs leaked all over the lab ceiling and we're simply going to have to turn Mrs.

DATE	LOCATION	FLIGHT TIME	FLIGHT NUMBER	AIRLINE
Sunday 2/11	Lv. Chicago Ar. Salt Lake City (overnight in S.L.C.)	3:15 P.M. 5:47 P.M.	# 77 (dinner flight)	Western
Monday	Lv. Salt Lake City Ar. San Francisco (overnight in San Francisco)	9:00 A.M. 11:35 A.M.	# 727	Western
Tuesday	Lv. San Francisco Ar. Portland (overnight in Portland)	10:15 A.M. 11:15 A.M.	# 726	Western
Wednesday	Lv. Portland Ar. Chicago	10:58 A.M. 2:30 P.M.	# 860 (lunch flight)	United Air Lines

Figure 14.2
A sample itinerary for a long trip.

Jones's account over to the collectors and Mr. Gray says he's going to sue" is not the greeting your dentist should receive. A chance to feel pleasant about the office before you discuss the problems that arose during the dentist's absence is important. Most of the problems will keep a few hours. Then present them—one at a time, please.

Arrangements for Meetings and Conferences

If your dentist happens to be deeply involved with organizational work, it may be necessary for you to make arrangements for meetings for large groups of people. Creating successful meetings begins with preplanning for them. The reservation of the meeting place on the proper date and at the proper time is the first step. Your dentist should tell you when the group is to meet and how many members are anticipated. He or she may specify the place where the meeting is to be held. He or she may ask you to find a large enough space for the meeting.

Call the hotel manager, or the resident manager if it is a meeting hall rather than a hotel, and state the name of the organization, the anticipated size of the group, and the date and time of the meeting. Ask for a written verification of the space, the cost, and any other information your dentist may need.

A small group will often meet in the library or study rooms of the local dental society. If this is the plan for the meeting for which you must obtain space, call the executive secretary of the local dental society and ask for the reservation for the time and date for which your dentist has made a request. Be sure you have written confirmation of the time and date for any meeting.

If you should be asked to make reservations for a very large meeting, the procedure is the same. However, very large meetings, such as state dental society meetings, are usually arranged by a special employee of the dental society.

The second step is to see that the notices of meetings are properly prepared. To accomplish this task, be sure you have the correct time and place of the meeting. If someone is to speak, be certain you have the correct spelling of the person's name and the topic. When you have the copy accurately prepared for reproduction, it is wise to check with your dentist for accuracy before the meeting notice is printed.

If the notices are to be sent to a small number of people—say ten—perhaps you may use a copier. However, it is possible that a letter service or a printer will be engaged to prepare enough copies of the notice. Be sure to have this order prepared in ample time.

The third step is to have an accurate mailing list of the correct names and addresses, including zip codes, of all the persons to whom the notice is to be sent. With the self-adhering mailing labels now available, it is probably easier to type the addresses on labels and attach them to the envelopes or postcards.

If your dentist is president of the meeting, it is usually necessary to have an agenda—a typed listing of what is to occur at the meeting. It begins with calling the meeting to order and proceeds through the order of business to be considered. Since this order is determined by the rules of order in conducting a meeting, it would be a good idea to have a reference copy of a rules-of-order book in your library. A sample agenda appears in figure 14.3.

If your dentist happens to be secretary of the organization, there will be minutes of the meeting to be prepared and usually distributed. He or she will bring you the notes or the tape of the meeting. You will transcribe it and have him or her read it for approval. Then it will be duplicated by whatever method is correct, depending on the number of copies to be made. If the number is large, perhaps the preparation will not be made in the office; that is, a printer will do this part of the work.

```
                        AGENDA
CALL TO ORDER
MINUTES OF THE LAST MEETING
TREASURER'S REPORT
OLD BUSINESS
     Report on school Examination program
NEW BUSINESS
     Consideration of new members' applications
     The Memorial Scholarship Fund
     Report of the Committee on Flouridation of the
        Water Supply
COMMITTEE REPORTS
     Finance
     Publications
ADJOURNMENT
```

Figure 14.3

A sample agenda.

The distribution of the minutes may be your job. If so, address another set of labels and mail out the minutes as soon as you are told to do so. Some organizations expect the members to pick up the minutes of the last meeting at the current meeting, avoiding the expense of mailing. If this is the case, you must see that the minutes of the last meeting are ready for your dentist to take to the meeting.

Summary

Special preparation for a meeting of a dental society includes proper reservation of time in the appointment book, preparation of any materials for which your dentist is responsible, preparation of the itinerary, and collection of reservations, ticket, and the like, should the meeting be in another city.

The preparation for the dentist's return should include special cleanup of the office, should this be possible, and light appointing of patients the first two or three days in order to give the dentist a chance to readjust to the workload.

Conference arrangements are made by the dental assistant should her or his dentist be in charge of some area of preparation for such a meeting. The dentist should be prepared with any papers for which he or she is responsible.

Study Questions

1. Describe an agenda. Under what circumstances might you be asked to prepare an agenda?
2. List the things you must do if your dentist attends a convention in another city.
3. What is an itinerary? Why should you have a copy?
4. What can you do while your dentist is away to make your work easier after his or her return?
5. Why should the schedule be light for the first two or three days after the dentist's return? Prior to the trip?
6. Your dentist is responsible for calling a meeting of ten members of a committee who will meet in the dental society rooms. What are your responsibilities?
7. Your dentist is secretary of the dental society. What are your responsibilities?

Vocabulary

agenda   plan of topics to be considered at a meeting
itinerary   route or proposed outline of a trip

Word Elements	
Word Element	*Example*
algia, alg suffix meaning: pain	***neuralgia*** pain that extends along a nerve
esthes combining form meaning: perceive, feel	***esthetic*** pertaining to beauty, the improvement of appearance
sens combining form meaning: to perceive, to feel	***sensitivity*** a state of responsiveness to things felt
plas, plast prefix meaning: mold, shape	***plastic*** material that can be molded
narco combining form meaning: relationship to numb, stupor	***narcotics*** a drug that tends to produce stupor, and that relieves pain
phobia suffix meaning: fear of	***odontophobia*** a morbid fear or abnormal dread of dental operations
sclero combining form meaning: hard	***sclerosis*** hardening, thickening, or increased density of tissue
stereo combining form meaning: firm, solid, having three dimensions	***stereoscope*** an instrument giving a three dimensional view from a photograph or radiograph
therm combining form meaning: heat	***thermoplastic*** a material that is rigid at normal temperature but becomes soft when heated
cale, calor combining form meaning: heat	***calorie*** a measure of heat

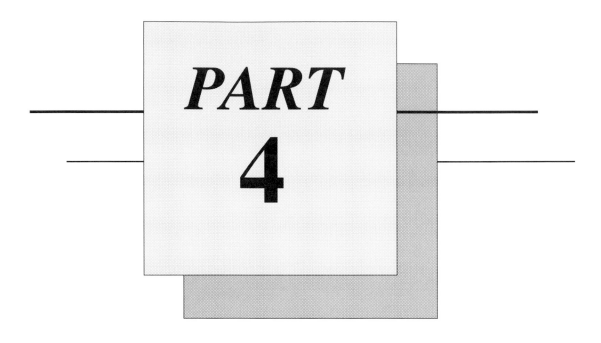

Professional and Business Records

Patients and dentists need accurate records of the dental services rendered and the financial transactions these services involve.

The dental assistant must understand how to keep such records, including all records concerning:

services rendered patients,
accounting of services rendered patients,
financial arrangements for patients,
credit and collections,
office operating expenses,
taxes,
insurance, and
office income.

The records that concern the rendering of dental services for patients are *professional* records. Sometimes this part of the record is spoken of as the patient's *clinical* record to distinguish it from a record of payment for the services received. The patient payment record is often called the *patient's account record*. The financial and professional records are usually kept separately.

Part Four is devoted to a comprehension of basic record-keeping.

CHAPTER 15

Clinical Records

The Purpose of Clinical Records
Patient Registration (Acquaintance Form)
Patient's Individual Record Card
Case History
Color-coding the Record of Special Patients
Radiographs (X Rays)
Study Models
Slides
Patient's Record Envelope
New Patient Examination and Diagnosis Card
Case Presentations

The Purpose of Clinical Records

Clinical records are vital to your dentist for his or her professional protection. Complete records are the best protection against professional liability claims. An accurate record of the previous treatment is an aid in providing the best care of the patient. In addition, dental records may be used in court on behalf of the patient. The records are preserved in order that all the information your dentist may need at some future date is available. These records include written notes, radiographs (X rays), study models, and photographs.

A wise dentist makes a thorough case study before beginning treatment in order to have a complete written record of the diagnosis of the case. The subsequent treatment or service record, the diagnostic records of the case study, the study models, radiographs, and the color slides together comprise the permanent record. This record is essential to the dentist for reference as he or she completes the prescribed dentistry for the patient. During the progress of the work, a patient may forget the original agreement and need to be shown records that will eliminate any misunderstanding that has developed.

Clinical records are considered legal records. Should a patient ever bring a court action against a dentist, the clinical records become vitally important in the dentist's defense. *Never alter entries on clinical records.* If an error has been made in an entry, draw one line through the incorrect entry and write the correct entry below. Be sure the incorrect entry can still be read. Initial both entries. Date your correction.

Accurate, complete, neat records, properly filed, will be invaluable to your dentist and thoroughly appreciated by him or her.

We will now discuss in detail the types of records that will be found in dental offices. Not all offices will keep all records, but some of these records, or similar forms, will be used in most dental offices.

Patient Registration (Acquaintance Form)

The procedures used in various dental offices for the registration of patients range from an extremely detailed personal history, with a signed permission for the dentist to treat a case as he or she decides is best, to no requests for information whatsoever. In the office of an oral surgeon or other specialist, there may be need for a detailed registration form. Every office will benefit from using some form of patient registration, however.

The **patient registration form** may be considered either a medical record or a business record since some of the information requested is used both by the dentist

for dental diagnosis and by the bookkeeper for financial arrangements. It also tells the office something about the patient's stability. The information to be found on a patient registration form usually includes:

1. Date
2. Patient's complete name
3. Patient's home and business addresses
4. Patient's home and business telephone numbers
5. Patient's employer and address
6. Patient's social security number
7. Patient's age, date of birth
8. Name of spouse of patient
9. Employer of spouse
10. Insurance carried by patient for health care
11. Number of insurance contract
12. Referral (name of person who referred patient to office)
13. Name of person legally responsible for the account if the patient is a minor
14. Person responsible for the account
15. Name of a relative or close friend and address of that person
16. Convenient time for appointments

Some dentists request this added information:

17. Name of patient's physician
18. Name of patient's former dentist

The information usually requested on a registration form serves to positively identify the patient, since the patient records the information. His or her name will be spelled correctly. If there is any question, the correct pronunciation of the name should be asked when the registration form is received by the assistant. The address will be the current one. Whatever information the particular office asks the patient to supply on such a form is more likely to be accurate because it is handwritten by the patient.

The information requested on a registration form should not be confused with that which the dentist may ask in the way of a dento-medical history before proceeding with examination and diagnosis. The registration form deals primarily with the information needed for effective conduct of the business requirements between the dental office and the patient.

When properly presented to the patient, a form with blanks provided for this information will be completed without question. "Proper presentation" means the manner used by the assistant to indicate that this form is routinely used by the office and is routinely filled out by all new patients.

One suggestion that has been made for the use of such a form is that it be headed Acquaintance Form rather than Registration Form or Patient's Registration. (See figure 15.1.)

ACQUAINTANCE FORM

Date _____

NAME _____
          FIRST NAME   MIDDLE INITIAL   LAST NAME

HOME ADDRESS _____ CITY _____

ZIP CODE _____ HOME PHONE _____ BIRTH DATE _____

EMPLOYED BY _____ BUSINESS PHONE _____

ADDRESS _____

OCCUPATION _____

REFERRED BY _____

PERSON RESPONSIBLE FOR ACCOUNT _____

SOCIAL SEC. NO. _____ DENTAL INSURANCE? _____

INSURANCE CO. _____ POLICY or GROUP NO. _____

HOW LONG SINCE YOU HAVE BEEN TO A DENTIST? _____

FORMER DENTIST _____

PURPOSE OF CALL _____

HEALTH QUESTIONS: Yes   No

Are You Under a Physician's Care Now? .... [ ]   [ ]
Are You Now Taking Pills, Drugs or Medication? .... [ ]   [ ]
Have You Ever Had:
    Abnormal Heart Condition?   .... [ ]   [ ]
    Rheumatic Fever?   .... [ ]   [ ]
    Diabetes?   .... [ ]   [ ]
    Abnormal Bleeding From a Cut?   .... [ ]   [ ]
    Unusual Reaction to Any Drug or Local Anesthetic?   .... [ ]   [ ]
    Tuberculosis or Hepatitis?   .... [ ]   [ ]
    Radiation Treatment?   .... [ ]   [ ]
    Abnormal Blood Pressure ?   .... [ ]   [ ]
Do You Have Any Allergies or Asthma?   .... [ ]   [ ]

Is There Any Other Information About Your Health That Should Be Known?

_____

_____ Signature _____

RF-A-REV. 3-89   SPILLANE'S, INC., MINNEAPOLIS, MN.

Figure 15.1
An acquaintance form.

Patient's Individual Record Card

The patient records maintained by dental offices vary from extremely simple records to properly detailed and maintained records of dental services.

For the purposes of training, one type of record-keeping will be discussed here. It remains for any new dental assistant to adapt herself or himself to the particular method of recording patient services, and all record-keeping in general, used in the office in which he or she is employed.

The **patient's individual record card,** 8½-by-11 inches in size, has headings across the top that should be carefully completed by the assistant. Information that is apt to be permanent is typed or written in ink. Temporary information is written in pencil. Thus, in the proper spaces type or write in ink these items:

1. Patient's name: last name first, then first name, middle name or initial, and any title in parentheses

2. Birth date
3. Name of person who referred patient, preceded by the words "Referred by"
4. Insurance company and policy number

In pencil enter these items:

1. Home address and telephone
2. Business address and telephone

The body of the patient's record card contains ruled columns and lines that provide space for the following information relating to the dental services performed for that patient: (1) year, month, and day; (2) service rendered (should be detailed well); (3) chair time and/or laboratory time required for the service; and (4) fee charged. Frequently there is also room for amounts paid and the balance owing on the account. In some offices the dentist will complete the entries on this record; in others, the assistant is expected to copy the required information. In either case, completion of the record should be accomplished as soon as possible after the service is given to the patient because the information is remembered and can be entered in good detail at that time.

Notes should be made on patient's records of emergency treatment, surgical procedures, and treatment of infections. Further, note any warnings of possible complications or any instructions to report to the office on a specific date for observation, which were given by the dentist or staff. Should any legal action be started by a patient, these records are invaluable. Details of treatment should be complete, even though abbreviated wording is used.

Case History

Case history is a term applied to a collection of pertinent facts related to the examination, diagnosis, prognosis, and treatment of the patient. The examination portion may include such information as age, sex, marital status, nationality, occupation, spouse's occupation, educational level, history of systemic and oral diseases, medications, allergies, weight, height, complexion, physical infirmities, temperament, diet, dental history, and habits. It is common practice to do a thorough case history in university dental school clinics, dental public health clinics, and hospitals. In private dental practice, however, this questioning of the patient regarding his or her physical history is frequently reduced to a minimum. Six or seven questions can usually satisfy the important points of physical condition required by the dentist. The circumstances in private dental practice usually do not necessitate the detailed physical history, since most patients seen in a dental office are ambulatory and their physical condition is usually good. When the reverse is true, it is quite easily discovered by a condensed version, and further information can be elicited from the patient. A consultation with the patient's physician will be requested if the dentist deems it necessary or desirable for the patient's welfare.

Color-coding the Record of Special Patients

Regardless of what other information is sought, of utmost importance on any case history in a dental office is information relating to conditions that may require special medical attention. Routinely, the dentist must know these facts:

1. Does the patient have an allergic reaction? If so, what causes the reaction and what drug or drugs must be avoided for the patient's safety and comfort? (If the patient is vague about allergies, consult the patient's physician.)
2. Does the patient take a "maintenance dosage" of any drug? This drug may affect the individual's ability to tolerate certain dental treatment, may require the administration of some medication to make dental treatment possible, or may create a problem for even the most routine dental procedures. For example, cardiovascular patients commonly take anticoagulant drugs, which prevent blood from clotting. Special treatments must be instituted with these patients before any dental surgery is performed.
3. Does the patient have any chronic condition that may develop into an emergency in the dental office? For example, the patient may be subject to epileptic seizures or may be a diabetic and, therefore, subject to insulin shock. Prompt medical attention is essential under certain circumstances.

Some dentists use an arresting color to mark the records of patients who may require special medical attention. On the top of the record, the physician's telephone number is written boldly in a color that can be seen easily. Should an emergency arise, the physician can be contacted quickly because the number is easy to locate. The color-coding of the record envelope and patient's service card reminds the staff that this patient may develop an emergency requiring immediate attention. Should color-coding be used, each new page of patient record must be marked.

Radiographs (X Rays)

Patient records are the property of the dentist. X rays are a part of those records, although many patients misunderstand this relationship because many dentists state a charge "for X rays," rather than stating that the charge is for the "Examination" in its entirety. If any treatment beyond examination and diagnosis is performed for a patient, the X rays should be retained as a part of the legal record of the office. In circumstances involving a request for the X rays by the patient, many dentists will send the X rays to another dentist for the patient if no actual treatment was involved beyond examination and diagnosis. If regular patients find they are to be transferred to another city, it is not unusual to supply them with their most recent X rays as a gesture of courtesy. It is preferable, however, to forward radiographs by mail directly to the dentist named by the patients as their new practitioner.

Radiographs must be placed in an X-ray mount to be properly examined. The name of the patient and the date of X rays are written in pencil on the mount. This provides for neat reuse of the mount when radiographs are made later. Mounts containing radiographs that are sent out of the office—for the use of a specialist, for example—should have the name of your dentist and all other data written in ink.

When X rays are no longer current, they are usually removed from the mount and placed in a coin envelope with the date and the patient's name on it. They can then be filed in the patient's record envelope or a separate X-ray file. How long they should be kept as a clinical record is a matter of your dentist's choice.

Mounted X rays are usually filed separately. One of three plans is used for filing. (1) They can be numbered and filed by number. A 3-by-5 inch file of the patients' names in alphabetical order lists the numbers of their X rays on the cards. The assistant refers to the name file for the number of the X ray, then locates and removes the X rays from the numeric file. (2) The information may be kept in an X-ray guidebook, which lists the patients' names and the numbers of the X rays. (3) Radiographs may be kept in the patient's record envelope.

Study Models

A dentist may use study models of a patient's mouth in order to study and diagnose the problems of the individual patient more accurately. These **study models** are casts made from impressions taken of a patient's mouth. They are carefully labeled with the patient's name and the date. After the dentist has made the diagnosis, they are stored safely for future reference, usually in model boxes on which the patient's name is written.

Slides

Many dentists are aware of the importance of intraoral and extraoral photography and use both before and after color slides of patients who have a prosthesis or a mouth reconstruction that affects their appearance.

The slides, both extraoral and intraoral, are filed by number. A number is placed on the slide mounting itself or on a gummed label. The gummed label is glued to the slide mount. The number of the slide is written on the patient's record. The slides are then filed in numerical order. A slide number book may also be used. In this book the patients' names are listed alphabetically, with the slide number after the name.

Patient's Record Envelope

The envelope that is used to contain and protect the patient's record card and X-ray mounts is slightly larger than the record card. Whether or not it has ruled lines for entry of the various details required, it is important that this information be entered in exactly the same manner and in the same position on each patient's record envelope. The form used is the same as that used on the heading of the record card: patient's last name, first name, and middle name or initial, in ink or typed, in the upper-left-hand area of the envelope. This is followed on the same line by the home address, telephone number, city, and zip code in pencil. The second line has no entry under the name of the patient but has the business address below the residence address, and business phone below the home telephone number, all in pencil. A 3-H or 4-H pencil is good for such entries. The use of an art-gum eraser will permit the envelopes and cards to last through many changes of address.

A minor's birth date is entered in ink on the third line, center, of the patient's record envelope. The name of the father or responsible adult is entered in ink in a routine place in the heading section of the patient's record card, and just below the minor's name on the record envelope, in ink. Since the statement must go to the responsible individual, not to the minor, the information is necessary for billing.

The use of Ms., Miss, Mrs., and Mr. provides a simple method of indicating a self-supporting minor.

Yearly number: Many dental offices like to keep some additional information on the patient's record envelope. One item is the *yearly number* of each patient. The first time a patient is seen during a year, he or she is assigned a number. Beginning with the first workday in January of each year, the first patient receives the number *1*, entered in ink on the left side of the patient's record envelope, below the top three-line area, thus: 1992–1. The sequence of numbers is kept in order by noting the next number to be used on the day sheet. For example, after placing 1992–1 on the first patient's record envelope, the number *1* in the bottom margin of the day sheet is crossed off and the number *2* written after it. When number *2* has been assigned to the second patient's record envelope, it in turn is crossed off at the bottom of the day sheet, and the number *3* is written. At the end of each day the next number to be used is transferred to the day sheet for the next day. Thus the final workday in December will carry the figure indicating the total number of patients seen in the course of the year. The increase each month can be entered as a separate figure in that month's reports for comparison with previous months or previous years. A patient of some years' standing would have a vertical column

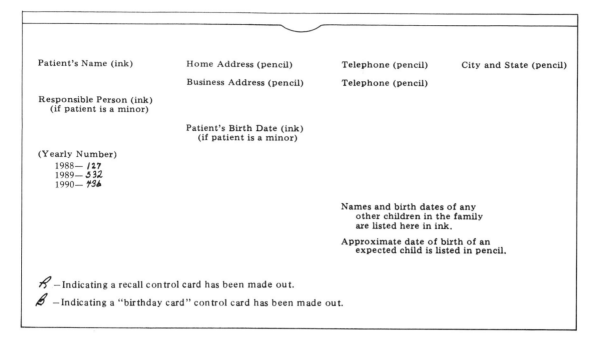

Figure 15.2
Patient's record envelope.

of figures representing the first year he or she became a patient in the practice and each year he or she has been in as a patient thereafter. It indicates, in general, how regular his or her attendance has been. The total figures are of use statistically to the dentist and, if kept at all, should be kept accurately.

Family records: Some dentists like to have the children's names and birth dates entered on the record envelope of a parent as a means of keeping up with the family and encouraging their entry into the practice at the proper time. Those entries are made in ink in the lower right quarter of the patient's record envelope.

Recall and birthday records: If a separate recall card system is used in a come-up card file, the fact that a recall card has been made out from the patient's record envelope information can be so indicated by writing the letter *R* in the lower-left-hand corner of the envelope. If the dentist sends birthday cards to his or her young patients, a similar card for the birthday come-up file is necessary, and a letter *B* in the lower left corner of the envelope indicates that this card has been made out and is in the birthday card file (fig. 15.2).

New Patient Examination and Diagnosis Card

Another card that is often used in conjunction with the patient's record card is the new patient's examination and diagnosis card, also 8½-by-11 inches in size (fig.

15.3). This card usually includes a diagram of the teeth for entry of the necessary treatment pictorially, several entries for a history of the patient, space for entry of results of vitality tests of the teeth, and usually space for a written summary of the required dental work with the fees to be charged for the services. The information at the top of the card is completed by the assistant before the examination. The diagnostic part of the record might be completed either by the dentist, who enters the information during the examination, or by the assistant as the dentist dictates the information. The estimate portion may be made up by the dentist; or if the assistant has developed a familiarity with the procedures, the dentist may delegate the work of making up the listings and estimates.

Case Presentations

Now that all the patient records are gathered—including radiographs, models, case histories, and photographs—the dentist may have an appointment with the patient for case presentation to help the patient understand his or her dental needs.

The **case-presentation** appointment is an appointment for the express purpose of discussing the dental needs and the treatment to be instituted with the patient or other responsible person. The required dental work, the various ways of accomplishing the desired results, the recommendations of the dentist, and the costs

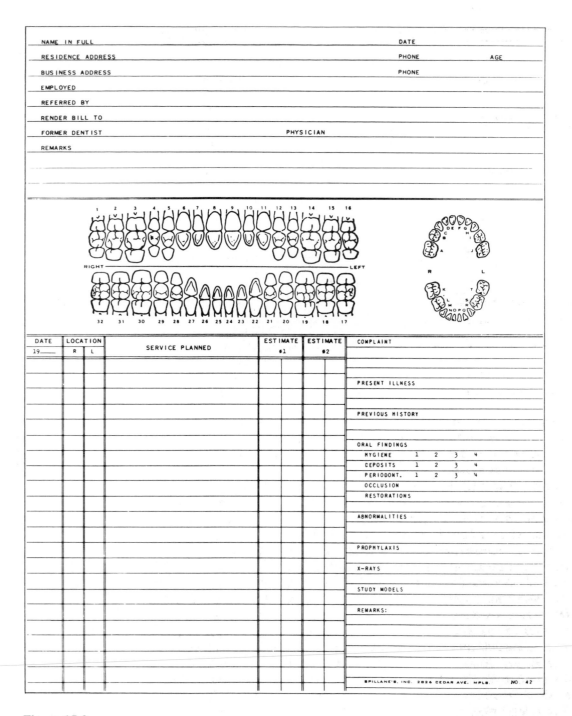

Figure 15.3

Combination examination and estimate form.

involved in the various methods of treatment are discussed. Some offices vary this routine by doing only the full-mouth X rays, bitewing X rays, and study models, if desired, on the first visit. The second appointment is a prophylaxis and oral examination, followed by a discussion with the patient or other responsible person of the dental needs and treatment.

Such procedures are not used by all dental offices, of course. The assistant should familiarize herself or himself with the wishes of the dentist and should perform all phases of office routine as her or his employer prefers.

It is necessary that a case presentation be protected from any outside interference, such as other members of the office staff moving around, telephone calls for the dentist, or any distracting degree of noise. If a private office is available, it is usually the place selected for these discussions. Some dentists prefer using an operatory, however.

Everything pertaining to the patient's examination and diagnosis is made available beforehand, including X rays and a method for viewing them. Any models your dentist has that might be applicable to the case are placed with the patient records. Frequently, seating space is required for another person in addition to the patient.

Many methods of presenting cases to patients exist. Variations in the part that the dental assistant is to play in this procedure also exist. Your dentist may teach you to take over all arrangements once the patient has made a decision about the dental work to be performed. In that event, you will be instructed in arranging payment and scheduling appointments for the work.

If the patient is a minor, the dental office must be sure that the parent gives written consent to the planned course of treatment in all cases.

In summary, then, be sure that no one disturbs the dentist and patient during a case presentation. When the dentist has finished his or her part of the conference, be ready with your appointment book and other materials that you may need to complete the presentation as your dentist desires. It is well to memorize thoroughly any instructions that he or she wishes to give the patient. Use notes, if necessary, to be certain nothing is omitted during case presentation.

Summary

Clinical records are vital to your dentist for patient treatment and professional protection. The records include complete studies of the patient's dental health, diagnosis, and treatment.

The *patient registration form* includes the patient's name, address, telephone number, person responsible for the account, and the individual who referred the patient to the dentist.

The *patient's individual record card* is a detailed record of the services performed. It also has the necessary information about the patient's name, address, telephone, birth, etc., entered at the top of the card. The detailed service record is to be completed as soon after service as possible. Be sure to write the date of service.

A *case history* is a detailed physical examination record that is usually used only in clinics or university dental schools. A condensed version is more applicable to the dental office because patients who enter the dental office ordinarily are ambulatory.

Radiographs are identified on the mount, with the patient's name in pencil. If the radiographs are kept in a coin envelope, the patient's name and the date of X rays are listed on the envelope.

Study models are used to help diagnose dental ills. They are made from impressions taken of the patient's mouth.

Slides of "before" and "after" appearance of the patient are sometimes used when prosthetics or mouth reconstruction is performed.

The *patient's record envelope* is used to protect records. It carries identifying information on the exterior: name, address, telephone, minor's birth date, and other pertinent data.

The *new patient examination and diagnosis card* is used in some offices for each new patient. It is similar to the patient's individual record card and contains room for dental history and diagnosis.

Case presentations are conducted by many dentists to enlighten patients about the conditions of their mouths and which services are actually necessary. During this important interview, the dentist and patient should be undisturbed.

Study Questions

1. What are clinical records and what is their purpose?
2. Discuss the minimum requirements for patient registration.
3. Why are complete records of a patient desirable?
4. Who usually makes entries on a patient record card?
5. What is a case history?
6. To whom do X rays belong?
7. How are X rays stored?
8. What are study models and what does the assistant do with them before use and after use?
9. If your dentist uses slides, how do you care for them?
10. What information is usually found on a patient's record envelope?
11. What is a new patient examination and diagnosis card?
12. What is a case-presentation appointment? What is the usual responsibility of the staff during such an appointment?

Word Elements

Word Element	Example
artero combining form meaning: relationship to an artery	**arteriosclerosis** hardening of the arteries
arthr, arthro combining form meaning: relationship to a joint	**arthralgia** pain in a joint
angio combining form meaning: relationship to a vessel	**angiology** scientific study of blood vessels
phlebo, phleb combining form meaning: relationship to the veins	**phlebectasia** dilation of a vessel
thermo combining form meaning: relationship to heat	**thermometer** a device for measuring changes in temperature
chemo combining form meaning: relating to chemistry	**chemotherapy** treatment of disease with chemicals
nomo combining form meaning: relationship to law, custom	**taxonomy** orderly classification
radio combining form meaning: relationship to ray or radiation	**radiography** photography with X rays or radiation
philia combining form meaning: affinity for	**hemophilia** a genetic disease of males characterized by excessive hermorrhaging
sarco combining form meaning: relationship to flesh	**sarcoma** a tumor composed of connective tissue elements

CHAPTER 16

Financial Records: Part One, Receipts

Records Are Important
Business Services for Dentists
The "Why" of Record-keeping
Basic Requirements in Financial Records
Receipt Book
Office Change Fund
Patient's Service and Account Records
   Patient's Service Record
   Patient's Account Record (or Ledger Card)
The Day Sheet or Daily Record Sheet
Discounts
Patient Records and Governmental Third-Party
      Payment
Statements for Patients
Payments by Check from Patients
Accounts Receivable Control

Records Are Important

The financial records detailing the dentist's income and expenditures are just as important as the clinical records detailing the care given to patients. Remember, the patient will expect the same accuracy in billing as in dental treatment. From the patient's perspective, clinical records and financial records reflect one and the same capacity—that is, either accuracy or inaccuracy. It may be illogical, but accuracy in bookkeeping equals accuracy in dental treatment in the minds of many patients.

Business Services for Dentists

In addition to being professionally competent to practice dentistry, a dentist must also operate a business in order to be properly remunerated for professional services and to provide the necessary organization to treat patients. In the lengthy education of a dentist, little time can be devoted to business education. At the same time, our society has become more complex, and comprehension of business procedures is a necessity. The result is that dentists are increasingly hiring accountants to design and manage a method of keeping their business records. An accountant (hopefully a certified public accountant) is a person who has studied management and record-keeping. A certified public accountant (CPA) has served a period of apprenticeship, has passed difficult examinations, and then is certified much as a dental assistant is certified after passing registration examinations. The initials *CPA* are then used after the accountant's name to indicate skill in accounting.

A dentist may employ the services of a dental CPA firm. These firms, whose owners are usually CPAs, perform all types of financial recording for dental offices. Usually a dentist has a choice of several services. The CPAs may prepare only the tax returns if the dentist so desires, or the firm may contract to furnish accounting for the office. The dental assistant will make receipts for money received and post the charges on the patients' account records. The CPA firm will assume responsibility at that point, and no further accounting is performed by any employee of the dentist. There are many "packages" of service offered by CPAs, between the two extremes of minimal service to complete responsibility. The amount of outside assistance is determined by the dentist, who decides how much accounting service to purchase. If the dentist plans to have an accountant prepare income tax statements, the dentist probably has the accountant supervise the accounting during the year.

Another person a dentist might employ is a **management consultant** who may or may not be a CPA. The management consultant advises the dentist about business matters and sometimes about investments. Initially the consultant studies the dentist's way of practicing dentistry and keeping records. Next, the consultant sets up a system of accurate bookkeeping for the maintenance of proper records, following through and working with the dentist on a monthly basis. The consultant trains each new assistant in the type of record-keeping to be performed in the office. The consultant trains the dentist's office employees to maintain the office records exactly as the consultant wishes for use in evaluating the business operation of the office, in preparing tax forms, and in periodically examining, analyzing, and reporting to the dentist.

In addition to the accountant services, there are systems such as the Write-It-Once bookkeeping systems promoted by such firms as Burroughs, and the pegboard systems made by a number of firms including Little Press, Inc., of Minneapolis, and National Cash Register. These services ease the complicated problems of accurately keeping records and writing the same information several times.

With computers and rapid office machines, mechanization is overtaking the bookkeeping of the professional office. It appears that data processing (the name given the mechanized form of office accounting) may be responsible for the major part of accounting procedures in dental offices because these offices are being computerized.

The "Why" of Record-keeping

No matter how mechanized data processing becomes, each office must still have some method of maintaining day-by-day records that, in turn, can be stored in the computer. The initial data must be prepared by hand by some employee who is accurate in the preparation of these records. This employee's responsibilities include orderliness and accuracy. An accountant or management consultant will usually supervise the overall plan of keeping records. The record-keeper will be told exactly what to do and how to do it.

Everything that exists in a business can be divided into:

    things that are *owned;*

    things that are *owed;* and

    that which is left over after these two are equaled.

That which is left over belongs to the owner of the business.

Things that are owned are called **assets.** They could be converted to cash. Things that are owed are called **liabilities.** They represent money owed and are claims against the business. The **cash value** of the difference between assets and liabilities is called **proprietorship** because the owner of a business is a proprietor, and this extra cash value belongs to the owner.

No matter what system of bookkeeping is used, every set of books (record-keeping) has to reflect the fact that whenever you get something you give something, and whenever you give something you get something. Two things happen in every transaction. You get a box of X-ray film and you give cash; or you give a patient a treatment and you get cash.

Assets in a dental office include:

1. Any property owned by the dentist
2. Accounts receivable
3. Money in bank accounts
4. Money already received but not yet deposited
5. Cash on hand (petty cash and office change fund are examples)

Liabilities in a dental office include:

1. Obligations to pay for goods already received (for example, supplies to be used during the month)
2. Accounts payable (such as rent on a monthly basis)
3. Interest on debts
4. Notes (such as a promise to pay for equipment over a period of time)
5. Bad debts (bills that are owed by, but will not be paid by, patients)

Proprietorship (net worth) refers to what the dentist owns after his or her assets and liabilities are balanced. If the dentist has $1,000 in liabilities and $2,000 cash on hand and in accounts receivable, he or she has a proprietorship of $1,000.

Assets equal liabilities plus proprietorship. This information is carefully recorded and studied by the accountant who sets up the bookkeeping system so that he or she can watch the factors in this formula. Ordinarily the bookkeeping cycle that is used is called **double entry bookkeeping.** It starts with the keeping of a journal and proceeds through posting, adjusting, closing, and issuing financial statements. Some form of this system will be used in the office in which you work. If there is an accountant or management consultant, your work will be simplified. If you are expected to manage the entire matter yourself, you will need special training in bookkeeping and accounting prior to assuming such responsibilities.

Regardless of what system of bookkeeping is used, every assistant who works with the office records should be sure he or she keeps careful formal written records of:

that which the office owes to others;
that which others owe to the office;
all money received; and
all money spent.

As a dental assistant, you should be aware that you must acquire and keep all source documents. (**Source documents** are the records of proof of billing or proof of payment.) If you order some impression material from the supply house, you must find and keep the invoice, which either comes in the package or is mailed to you separately. This is a source document. (Figure 11.5 in chapter 11, "Supplies and Their Control," is a source document.)

When a patient visits the office, charges for the services rendered are recorded for the first time on the patient's service record and/or on a charge slip if a Write-It-Once bookkeeping system is used. This first record is a source document and must be kept permanently. Invoices for supplies received are also source documents. The record-keeper must know where these source documents are. They are the "backup" documents—the proof that a service actually was performed or that a supply actually was received.

If your office uses the services of an accountant or management consultant, he or she will expect you to have these documents available for proof. Be certain that you know which are your source documents and their location.

Sometimes by paying a bill from the invoice you can save money. Some firms offer a 1 or 2 percent discount for paying from the invoice rather than from the monthly statement. It saves them bookkeeping expense, and they are willing to pass the savings on to encourage prompt payment. An alert dental assistant watches for notes of such discount written on the invoices that come to the office.

Whatever system of bookkeeping is used in the office in which you work, be sure to ask questions and be certain that you follow directions. It is better to ask questions than to guess and do your work incorrectly.

It is also wise to ask your supervisor how you can check periodically to see how well you are doing. Write down any questions that occur to you during the first week you are working with a bookkeeping system and have them available for your supervisor when he or she comes to verify your work at the end of the week. Ask the supervisor for evaluation if he or she does not regularly inspect your work.

assets   things that are owned (could be converted to cash)

liabilities   things that are owed (claims against the business)

cash value   monetary value of something (what an item is worth in dollars)

proprietorship   cash value of the difference between assets and liabilities (net worth)

double entry bookkeeping   a system that records both the receiving and giving (owning and owing) aspects of a business, so that the assets, liabilities, and proprietorship values are immediately obvious

source document   the original written proof of purchase or proof of payment

transactions   a piece of business completed between two or more persons (i.e., a patient receives dental treatment from the dentist for a fee; the service and payment constitute a transaction.)

ledger   a book containing accounts showing both the debits and credits listed (posted) to each account (A ledger is not used as frequently as a ledger card system in dental offices.)

ledger card   a card for each patient on which is recorded charges for services rendered, payments received, and balance of account (It is a permanent record maintained in the office.)

post   to transfer entries from one record to another, as transferring receipts from the receipt book to the day sheet and to the patient's account record (also called the ledger card)

debit   (charge) an amount owed (Service is rendered the patient, and the amount charged for the service is debited to the account of the patient who now owes that amount. The entry is made in the charges column.)

credit   an amount paid (The patient sends the money due for service rendered and the patient's account is credited. Hopefully the debit and credit balance, and now nothing is owed. The entry is made in the receipt column.)

income, gross   the total income received before any business expenses are deducted

income, net   the amount left after business expenditures are deducted (Net income is the amount on which taxes are computed.)

You are not expected to be able to set up books for the running of a dental practice. You are expected to be able to follow directions and keep the records exactly as your dentist wishes to have them kept.

Basic Requirements in Financial Records

While it is likely that the majority of dental offices may be mechanized, there still will be many offices throughout the country in which the assistant will be managing the financial records. The basic requirements for adequate financial records must be met. The successful management of a dental practice requires a bookkeeping system that is fundamentally sound in all its phases, able to provide the information the dentist desires, and able to provide the necessary information for income tax returns.

This section will present one way of meeting these complete basic requirements for the dentist who does not employ an accounting service.[1]

We stated that every record-keeper must maintain careful records of the following:

1. Money received and spent.
2. All things for which the office owes others.
3. All things others owe the office.

Records of importance for these classifications include:

1. Records of receipts.
2. An office change fund.

3. Patient service and account records (transactions with individual patients).
4. A day sheet (records of all service rendered and all financial transactions).
5. Discount records.
6. Statements to patients for services rendered.
7. Accounts receivable control to verify the record-keeping.
8. Records of petty cash expenditures.
9. Invoices and statements for office purchases.
10. Disbursement records (where the money went).
11. A yearly summary of the entire business operation of the office.

In addition to understanding these records, the process of banking and using the checkbook correctly must be thoroughly comprehended.

We will divide financial records into two groups: (1) records about money received for service rendered, and (2) records about expenditures, including banking records.

The Write-It-Once bookkeeping system will be described in chapter 17. Tax records, insurance records, health care plan records, and credit and collections, which must also be considered, will comprise other chapters. The rest of chapter 16 is devoted to a discussion of records about money received for services rendered.

Receipt Book

A **receipt** (ree-*seat*) is written acknowledgment of anything, such as money or goods, obtained from another person. In the dental office a receipt should be made out for every payment that is received by that office.

Receipts should be made in duplicate. The original copy is given to the patient; the carbon copy remains bound in the book as part of the permanent record for the year. The receipt book of carbons must show every payment that has been made in the dental office during the year; therefore, it is necessary to make a receipt for every payment (regardless of whether the payment is by check or cash). The total amount of money shown on the carbon receipts for a year should equal the gross income of the dental office for that year.

Patients need receipts as proof of payment if they pay for these services by cash. Receipts are not so essential to them if they pay by check, although it is desirable to have proof for income tax purposes that they actually paid the dentist the amount that they stated they paid.

When the patient makes a payment in person, give him or her a receipt at that time. Daily, when time is available, the payments received through the mail are entered in the receipt book. It generally is not necessary to send the original receipts to the patients whose payments were by check or money order, but some of them may request it. In any event, every payment must be entered in the receipt book. The bound receipt book, then, is an accurate, permanent record of the gross income received.

The receipt should be made out to the individual to whom the account was billed. If the charge was made for six-year-old John and the account was billed to his father, Mr. James Jones, the receipt should be made out to "Mr. James Jones, for John." To insure against errors in crediting an account, the name on the receipt should be followed by the address on the next line. Indicate whether the payment was by check or by cash. When balancing the books at the close of the day, you will find it helpful to know which payments were cash and how much cash was actually received.

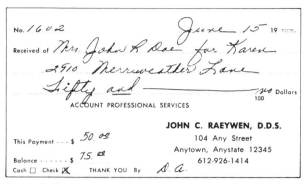

Courtesy Spillane's, Inc., Minneapolis

Figure 16.1
A sample receipt.

Be sure that the carbon copy is always legible. It is your permanent record. A few suggestions can help insure legible carbon copies. Use a good ball-point pen for writing receipts and write firmly. If your office uses receipts for which carbon paper is furnished, buy extra pencil carbon paper and change the carbon frequently. (Some offices now have receipts with carbon paper furnished for each receipt, or paper that duplicates without carbon.)

Office Change Fund

Patients who pay their bills by cash sometimes need change. It is desirable to keep ten to fifteen dollars in small bills in an office cash box—separate from the petty cash fund. (See Terms to Be Understood.)

The dentist writes a check for the office change fund once. The money is permanently available; therefore, the record-keeper must always remember to set this amount aside when totaling the cash received during the day. If it is included with the cash received during the day, the total will be greater by exactly the amount that should be in the office change fund.

Another difficulty commonly experienced is illustrated by this example: suppose Mr. Johnson offers the record-keeper, Miss Patrick, a twenty dollar bill and states that he wishes to pay fifteen dollars on account. Miss Patrick makes a receipt for fifteen dollars cash for Mr. Johnson. She now has a twenty dollar bill in her cash receipts, but five of it belongs in the office change fund. It will be necessary for her to make change during the day and replace the five dollars in the office change fund, or at the close of the day Miss Patrick will have five dollars more in the day's receipts than she has actually collected.

Business Address: Housewife | Business Telephone: | NAME: Doe, Mrs. T. K. (Mary) | Residence Telephone: 826-9172

Address: 6152 Alphonso Street, Anytown, Anystate 12345

Send Bill To: Doe, Mr. Thomas K.

DATE 19__		Tooth Number	Cavity Location	OPERATION Chair	DEBIT	CREDIT	BALANCE	DATE 19__		Tooth Number	Cavity Location	OPERATION	DEBIT	CREDIT	BALANCE
6	2	L5	MOD	Amal. Nav. 45	56 -		56 -								
6	10	R5	Full cov	Prep. Nav. 55	150		206 -								

Figure 16.2
Patient's service record.

Patient's Service and Account Records

Each day several patients receive dental care for which they are to pay either immediately or within the near future, and some records of the dental service, the charges, and the payments received are necessary. These records are called the **patient's service record** and the **patient's account record.** Each is a record for an individual patient.

Some offices combine the patient's service record and the patient's account record and call it the **patient's service and account record.** With such a system the dentist enters in detail the services performed and the charges for them. The assistant enters the payments received and figures the balance. A special filing arrangement is used to keep all records of patients who still owe money in an active file (see chap. 12).

For purposes of understanding these records more easily, the two types will be discussed separately. They may be maintained as separate records in your office—or combined on one record.

Patient's Service Record

The patient's service record shows the patient's name, address, and telephone number at the top. It may show both home and business telephones and addresses. If the patient is a minor, there is space for his or her parent's name or other guarantor of the account.

The card provides space for the date and for detailed entry of services rendered. Each time a patient receives a service, the specific service is entered in detail, usually by the dentist. This card is kept in the patient's envelope.

Study the entries on the patient's service record in figure 16.2.

Patient's Account Record (or Ledger Card)

A card is used with the patient's name, address, and telephone number at the top. It has spaces for date, item, charges, receipts, and balance (fig. 16.3).

When the patient receives services, the charge for these services is entered with the date. When the patient pays on account, the amount paid is entered in the receipts column, the balance in the balance column, and the date in its column.

When you transfer the services and charges from the patient's service record, you put a check mark on the patient's service record to indicate that the charge has been posted (transferred) to the account record. Each day you transfer from your receipt book to the patient's account records all payments for which you have written receipts. As soon as you copy the figure on a patient's account record, you put a check mark on the carbon receipt to indicate that you have posted the payment. The balance is figured each time you post an entry (charge or payment) in order to have all patient account record balances current.

The Day Sheet or Daily Record Sheet

The dentist must have a detailed record of services rendered, the charges for those services, and the money received from patients. This complete, detailed record, professional as well as financial, of the day's activities relating to patients is called a **day sheet.** Some dentists use a book called a "Daily Log," others a printed sheet or card called a "Daily Record"; but they are all classified as a day sheet.

The name of each patient, the service received, and the charge for this service are written in the proper columns. Some dentists ask that the chair-time be entered also. (Chair-time is the actual working time of the dentist while the patient is in the dental chair.)

In addition to the work performed during the day, payments are received, usually through the mail, for patients who do not have any dentistry performed that day. These receipts must be entered on the day sheet as well as in the receipt book since all the money received during the day must be accounted for on the day sheet. Your dentist's preference will determine the method of entry. One method is: moneys received from patients who have appointments and therefore pay in person are entered on the same line as the record of the dentistry performed. (See Johnson, Mary, in figure 16.4.) All the moneys received in the mail and from persons who drop in to pay a bill but do not have dentistry performed are totaled from the receipts you issued. The total amount is listed as receipts for the day (fig. 16.4).

Another method identifies the amount of money each person pays by listing on the day sheet the name of the patient and the amount received. Thus, if a patient has dentistry performed and pays for all or part of it, the entry is made as the Johnson, Mary, item in figure 16.4. However, the receipts for the day are not totaled and made as one entry, but entered individually as in figure 16.5—Mason, T.K., $20, etc.

In either case, at the close of the day, total the *Charge* and *Received on Account* columns. The *Charge* column is the total dentistry performed during the day.

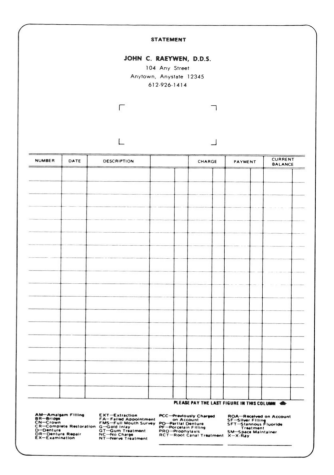

Figure 16.3
A patient's ledger card.

PATIENT	SERVICE	TIME CHAIR	TIME LAB	CHARGE	REC'D ON ACCOUNT
Johnson, Mary	#4 MOD amal. nov.	30		56⁰⁰	56⁰⁰
Smith, Robert	#16 removal nov.	45		41⁰⁰	
Zambolini, Jim	#19 full crn. prep. nov.	90		150⁰⁰	
Morgan, E.R.	dent. adj.	10		—	
Eklund, A.T.	lower part. imps.	30	60	400⁰⁰	
Oppen, Olive	#8 fil. nov.	30		40⁰⁰	
Franklin, B.J.	case pres.	30		40⁰⁰	
Receipts for day (by mail)					485⁰⁰
Total				727⁰⁰	541⁰⁰

Figure 16.4
A sample day sheet.

PATIENT	SERVICE	TIME CHAIR	LAB	CHARGE	REC'D ON ACCOUNT
Mason, J. K.					20.00
Andrews, John					150.00
Peterson, Roy					200.00
Smith, Mary					30.00
Quiggley, Sam					35.00
Total				400.00	455.00

Figure 16.5

An alternative method of listing on the day sheet, payments received through the mail.

SUMMARY FOR THE MONTH OF *January* YEAR *19 XX*

DAY OF MONTH	CHARGES	DISCOUNTS	PAYMENTS
1	220.00	20.00	435.00
2	509.00	—	820.00
3	659.00	5.00	650.00
4	420.00	17.00	420.00
31	330.00	—	135.00
TOTAL	54,400.00	325.00	11,300.00

Figure 16.6

A monthly summary sheet.

The *Received on Account* column is the total receipts for the day.

These totals are listed on the monthly summary sheet (fig. 16.6) in their appropriate columns. The monthly totals are listed in the yearly summary sheet at the close of each month. On December 31 you know exactly how much dentistry was performed during the year and how much money was collected during the year—two very important factors in working with tax reports.

Discounts

A discount is a reduction in fee or price offered to a specified person in specified circumstances, i.e., a patient who qualifies receives a discount. (The dentist determines the qualifications: poverty, old age, religious order, and employee are some.) A business firm may offer a reduced price if the amount owed is paid within a specified time limit. Discounts are purely voluntary and are given by the person who desires to do so. Thus, the dentist decides whether or not to give a discount in cirumstances he or she specifies. One of his or her employees may not decide to give a discount. The discount policy is established in writing by the dentist. A discount must be properly entered in the bookkeeping system to show as a discount. (One of the pegboard systems has a special column for the express purpose of listing such discounts.) The books should not read that Mrs. Gray paid twenty-five dollars for complete X rays and Mrs. Jones paid fifteen dollars for the same service. Mrs. Jones's account must show the charge as twenty-five dollars. An entry must be made for a discount of ten dollars, and the balance will appear as fifteen dollars.

Patient Records and Governmental Third-Party Payment

A dentist may perform dental services for patients whose bills are paid by one of several governmental agencies: Aid for Dependent Children, Family Welfare, County Relief Boards, and the Veterans' Administration. Most of these organizations have a set fee scale by which they pay for dentistry. It is necessary to contact them for the proper forms prior to performing the dentistry and to return to them an estimate of the work to be done and the cost. When the dentist has written permission to perform the dentistry as designated on the form, he or she is able to appoint the patient and perform the dentistry explicitly stated on the estimate form—and no more, unless approval is requested of the agency.

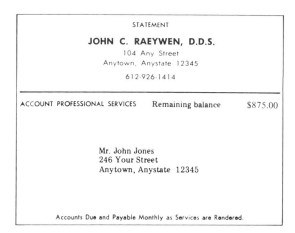

Figure 16.7
A simplified statement form.

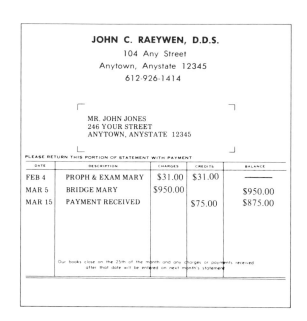

Figure 16.8
An itemized statement form.

Should your dentist work for one of these agencies, become familiar with the forms to be completed for that agency and any instructions regarding their use and the patient's care.

Statements for Patients

A **statement** is a bill sent to the patient at the end of the month that states the amount the patient owes the dentist for dentistry performed.

It is important that these statements be mailed on time every month—the same time. It is wise to pick a date for closing accounts (such as the twenty-fifth of the month) and state that all charges and credits after that date will appear on the next month's statement. If the twenty-fifth is chosen, the dental assistant is allowed time to prepare the statements and have them mailed several days before the end of the month in order that all statements are received by patients on or before the first of the following month. In modern-day billing procedures of large stores, accounts for names beginning with different letters of the alphabet are closed on various dates throughout the month. People are quite accustomed to receiving bills during the month. The main purpose in closing the books early is to be certain that statements go out on the same date each month. Patients are less likely to treat payments of your statements in a haphazard manner if you are exacting in your habit of mailing the statement at the same time each month.

Statements, of course, achieve a more business-like impression if they are typed rather than handwritten. The entire statement and envelope should present a neat and attractive appearance (figures 16.7 and 16.8).

Payments by Check from Patients

Checks received from patients should be immediately endorsed. The assistant may endorse the check by simply writing "For deposit only" on the back and signing the dentist's name. Many dentists have a stamp that is used for endorsing a check. Once a check has been stamped with this marking, it can be deposited only to the dentist's account.

Occasionally you deposit a check from a patient and in a few days you receive the check back from the bank, with a note saying it is not acceptable because the patient does not have sufficient funds in his or her account to pay the amount of the check. Some people refer to this as "insufficient funds" or a "rubber check" (because it bounces). Whatever its label, it means that you have not received that money which the patient says he or she paid you. There are several methods of collecting when this happens. One is to call the patient and explain that the check was returned for insufficient funds. The patient will then tell you the funds are now available or give you a date when the check can be represented. At such time you redeposit the check and hopefully you receive credit for it. Or perhaps the patient will prefer to send you another check or a cashier's check.

Suppose you find the patient uncooperative, and it is impossible for you to collect the amount in this manner. The next step is to enter the check for collection with your bank. There is a charge for this service, depending on the size of the check. The bank will attempt to collect it for you. Should this method fail, it is time to turn the matter over to your attorney or your collection agency.

If a receipt has been given to the patient for a payment by check, you will be wise to write the patient a letter immediately, stating that the check has been returned for insufficient funds and that the receipt that had been issued is not valid. This letter should be sent by registered mail with a return receipt requested.

Accounts Receivable Control

Statements must be sent to patients each month indicating the amount of money they owe and, in some offices, the services rendered. How can you know that you are sending statements to all the patients who owe money? The **accounts receivable control** permits a verification of these records.

Each patient account record shows the balance the patient owes. Therefore, total all the patient account record balances. Now total the amounts on all the statements to be sent. These two totals should agree. If they do not agree, it is necessary to recheck all records and arithmetic.

An accounts receivable control is figured thus:

To
Total accounts receivable
   from previous month: $43,300.00
Add
Charges for dentistry
   performed during
   current month: $11,100.00
                                $54,400.00

Subtract
Current month's
   receipts: $11,300.00
   and
Discounts given during
   month: $ 325.00
                  $11,625.00 $11,625.00
Total accounts receivable
   at end of current
   month: $42,775.00

Terms to Be Understood

accounts receivable control a method of verifying that all outstanding charges have been billed to the persons owing money

day sheet a complete detailed record of professional and financial activities completed during one day

discount a reduction in fee or price offered in specified circumstances

invoice an itemized record of materials purchased from a firm (The invoice usually accompanies the merchandise. It is a source document and must be filed for later verification with the monthly statement from that firm, and then refiled permanently as the proof of purchase of that specific item.)

office change fund money kept separately in the office to make change for patients who pay with cash and do not have the correct change

patient's account record a detailed permanent record of all charges for dental work performed for a specific patient and all payments received from that patient (Sometimes the patient account record is a family account and the transactions with the entire family are recorded on one card.)

patient's service record a detailed permanent record of all dental work performed for the specific patient

petty cash fund a special cash fund available in the office for expenditures of a minor nature—amounts so small that writing a check is not feasible

receipt a written record acknowledging that the stated sum of money or goods has been received from the person named on the receipt

statement a summary report at the end of the billing period sent to persons who have charged goods or services during that billing period (The statement lists, usually by number or department, the purchases made and the charge for each with the total amount owed.)

The total amount of money billed on the statements should equal the final figure, $42,775.00. If there is a discrepancy between your statements and this control, there has been an error in (1) posting, (2) subtracting, or (3) adding. The error must be located and corrected. If the error is an error in posting, look first for transposition in figures. For example, you have recorded a check for $502. When you recheck, you discover it should have been for $520. The second item to check is to see whether you have put the amount in the wrong column. If it is an asset, it should not be placed in the liability column, and vice versa. The total of accounts receivable figures should coincide when calculated in each method. Keeping this control assures that postings are being done accurately and that account balances are correct.

This control is necessary to ascertain that patients are being charged for the services they receive. Without accuracy in billing it is conceivable that a dentist would soon be unable to pay the salaries of the staff.

Summary

The Summary and Study Questions for this chapter will be found at the end of chapter 17.

Vocabulary

Many new words were used in this chapter. Study the boxed definitions for review.

Word Elements	
Word Element	*Example*
dorsi, dorse combining form meaning: relationship to the back	*dorsal* pertaining to the back or posterior part of an organ
latero, lati combining form meaning: relationship to the side	*lateral* to the side
neur, neuro combining form meaning: relationship to the nerves or nervous system	*neuritis* inflammation of a nerve
phago combining form meaning: relationship to eating	*phagocyte* a cell that engulfs or devours microbes, cells, debris, and other substances
pleura combining form meaning: relationship to the side, rib, or pleura	*pleurisy* inflammation of the pleura with exudation into the cavity and on its surface
pod combining form meaning: relationship to the foot	*podiatrist* one who treats the feet
sangui combining form meaning: relationship to the blood	*sanguine* abounding in blood
tax combining form meaning: order, arrange	*ataxia* failure of muscular coordination
ventro combining form meaning: to the front, abdomen	*ventrolateral* both front and side

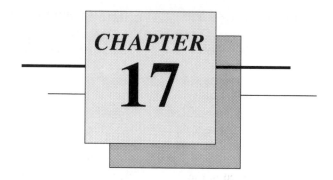

Financial Records:
Part Two, Disbursements

Records About Money Spent (Expenditures)
Petty Cash Fund
Dental Office Charge Accounts—Payment by Check
  Invoices for Dental Office Purchases
  Statements for Dental Office Purchases
Disbursement Record
  Preparing the Disbursement Record
Yearly Summary
Banking Procedures
  Deposit Slips
  Checkbook
  Check-writing Procedure
  Checkbook Reconciliation
    Checkbook Reconciliation Procedure
Monthly Record-keeping Responsibilities—
        A Summary
The Write-It-Once or Pegboard Bookkeeping
        Systems
  How Pegboard Systems Differ
Computers in the Dental Office
  Computer Systems at Service Bureaus
  Computer Systems in the Office
  The Magic Box Concept
Additional Banking Services
Power of Attorney
Notary Public

Records About Money Spent (Expenditures)

Records discussed in chapter 16 were records about money received. It is also necessary to spend money in the dental office. Records of these expenditures are very important. There are petty cash expenditures and charge account expenditures paid by check. There are also salary checks to be written.

Petty Cash Fund

Every dental office has some expenditures of a minor nature that do not warrant the writing of a check. Cash kept in the office for these expenditures is called a **petty cash fund.** To begin such a fund, a check is written to the dentist and endorsed by him or her. "Disbursement to the petty cash fund" is recorded on the stub, and the check is cashed. The cash should be kept separately from all other cash that comes into the office so that there will be no confusion of money. A small notebook or journal may be purchased for the year's record; or a ruled sheet may be used for each month's record of the petty cash fund. A page is headed "Petty Cash Fund." The name of the month is written at the top of the sheet. The next line is to show the headings for the columns. Divide the page into five columns. Make a narrow column on the left, headed "Date." Next, make a wide column for "Detailed Itemizations." Then make three equal columns headed "Disbursements," "Receipts," and "Balance." The amount used in this fund will vary in different dental offices, but it should be sufficient to cover the largest month's minor expenses so that only one check need be issued each month.

The first entry on this sheet would be dated the first of the month. The detail entry would be "Check No. xxxx." The amount of the check would be written in the "Receipts" column.

For example, suppose that on the tenth of the month a ball-point pen was purchased at the stationery store. This entry, dated the tenth, would be made as, "ball-point pen"; and under "Disbursements" the cost would be entered. A receipt for the pen should be clipped to the petty cash sheet. This receipt is your **source document.** The balance remaining in the petty cash fund should be entered in the "Balance" column (fig. 17.1).

At the end of the month, the actual cash in the petty cash fund is counted and checked against the petty cash sheet indication of "Balance." The amount of money in your fund and the figure in the balance column should agree. An office check is made out for the amount necessary to return the petty cash fund to its original balance. The petty cash expenditures for each month are written on a separate page of the ledger. On the new sheet made out for the next month, the first entry carries forward the balance remaining in the petty cash fund at the end of the previous month, the second entry is for the check (and its number), the amount entered under "Receipts" and the new balance written in, which should be the original established for the petty cash fund.

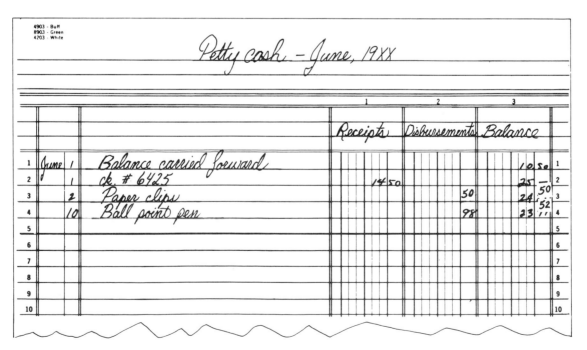

Figure 17.1

A three column ruled account sheet for petty cash records.

There should be no cash expenditures from the office except through a petty cash fund. For every petty cash disbursement there must be a receipt.

Dental Office Charge Accounts— Payment by Check

When a dental supply is charged, the payment is usually made at the end of the month. For charge accounts there will be both *invoices* and *statements* for office purchases. The invoices will be sent with the supply at the time it is ordered; the statement will follow at the close of the month.

Invoices for Dental Office Purchases

An **invoice** is a form included with an order of supplies. It usually has a number on it, the date, the name and address of the firm sending the supplies, the name and address of the dentist receiving them, how many and what supplies they are, and the price. This invoice is a source document.

During the month, you receive invoices from various firms from whom you have ordered supplies. Verify them when received to be certain (1) that the charge is correct for the material you have received, and (2) that you have received all material listed. File them in a folder marked "Current Invoices." Clip all invoices of each firm together in the file as they are received.

Statements for Dental Office Purchases

At the end of the month, each firm sends a **statement** listing all the items (sometimes by invoice number) that you have ordered and giving the total amount you owe the firm.

Upon the receipt of a firm's statement, proceed as follows:

1. Remove the invoices for that firm from the current invoices file.
2. Compare the invoices with the statement to be certain that you have received the materials as charged and that the charges are correct.
3. Clip to this statement the invoices you have received since the previous billing.
4. Write a check for the correct amount.
5. Write the check number and the date on which you write the check on the lower half of the statement from the firm.
6. Tear off the upper half (which lists the firm name and your dentist's name).

7. Clip the upper half of the statement to the check.
8. Address an envelope if one is not furnished with the statement.
9. Put the statement, check, and envelope on your dentist's desk if he or she is to sign the check.
10. When the check has been signed, insert the check and statement in the envelope and mail it.
11. Staple the lower half of the statement to the invoices for that month and file this packet in the permanent record section of the file. A file folder for the firm or for the month is commonly used.
12. At the end of the year, these statements are bundled, either by firm name or by month, and packaged in dead storage for future reference. The packages are clearly labeled.

Figure 17.2 shows a statement and invoice from a supply firm.

Disbursement Record

The expenditures in the dental office must be recorded in permanent form much like the day sheet record of services for patients and moneys received. The record of the expenditures is called a **disbursement record.**

A disbursement record is composed of columns for recording certain information. Usually the column headings read Date, Name of Firm (or Person) Paid, Object Purchased, Check Number, Amount of Check, Deposits, and Bank Balance.

In addition, most disbursement records have columns for classifying the purchases. The disbursement record will then continue on, after the Bank Balance, with columns headed Taxes, Insurance, Rent, Laboratory Expense, Dental Supplies, Dental Equipment, Household Drawing, Contributions, and so on.

A common form for a disbursement record is a thirteen-column ruled tablet on which the individual can write the headings he or she desires to use.

The Internal Revenue Service recommends a separate checking account for a dentist's personal expenses. It recommends that once or twice a month a check be deposited to the personal checking account and that all personal expenditures be paid from this account. The business expenses, which are legally deductible before the dentist's income is figured for tax purposes, are then clearly separated from those expenses that must be paid from his or her own income,

STATEMENT

John Marcus Dental Supply Co.

3037 Lyndale Avenue South, Minneapolis, Minnesota 55408

Phone: 827-6125

John C. Raeywen, D.D.S.
104 Any Street
Anytown, Anystate 12345

DATE	INVOICE NO.	CHARGES	CREDITS	BALANCE
			BALANCE FORWARD	$120.50
Apr 2	330007	$161.06		$281.56
Apr 8	330121	90.63		$372.19
Apr 10	Check 2501		$120.50	$251.69
Apr 15	330392	76.50		$328.19

John Marcus Dental Supply Co. TERMS: NET 10TH

a

John Marcus Dental Supply Company

3037 LYNDALE AVE. SO. • MINNEAPOLIS MINNESOTA 55408 • PHONE 827-6125

Invoice # 330121
Salesman Dick
Customer
Date April 8, 19—

TO John C. Raeywen, D.D.S.
104 Any Street
Anytown, Anystate 12345

MANUFACTURER	BACK ORDERED	QUAN. ORDERED	QUAN. SHIPPED	DESCRIPTION	UNIT PRICE	AMOUNT
K.P.		3	3	Bib (rate for 3 or more cartons)	$28.50	$85.50
					SUB TOTAL	$85.50
					SHIPPING	1.50
					TAX	$5.13
					TOTAL	$90.63

ITEMS APPEARING IN BACK ORDER COLUMN WILL FOLLOW SHORTLY

b

Figure 17.2
a) Statement for dental office purchases; and b) one of the invoices listed on the statement.

such as clothing, house payments or home rent, and medical bills. A column in the business disbursement record titled "Personal Account" or "Household Drawing Account," in which checks to the personal drawing account may be entered, keeps the business and personal expenses separated satisfactorily.

Usually there is a column on the disbursement record headed "Personal Deductions" or "Donations" separate from "Personal Account" or "Household Drawing Account," because this information is needed for tax purposes and is readily found if it is in a separate column. Generally speaking, personal donations are not deductible as a business expense but may be deducted from personal income taxes. However, some donations are properly considered business expenses—for example, contributions to a dental charity (assuming it is on the Internal Revenue Service approved list of deductible items) or a memorial to a recognized charity for a patient, etc. Sometimes it is necessary to make donations from the office which are not deductible as a business expense. It is customary to put all donations made from the office in the "Personal Deductions" column in the disbursement record.

Preparing the Disbursement Record

After the checks for office expenditures have been written, the disbursement record can be completed, using the check register. (Checking procedures will be discussed later in this chapter.) Fill in the columns on the disbursement record as required by the particular check being recorded.

1. Start with the first check written in January.
2. Enter the date, check number, description (to whom and for what), and amount in the columns provided.
3. Now look across the headings and see what column describes this check. If it is a rent check and there is a column for rent, write the amount in that column (fig. 17.3).
4. Continue this process until all the checks written have been recorded. It is possible to use a code system to be certain that each check has been recorded on the disbursement record.
5. Sometimes a check is written for an amount that must be divided on the disbursement record. For example, your dentist may purchase supplies and equipment from the same dental firm and make a payment by one check. It will be necessary to divide the payment on the disbursement record. For example, equipment costing $100 is purchased along with supplies totaling $52. The entire $152 is entered as the amount of the check the first time it is recorded on the disbursement sheet. Enter the $100 under "Equipment" and the $52 under "Supplies" in the disbursement record.
6. Divide the petty cash expenditures into their proper categories. When the petty cash fund is reimbursed, write the total amount of the check in the "Check Amount" column and write the amount of each type of expenditure in the proper column in the disbursement record.
7. At the end of the month, total each disbursement column.
8. Total the *totals* of the disbursement columns.
9. Total the check column. The total of the check column and the total of all the disbursement totals should agree.
10. The totals can be carried forward each month, and the dentist can know at the end of any month exactly what his or her expenses have been in relation to his or her income for the year or for any particular month.

Yearly Summary

At the close of the year, all income and expenditures must be summarized. A summary sheet, maintained monthly, brings the record up-to-date. Usually these forms have spaces for listing fees or charges, unpaid balance on accounts, and money collected in order to figure the gross income of the dental practice. There are also spaces for totals from the disbursement records, showing expenses such as materials, laboratory bills, general expenses, personal account, personal deductions, and permanent equipment. The total disbursements of a business nature (excepting personal accounts) are deducted from the total receipts to find the net income on which personal income tax is figured. Most yearly summaries have a section where general expenses may be broken down for further study. Depreciation on permanent equipment is usually figured when the tax returns are prepared.

Banking Procedures

Possibly the most familiar area of banking service for the dental assistant is the **checking account.** A checking account is simply a way of transferring money to other people for the things you wish to buy. A check cannot be cashed except by the person to whom it is drawn (made out). This means that it is safe to send a check through the mail. It is more difficult to steal.

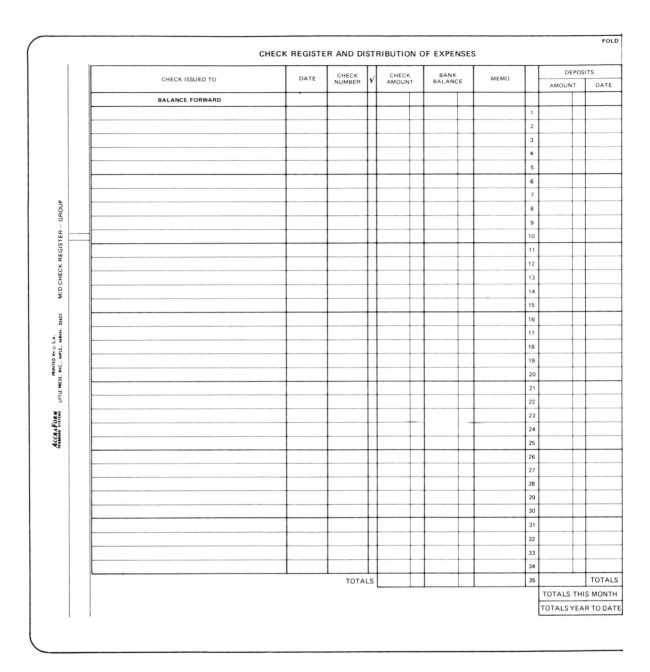

Figure 17.3

A disbursement record.

Basically, the checking account simply means that the owner has gone to the bank, signed a card with his signature, deposited some money, and has been given some checks to use. In today's mechanized banking world, almost all checks have an account number printed on each check. The owner of a checking account has his or her own account number. All his or her banking transactions (deposits and withdrawals by means of check-writing) are performed on checks and deposit slips that have his or her number printed on them. These numbers are usually sensitized, and a machine automatically enters the transaction on the correct account.

A business checking account balance may not earn interest as a savings account does. If the owner keeps enough money in the checking account (an amount specified by the bank), the account costs him or her little or nothing to operate. However, if the balance falls below this specified amount, a charge is made for each check written. This is called a **service charge.**

BANK _____									ACCOUNT NAME _____						
ACCOUNT NO. _____			MONTH _____				19 ___ PAGE NO. _____								
	RENT & UTILITIES	TELEPHONE	PROF. SUPPLIES & DRUGS	OUTSIDE PROF. LAB. SERVICES	BUSINESS OFFICE SUPPLIES	BUSINESS TAXES	BUSINESS INSURANCE	FEES	BUSINESS AUTO & TRAVEL	CONVEN- TIONS & MEETINGS	PROF. DUES AND JOURNALS	RETIRE- MENT PLANS	EMPLOYEE FRINGE BENEFITS	

A checking account is maintained for the office. It is a business checking account into which any money received from patients must be deposited.

Only by depositing every penny of income in the **office checking account** is it possible to have an accountant verify the income in the office. Internal Revenue Service agents are particular about accounting for income whenever money is collected in a business. A person who receives a salary check is a less likely object of concern than a person whose income is irregular. A dentist has an irregular income, which can facilitate inaccurate income reporting to the government. Therefore, a dentist must be especially careful to so conduct the accounting that there can be no question about the fact that all income has been reported. The easiest way to do this is to deposit all income in an office checking account. Checks can then be written for personal drawing accounts on whatever basis the dentist wishes.

Each day's receipts should be deposited as a unit. Verification of the accuracy of the day's receipts is thus provided.

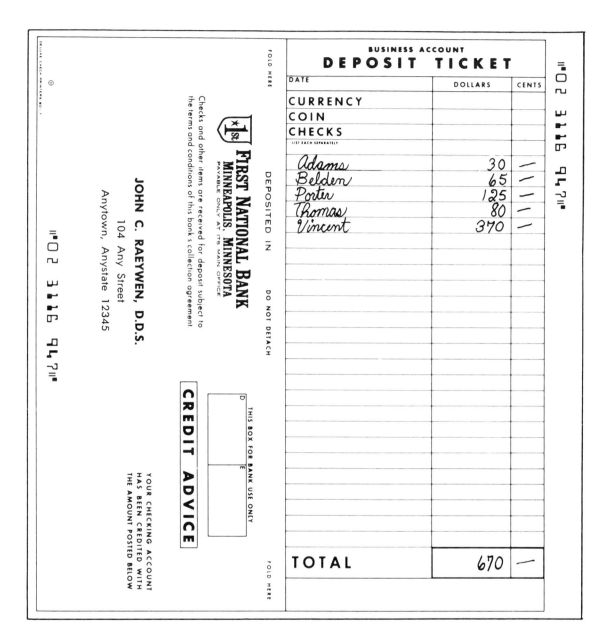

Figure 17.4

A deposit slip.

Deposit Slips

At the close of each day, the total receipts on the day sheet should equal exactly the total of the cash and checks on hand. A deposit slip is then made out for the day's receipts, and the cash and checks are clipped to it. The deposit is made as soon as convenient. It is preferable to make a deposit for each day, but if this is not convenient or necessary, deposits should be made frequently enough to prevent the accumulation of checks or cash in the office. More frequent deposits are helpful in showing errors as soon as possible after they occur.

Deposit slip books are available from most banks in numbered, *duplicate* pages. This is the type that should be used for the office. Each deposit slip is used consecutively. It is recommended that the bank teller stamp the duplicate deposit slip at the time the deposit is made (fig. 17.4).

Final deposits are made to cover any payments made through the last day of each month. While this deposit will usually be made on the first day of the new month, it is nevertheless made out as an individual deposit to close the preceding month. Any additional moneys for deposit at that time (money collected on the first day of the new month) are listed on a separate deposit slip—the next consecutively numbered slip.

A new deposit slip book should be started with the first of each year in order that all records for the year just completed may be stored together.

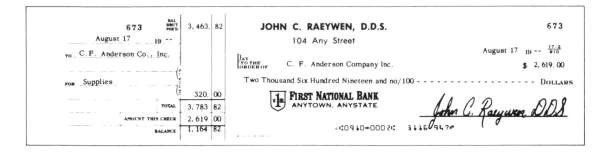

Figure 17.5
A check and check stub properly filled out.

CHECK NO.	DATE	CHECK ISSUED TO	IN PAYMENT OF	AMOUNT OF CHECK	✓	DATE OF DEPOSIT	AMOUNT OF DEPOSIT	BALANCE
			5/31/-			BALANCE BROUGHT FORWARD →		5240 —
2085	6/1/-	ABC Dental Laboratory	Case #3264	300 00				4940 -
2086	6/1/-	Jafa Morgan Dentl Supply	Supplies	35 50				4904 50
2087	6/1/-	Dahl Pharmacy	Drugs	48 50				4856 —
2088	6/1/-	Dr. John C. Raeywen	W W Draw	500 -				4356 -
						6/4/-	350 —	4706 —
2089	6/5/-	Minn. Natural Gas Co.	Service	6 48				4699 52
2090	6/5/-	Northern State Power Co.	Elec Service	42 58				4656 94
2091	6/5/-	N.W. Bell Telephone Co.	Telephone Ser.	48 50				4608 44

Figure 17.6
A check register correctly maintained.

Checkbook

The business checking account should be used only for the business receipts and expenses. The dentist should receive a check from the business checking account once or twice a month. This check is deposited in the dentist's personal or household checking account.

A **check** is an authorization to the bank to pay a specified amount of money to the person named on the check from the account of the person who signs the check. Sometimes the person signs for a firm, and then the authorization is for the firm rather than the individual (fig. 17.5).

The dental assistant is generally given the duty of making out checks for the payment of the various bills against the dental office and may or may not have her or his signature authorized for the checking account. If the assistant's signature is authorized by the dentist and entered at the bank in their records, the assistant may complete the entire procedure of paying bills for the office. If the assistant's signature is not authorized for the checking account, the dentist must sign the checks.

Dental office records, including the checkbook, should be written with a permanent ink. The only exception to this rule is that receipts and deposit slips that require carbon copies are made with a ball-point pen.

The **check stub** or **check register** is a record retained in the office. It includes this information, either on each individual check stub or on each page of the check register: (1) the number of the check; (2) the date; (3) to whom the check is written; (4) for what the check is written; (5) the checkbook balance; (6) recording of any deposits; (7) date of deposits; (8) total of the checkbook balance and deposit combined; (9) amount of the check just written; and (10) new checkbook balance (subtract the amount of the check from the previous balance). Thus, after writing a check it is possible to know how much money is still available in the checking account.

It is highly recommended that the check stub or register be completed first, then the check, and that both these forms be verified with the statement of the bill being paid. Accuracy is essential.

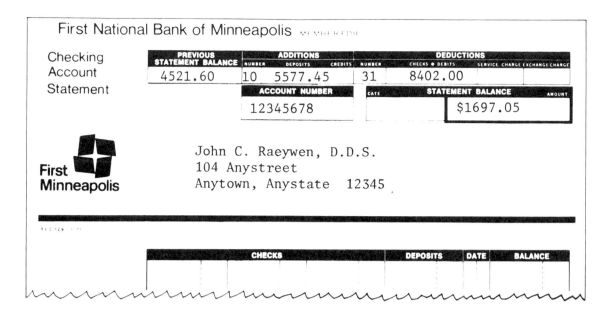

Figure 17.7
Bank statement for checking account.

Check-writing Procedure

It is the first day of the month. You have received a statement for rent, perhaps including charges for services such as electricity and heat, and a statement from a dental supply company. You have verified each invoice of materials purchased from them throughout the month against this statement and found it to be correct. You write the necessary information on the check stub, or in the check register, then write out a check to the Medical Arts Building Enterprises, Inc., for the amount of the statement that they sent you. You fill in the number if it is not already printed on the check, the date, the name, and the amount (handwritten numerically and also written as words). You do the same for the dental supply company. These checks, with the statements and envelopes, are then placed on the dentist's desk for his or her signature. After the checks have been signed, place the top half of the statement in the envelope with the check, seal the envelope, mail it, and file the bottom half of the statement with the invoices (as previously mentioned in this chapter).

If a dentist uses a Write-It-Once system of bookkeeping, he or she may also use the checks of such a system. The register (or stub) is a page, and the checks with carbon lines are placed over the page in the same way as the charge/receipt slip. One writing completes the check and register entries. (A discussion of the details of Write-It-Once bookkeeping occurs later in this chapter.)

Your dentist may rent the use of a check-writing machine. This is a device which is rented from a firm for a nominal sum. It is protection against alteration of the check amount. The machine writes in the amount of the check with finely punched holes and much red and blue ink around the writing. It is impossible for anyone to alter the amount of the check. It is simple to learn to operate this machine, and should there be one in the office in which you work, it will save you the necessity of writing out the amount in longhand. The rest of the check is prepared like any other check.

Some dentists may prefer to have you type the checks. This also is protection against alteration of the check because it is impossible to erase the typed figures and it is more difficult to alter a typed figure than a handwritten one.

Checkbook Reconciliation

At or near the close of each month, a statement of the account, together with the cancelled checks listed on the statement, is received from the bank. The balance in the checking account as shown on the bank statement will not agree with the balance shown on the last stub in the checkbook.

These figures must be checked to determine whether they are correct. This is known as **reconciliation** of the bank statement balance with the checkbook balance. This reconciliation process is not confusing if you follow a set procedure in accomplishing it.

Cancelled checks are those originally made out to pay a dental office account. The check was received by the company to which it was sent. The company endorsed the check for deposit to their account at their bank. Their bank put the check through a "clearing house" procedure, which ultimately meant that the money from your office's bank, on which the check was drawn, was transferred to the bank of the company to which the check was sent. In exchange for transferring this money, your bank received the check itself. Since the purpose for which it was written has been accomplished, the check is cancelled by means of a stamp placed on it (usually punching tiny holes) stating that the check has been paid. These paid or cancelled checks are then listed on your bank statement and are deducted from the balance you have on record at the bank. In addition to deducting the paid checks, the bank will deduct bank charges and, in some cases, charges for "exchange"—a service charge for handling checks drawn on certain types of banks.

Some banks do not return your cancelled checks. The bank statement shows the date, check number, and amount of each check that has cleared. You must verify these figures with your check register.

As you issued checks during the month, you will have deducted the amount of each check from your balance. However, on the bank statement there may be bank service charges or exchange charges that you will not have listed in your check register.

You will have added, on your checkbook stubs or register, the deposits that you made. The bank statement covers through only a certain day of the month, and deposits made on or after that closing day are not included in the balance that the bank statement will show.

You may have had an office account, which you paid by check, with a firm located in some other city, or some firm to which you sent a check may not have deposited that check immediately. Thus, it may not be cancelled in time to appear on your statement. This check, of course, will not be deducted from the balance according to the bank's figures. You deducted it, however, when you wrote it.

For this reason, the bank's monthly statement of your checking account is not always the exact figure you have listed as the balance according to your last check stub. There are many figures to be carefully and accurately checked. *Do not permit the bank statement to go unreconciled.* Keep checking until it does correspond with your check stubs or register. Banks can make errors, and an error must be called to their attention within a specified time or the bank statement is assumed to be correct.

Checkbook Reconciliation Procedure

1. If you receive cancelled checks, arrange them in numerical sequence.
2. Verify each cancelled check or each check number on the bank statement with your check register. Place a check mark by the number on the register for each check that has cleared. If the bank statement does not list a check, do not place a check mark by that number on the register or stub.
3. Note the number of the last check listed on the bank statement. On your check register draw a line just below that check. This is the point at which you will reconcile your checking statement.
4. Verify that the amount listed for each check on your bank statement is the same as the amount listed on your check register. (If they are not the same, note the difference on a sheet of paper and copy the rest of the information from the check. It may be necessary to call the bank and have them correct their records.)
5. Note each check number in your register that has no check mark beside it. These checks will be the outstanding checks— those which have not yet cleared the bank. Do not go beyond the line you drew. That line indicates the place at which the checkbook should "reconcile" with the bank.

   On the back of the bank statement (fig. 17.8), write the number of each outstanding check and the amount of the check in the appropriate columns in item 3. Total these checks as instructed on the statement.
6. Now verify that each deposit has been recorded by the bank. If the bank has not sent you the receipt for some of the deposits you have already made, list each deposit. Write the total of these deposits in the appropriate column on the bank form.
7. Write the current balance, shown by the bank on the face of the statement, in the proper place on the back of the statement.
8. Total the bank's balance of your account and any outstanding *deposits.*
9. Subtract the outstanding checks from this amount.
10. Note any charges for bank services. Subtract this amount from the balance in your checkbook at the point at which you drew the line.

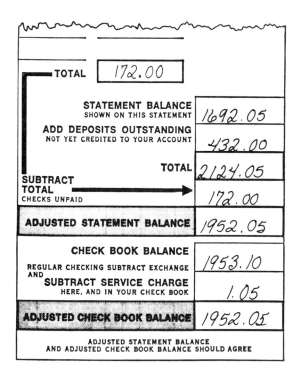

TO BALANCE YOUR ACCOUNT

1. SORT CHECKS INTO NUMERICAL ORDER.
2. CHECK OFF ALL CHECKS RETURNED WITH **THIS** STATEMENT IN YOUR CHECK REGISTER.

CHECK NO.	CHECK AMOUNT
4236	50.00
4251	100.50
4289	21.50

3. LIST CHECKS UNPAID.

WRITTEN BUT NOT YET CHARGED TO YOUR ACCOUNT

TOTAL	172.00
STATEMENT BALANCE SHOWN ON THIS STATEMENT	1692.05
ADD DEPOSITS OUTSTANDING NOT YET CREDITED TO YOUR ACCOUNT	432.00
TOTAL	2124.05
SUBTRACT TOTAL CHECKS UNPAID	172.00
ADJUSTED STATEMENT BALANCE	1952.05
CHECK BOOK BALANCE REGULAR CHECKING SUBTRACT EXCHANGE AND	1953.10
SUBTRACT SERVICE CHARGE HERE, AND IN YOUR CHECK BOOK	1.05
ADJUSTED CHECK BOOK BALANCE	1952.05

ADJUSTED STATEMENT BALANCE AND ADJUSTED CHECK BOOK BALANCE SHOULD AGREE

Figure 17.8
Reverse side of statement shown in Figure 17.7.

11. This amount and the bank statement of current balance should agree. For example:

Bank balance:	$1,692.05	Your checkbook balance:	$1,953.10
Plus outstanding deposits:	432.00	Less service charges:	1.05
	$2,124.05		$1,952.05
Less outstanding checks:	$ 172.00		
	$1,952.05		

(A detailed practice example of checkbook reconciliation will be found in the workbook to accompany *Effective Dental Assisting*.)

Monthly Record-keeping Responsibilities—A Summary

Your record-keeping responsibilities, then, include these steps:

1. For payments received:
   a. Write a receipt for every payment made.
   b. Enter the payment on the patient's account record.
2. For services to patients:
   a. Enter on the day sheet the name of each patient for whom service is performed, the service, and the charge.
   b. Check to see whether the dentist has entered the information on the patient's service record. See that it is entered.
   c. Enter the charges for this service on the patient's account record.
3. For money disbursed:
   a. Collect a receipt and write an entry in the petty cash fund book for every penny of cash that is spent through your office.
   b. Write any disbursements, other than petty cash, in the disbursement record. (If you are writing a check to reimburse petty cash, as must be done once a month or as needed, enter that check on the disbursement record and properly disburse the money so spent.)
   c. Once a month check the statements from firms against the invoices received during that month, and pay the bills.
4. Once a month put your totals on the yearly summary sheet.

5. Check all invoices as they come to your attention.
6. Reconcile the checkbook once a month.
7. Make deposits on a daily, biweekly, or weekly basis, or as your dentist directs.
8. Prepare and send statements to patients for services rendered.

The Write-It-Once or Pegboard Bookkeeping Systems

If you work in an office that employs a mechanized bookkeeping system, you will be given specific instructions about its operation and your responsibilities for that system. However, a brief résumé may be helpful. This system is referred to as **instant bookkeeping.** It is so designed that one writing of information by the assistant enters the information everywhere it is needed. It records all necessary records with proof of accuracy (because they are all written at the same time). There can be no transposing of figures or miscopying of names or services. You simply write it once. It records all these records at once: patient's receipt-statement (record of today's charge), patient's monthly statement, patient's financial card, record of charges and receipts (daily log), and the bank deposit record.

A pegboard system of record-keeping differs in the following ways from the explanation of the basics of record-keeping.

1. The **patient account card** is a special form (fig. 17.9). As in other systems, all the charges and payments must be entered on this card. It may be a *family* card; that is, the responsible adult has a card, and all the charges for dentistry for the family are entered on the card. It may be an *individual* card if for only one person.

    Type at the top of the card the name and address of the person responsible for the account. These cards are kept in a tray, alphabetically arranged.

    At the time chosen by your dentist for sending out statements, the account cards are run through a copying machine, and the copy is sent to the patient.
2. The day sheet is mounted on the pegboard (fig. 17.10). It is a special sheet furnished by the company that manufactures the pegboard system used in your office. The pegboard is a flat board usually made of some kind of composition board. It has a row of pegs on the left side designed to hold two or three papers in a certain position. The day sheet is on the bottom

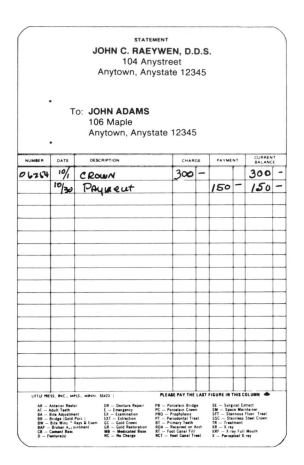

Figure 17.9
A patient account card.

and a carbon is placed over it. The charge/receipt slip (fig. 17.11) is carefully placed on the pegs so that the entry on the charge/receipt slip will be entered on the day sheet on the proper line. Now the patient's account card (also called a ledger card) is inserted between the carbon paper that was placed over the day sheet and the charge/receipt slip. Since the charge/receipt slip and the day sheet are held in place by the pegs, they cannot slip.

Position the patient's account card so the entry written on the charge/receipt slip will appear on the correct line of the patient's account card. The carbon on the back of the charge/receipt slip will cause the entry to appear on the patient's account card; the carbon paper beneath the patient's account card will cause the entry to be made on the day sheet.

The charge/receipt slip may be used as a receipt or a statement for the patient. The stub of the charge/receipt slip becomes a communication channel between the dentist, receptionist, and patient.

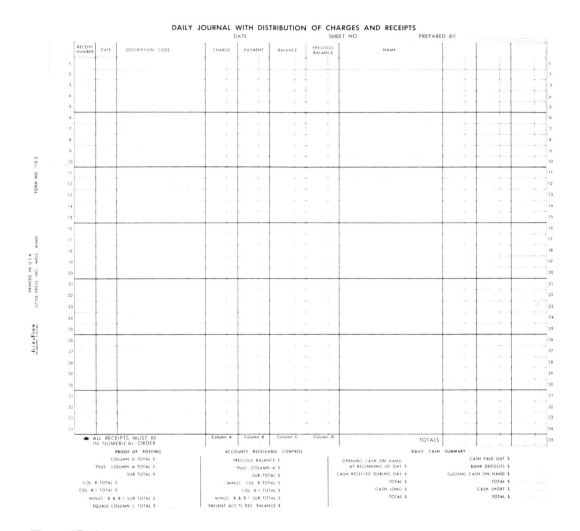

Figure 17.10
A pegboard day sheet.

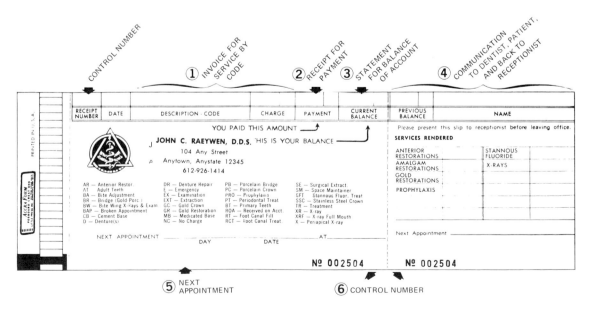

Figure 17.11
Pegboard charge/receipt slip.

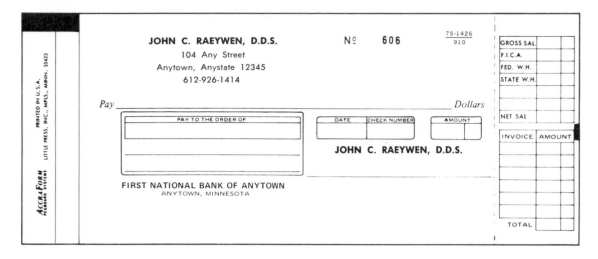

Figure 17.12
Pegboard check form.

How Pegboard Systems Differ

Pegboard systems differ somewhat depending on the arrangements offered by the several manufacturers. Basically, the record-keeping duties are the same regardless of the system used.

The day sheet contains all the necessary entries for the tax records. Every charge and every payment are recorded as they occur during the day. One writing makes the receipt for the patient and the entry on the day sheet. Thus, there is no separate receipt book. Each item is recorded by a printed control number (recopied by the assistant onto the day sheet), and the name of the patient. The day sheet (fig. 17.10) also has space for Proof of Posting (to determine the accuracy of the bookkeeping), the Accounts Receivable Control, and the Daily Cash Summary. Thus, on one sheet all the information regarding dentistry performed and cash received is summarized. Each day the totals are carried forward to the new day sheet so that at any time the dentist knows how much dentistry has been performed, how much money has been collected, and how much money is outstanding.

Figure 17.12 is a check form often used with a pegboard system. The check is placed over the check register, and the information transfers to the register by carbon as the check is written.

Computers in the Dental Office
(Kay Schwarzrock, B.A.)

There are two major categories of computer systems available for use in dental offices: systems where the computer is in the dental office and systems where the computer is somewhere else, usually at a service bureau.

There are three types of systems in use at service bureaus: batch systems, remote data entry systems, and remote online systems. If the computer is in the dental office, it is highly likely that the system is an online system.

Computer Systems at Service Bureaus

The simplest service bureau system is a **batch system,** in which the office personnel fill out charge forms for all work done each day and also account maintenance forms to add, change, or delete account information. The forms are sent to a service bureau where they are entered and processed by the service bureau's computer. Either daily, or at scheduled times during the month, computer printed statements are produced for the dental office. Some service bureaus mail the statements to patients while others give them to the dental office for verification and mailing. A batch system may produce billing statements only or may also produce other types of financial reports.

The **remote data entry system** is similar to a batch system. Instead of writing out the day's charges by hand on a form, the charges and other information are keyed at a *remote data entry terminal.* This terminal is referred to as remote because it is in the dental office while the computer is somewhere else, connected to the terminal by telephone lines. A *data entry terminal* is a device used to feed information (data) into a computer system. Sometimes this terminal is referred to as a *dumb tube* because you key information in but cannot ask the computer system to give information to you on the terminal. The data either is entered directly into the service bureau computer or it is stored in memory in the dental office and transmitted to the service bureau at scheduled times. The computer system then produces billing statements and financial reports in the same manner as a batch system.

A **remote online system,** sometimes referred to as a time-share system, is more sophisticated than either a batch or a dumb tube system. With an online system, you can look at the information that is stored any time you request it at a CRT. (CRT is the commonly used term for *cathode ray tube:* a TV screen with a typewriter keyboard attached to it so that when you type, letters appear on the screen). The dental office will have one or more printers and one or more CRTs. Time-share systems vary in the amount of service they provide. Some are as simple as a batch or dumb tube system. The more sophisticated systems will keep account history, provide financial reports, prepare tax information and patient-insurance claims, produce statements, or even keep the appointment book. Reports are either printed on a printer in the dental office or on the service bureau's printer.

Large computers are very expensive. Time-sharing systems were developed to provide small businesses access to computers with minimal cost. A company owning a large computer will sell computer time to a small business, usually providing all the business programs (instructions that tell the computer what to do with the data you enter). In this way, a small dental office can afford to use a computer system.

Computer Systems in the Office

In the last few years, advances have been made in cutting the cost of producing computers and smaller computers have been designed for smaller businesses. The computers commonly used in dental offices are called **personal computers.** They are modular systems, which means they can be expanded by purchasing additional hardware such as CRTs, printers, or memory. The smallest system would have one CRT and one printer. In a clinic environment, the system would have multiple CRTs and printers. It might even have two or more CPUs linked together to handle more processing, like a train which has more than one engine. (A CPU is the commonly used term for *central processing unit:* the brain of the computer which controls the computer and does all the processing or thinking.) In a dental office with two or more physical locations, the physical locations can be linked together on one computer system network or they can have independent systems. Regardless of the size of the computer system, the functionality is the same. The software can be purchased separately or in a package with the hardware. In either case, instruction manuals are furnished.

These systems can provide sophisticated tools for the office, including patient history, account history, a wide range of financial reports, and specialized packages such as an orthognathic planner for an oral surgeon or a general ledger system. In addition, they can keep the appointment book, provide the daily patient lists for every member of the office staff, print statements, prepare tax information and patient insurance claims, and track the financial affairs of the office for an entire year or more. It is also possible to access data from a remote location so that the dentist can verify patient information from home during off hours if he or she has a personal computer and *dial-up* capabilities (the ability to call one computer from another computer using telephone lines).

The services provided can vary considerably depending on the sophistication of the system purchased. Online systems allow immediate access to information stored on the computer. Batch and remote data entry systems do not because they are not online. Keeping the appointment book on the computer is only practical in an online environment. Other than that difference, all of the systems *can* be programmed to perform the same functions. The functional range of a specific system depends on how the system was designed and has a direct impact on its cost.

The paper on which most computer systems print reports differs from regular paper in two respects: the forms are continuous, and the left and right margins each have a row of perforations used to control the flow of paper through the printer. On preprinted forms, such as statements, the computer is programmed to print information in the appropriate areas. It is also possible to print on blank paper (like typing paper). Computer paper can be 8½″ × 11″ or 15″ × 11″. It can be blank or have horizontal bands of pale color to improve readability. Computerized statements can be printed on forms that could be used for hand-written or typed statements or they can be printed on forms that become a complete mailer-envelope.

The Magic Box Concept

People tend to think of a computer as a magic box. Computers are not magic, they are just *completely logical.* They do exactly what you tell them to do. If the computer does not do what you thought you told it to do, your directions were probably incorrect or inadequate. The remedy is to reread the instructions for your system and try again. People also tend to feel that if they do something wrong, the computer will be destroyed. This probably stems from the phrase "my program blew up," which is computer industry jargon for indicating that the program didn't work correctly. It does not refer to blowing up in the sense of an explosion. On the systems available for dental offices, there is virtually nothing you can do to destroy the machine.

```
                  ROUTING SLIP

PATIENT'S NAME_____

  CHARGES IN COMPUTER_____

  PRIOR AUTH. SUBMITTED_____

  PRIOR AUTH. OK_____

  DENTAL INS.  PRINTED_____
               MAILED_____

  MEDICAL INS. PRINTED_____
               MAILED_____

  REFERRAL TO D.D.S.
     PRIMARY   PRINTED_____
              MAILED_____
               X-RAY RETURNED_____

     SECONDARY PRINTED_____
              MAILED_____
               X-RAY RETURNED_____

  INSURANCE INFO REQUESTED_____
                 MAILED_____

  DICTATION_____
  OTHER_____
```

Figure 17.13
An oral surgeon's routing slip used with computers.

If you type in the wrong direction, the computer will tell you it is wrong or do something other than what you planned.

The specific operating instructions for computer systems vary widely due to the variety of systems available. Consequently, it is not possible to provide specific directions in this textbook. In any dental office in which the assistant's duties include operation of a computer, training for that specific system will be provided in the dental office.

Figure 17.13 illustrates a routing slip that is used by an oral surgeon to be certain that all the necessary information forms are properly completed for each patient. Figure 17.14 is part of an oral surgeon's computer form for indicating procedures performed. The surgeon marks the procedures performed; the assistant enters the code number by all marked procedures; the computer registers the charge and completes the bookkeeping.

Computer Vocabulary

backup   Periodically (daily or every other day), all the information stored on the computer is copied onto an extra storage device. In the event of a malfunction that causes data to be lost, the backup device can be used to recover lost data up to the point of the last backup, minimizing the need for re-entering data.

boot up   All of the activities required to take a computer from a power-off condition to a fully functional condition.

CPU   Central processing unit. The brain of the computer. It specifies which tasks are to be done, in what sequence, and does all the processing (thinking).

core   The central memory of the CPU on which data is stored magnetically by use of electrical charges.

disc   A storage unit for information. It is a flat, circular plate (like a record) with a magnetizable surface. Magnetic charges on the disc represent data.

downtime   The time a computer is not functional when it is supposed to be.

hardware   The mechanical components of a computer: the discs, the printer, the CRTs, the CPU, etc.

program   The instructions that tell the computer what to do with the data you enter. The instructions are written in a language the computer can understand.

security code   A code that prevents unauthorized access to information in the system. The terminal operator must key in the correct security code in order to use a protected function.

software   All the programs the computer executes.

terminal   Any piece of hardware, attached to the CPU, that is used to input or output data.

Additional Banking Services

There are many services offered by banks, and an assistant should be familiar with them. One such service is a **safe deposit box,** which may be rented for an annual fee. This box is in a vault, assuring protection against theft, fire, or almost any type of catastrophe. Usually, valuable papers are kept in a safe deposit box. Only the person or persons whose names are recorded at the Safe Deposit Registry are permitted to use the box, and each time the box is used, the user must sign a request to enter the box and must write his or her key number on the slip. This slip is then verified by a clerk to be sure it compares with the information recorded when the box was rented. The person is given permission to enter the vault area where an attendant takes the registration slip

ATTENDING ORAL SURGEON'S STATEMENT A.D.A. Procedures and Nomenclature

A–DIAGNOSIS	FEE
Examination - Office	00110 ____
Periodic Exam	00120 ____
Consultation	09310 ____
☐ Brief ☐ Inter. ☐ Extended	
Hospital Visit	09420 ____
Office Visit After Hours	09440 ____
X-Ray - Single Intraoral	00220 ____
X-Ray - Add'l Intraoral	00230 ____
X-Ray - Occlusal	00240 ____
X-Ray - TMJ	00321 ____
X-Ray - Panoramic	00330 ____
Bacteriologic Culture	00410 ____
Biopsy of Hard Tissue	07285 ____
Biopsy of Soft Tissue	07286 ____
Pulp Vitality Tests	00460 ____
Diagnostic Models	00470 ____

B–ANESTHESIA	
Anesthesia-Local Non-Surgical	09210 ____
Anesthesia - General or IV	09220 ____
Analgesia	09230 ____

C–EXODONTIA	
Extraction - Single _____	07110 ____
Ext. Sing. Other Sext. _____	07110 ____
Extractions - Add'l _____	07120 ____
Surgical Extractions _____	07210 ____
Surg. Removal Impact. By Incision & Elevation _____	07220 ____
Surg. Removal Impact. By Incision. Remove Bone or Section Tooth	07230 ____
Surg. Removal Impact. By Incision. Remove Bone and Section Tooth	07240 ____
Surg. Removal Impact. By Incision. Remove Bone and Section Tooth - Unusual Difficulty	07241 ____
Surgical Removal Retained Root	07250 ____
Surgical Exposure	
Tissue Impaction _____	07280 ____
Partial Bony Impaction _____	07281 ____
Full Bony Impaction _____	07282 ____
Tooth Replantation _____	07270 ____
Tooth Transplantation _____	07272 ____

D–ALVEOPLOPLASTY	
Alveoloplasty per sextant w/ext	07310 ____
Alveoloplasty per sex. wo/ext	07320 ____
Alveoloplasty Cusp.-Custp. w/ext	07330 ____

E–ENDODONTIA		FEE
Rct 1 canal 03310	2 canal 03320	
Apicoectomy. per tooth. 1st root	03410 ____	
Apicoectomy. per tooth. each add'l	03411 ____	
Apicoectomy w/Retrofill _____	03430 ____	
Apical Curettage	03440 ____	
Root Amputation _____	03450 ____	

F–SOFT TISSUE SURGERY & REPAIR	
Gingivectomy. per quadrant _____	04210 ____
Vestibuloplasty-ridge extension	07340 ____
Vestibuloplasty-ridge extension (Including grafts. re-attachments. etc.)	07350 ____
Excision Hyperplastic Tissue	07970 ____
Freqenctomy-Labial. Lingual	07960 ____
Sialolithotomy	07980 ____
Oral Antral Fistula Closure	07260 ____
Maxillary Sinusotomy _____	09999 ____
Suture Wounds-	
Uncomplicated to 6.0cm	07910 ____
Complicated to 6.0cm	07911 ____
Complicated over 6.0cm	07912 ____
Graft to Mandible	07950 ____

G–SURGICAL EXCISION	
Rad. Excis. Lesion Up to 1.0cm	07410 ____
Rad. Excis. lesion Over 1.0cm	07420 ____
Excise Tum -Ben. Up to 1.0cm	07430 ____
Excise Tum -Ben. Over 1.0cm	07431 ____
Exc. Tum -Malig. Up to 1.0cm	07440 ____
Exc. Tum -Malig. Over 1.0cm	07441 ____
Excise Odontogenic Tumor/Cyst	
Up to 1.0cm	07450 ____
Over 1.0cm	07451 ____
Excise Nonodontogenic Tumor/Cyst	
Up to 1.0cm	07460 ____
Over 1.0cm	07461 ____
Remove Exostosis Max/Mand	07470 ____
Partial Ostectomy	07480 ____
Radical Resection Mandible w/Bone Graft	07490 ____

H–SURGICAL INCISION	
I & D Intraoral _____	07510 ____
I & D Extraoral _____	07520 ____
Sequestrectomy	07550 ____

I–ORTHOGNATHIC SURGERY	
Osteoplasty for Retrognathia	
Prognathism	07940 ____

J–REDUCTIONS FRACTURES. DISLOCATIONS		
Reduction Fractures - Simple		
Maxilla-Open 07610	Closed 07620 ____	
Mandible-Open 07630	Closed 07640 ____	

NAME _____

Date of Service _____

SURGERY – DIAGNOSIS OR SYMPTOMS

_____

_____

PLACE OF SERVICE:

☐ Office ☐ Hospital ☐ Emer. Rm. ☐ _____

J–REDUCTION FRACTURE-SIMPLE-CONT.		FEE
Malar Open 07650	Closed 07660 ____	
Alveolar	07670 ____	
Facial Bones - Complicated	07680 ____	
Reduction Fractures - Compound		
Maxilla Open 07710	Closed 07720 ____	
Mandible Open 07730	Closed 07740 ____	
Malar Open 07750	Closed 07760 ____	
Alveolar	07770 ____	
Closed Reduction TMJ Dislocation	07820 ____	
TMJ Condylectomy	07840 ____	
TMJ Arthrotomy	07860 ____	
TMJ Dysfunction	07800 ____	

K–OTHER SERVICES	
Palliative Treatment	09110 ____
Therapeutic Drug Injection	09610 ____
Drugs & Medications	09630 ____
Tissue Conditioning	05850 ____

_____

_____

☐ THIS IS A PRE-TREATMENT ESTIMATE
CIRCLED FEES ARE FOR SERVICES PERFORMED
Today's   Treatment
Charges $ _____   Estimate $ _____

INSURANCE CARRIERS—This form has been adopted to keep paper work costs down. If any add'l form or itemized bill is required, they will be completed on receipt of $10.00.

ORAL AND MAXILOFACIAL SURGERY

☐ F.P. Robal, D.D.S. ☐ M.C. Raeywen, D.D.S.

Meadow brook Medical Building
Anytown, Anystate 12345
(612) 962 1414

I authorize the release of information regarding examination or treatment related to this claim & permit payment directly to the Oral Surgeon of any benefits due. I accept personal responsibility for payment of fees at time services rendered.

Signed-Patient or
Parent of Insured _____   Date ____/____/____

Figure 17.14

An oral surgeon's computer form for indicating procedures performed.

and the person's key to the box. The attendant unlocks the safe deposit box, using two keys: the bank's and the key of the box renter. The box is given to the renter, who then goes to a private booth to insert or remove papers or valuables. The renter then returns the box to the attendant, and the attendant again uses the two keys to relock the box.

Loans are made by banks for a number of purposes. The bank investigates the individual who applies for a loan. If that individual meets certain standards, the bank will loan the individual a designated amount of money to be repaid on a specified schedule for a certain percentage of interest plus the charges for the paper work of making out the loan. These standards mean the borrower has something of value for collateral (something the bank could sell if the borrower doesn't pay

the money owed as agreed) or the bank administrators decide a certain individual is a good risk for repayment for some other reason.

Loans are made for small amounts of money, some under a hundred dollars, and also are made for large sums, hundreds of thousands of dollars, depending on the purpose of the loan, the reputation of the borrower, and the risk involved. To begin to practice dentistry, a dentist may find it necessary to borrow several thousand dollars to be repaid with interest from the income earned practicing dentistry.

As a dentist acquires more patients and his or her income increases, the dentist not only pays off any loans, but may be in a position to begin saving money. Since a dentist works for himself or herself without the protection of a large firm to provide a retirement fund, it is necessary to build one. Wise investments become a necessity. (Investments are those business transactions in which an individual puts money into some venture he or she believes will increase his or her money or will at least pay for the use of it.) Perhaps the dentist invests in the stock market in some "blue chip" stocks (those which are considered very safe investments). These stocks pay a dividend (interest for the use of his or her money). The dentist has become a lender, in a sense, like the bank that loaned the money to start a practice. The dentist may also discover that these investments become so good—increase in value, both because money was added to the investment account over the years and the stocks themselves increased in value— that the dentist decides to establish a trust fund.

A **trust** is the setting up of an arrangement whereby someone, usually a bank, holds your investments for you, and when you reach the age you have specified, they begin to pay you a monthly income from these investments. Should a dentist die prematurely, the trust may begin to pay the heirs an income immediately and provide for his or her children's education. Trusts have many advantages and are very complicated. There are numerous choices one can make in arranging a trust. It has some definite inheritance tax advantages. As a dental assistant, you may be expected to write checks for deposit in a trust fund.

The bank also issues **cashier's checks** and **certified checks.** These checks are important for you to understand. If a patient presents you with one of these checks, you know the bill is paid. This check cannot be returned marked "insufficient funds" because the person drawing the check must go to the bank and pay the money before the bank makes out the check. The funds are then held in reserve by the bank until the check is cashed. These checks are sometimes necessary to use when you wish to pay a bill in some distant city. Some firms insist that all out-of-town accounts be paid by cashier's checks or certified checks.

Power of Attorney

A **power of attorney** is a legal device by which a person authorizes someone else to act for him or her in legal matters. If a patient is to undergo surgery, for example, and expects to be incapacitated for a period of time, he or she may decide to have someone handle his or her legal affairs. It would mean that someone else could pay the bills, and so on. Many husbands and wives have power of attorney drawn for each other so they can take care of each other's business as the occasion arises. Sometimes an elderly person will have someone younger help in this way.

As you know, the only person who can request disclosure of a patient record is the patient. If the patient is incapacitated and the information is necessary for his or her welfare, someone who has power of attorney can make the request or even pay a bill with the patient's funds.

Whenever you see a request with a power of attorney attached (a letter properly signed and notarized), consult the attorney of your dentist to be certain that you do have the legal privilege of conforming with the request.

Notary Public

A **notary public** is an individual who has been given power by the courts to legalize certain documents. If a person has to sign certain papers witnessed by a notary, the signature and the seal of the notary must be on the document. Since frequently it is necessary for documents in the dental office to be notarized, a dentist may request that an employee be a notary public. A fee is paid for this privilege. Usually a charge is made when you use the services of a notary public outside your office.

Summary

Financial records are as important as clinical records to the dentist and the patients. The recordkeeper should maintain careful records of that which the office owes others, that which others owe the office, all money that is received, and all money that is spent.

Basic bookkeeping requirements include:

1. *Source documents* (records of proof of billing or proof of payment which must be permanently filed).
2. *Records of receipts* issued by the office. (A receipt must be written for each payment received.)
3. An *office change fund* (necessary to make change for patients who pay cash).
4. A *patient's service record* (to show the dentistry performed).
5. A *patient's account record* (to show the financial transactions for the services performed).
6. The *day sheet* (to show all the activity in dentistry and finance for a single day).
7. *Discounts* (must be shown as discounts on the records).

8. *Statements* (must be sent to patients and should indicate the dentistry performed and the charges to be paid. These statements should be mailed on the same date each month).

9. *Checks received* (should be endorsed immediately with the words "For deposit only" or should be endorsed with a bank stamp).

10. *Third-party payment records* (must be maintained as required by the third party whether it be a government agency or an insurance firm or any other organization. It is important to follow the regulations of the particular agency to assure payment for the services performed).

11. An *accounts receivable control* (to permit verification of the outstanding accounts so the record-keeper knows whether or not the correct number of statements are being sent to patients).

Records about money spent include:

1. A *petty cash fund* for minor office expenditures.

2. *Invoices* for dental office charge accounts.

3. *Statements* for dental office charge accounts which are verified against the invoices prior to payment of the statement. Invoices and the lower half of the statement are then filed by firm name.

4. A *disbursement record* shows the classification of purchases during the month.

5. A *yearly summary* shows the income and expenditures for an entire year.

All money received is deposited in the office checking account.

Deposit slips are made in duplicate.

The *business checking account* is used only for business.

A *check* is an authorization to the bank to pay a specified amount of money to the person named on the check from the account of the person who signs the check.

A *check stub* or *check register* is a record retained in the office and gives information found on the check as well as the bank balance.

Checkbook reconciliation is a procedure to ascertain that the bank records and the office records agree about the amount of money in the checking account.

Write-It-Once or *pegboard bookkeeping systems* offer a method of record-keeping that avoids errors in copying figures because items are written only once.

Many dental offices are now using *computers.* Special routines are followed in these offices. Learn the computer vocabulary for your work in such an office.

Banks offer services including *safe deposit boxes, loans, trusts, certified* and *cashier's checks,* as well as *savings accounts* and *personal checking accounts.*

A *power of attorney* is a legal device that permits an adult to allow someone else to act for him or her in legal matters.

A *notary public* is a person who has been given power by the courts to legalize certain documents. Sometimes it is necessary to use a notary public in preparing papers.

Study Questions

1. Describe the records that are essential for operating the dental office effectively.

2. Explain these terms:

source documents	patient's account record
day sheet	accounts receivable
discount	control
statement	third-party payment
receipt	patient's service record
invoice	disbursement record
boot up	yearly summary
disc	
backup	
CPR	

3. Distinguish between an office change fund and a petty cash fund.

4. Describe a checkbook reconciliation procedure. Why is it important?

5. What is the difference between an online and a batch system?

6. What is a dumb tube? a security code?

Vocabulary

Many new words are found in the last two chapters. Study the boxed definitions for review.

Word Elements

Word Element	Example
auto, aut prefix meaning: self, relationship	**autoclave** self-regulated sterilizer
and, andro combining form meaning: relationship to man, male	**androgenic** producing masculine characteristics
anthrop combining form meaning: relationship to man, mankind	**anthropology** science of man and his origins
gyn, gyne, gyneco combining form meaning: relationship to woman	**gynopathy** any disease of women
hetero combining form meaning: relationship to others	**heterograft** a graft of tissue taken from one species and used in another species
pedo combining form meaning: relationship to child	**pedodontics** branch of dentistry that studies and treats children's dental needs
clus, clud combining form meaning: relationship to close, shut	**occlude** to fit closely together, to shut
dextro combining form meaning: relationship to the right	**dexter** relating to or situated on the right
phagy, phagia suffix meaning: relationship to eating, swallowing	**phagocytosis** engulfing and destroying of microorganisms, cells, or other substances by a cell called a phagocyte
rhin combining form meaning: relationship to the nose	**rhinoanemometer** apparatus for measuring air passing through nose during respiration

CHAPTER 18

Records for Taxes, Insurance, and Prepaid Care Programs

Part One: Records for Taxes
Complete, Accurate Records
Office Salary and Tax Records
Tax Forms
    Payment to Internal Revenue Service
    State Unemployment Tax Form
Part Two: Insurance and Prepaid Care Programs
The Principle of Insurance
Dental Insurance Programs
Types of Insurances
Delta Dental Plans
Other Plans
Procedures for Managing Insurance Cases
Determination of Reasonable Charge
Insurance Terminology

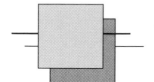

Part One: Records For Taxes

Complete, Accurate Records

It is to your dentist's advantage that complete, accurate records be kept of *all* transactions involving money. It is also wise to use the services of a CPA in the preparation of tax returns. The Internal Revenue Service is more likely to accept the statement of earnings made by a CPA because a CPA's record is built on training and knowledge in business and tax matters. Accurate record-keeping is also a necessity.

If your office uses the services of a CPA or management consultant, the area of record-keeping for tax purposes will be designed for you, and it will be necessary for you to keep only such records as the service directs.

If you are expected to keep records for the state and federal taxes, you should be familiar with the material in this chapter.

Every employee in the office must have social security tax, federal income tax, and in some states, state income tax withheld from his or her salary. In addition, federal unemployment taxes must be paid by each employer. Some states also collect unemployment taxes from employers.

Most of these taxes are paid quarterly, and special forms are required for each tax. Some forms are mailed to the office, but in certain states it is necessary to send for the unemployment compensation forms.

Records must be kept of the total salary of each employee and the amount withheld for each individual tax, and must specify the purpose for which other amounts are withheld. At the end of the year, special forms that list all taxes withheld and the total salary paid must be completed.

Any inaccuracies or omissions in these reports can lead to a penalty payment of a percentage of the amount not reported, so take care that you prepare them accurately and on time. If your dentist has not made tax reports (perhaps you are the first employee), you must secure the forms from your nearest federal and state offices. If the dentist has previously submitted tax reports, the forms will be sent directly to your office each quarter.

Office Salary and Tax Records

A record must be maintained concerning every paycheck prepared. A sheet is maintained for each employee. It contains the entire record of salary paid and amounts withheld (fig. 18.1).

Since no employee is able to take home all money earned, records must be kept of the taxes and amounts withheld from the take-home pay. The example shows FICA (also referred to as social security or old age benefits (OAB) on some forms), federal and state withholding taxes, and net paid (fig. 18.1).

Some states have other taxes that are also withheld. In most states, unemployment compensation is not withheld from an employee's wages. It is a tax paid by the employer only. For every item to be withheld in your particular locality, there should be a column so listed on the office salary and tax record for each employee.

Tax Forms

The most commonly used federal government tax forms are illustrated in the sections that follow. If you can understand how to prepare these forms, you will be able to master the state forms required in your state. Since most states have withholding taxes and some form of unemployment insurance compensation, it is wise to investigate before you are penalized for nonpayment.

Because some reports are filed on a quarterly basis, it is easier to complete reports if you keep regular bookkeeping records from which you can summarize the quarterly information.

All tax forms are said to have complete, clear directions for their preparation. Since these directions change frequently and the amounts of money that are required for payment also change, it is impossible for us to give you accurate information concerning the use of these forms. However, if you will read the text material describing the forms and note the illustrations, you will be aware of the forms to complete for your office. By following the directions on each form, you will be able to comply with the tax laws and thus will not be penalized for failure to pay taxes.

SALARY AND TAX RECORD

Employee's Name: Mary M. Smith   Number of Exemptions: 0

Address: 215 Elm Street   Marital Status: S

                    Anytown, Anystate, 12345   Social Security Number: 123-11-2345

DATE	TOTAL EARNINGS	SOCIAL SECURITY TAX	FEDERAL WITHHOLDING TAX	STATE WITHHOLDING TAX	OTHER DEDUCTIONS	NET PAY
6 1	720 0.00	54.00	90.00	37.00	—	539.00
6 15	720 0.00	54.00	90.00	37.00	—	539.00

Figure 18.1
Office salary and tax record.

Tax forms that do not require payment, but must be completed and filed annually or kept on file in the office, are:

The **Withholding Tax Statement, Form W-2** (fig. 18.2) which must be filed at the close of the year. There are four copies, each labeled for a specific purpose: one for the district director, one for the employer's records, and two for the employee: one to keep and one to file with the annual tax return.

The **Employee's Withholding Exemption Certificate, Form W-4** (fig. 18.3) which each new employee must complete. It is kept on file as long as the person is employed in the office and can be amended whenever the employee changes the number of allowances claimed.

Tax forms you may need to file with payments are:

U.S. Tax Form No. 941: Employers Quarterly Federal Tax Return (fig. 18.4). The taxes that are required are paid on a quarterly or monthly basis, determined by the dollar amount your dentist must pay. The taxes covered are Social Security or old age benefits (FICA or OAB) and withheld income taxes.

If payments are to be made on a monthly basis, you will receive a form called a **Federal Depositary Receipt, Form 8109** (fig. 18.5). This form is to accompany your monthly check.

Whether you pay monthly or quarterly, Form 941 must be completed and sent to the Internal Revenue Service each quarter with a check for the amount due.

Another form to be used quarterly is the **Transmittal of Wage and Tax Statements, Form W-3** (fig. 18.6).

Annually the **U.S. Tax Form 940, Employer's Annual Federal Unemployment Tax Report** (fig. 18.7) must also be completed and filed.

Payment to Internal Revenue Service

These forms require payment with the form. A check, payable to the Internal Revenue Service, must be sent with each form. The check and form should be sent in the same envelope on or before the last day of the first month following the close of the quarter for taxes paid quarterly. Instructions on the Federal Depository Receipt will explain when the monthly payment is due for those who must pay by the month.

State Unemployment Tax Form

The state unemployment form will also require a check sent with it for the entire amount owed by your office. Usually a percentage is determined by the use your office has made of the state unemployment insurance funds. If, for example, no one has filed a claim against your office for unemployment compensation (in other words, your dentist has never fired an employee), the rate may be the lowest the state collects. If, however, the office has had one or two claims filed against it, the rate is immediately higher. As the number of claims increases, the rate of the tax increases. If a period of time, such as three years, has elapsed and no claims have been filed, the tax rate may again drop to its lowest point.

The form that your office receives from the unemployment compensation fund will state the rate that your office is required to pay.

1 Control number			
		OMB No. 1545-0008	

2 Employer's name, address, and ZIP code		3 Employer's identification number	4 Employer's state I.D. number

| 5 Statutory employee ☐ | Deceased ☐ | Pension plan ☐ | Legal rep. ☐ | 942 emp. ☐ | Subtotal ☐ | Deferred compensation ☐ | Void ☐ |

6 Allocated tips	7 Advance EIC payment

8 Employee's social security number	9 Federal income tax withheld	10 Wages, tips, other compensation	11 Social security tax withheld

12 Employee's name, address, and ZIP code	13 Social security wages	14 Social security tips

16	16a Fringe benefits incl. in Box 10

17 State income tax	18 State wages, tips, etc.	19 Name of state
20 Local income tax	21 Local wages, tips, etc.	22 Name of locality

Form **W-2 Wage and Tax Statement**   **1989**

Employee's and employer's copy compared ☐

Copy 1 For State, City, or Local Tax Department

Figure 18.2

U.S. Tax Form W-2, Withholding Tax Statement.

19**89** Form W-4

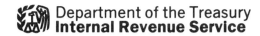
Department of the Treasury
Internal Revenue Service

Purpose. Complete Form W-4 so that your employer can withhold the correct amount of Federal income tax from your pay.

Exemption From Withholding. Read line 6 of the certificate below to see if you can claim exempt status. If exempt, only complete the certificate; but do not complete lines 4 and 5. No Federal income tax will be withheld from your pay.

Basic Instructions. Employees who are not exempt should complete the Personal Allowances Worksheet. Additional worksheets are provided on page 2 for employees to adjust their withholding allowances based on itemized deductions, adjustments to income, or two-earner/two-job situations. Complete all worksheets that apply to your situation. The worksheets will help you figure the number of withholding allowances you are

entitled to claim. However, you may claim fewer allowances than this.

Head of Household. Generally, you may claim head of household filing status on your tax return only if you are unmarried and pay more than 50% of the costs of keeping up a home for yourself and your dependent(s) or other qualifying individuals.

Nonwage Income. If you have a large amount of nonwage income, such as interest or dividends, you should consider making estimated tax payments using Form 1040-ES. Otherwise, you may find that you owe additional tax at the end of the year.

Two-Earner/Two-Jobs. If you have a working spouse or more than one job, figure the total number of allowances you are entitled to claim on all jobs using worksheets from only one Form

W-4. This total should be divided among all jobs. Your withholding will usually be most accurate when all allowances are claimed on the W-4 filed for the highest paying job and zero allowances are claimed for the others.

Advance Earned Income Credit. If you are eligible for this credit, you can receive it added to your paycheck throughout the year. For details, obtain Form W-5 from your employer.

Check Your Withholding. After your W-4 takes effect, you can use **Publication 919,** Is My Withholding Correct for 1989?, to see how the dollar amount you are having withheld compares to your estimated total annual tax. Call 1-800-424-3676 (in Hawaii and Alaska, check your local telephone directory) to obtain this publication.

Personal Allowances Worksheet

A Enter "1" for **yourself** if no one else can claim you as a dependent . . . . **A** ____

B Enter "1" if: { **1.** You are single and have only one job; or
2. You are married, have only one job, and your spouse does not work; or } . . . . **B** ____
3. Your wages from a second job or your spouse's wages (or the total of both) are $2,500 or less.

C Enter "1" for your **spouse.** But, you may choose to enter "0" if you are married and have either a working spouse or more than one job (this may help you avoid having too little tax withheld) . . . . **C** ____

D Enter number of **dependents** (other than your spouse or yourself) whom you will claim on your tax return . . . . . . **D** ____

E Enter "1" if you will file as a **head of household** on your tax return (see conditions under "Head of Household," above) . . **E** ____

F Enter "1" if you have at least $1,500 of **child or dependent care expenses** for which you plan to claim a credit . . . . **F** ____

G Add lines A through F and enter total here . . . . ▶ **G** ____

For accuracy, do all worksheets that apply.
{
- If you plan to **itemize or claim adjustments to income** and want to reduce your withholding, turn to the Deductions and Adjustments Worksheet on page 2.
- If you are **single** and have **more than one job** and your combined earnings from all jobs exceed $25,000 OR if you are **married** and have a **working spouse or more than one job,** and the combined earnings from all jobs exceed $40,000, then turn to the Two-Earner/Two-Job Worksheet on page 2 if you want to avoid having too little tax withheld.
- If **neither** of the above situations applies to you, **stop here** and enter the number from line G on line 4 of Form W-4 below.
}

- **Cut here and give the certificate to your employer. Keep the top portion for your records.** -

Form **W-4** Department of the Treasury Internal Revenue Service	**Employee's Withholding Allowance Certificate** ▶ **For Privacy Act and Paperwork Reduction Act Notice, see reverse.**	OMB No. 1545-0010 19**89**

1 Type or print your first name and middle initial	Last name	**2** Your social security number

Home address (number and street or rural route)	**3** Marital Status	☐ Single ☐ Married ☐ Married, but withhold at higher Single rate.
City or town, state, and ZIP code		**Note:** If married, but legally separated, or spouse is a nonresident alien, check the Single box.

4 Total number of allowances you are claiming (from line G above or from the Worksheets on back if they apply) . . . **4** ____

5 Additional amount, if any, you want deducted from each pay . . . . **5** $ ____

6 I claim exemption from withholding and I certify that I meet **ALL** of the following conditions for exemption:
- Last year I had a right to a refund of **ALL** Federal income tax withheld because I had **NO** tax liability; **AND**
- This year I expect a refund of **ALL** Federal income tax withheld because I expect to have **NO** tax liability; **AND**
- This year if my income exceeds $500 and includes nonwage income, another person cannot claim me as a dependent.

If you meet all of the above conditions, enter the year effective and "EXEMPT" here . . . . . ▶ **6** | 19

7 Are you a full-time student? (Note: Full-time students are not automatically exempt.) . . . . **7** ☐Yes ☐No

Under penalties of perjury, I certify that I am entitled to the number of withholding allowances claimed on this certificate or entitled to claim exempt status.

Employee's signature ▶ _____ Date ▶ _____ , 198__

8 Employer's name and address (**Employer:** Complete 8 and 10 **only if sending to IRS**)	**9** Office code (optional)	**10** Employer identification number

---

Figure 18.3
Employee's Withholding Exemption Certificate.

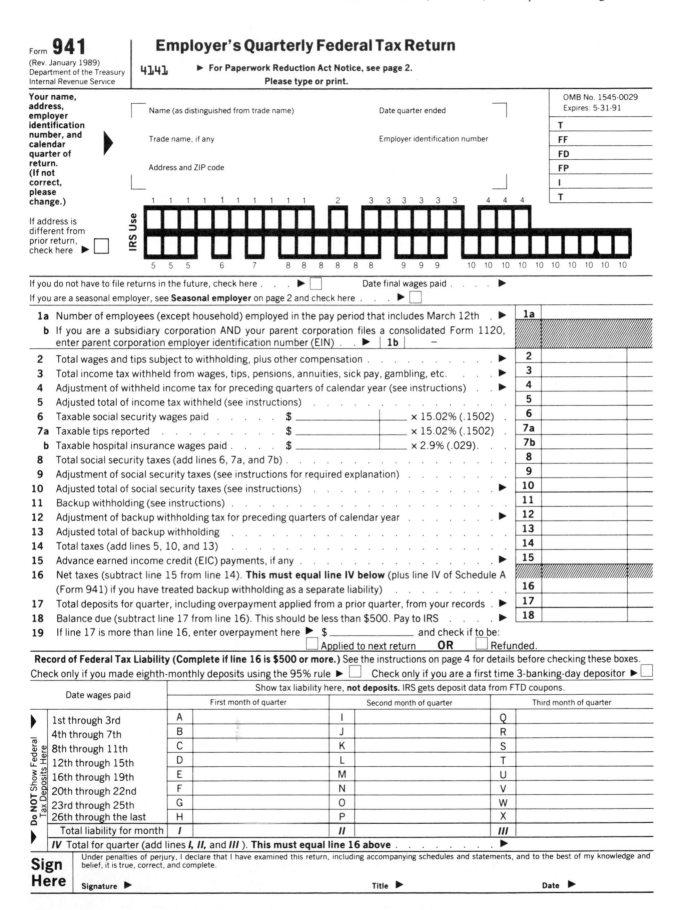

Figure 18.4

U.S. Tax Form No. 941, Employer's Quarterly Federal Tax Return.

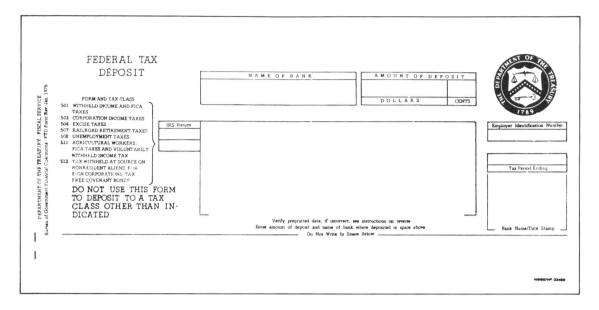

Figure 18.5
Federal Depositary Receipt.

DO NOT STAPLE

1 Control number	33333	For Official Use Only ▶ OMB No. 1545-0008			
☐ **Kind of Payer** ▶	2 941/941E ☐ Military ☐ 943 ☐ CT-1 ☐ 942 ☐ Medicare gov't. emp. ☐		3 ▨▨▨	4 ▨▨▨	5 Total number of statements
6 Allocated tips	7 Advance EIC payments		8 Establishment number		
9 Federal income tax withheld	10 Wages, tips, and other compensation		11 Social security tax withheld		
12 Employer's state I.D. number	13 Social security wages		14 Social security tips		
15 Employer's identification number			16 Other EIN used this year		
17 Employer's name			18 Gross annuity, pension, etc. (Form W-2P)		
			20 Taxable amount (Form W-2P)		
19 Employer's address and ZIP code (If available, place label over boxes 15, 17, and 19.)			21 Income tax withheld by third-party payer		

Under penalties of perjury, I declare that I have examined this return and accompanying documents, and to the best of my knowledge and belief they are true, correct, and complete.

Signature ▶   Title ▶   Date ▶

Telephone number (optional)_____

Form **W-3 Transmittal of Income and Tax Statements** 1990   Department of the Treasury Internal Revenue Service

Figure 18.6
U.S. Tax Form W-3, Transmittal of Income and Tax Statements.

Form **940**	**Employer's Annual Federal Unemployment (FUTA) Tax Return**	OMB No. 1545-0028
Department of the Treasury Internal Revenue Service	▶ For Paperwork Reduction Act Notice, see page 2.	19**88**

			T	
	⌐Name (as distinguished from trade name)	Calendar year	FF	
If incorrect, make any necessary change. ▶	Trade name, if any		FD	
			FP	
			I	
	Address and ZIP code ∟	Employer identification number [—]	T	

A Did you pay all required contributions to state unemployment funds by the due date of Form 940? (See instructions if none required.) . . . ☐ **Yes** ☐ **No**

    If you checked the "Yes" box, enter the amount of contributions paid to state unemployment funds . . . . ▶ $ _____ |

B Are you required to pay contributions to only one state? . . . . ☐ **Yes** ☐ **No**

    If you checked the "Yes" box: (1) Enter the name of the state where you are required to pay contributions . . . . ▶ _____

    (2) Enter your state reporting number(s) as shown on state unemployment tax return. ▶ _____

C If any part of wages taxable for FUTA tax is exempt from state unemployment tax, check the box. (See the Specific Instructions on page 2.) . . . . . ☐

Part I   Computation of Taxable Wages and Credit Reduction (to be completed by all taxpayers)

1	Total payments (including exempt payments) during the calendar year for services of employees	**1**	▨
2	Exempt payments. (Explain each exemption shown, attaching additional sheets if necessary.) ▶ _____	Amount paid **2**	▨
3	Payments for services of more than $7,000. Enter only the excess over the first $7,000 paid to individual employees not including exempt amounts shown on line 2. Do not use the state wage limitation.	**3**	▨
4	Total exempt payments (add lines 2 and 3)	**4**	
5	**Total taxable wages** (subtract line 4 from line 1). (If any part is exempt from state contributions, see instructions.) ▶	**5**	

Part II   Tax Due or Refund (Complete if you checked the "Yes" boxes in both questions A and B and did not check the box in C above.)

1	**Total FUTA tax.** Multiply the wages in Part I, line 5, by .008 and enter here.	**1**	
2	Minus: Total FUTA tax deposited for the year, including any overpayment applied from a prior year (from your records)	**2**	
3	**Balance due** (subtract line 2 from line 1). This should be $100 or less. Pay to IRS . . . . . . ▶	**3**	
4	**Overpayment** (subtract line 1 from line 2). Check if it is to be: ☐ Applied to next return, or ☐ Refunded . ▶	**4**	

Part III   Tax Due or Refund (Complete if you checked the "No" box in either question A or B or you checked the box in C above. Also complete Part V.)

1	Gross FUTA tax. Multiply the wages in Part I, line 5, by .062	**1**	
2	Maximum credit. Multiply the wages in Part I, line 5, by .054	**2**	▨
3	**Credit allowable:** Enter the smaller of the amount in Part V, line 11, or Part III, line 2 . . .	**3**	▨
4	**Total FUTA tax** (subtract line 3 from line 1)	**4**	
5	Minus: Total FUTA tax deposited for the year, including any overpayment applied from a prior year (from your records)	**5**	
6	**Balance due** (subtract line 5 from line 4). This should be $100 or less. Pay to IRS . . . . . ▶	**6**	
7	**Overpayment** (subtract line 4 from line 5). Check if it is to be: ☐ Applied to next return, or ☐ Refunded . ▶	**7**	

Part IV   Record of Quarterly Federal Tax Liability for Unemployment Tax (Do not include state liability.)

Quarter	First	Second	Third	Fourth	Total for Year
Liability for quarter					

Part V   Computation of Tentative Credit (Complete if you checked the "No" box in either question A or B or you checked the box in C, on page 1—see instructions.)

Name of state **1**	State reporting number(s) as shown on employer's state contribution returns **2**	Taxable payroll (as defined in state act) **3**	State experience rate period **4** From— To—	State experience rate **5**	Contributions if rate had been 5.4% (col. 3 x .054) **6**	Contributions payable at experience rate (col. 3 x col. 5) **7**	Additional credit (col. 6 minus col. 7) If 0 or less, enter 0. **8**	Contributions actually paid to the state **9**

10 Totals . . . . ▶   (columns 6 and 7 shaded)

11 Total tentative credit (add line 10, columns 8 and 9—see instructions for limitations) . . . . ▶

If you will not have to file returns in the future, write "Final" here (see general instruction "Who Must File") and sign the return. ▶

Under penalties of perjury, I declare that I have examined this return, including accompanying schedules and statements, and to the best of my knowledge and belief, it is true, correct, and complete, and that no part of any payment made to a state unemployment fund claimed as a credit was or is to be deducted from the payments to employees.

Signature ▶   Title (Owner, etc.) ▶   Date ▶

Form **940** (1988)

Figure 18.7

U.S. Tax Form 940, Employer's Annual Federal Unemployment Tax Report.

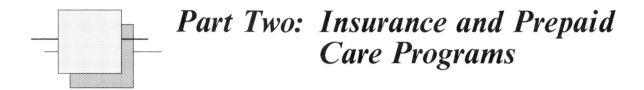

Part Two: Insurance and Prepaid Care Programs

The Principle of Insurance

Insurance was developed a long time ago based on the idea that a group can better manage catastrophe than an individual. When all the neighbors would try to help put out a fire on someone's farm, this was a form of insurance. "We help each other." When the neighbors formed a crew to help harvest the crops of a sick farmer, this was insurance. Gradually the idea grew that it would be possible to use the same principle to handle many catastrophes that occur. A hail storm or a tornado might wreck a house. Who would rebuild it? For a time the immediate neighbors would cooperate, lending their skills and services in the rebuilding. Gradually it became popular to take out an insurance policy. If 100 persons bought a tornado insurance policy and one home was devastated by a tornado, the premiums (amount of money paid in by the subscribers) were used to pay the bills to reconstruct the demolished house. Each family that had been spared the demolishing would be grateful that their house had been spared.

This principle, that we can all pay a little something to insure ourselves against a catastrophic major loss, is the idea that gave rise to the hundreds of insurance companies in existence today. First it was life insurance. Later, health and accident insurance became very popular. Today we have hundreds of programs—Blue Cross/Blue Shield, Delta Dental Plan, Medicare, government-sponsored insurance, nonprofit dental care, prepaid dental care, health and accident insurance, workmen's compensation insurance, and group prepaid dental insurance plans.

Insurance is based on the law of probability, which is figured carefully by **actuaries** (persons who figure the necessary premium needed to provide the coverage in insurance offered to any group of persons). Life insurance premiums are based on the life expectancy table prepared by actuaries. Insurance is so much a part of our lives today that groups of persons are insured who have some common factor in their lives (it may be religion or the same employer). For example, Blue Cross/Blue Shield contracts are offered to groups of persons working for the same employer. The **premium** (amount necessary to pay each year) depends on the size of the

group and the conditions that the actuaries have determined about that group. The rates are the lowest possible for persons working at that occupation, in that particular office or area of the country. Dentists and physicians have special group insurance policies to which they can subscribe. This is true of almost every profession and every business.

Dental Insurance Programs

Increasingly, dental bills are being paid by insurance and dental care programs. Some of these are group insurance programs, some private and some government. This type of dental care requires special handling of billing procedures because insurance companies have special forms which must be completed before they will pay any dental bill. The procedure can become very complex since some types of insurance pay all the expenses, some pay part, and some pay part depending on certain circumstances. *It is important that you understand exactly what is expected of the office and the patient for each insurance form that must be completed.* It is helpful if you understand what part of the bill the insurance company will pay. It may save confusion and irritation on the part of the patient.

Your patient registration information form should contain all information that you may eventually need in preparing insurance papers. Name of the insurance company, type of benefits, the patient's insurance policy number, the type of insurance carried, and the employer's name and group number (if it is group insurance) should all be in the file for each patient.

When you have an insurance form to complete, attempt to have your dentist complete the dental part of the report at the time of the examination. Dental terminology is very important on the insurance form, and you must be certain you know what you are writing. If there is any question, ask your dentist.

It will be your duty to check the fee schedules issued by the insurance companies to be certain that you list on an itemized statement all the items for which charges are acceptable under the insurance plan. (For example, the insurance firm may break down the charges for services in the office so that it is necessary to list two or three items.)

You can see why this is complicated. Each insurance firm may handle claims differently and may pay for different services. It is your responsibility to see that the correct information reaches the insurance firm so that you will receive full payment from the insurance company. Read the fine print on each form you must complete!

Types of Insurances

Health insurances vary from: nonprofit organizations to commercial insurance companies, individual policies to group policies, prepaid dental care to care only when qualified by terms of the insurance policy.

In prepaid policies, the insurance firm has an arrangement with a dentist so that all the patients carrying the insurance receive their care without paying the dentist. They simply pay the insurance firm an annual premium. The dentist is paid by the insurance company.

The insurance companies state in their policies:

the fee regulations by which the dentist is to be paid,
the method of payment (that is, whether they pay the dentist directly or whether they pay the patient and the patient pays the dentist), any exclusions or special provisions.

Policies must be read carefully because the insurance company pays only if the terms of the insurance policy are met.

The assistant to a dentist who is affiliated with any prepaid dental plan must be very certain that she or he understands the terms of the insurance and that each patient who claims membership in such a group is actually enrolled at the time of the dental care. (The membership card may have expired.)

Delta Dental Plans

The nonprofit Delta Dental Plan of the ADA has been developed as a result of the growing interest in prepaid dental care. The national association of Delta Dental Plan has its office in the headquarters building of the American Dental Association in Chicago and is approved by the ADA as well as the states in which the plan operates.

The purpose of this type of insurance is to provide basic dental care. Options allow partial payment of other, more extensive dentistry. Firms and unions join. Their employees and/or members are then insured under the group plan. The families who are insured go to the dentist of their choice, and the bill is prepaid through their group. The family either pays a monthly premium or the union or employer furnishes this care as a fringe benefit.

Figure 18.8 shows the Delta Dental Plan of Minnesota Examination and Treatment Plan Form.

Other Plans

There are other plans whereby a family may receive complete care by belonging to a group that employs a clinic of dentists to care for them. Almost all their dental care is covered by their annual premium payment. There are many plans of this nature throughout the United States, including some established by unions. The dentist is paid a definite amount annually for each person who places himself or herself in the dentist's care. The dentist must then provide complete service with certain listed exclusions.

If the patient has a private insurance policy—not a group policy—it is usually one in which the insurance company pays the patient and the patient pays the dentist.

Procedures for Managing Insurance Cases

It is very important that you keep *all* the necessary records. Be alert to educating patients to just how much their insurance covers and what their responsibilities are. See that you send accurate reports to the insurance firms on time.

There are two ways in which dentists are paid by insurance. If they agree to participate, they agree to serve for a minimum fee for families whose income falls below a set amount established in the Schedule of Allowances. If the income of the family is above that amount, the dentist is free to charge his or her usual fee. The patient pays everything above the basic amount indicated by the insurance company. It is important for the secretary to be certain that the patient who uses such an insurance plan understands exactly his or her financial obligations to the dentist. Some people are very confused by insurance terms.

Have necessary information about the patient's insurance records on the acquaintance card.

A nice way to approach the patient is to say "Mr. Jones, if you care to, you may sign this form from your insurance company, and then we can collect your bill directly from them."

Be sure to add, "You know they may not pay the entire bill, but when we have received the payment from them, we shall send you a statement showing what they paid and what you still owe us."

If he agrees to this method, he signs the form and your office assumes the responsibility for completing and mailing the form to the office that processes these claims for your city or state.

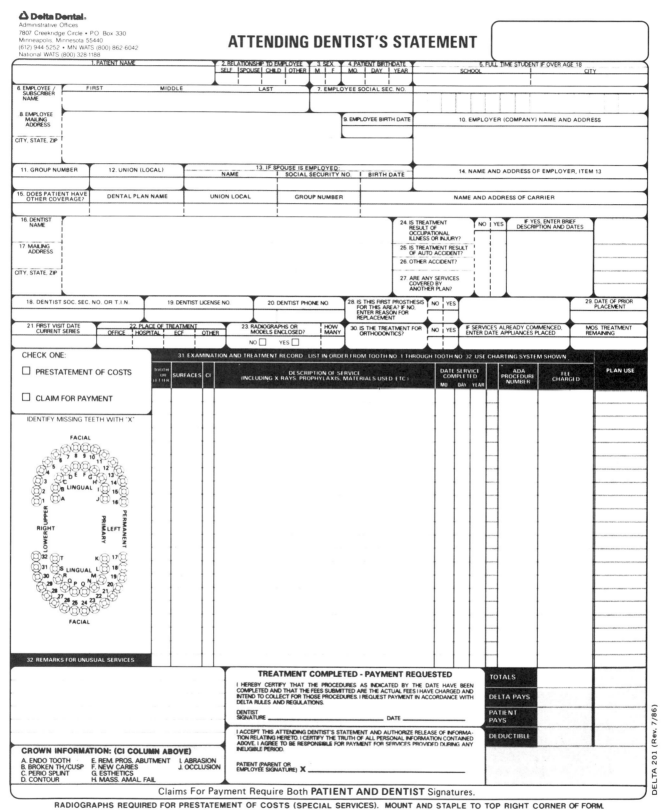

Figure 18.8
*Delta Dental Plan Examination and Treatment Plan Form. (Each state has its own form as
this plan is ADA sponsored and is nationwide.)*

The information that the insurance company needs, in this case, includes:

1. Dentist's name
2. Patient's name
3. Each date services were provided
4. Place services were provided
5. Description of the services provided on each occasion (It is important to document special circumstances that would explain a higher than normal charge for a specific service.)
6. Charges for each service
7. Amount the patient has paid

Determination of Reasonable Charge

Payment for services of the dentist is made on the basis of **reasonable charges.** The reasonable charge is determined by:

1. The customary charges for similar services generally made by the dentist
2. The prevailing charges in the locality for similar service

A **customary charge** is one that a dentist most frequently charges for that particular service.

A **prevailing charge** is a range of charges most frequently and widely charged in a specific community. In one community the prevailing charge for a crown might range from $300 to $600. In another community the range might be from $400 to $800. Population density, economic levels, and other major differences in communities will affect the determination of prevailing charges.

To understand reasonable charges, let us cite four examples of dental fees. The prevailing charge for this specific service in this community is $30 to $75.

Dr. James Jones charges this particular patient $25, although he usually charges $35. He will receive $25 because he cannot charge the insurance firm more than he actually charged the patient. (Note that $25 is less than the prevailing charge range.) The reasonable charge cannot be more than the actual charge.

Dr. Sally Knudsen charges $50, her usual fee. She will receive $50 from the insurance firm because it is her usual charge and it is within the range of the prevailing charge for the community.

Dr. Robert Myers charges $75 although he usually charges $50. There were no unusual circumstances to warrant the additional charge. Dr. Myers will receive $50 from the insurance firm because that is his customary charge for the service. He cannot collect more for the service simply because an insurance firm is involved.

Dr. Donna Lawson charges her customary $100. The insurance coverage will only pay $75—the top of the prevailing charge range. If Dr. Lawson had made an arrangement with her patient whereby the patient paid Dr. Lawson and then collected from the insurance company, Dr. Lawson would have received her customary $100, with the patient paying the balance refused by the insurance company.

If dentists do not wish to be bound by the prevailing fees, they must have the patient pay them in full and have the patient collect from the insurance company whatever part of the charge the insurance company will pay. Be sure both you and your patients understand what portion of the total charges will be paid by an insurance firm.

Insurance Terminology

The following words are frequently used in working with insurance. The dental assistant can facilitate the work in preparing insurance forms by understanding this insurance terminology.

assignment of insurance benefits   authorization to the insurance company by the insured to pay policy benefits to someone other than the insured

assistant   a person trained in oral health care who is supervised by a dentist

beneficiary   the person named in the insurance policy to receive benefit payment

claim   a formal request to an insurance company to make payment under the terms of its policy

co-insurance (COB)   an arrangement whereby the insured pays part of a loss (is a co-insurer)

deductible   a specified dollar amount to be paid by the insured before the insurance company participates in a claim

dentist's profile   the overall oral health condition of a patient as seen by the dentist after a thorough oral examination

disability   the inability to perform the duties of your occupation as a result of an accident or illness

effective date   the date on which an insurance policy goes into force

eligible members   those persons in a group who qualify for a group insurance plan, or in a family who qualify for a family insurance plan

emergency care   treatment required in the first twenty-four hours after an accident or sudden illness

exclusions or **exceptions**   those occurrences, stated in the insurance policy, for which no coverage is provided

extended care   health care provided for inpatients by a health facility other than a hospital

fee or benefit schedules   a listing in an insurance policy of the flat payment to be made for certain losses

income limit   (1) the maximum income a person can earn and still qualify for health insurance, or (2) the maximum amount of income protection an insurance company will issue

inpatient   a patient in the hospital who is charged for at least one day of room and board

insuring clause   the portion of the policy stating the purpose of the policy, setting forth the terms applying to benefits and specifying how the loss insured against must occur

lapse   nonrenewal of a policy

other benefits   benefits paid by other insurance policies, workers compensation, or government agencies

outpatient   a patient who comes to the hospital for treatment and returns home; the patient does not stay at the hospital overnight and there is no charge for room and board

participating dentist   a dentist who is a member of a group or organization providing health care, such as Blue Shield, health maintenance organizations, and so on

patient services   those services provided by a dentist, physician, or health care facility which are covered by the insurance policy

pre-existing conditions   an abnormal physical or mental condition that existed prior to the effective date of an insurance policy

premium   the cost of an insurance policy, computed for a specific period of time, such as annually, quarterly, and so on

primary dentist   dentist who first sees the patient

referring dentist   the dentist who authorizes admittance to a hospital or who suggests that the patient see another dentist

release of information   a health report about a patient made by a dentist, physician, hospital, or other health care facility; the patient must sign a form granting permission for the release of this information unless the patient has been examined by a dentist or physician employed by an insurance company to determine eligibility for an insurance policy

retroactive   made effective to an earlier date

usual and customary   charges normally made for the service

Summary

Tax records must be kept for the state and federal taxes which every business must pay. Records to keep include office salary and tax record, employer's quarterly federal tax return and quarterly report of wages taxable under the federal insurance contributions act (FICA), withholding tax statements, transmittal of wage and tax statements, federal depositary receipt, and the federal unemployment tax record. If an error in the report is made, a special form should be mailed promptly.

Insurance and dental care programs are paying an increasingly large share of dental bills. When you have an insurance form to complete, be sure that it is accurately prepared. Have your dentist prepare the dental report.

Insurances vary in coverages and types of policies.

Insurances similar to the Blue Cross/Blue Shield are common throughout the country. They provide prepaid insurance, with certain exclusions. It is necessary for the assistant to know the basic data for collecting fees from the insurance companies.

It is important to collect the necessary insurance information from the patient at the time of registration.

Payment for dentistry performed is made on the basis of a "reasonable charge" that is determined by customary and prevailing fees.

Study Questions
1.   Why is it important for a dental office to have complete and accurate records of all income and outgo?
2.   Why is it advisable to employ a CPA?
3.   What taxes must be withheld from each employee's pay?
4.   What happens if your office is late in paying the taxes withheld?
5.   Describe an office salary and tax record.
6.   When and for what reason is a federal depositary receipt issued?
7.   Why is it necessary to be certain that the insurance reports are accurately prepared?
8.   What is prepaid insurance?
9.   What added information should the dental assistant record on the patient's Acquaintance Form?
10.   Discuss reasonable charge.

Vocabulary
Study the "Insurance Terminology" section of this chapter.

Word Elements	
Word Element	*Example*
laryn combining form meaning: relationship to the larynx	*laryngitis* inflammation of the larynx
oto combining form meaning: relationship to the ear	*otology* branch of medicine that studies and treats the ear
oro combining form meaning: relationship to the mouth	*orolingual* pertaining to the mouth and tongue
odonto combining form meaning: relationship to a tooth	*odontoma* a tumor that is toothlike in structure
ophthalm combining form meaning: relationship to the eye	*ophthalmology* branch of medicine that studies and treats the eye
pharyngo combining form meaning: relationship to the pharynx	*pharyngitis* inflammation of the pharynx
sialo combining form meaning: relationship to saliva, salivary glands	*sialolithiasis* formation of salivary calculi within the ducts of the salivary glands
tracheo combining form meaning: relationship to the trachea	*tracheotomy* cutting into the trachea to give a patient an airway when the airway has been blocked
trachelo combining form meaning: relationship to the neck or a necklike structure	*trachelomyitis* inflammation of the muscles of the neck
viscero combining form meaning: relationship to organs of the body	*visceromegaly* enlargement of the viscera

CHAPTER 19

Credit and Collections

Collecting Remuneration
Credit
   Consumer Credit
   Dental Credit
Federal Regulation of Credit
   Truth-in-Lending Laws
How the Patient Pays for Services
Depreciation of Accounts Receivable
Age Analysis
Collection Ratio
Good Management of Credit
   Patient Registration
   Acquiring Patient Registration Information
Credit Control
Collection Follow-Up Procedure
   Routine for Follow-Up Procedure
Procedures without Collection Agencies
   The Telephone
   The Letter
   The Personal Interview
Procedures with Collection Agencies
Collection Advice from the American Collectors
      Association
   When to Seek Help
   What to Look for in Selecting a Collection
      Agency

Collecting Remuneration

"You give something and you get something." You perform dental service for a patient, and you receive money for the service—or do you? With most people the answer is yes, but there are a few who do not part with money unless coerced. Many more people are inclined to pay the doctor last, while others intend to pay, but unless reminded to do so, they just forget.

Years ago it was considered too commercial to discuss fees for dental and medical services. Today this is no longer true. Society recognizes that dentists and their staffs deserve remuneration for their services. Dentists recognize that patients need to understand exactly what service they are paying for and how much that service will cost. It is also true that patients frequently need to arrange for payments extended over a period of time.

Thus it is recognized that *both the dentist and the patient have need for a clear understanding of the financial arrangements for dental service.*

Credit and collections are a significant part of a dental practice. They involve important work for the dental assistant because she or he is the individual who must complete all records of services rendered and payments received. The dental assistant must also be certain that amounts are actually paid.

Payment for dentistry performed may be received from several sources.

1. The patient pays the bill either as cash or on a monthly budget.
2. A third party pays the bill in part or in total for the patient. The insurance company, the employer, and the union to which the patient belongs are all examples of payment by a third party.
3. The welfare agency of the city or state may pay the bill for an eligible patient.
4. The federal government pays the bill for certain classes of patients.

It is necessary that the dental assistant know what method of payment is used by each patient.

Credit

Exactly what is *credit?* The word *credit* comes from the Latin *credere,* meaning "to believe." In the sense in which we use the word, it means a trust in an individual's business integrity and in his or her financial capacity to meet all obligations when they become due.

There are many kinds of credit. Credit for professional services is classified under the general heading "Consumer Credit," and this is the area dental assistants must understand thoroughly.

Consumer Credit

Credit has become a tool for modern and better living. Gone are the days when only a few socially prominent persons could get credit. Today most people are not only able to purchase things on credit, but are eagerly urged by moneylenders to buy "on time." In fact, some firms are so aware of the interest they can earn by selling goods on credit that they discourage cash customers.

At least 90 percent of all business transactions today are based entirely or partly on the use of credit. Readily available consumer credit has had much to do with the development of the high standard of living we enjoy in America. If all forms of consumer credit were suddenly to be abolished, our entire economy would slow down very markedly, if not collapse.

Credit is not only a substitute for money; credit multiplies the effective value of money. Credit, therefore, is creative. When a seller of either merchandise or professional services invites customers or patients to use credit facilities, he or she is merely employing a business principle, advantageous to buyer and seller alike when rightly used, but a principle that could be a detriment to them both if abused.

Dental Credit

Good management of credit in the dental office is essential. The professional who provides services for the public must be properly paid for those services. Once the service is performed, there is no way to remove it from the receiver. (If a person buys material possessions such as a TV or car, these items can be repossessed by the seller, should payment not be forthcoming. However, dental restoration or periodontal surgery, for example, cannot be repossessed.) Thus, collection of money due for services rendered is highly important. Either the fee is collected, or the service performed becomes a bad debt. Bad debts in the dental office can mean lessened income with which to pay salaries to team members. Proper management of credit and collections in the dental office is just as ethical and important as proper management of any phase of dental treatment for the patient. It is the responsibility of the dental assistant to provide the follow-through of credit management.

Credit in the dental office is a business arrangement based on the ability and willingness of the patient to pay bills according to a predetermined agreement. Credit-granting in the dental office, therefore, should follow correct procedures.

The necessary steps before granting credit are:

1. Have a complete registration record of your patient. You will know how payment is to be made and whether the patient has dental insurance.

2. Tell the patient what the charges will be.
3. If the patient does not have insurance, make a definite arrangement for payment before services are performed. Know, and have in writing, whether the payment plan is one total payment, one-half down and the balance on a certain date, or a budget payment of a certain amount on or before a specified date each month.

The ability of the patient to pay for the dental services can be fairly well determined if the above-mentioned steps are followed. The complete registration information will detail the patient's financial stability and offer information that will permit further verification through a Retail Credit Association report if necessary. Except for unforeseen financial complications (with which your office can be cooperative), payments can be expected as promised.

The willingness to pay is more difficult to pinpoint. The patient must be given the best possible service and attention in both the professional and the business functions of the dental office. That is to say, the patient must feel that his or her needs have been sympathetically and competently met. If the patient likes the dentist and staff—has found them to be cooperative, friendly, and pleasant—the patient will be more willing to pay the bill promptly as agreed.

On the other hand, if the patient is dissatisfied or if he or she feels that the services in the office are inadequate in any area—business, professional, or public relations—that patient will lack willingness to pay.

Your dentist must assume the responsibility for the professional service given and be certain unwarranted promises are not made. The staff must provide an interested, friendly, cooperative, and competent atmosphere for the patient. If the patient is dissatisfied, he or she may become a collection problem. That is one reason why good public relations are important. The atmosphere of the office and the attitudes of the staff have much to do with success in gaining confidence, in winning cooperation, and in bringing about prompt payment of accounts. A hostile or generally suspicious attitude is to be avoided by the person who arranges financial payments with patients.

Federal Regulation of Credit

Credit-granting can offer the grantor an opportunity to increase his or her income by the interest fees charged for the service. Often persons who buy "on time" have unknowingly paid exorbitant interest fees. Thus, the federal government passed a law (the truth-in-lending law) which states that the true interest rates must be clearly delineated.

FEDERAL TRUTH IN LENDING DISCLOSURE STATEMENT
FOR PROFESSIONAL SERVICES RENDERED

Date: ____________

Patient Name ____________ Parent Name ____________ (IF MINOR)

Address ____________

____

John C. Raeywen, D.D.S.
104 Any Street
Anytown, Anystate 12345
(612) 926-1414

Services performed or to be performed:

Date of Services ____________

1. Cash Price (Professional Fee) $ ____________
2. Less: Cash Down Payment (Initial Fee) $ ____________
3. Unpaid Balance of Cash Price $ ____________
4. Amount Financed $ ____________
5. FINANCE CHARGE ____________
6. Total of Payments (4 + 5 above) $ ____________
7. Deferred Payment Price (1 + 5 above) $ ____________
8. ANNUAL PERCENTAGE RATE ____________

Patient hereby agrees to pay to ____________ (DOCTOR'S NAME) at his office shown above the "Total of Payments" shown above in ______ equal monthly installments of $ ______, the first installment being payable ____________ 19____, and all subsequent installments on the same day of each consecutive month until paid in full.

I HEREBY CERTIFY, that I have read and received a copy of the foregoing Disclosure Statement this ______ day of ____________ 19______.

Mr. ____________

Mrs. ____________

(SIGNATURE OF PATIENT OR PARENT IF PATIENT IS A MINOR)

TIL-101
Spillane's, Inc., 2826 Cedar Ave., Mpls, Minn.

Figure 19.1
A truth-in-lending statement.

Truth-in-Lending Laws

Normally, dentists do not charge interest for carrying patients' accounts over a period of months. However, the national truth-in-lending laws pose a problem. Any account carried over three months is assumed by the Internal Revenue Service to carry interest, regardless of whether or not an interest charge is stated. It may surprise some dental assistants and dentists to discover that this law applies to dentists as well as to retail business.

The dentist is apt to exclaim, "But I have never charged interest! That is my fee for the work done." The Internal Revenue Service will assume that there is hidden interest unless a written statement appears that there is no interest charged. Any dentist who wishes to carry patients' accounts for three months or longer may do so, therefore, by posting a written statement that there are no interest charges. Once this statement is made, the office credit arrangements can proceed as before.

How the Patient Pays for Services

Because many patients do pay over a period of months, it is necessary to understand the ways such payment can be arranged—and the effect of this procedure on dental office routines.

A dentist can supply the credit. If a patient pays in thirty days, the dentist is in essence supplying credit for thirty days. If the patient (or a family) requires a larger amount of service (incurring a debt of several hundred dollars), the patient may wish to pay a set amount each month until the total has been paid.

If the dentist desires to carry these accounts, one of the many budget plans is used. The patient agrees to pay a predetermined amount each month until the total has been paid. Often the patient selects the date each month on which the payment will be made. Usually the payment is made soon after the patient receives a paycheck. The date on which the payment is due each month is written into the contract the patient signs. Then the responsibility falls on the dental assistant to see that the payment is received as scheduled. Normally no interest is charged by the dentist for carrying budget accounts.

Dental insurance often provides the fee. The popularity of dental insurance indicates the necessity for each member of the oral health care team to understand the prevalent insurance regulations. Insurance policies differ widely, and it is important to understand the terms of each policy that involves your office. Thus, the dentist and dental assistant must review the policy terms of each individual patient before dentistry is performed.

The contract for dentistry is between the dentist and the patient. If a third party is to be involved with payment, the terms of that payment must be clearly understood by the dentist and the patient. The dentist or assistant must not assume that the patient understands his or her own policy.

Some policies pay all costs, others have certain limitations. Commonly there may be a deductible amount (such as the first fifty dollars). Often the insurance carrier has a fee scale, stating specifically how much will be paid for each dental operation. Should the scale be less than the usual and customary fee of the dentist, he or she must collect the rest from the patient. The patient should be told exactly what his or her personal expense will be before any dental service is performed. It may be necessary to review the terms of the policy with him or her. Usually the insurance is paid in one sum on completion of the dental service.

Depreciation of Accounts Receivable

The cost of collecting the money due the office for services rendered affects the income of the office. Every penny of cost takes away from the total amount available with which to pay expenses. When you bill a patient for the total amount of the services he or she received, the cost includes: the price of the statement and envelope, the price of postage, and the salary of the employee who prepares the statement. When the check is received, there is additional cost involved in recording the payment.

If the patient fails to pay the bill within thirty days, a second statement must be prepared. The amount of dollars to be received remains the same, but the cost of preparing the second statement has to be subtracted from the money you will receive for that statement. Let us assume the first month's billing cost is five dollars. The amount now lost out of the total amount owed is not five, but ten dollars. Every time a statement is mailed, the actual value of the money collected depreciates (is less).

In addition, with rising costs the expenses are not the same each month. They rise as the cost of paper, postage, and salaries rise. Other factors to consider are:

1. Inflation makes money less valuable.
2. If the money had been paid on time, that money could have earned interest. Thus, loss of income (interest) on the money which should have been yours also decreases the value of the account.
3. If it is necessary to have a collection agency take over the account, the collection agency must be paid—usually one-third or one-half the amount collected. Thus, the dollar you fail to receive after thirty days becomes much less with each passing month until shortly it is worth less than fifty cents and finally worth nothing at all.

Therefore, systematic and regular follow-up of accounts is essential. The rapid depreciation of professional accounts is even more marked because services, not tangible goods such as a car or TV set, are involved. The gratitude felt by the patient on being restored to good oral health soon evaporates. Try to collect as near to the peak of gratitude as possible. It takes a surprisingly short time to drop from the peak of gratitude to the valley of cost-consciousness and irritation at having to pay.

Age Analysis

One way to keep abreast of the length of time an account has been owing is to prepare an age analysis of all accounts. An **age analysis** is simply a summary form that shows who has and who has not been paying his or her bills. This analysis should be prepared during the first week of each month. It is a preliminary step in recommended collection follow-up, and it also gives a comprehensive and easily understood analysis of all money owing. Age analysis is an essential tool of sound credit management.

AGE ANALYSIS OF ACCOUNTS RECEIVABLE					
ACCOUNT NAME	TOTAL BALANCE	CURRENT MONTH	OWING 30-60 DAYS	OWING OVER 60 DAYS	COMMENTS
Adams, John	150	—	150	—	Will pay 1/15. Get loan if necessary.
Brown, Kay	50	50	—	—	
Crandall, Don	500	—	—	500	a skip - turn over to a collection agency (1/15)
Cupersmith, Eric	25	25	—	—	
Davenport, Pat	150	75	75	—	Daughter in hospital. Will pay $50/month (12/15)
MONTHLY TOTALS	22,875	10,575	7,300	5,000	

Figure 19.2

Age analysis of accounts receivable.

Prepare a sheet (as in fig. 19.2). The name of the person who is responsible for the account is entered in the first column. The second column shows the total balance owed. The third column shows the charge for dentistry performed during the current month. The fourth column shows the part owing for thirty to sixty days. The fifth column shows the part owing for over sixty days. In other words, if the current month is January, the *Total Balance* shows the entire amount the patient owes. The *Current Month* is the charges for dentistry performed in January. The *Owing 30–60 Days* column shows only those charges for dentistry performed during December and still owing, and so on. If no dentistry was performed during November, the next column is blank. Therefore, the total of all columns, except the *Total Balance* column, should equal the *Total Balance* column. In the space after the last column, notes are made about collection arrangements, such as "Promised to send $100 by 3/15/90."

By checking the age analysis file it is possible to know how much money is owed by each individual patient—and for how long. The total of each column tells you how much money is outstanding each month—and for how long is has been outstanding. This means that the monthly age analysis can be utilized as your collection sheet.

The age analysis figures can also be used as indications of collection trends. The various totals in the separate columns can be compared with totals for different periods. These comparisons give a good picture of whether payments are being held to a previous level,

are improving, or are getting worse. By keeping this analysis, you will also begin to see a definite pattern of payment habits for individual patients.

Collection Ratio

The **collection ratio** is obtained by dividing the amount of receipts from patients by the amount billed during the same period. Thus, if $10,500 were billed during the month of October and $9,660 were collected, the collection ratio would be 92 percent.

A cumulative record of the year-to-date gives the accountant a fairly accurate collection ratio. That is, all the monthly ratios would be considered for one year. If this were October 1, the ratios from November 1 of the previous year through October 1 of this year would be totaled and divided by twelve to get an annual collection ratio. On November 1 the ratio would begin with December 1 of the previous year—and so on, dropping the oldest month as the new month is added; thus always having a ratio based on twelve months of collections.

This collection ratio can be an indication of the soundness of your collection procedures. Today anything below 90 percent is considered poor.

Good Management of Credit

The professional aspect of the office should be separated from the business aspect of the office, if possible. The dentist should be encouraged to give the full benefit of his or her skill and knowledge in providing dental services for patients, up to and including the determination of the cost of those services. Originally the dentist determines the policies for credit and collections for the office. Once the dentist has indicated the cost for an individual patient's dentistry, the financial arrangements from this point on are best handled entirely by the secretary or financial assistant.

The credit policy, stating the credit regulations, who is responsible for follow-up of delinquent accounts, how the follow-up is to be managed, and the order of steps to be taken should be written and followed. No exceptions in applying the regulations should be allowed—even for the dentist's best friend.

With the policy and routines in writing, the dental assistant is now ready to apply the three tested procedures to achieve good management of credit.

1. The patient is told what the charges will be.
2. Arrangement for payment is made before dentistry is performed.
3. Accurate records are made—and used.

Patient Registration[1]

Taking a complete registration record on a new patient is the first step in good management of credit and collections. The education of the patient begins, therefore, with the patient's first visit to the dental office.

The Acquaintance Form is illustrated in chapter 15. We shall discuss the information requested on this form.[2]

Name: If a patient is married, the name of the spouse is often included. A married woman may be listed as *Johnson, Mrs. George W. (Grace)*—or she may be listed as *Johnson, Grace (Mrs. George W.).* She may also use her maiden name or a hyphenated name as Smith-Johnson, using her maiden name and her husband's name. Should she no longer be married (e.g., separated, divorced, widowed) she may wish to be listed as *Johnson, Grace L.* She may or may not wish to have the title, *Mrs.,* added. When an office has thousands of records on file, a completely detailed name helps identify the patient more easily. Several patients may have names very similar, if not identical, and then the address must be checked to completely identify the individual.

Date of Birth: Correct diagnosis of conditions in the mouth and decisions about the best method of treatment are often affected by the age of the patient. The amount of wear and the relationship of the mandible (lower jaw) to the maxilla (upper jaw) will also vary with age. Age is sometimes important in indicating possible psychological complications in undertaking certain types of treatment.

Person Responsible for Account: Naturally you and your dentist are interested in who is going to pay the bill for the dental services your office performs. All statements must be sent to the person who is legally responsible for the services rendered. It is wise for the dental staff to be alert to all the unintentional indicators which may reveal valuable information about patients and their abilities and intentions concerning the payment of fees for services rendered.

Be sure the person listed as responsible for the account is actually responsible. Problems in collection can arise from ignorance in this area. For example, an employed minor, living at home, may not be responsible for the account should he or she stop working; or an unmarried woman may quit her job and marry. Who is responsible for the dental work she had charged while she was working? When a divorce is pending, who is responsible for the wife's dental care?

These and other difficulties concerning the person legally responsible for the account should be consciously considered as you study a patient's registration information.

Investigate the legal aspects of various typical situations under the laws of the state in which you are employed so that you are better equipped to protect the investment that the oral health care delivery team will make in providing dental treatment to patients.

Residence Address and Telephone: Obviously a neccessity.

Business Address and Telephone: There may be times when the residence address may change while the individual is still working at the same place of employment. Your office may or may not be notified of the change of residence. If you are not notified, this will give you a place with which to check. In other words, if you are registering a married person, the place of employment of the spouse should be given. In the event of difficulty with the account at a later date, a means of following up the collection of the account is available. It also may provide a means of appointment notification in an emergency, when no one is available at the residence address. If this place of employment is with a firm of considerable size, you should secure information as to which department employs the individual.

Occupation: There are many occupational diseases which may be demonstrated in the mouth. Lead poisoning may be developing in a painter or lead worker. Some occupations may be more inclined to develop tensions than others, which may affect the choice of materials for a dental procedure, the design of a dental replacement, or the method of dental treatment. Knowing the occupation is also helpful in judging the acceptability of the patient as a credit risk.

How Long in Present Place of Employment: This information is helpful in its relationship to the previous item insofar as possible dental complications are concerned. It is also one of the most important individual factors in relation to the extension of credit. A person who has been with the same firm for six years is obviously a better risk than one who started with a company last week and has not worked with one firm or on one job for any length of time. Previous length of employment should be determined if the present employment period has been short. In addition, if employment and working hours have been established for some time, it is easier for you to plan appointment time with the patient, and generally it is easier for the patient to arrange to keep appointments.

Physician: Many systemic diseases have effects that are apparent in the mouth. Cancer occurs with frequency in the area under the dentist's observation. Dentists often check with the patient's physician before making a definite diagnosis and plan of treatment. Frequently the dentist and the physician work together to solve a patient's difficulties.

Referred By: Your office should be sure to send a note of appreciation, preferably handwritten by the dentist, to every individual who refers a patient to your office. It is frequently true that patients refer others who are quite like themselves in socioeconomic status and dependability.

Relative or Close Friend: Should your office have to change an appointment suddenly for reasons beyond your control, or should you wish to call the patient to change an appointment, you may not be able to reach the patient. A relative or close friend can sometimes take the message or tell you where the patient may be reached. Should a patient leave town before paying a bill, having the name of a relative or friend gives you a means of locating the patient. Sometimes it is possible to obtain this information in casual conversation with the patient; however, if there is the least doubt in your mind about the patient's ability to pay his or her bills, be certain to obtain the name of a relative or close friend.

Former Dentist: It may be desirable to contact the former dentist, if the patient gives permission, to discover the exact treatment of a given condition. If the patient does not wish you to contact his or her previous dentist, carefully ascertain his or her dependability. This reluctance probably indicates embarrassment about informing the former dentist concerning the change in dentists, but this reluctance can also indicate trouble—and perhaps it was collection trouble.

Convenient Time for Appointments: For the convenience of the patient and for insurance against broken appointments, records should be made, and used, of the best time for that patient's appointment. The record should include the time of the week (early part or latter part); morning or afternoon; early or latter part of the morning or early or latter part of the afternoon. In some cases, it could be extended to include the preferred time during a given month.

Insurance Firm and Number of Policy: This information is very important when the insurance forms are to be completed. Having it on the registration is helpful in your work.

Acquiring Patient Registration Information

Whether the patient is given a registration form to fill out or whether you ask the questions is not important. How it is done, in either case, is important. All considerations must be given to the patient's self-respect.

If the patient is filling out the registration and does not fill in certain answers, you can quietly, gently, and with a smile explain why you wish such information on the record. If patients are approached with an attitude of genuine liking for people and a real desire to be of service to them, plus an indication that the process is one that is routinely performed with everyone who enters your practice, you usually will find that everything you wish to know is given freely. Those occasions in which the opposite is true deserve further investigation on your part to establish a good relationship.

It is possible for a patient to develop a lasting dislike for a dental office simply due to seemingly unfriendly, discourteous, or snobbish attitudes on the part of the office assistants. Clumsy and thoughtless handling of the business details can be damaging to the team no matter how excellent the professional services may be.

It is important for you to develop the ability to pick up impressions—of sensing the reaction of a patient to your conversation or questions. At times patients will, consciously or unconsciously, withhold certain essential information. Behavior, mannerisms, nervous gestures, and other characteristics will often give an alert, sensitive interviewer clues to possible financial or domestic irregularities. Such clues mean that you should keep gently probing until either the irregularities prove groundless or the true facts are brought out.

Very often difficulties in collections, when they occur, can be traced to the purchase of a new car, a new television set, or some other outlay rather than the dental payment itself, even though something about the dental service may be picked out by the patient as being the cause—too high a fee, the denture doesn't fit, etc. This can be the reason a long-time, regular patient suddenly develops trouble in paying the account.

Avoid developing a generally suspicious attitude, however, looking for hidden things that probably do not exist. The vast majority of people are honest. What is more, practically everyone wants to be honest. Patients are people.

In registering a new patient, you should aim for the following objectives:

1. Obtain complete details of name and address, sufficient for positive identification.
2. Secure as much personal history as is necessary to establish credit responsibility.
3. Make the registration a pleasant and agreeable experience for the patient.
4. Sell the office and its service.
5. Leave the patient with a friendly attitude toward the office so he or she will feel free to discuss personal financial problems at any time.

Credit Control

When the patient registration is complete, the next step in credit management occurs at the case presentation. The patient is told exactly what the charges will be. It is at this time that any insurance payment is discussed, clarifying for the patient exactly what the patient will pay over and above that paid by the insurance company. Perhaps the insurance pays the entire bill. If so, this fact should be stated. Once the patient knows and agrees to the financial obligation, the treatment is begun.

Accurate records must be maintained both of services rendered and payments received. Inability to substantiate by date and detail the various charges and credit, when required, weakens a claim against a patient. Minimum bookkeeping requirements are discussed elsewhere. Complete names, accurate dates, accurate data on the services rendered, and accurate figures are a basic requisite. With these carefully maintained, accurate records it is possible to establish a monthly billing procedure that assures regularity and accuracy in billing.

Of major importance in building a good dentist-patient relationship is accuracy. The name of the person to be billed should be recorded exactly. Few things cause greater annoyance to a person than to have his or her name mispronounced or misspelled. Accuracy in the address, including the zip code, leads to prompt delivery of statements. The amounts billed should be correct. Errors are embarrassing to both the patient and the dentist.

Whatever bookkeeping or accounting system is used in your office, it should provide for the quick and accurate determination of the amount owed by each patient at any given time. It should also yield detailed information about all accounts, such as the age of the account.

Collection Follow-Up Procedure

Now that the importance of collecting remuneration as promised has been established, the necessity for following up patient accounts is clear. Whenever credit is given, there will always be some collection problems. *Train yourself to accept the responsibility for following up accounts promptly when necessary.* The sooner you learn to do so, the easier your work will be in this phase of dental practice.

While collection problems are relatively few in number, they are important. Slow accounts lead to bad debts, and bad debts reduce office earnings. Fortunately, most patients are both able and willing to pay their bills promptly. They want to justify the confidence shown in them. Good professional collections depend, first, on the ability and willingness of the patient to pay promptly and, second, on the follow-up procedures used in that dental office.

Every effort should be made to get monthly statements out promptly on the same date. When this is not done, patients are inclined to treat their payments in the same haphazard manner. Set a definite date for mailing statements; make sure they go out on that date. Arrange your schedule of work so that this highly important task of billing your patients is accomplished.

Routine for Follow-Up Procedure

What is a program of collection follow-up? The first statement for amounts due should be mailed to the patient on the date you have chosen as your mailing date following the service for which a charge is being made. It can be expected that many patients will remit sometime during that month. These are the "prompt pay" people. Collection follow-up routine may begin with the second billing, with the third billing, or with whatever billing your dentist decides is appropriate for all accounts. *That is where care must be taken to make sure that the routine does begin.* And, having begun, it must be followed, step by step.

For example, let us say that we have decided to begin follow-up procedures with the third month's billing. A *reminder* notice should be attached to all those statements for professional service remaining unpaid at the time the third billing is prepared, unless specific arrangements have been made or extension of time granted. (It is recommended that impersonal types, such as a printed sticker or a stamp, be used for the first 120 days if begun at the second billing; for the first 90 days if begun at the third billing.) A set series to be used should be selected for your office. The first might be simply a large *PLEASE*. The following month this account, if still unpaid, would receive the second in the series—perhaps, *This account is overdue. May we hear from you?* Since our example begins to use an impersonal reminder on the third billing, it is continued for one more billing (90 days). The third reminder used routinely might be, *Unless this account is paid within ten days we shall be required to take further action.*

Each office should decide when to start the series on all accounts, which reminders to use, the order in which they are to be used, and how many are to be used. When the final sticker or stamp is placed on an account, that account should be given to a reputable collection agency, without fail, at the expiration of the promised number of days—as, in our example, after ten days.

You select your charities; don't let charities select your office for free dental work.

Procedures without Collection Agencies

If your office so chooses, instead of going to the collection-agency step after a certain number of billings have been made without result, you may end the impersonal sticker or stamp reminder and start a more personal phase of attention. No stated routine can be set forth. The problem is to discover why the bill has not been paid. In most cases there will have been some reaction from the patient to the collection reminders. From what is known about the patient and from what has been elicited by the collection procedure, the office assistant should be in a good position to decide the next step.

One common problem in collection work involves debtors who have moved and have neglected to give the office their forwarding addresses. These careless people are known by the descriptive title of *skips*.

The first realization that a patient has become a skip usually occurs with the return of mail addressed to him or her at the last known address. Such returned mail is cause for immediate action.

Reference should be made to the original registration blank. Now the value of the information secured is recognized. Telephoning to the personal references sometimes brings results. The place of employment as given should be called and inquiry made as to current employment or if the personnel office has any knowledge of where the person has moved.

Should your own efforts to locate the skip fail, you then turn to the credit bureau. Many bureaus have locating facilities.

Of course, it is always possible that the patient has innocently failed to tell the office about the change of address. In such cases, certainly, he or she is entitled to every cooperation in arrangements for payment. Usually, however, skips mean collection problems, and it is wise to allow the professional collector to handle them.

The collection system outlined will suffice for most of your accounts. It will bring money in without loss of goodwill. Success of the system will depend on regularity in carrying it out.

It is dangerous to think, for example, that for one reason or another collection work can be suspended without mattering too much. Once patients come to know that your office expects prompt payment, you will gain respect for your businesslike attitude.

It is unnecessary to be hard, hostile, or rude at any time. On the contrary, it is important to retain a good-tempered approach. The stubborn and selfish attitudes of many people will exasperate you, but do not allow your feelings to be revealed. *Patience, persistence, and courtesy* are the qualities that lead to success in collections.

The Telephone

The telephone is a valuable collection tool. Of course, do your telephoning at times when patients are not in the office, or at least not within hearing distance. When you are positive that you are talking with the patient, or the person responsible for the account, make no apology for calling, and in a friendly but emphatic manner say that you would like to have an understanding about the account. Before you complete the conversation try to secure a definite promise for payment. Note the date carefully on the age analysis form. Exactly on the date promised, call the patient if the payment has not been received. If the patient realizes that you are following promises closely, he or she will regard the matter with greater respect.

Your office has a hard-and-fast policy about collections; you talk it over frankly with the patient and establish a payment plan in the beginning if cash isn't possible by the time the work is finished. The plan is established, and all you have asked is cooperation. When unexpected problems arise—Johnny breaks his leg; Daddy is ill and hasn't been able to work for three weeks—adjustments can be made, of course, to help the family over a hard financial period. However, the alert dental assistant keeping constant watch over the accounts, allows no one to miss a payment without calling to find out why the payment has not been made and to arrange to have it made up. The constant "jacking up" of slow payers, or those who slip, often turns them into patients who pay their bills promptly. Handling them otherwise can just as well turn them into patients who never pay their bills until forced to—even when they are personal friends of the dentist!

Remember that no matter how much the patient may not like being called about an overdue account, you, the bookkeeper, are doing it as part of your job. There will be no feeling of resentment directed at the dentist, and this is important. The patient may feel sorry for the dentist who has such an employee, but the patient doesn't resent the dentist. Be a third party to the situation to absorb such feelings as a protection to your dentist's practice.

One value of telephoning is that the patient is almost obliged to say something, even if only to offer a vague assurance that the matter will be looked into. Patients may ignore notices and letters, and perhaps even say they were never received. The telephone offers no such easy escape. Always be courteous. Consider the patient. The telephone often rings in the home at most inconvenient times. Experienced telephone collectors, after having first made sure they have the right person on the line (an important point), ask if it is convenient for the patient to talk about the account. Should the patient indicate that it is not, ask when it would be convenient to call back. It is both smart and courteous, after announcing who is calling, to let the patient talk. Some grievances or details of unexpected circumstances may be discovered. Listen attentively and courteously to such stories, but toward the end of the conversation try for some definite assurance of specific payment. Even when calling a "problem" patient, who perhaps has made several promises and failed to keep them or ignored your polite collection reminders, remember that your job is to sell payment rather than to force it. Control your feelings, pause before you call the patient, study the best approach to make, and above all, retain your poise and charm.

The Letter

Another method of contacting patients who have not responded to the impersonal reminders on the statements is to write a personal letter.

There is no place in professional collections for the form letter as used in collection and other correspondence by business firms. Such form letters are often inaccurately and poorly filled in. Where a rubber stamp or printed facsimile signature is used, the effect is still less impressive.

Effective composition of letters is discussed in "Written Communications." The sample letters in that chapter are just that—samples. Write your own letters based on the personal patients in your office. The basic ideas to remember in writing a collection letter are these:

1. Remember the patient. Write something that appeals to her or him. Talk her or his language. Use the *you* approach.
2. Use some idea to motivate the patient to want to pay the bill. Show how paying the bill will benefit the patient.
3. Be sure the patient knows exactly what you expect. Give him or her a choice of two ways of paying, for example, but never give the idea that payment can be avoided.

No more than two such letters should be written to any patient. Other means of collection must follow the second letter, either a personal interview or a collection agency.

The Personal Interview

Perhaps you will prefer to use a personal interview with a delinquent account. Possibly you will wait until you have contacted the patient by mail and/or telephone. When the time comes for this personal interview, remember that it is an interview—an appointment with *you,* the assistant, not with the dentist.

Make an appointment with the patient and arrange to confer in private.

Your attitude is most important in this interview. It should be pleasant—one of sympathy and understanding. If you are sympathetic and ask for clarification of reasons why the account has not been paid, the patient is more likely to feel like confiding.

Your conduct following the patient's explanation is determined by the factors involved. If the patient has had an illness, an accident, or is unable to pay for some other reason, be sure that the arrangement made for monthly payments is one the patient can meet. Remember that you will have the same problem in a month or two if the new payment schedule is one the patient is unable to meet.

It is wise to verify the patient's statement that he or she cannot pay. The patient may have some assets that could be used, but either doesn't recognize them or doesn't want to recognize them as assets to be used. A lending agency, such as a bank, may loan money, provided the borrower has something the bank can hold until the loan is paid. This something is called collateral. For example, a person may have stock that could be held by the bank until the loan is repaid. The patient uses the stock as collateral to secure the loan to pay the dental bill, and it is the bank who extends credit—not the dentist.

Procedures with Collection Agencies

The collection agency you select to work on your accounts should be selected with the same care you use when you select your bank. Both handle your money. Some local credit bureaus associated with the International Consumer Credit Association have collection departments. Dentists who are members will find many advantages in using these services.

You may be approached by salespersons for certain collection agencies seeking your collection accounts. Some of these, unfortunately, are unreliable. Do not sign a contract with a collection salesperson before you have taken every precaution to establish the trustworthiness and responsibility of the agency represented.

After an account has been turned over to the collection agency, all further dealings with the patient should be left entirely in their hands. Professional collectors specialize in collecting accounts, and best results are gained when they have a free hand. Patients will often contact the office when they receive the first letter from the agency and will attempt to make arrangements or plead for an extension of time. The position of the office assistant in such cases is to tell the patient that the account is now being handled by the agency and that all discussion must be with that agency.

Give the agency the full information needed: complete name and address and an itemized statement of amounts owing, together with dates of all payments or other transactions. Do not send the patient any more monthly statements or letters. Should the patient call you, courteously refer him or her to the agency.

If the agency asks you to accept payments if offered, report them promptly. If any information comes to you that you believe would assist in effecting collection, report it to the agency immediately.

Collection Advice from the American Collectors Association

The American Collectors Association has some words of advice about the collection of accounts. When to seek help and what to look for in selecting a collection agency are quoted from one of their brochures.

When to Seek Help

Remember, time is the safest refuge of any delinquent debtor. The more he gets of it, the less likely he is to pay.

It can be stated, with near categorical certainty, that the time has arrived for professional assistance:

1. When the new patient does not respond to your letters or telephone calls
2. When payment terms fail for no valid reason
3. When repetitious unfounded complaints occur
4. When there is a denial of responsibility
5. When repeated delinquencies are concurrent with repeated changes of address and/or occupation
6. When a delinquency co-exists with serious marital difficulties

7. When an obvious financial irresponsibility is exposed
8. When a patient is a skip
9. When any delinquent patient fails to sustain communication

Other situations of equal urgency may occur, but when any of your past-due accounts meet any of these points, it is time to recognize that your further efforts on these claims will produce fewer positive results than the amount of effort expended in the professional side of your practice.

In summary, it can be said that you need the assistance of a professional collector "when you have lost effective contact with your patient." To ignore the patient's delinquency is to encourage him or her to continue bad paying habits. It also means that it is highly unlikely that he or she or any member of the family will return to you for further services. Every credit grantor has an obligation to insure that every patient who is financially able to pay does so.

What to Look for in Selecting a Collection Agency

Selecting an agency to work with you in collecting your past-due accounts is like selecting one's physician or dentist, or any business associate. One does it by reputation and by recommendation.

However, in selecting a collection agency, a few other guideposts are helpful.

1. In most cases the owners will be local, well-established business persons.
2. You will know them from their memberships in civic and business clubs and activities.
3. They will be members of a recognized national trade association such as the American Collectors Association. This assures you that they have met a rigid set of membership requirements and that they are able to offer complete collection service, not only locally, but through their thousands of fellow-members throughout this part of the world.
4. They will seldom use a written contract. Most agencies work on a "contingent fee basis" which means they get paid a percentage of what they collect. There is no charge for listing accounts with the agency for collection, and they make no charge for work on any claim they are not able to collect.
5. And finally, visit the collector's offices and become familiar with the procedures they use.

Once this working relationship is established, you have confidence in that agency to represent you in the way you want, and to recover for you as high a percentage as possible of your past-due accounts.

Summary

Patients need to understand the financial arrangements for their dental service. It is important for both the dentist and the patient to understand what the fee is and how it is to be paid. Careful control of credit is essential to any good dental practice.

Credit in the dental office is a business arrangement based on the ability and willingness of the patient to pay bills according to an arranged agreement. Procedures to achieve good credit management are: (1) have a complete registration of the patient, (2) tell the patient what the charges will be, (3) make a definite arrangement for payment *before* services are performed, and (4) follow up on patients who do not pay promptly.

Patients need to be educated to regard bills for dental services in the same light as other consumer credit obligations—to be paid promptly, as arranged.

Good bookkeeping is necessary to manage credit and collections.

Following up accounts of patients who fail to keep their agreement to pay at a certain time must be done promptly and with unvarying routine. An age analysis of accounts receivable shows the pattern of pay habits for individual patients.

A routine for following up slow accounts should be established and then followed. One such method advises an impersonal reminder on the statement beginning with the third month of billing and continuing for three months. After this length of time, the account should be turned over to a reliable collection agency. If you do not wish to use a collection agency, follow-up may be accomplished by telephone, letter, or personal interview.

Study Questions

1. What is credit?
2. Credit in the dental office is a business arrangement. What are three procedures which are effective in managing credit?
3. Discuss the items important to good patient registration and explain why they are important.
4. State the objectives in registering a new patient.
5. Discuss the ability and willingness of the patient to pay.
6. Discuss age analysis of accounts.
7. What is a collection percentage and how do you determine it?
8. Discuss follow-up procedures.
9. What procedures for collection are available if you do not use a collection agency?
10. Why should the dental office refuse to work with the patient on collection after the account has been given to a collection agency?

Vocabulary

age analysis a summary of account payments, indicating who has and who has not been paying their bills

collateral something of value given to the lender by the borrower to protect the interests of the lender

credit trust in an individual's business integrity and in his or her financial capacity to meet all obligations when they become due

truth-in-lending requirement by the federal government to state the percentage of interest charged when an account is carried over thirty days

Word Elements	
Word Element	*Example*
ectomy suffix meaning: surgical removal	*odontectomy* removal of a tooth
otomy suffix meaning: incision	*pulpotomy* an operation in which all or part of the pulp is removed from a tooth
cid, cis combining form meaning: relationship to kill, cut	*excision* removal by cutting
tomy, tome suffix meaning: cut, an instrument for cutting	*odontotomy* prophylactic cutting into a tooth for preventive treatment
scop suffix meaning: an instrument to examine or view	*laryngoscope* an instrument to view the larynx
syn prefix meaning: union, association	*synthesis* combination of parts to form a whole
sym prefix meaning: union, association	*symmetry* similar arrangement on each side
plegia suffix meaning: paralysis	*paraplegia* paralysis of the legs and lower part of the body
sacro combining form meaning: relationship to the sacrum	*sacrodynia* pain in the sacral region of the back
spondylo combining form meaning: relationship to vertebrae, spinal column	*spondylitis* inflammation of the vertebrae

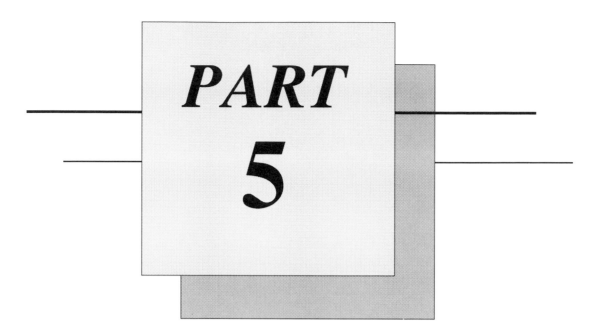

PART 5

Elementary Dental Knowledge

Basic information that the dental assistant knows as educational background will be found in this section of your text.

The basics—anatomy, anesthesia, annotating teeth, diet, microbiology, sterilization, oral pathology, caries, drugs, first aid, emergency care, oral hygiene, and some of the dental specialties with which you may be associated are discussed in succeeding chapters.

This section gives you an opportunity to saturate your mind with technical knowledge that will be invaluable to you in your work.

CHAPTER 20

The Systems of the Body[1]

The Patient as a Person
The Structure of the Body
  Cells
  Tissues
  Organs
  Body Cavities
  Body Planes
    Sagittal Plane
    Frontal Plane and Posterior Plane
    Transverse Plane
  Body Surfaces
  Review of Certain Body Structures
The Systems of the Body
  The Skeletal System
  Review of Skeletal System
  The Muscular System
    Muscular Action
  Review of Muscular System
  The Integumentary System
  Review of Integumentary System
  The Circulatory System
    The Heart
    The Course of the Blood

    Blood Circulating Systems
  Review of the Circulatory System
  The Lymphatic System
  Review of the Lymphatic System
  The Hemic or Blood System
  Review of the Hemic System
  The Respiratory System
  Review of the Respiratory System
  The Nervous System
    The Central Nervous System
    The Peripheral Nervous System
    The Autonomic Nervous System
    The Sense Organs
  Review of the Nervous System
  The Endocrine System
  Review of the Endocrine System
  The Digestive System
    Excretion
  Review of the Digestive System
  The Genitourinary System
    The Urinary System
  Review of the Urinary System
  The Reproductive System
  Review of the Reproductive System

The Patient as a Person

Dentistry has advanced from the mechanics of removing a decayed tooth to the fine art of preventing problems, preserving what can be preserved, restoring the entire mouth to health, and maintaining that health.

The health of the mouth involves the entire body. Thus, dental treatment must consider the person as a whole: including mental, emotional, and physical aspects as well as moral values that affect each individual's health. A person responds to the responsibilities in the socioeconomic environment in which he or she lives. When a person is faced with dentistry, he or she may develop apprehensions not only about the treatment to be experienced, but about financial obligations concerning that treatment—whether the treatment is worth the expense. That is, that person might be wondering, a) what will this dentistry do for my health and well being? or b) what might it do for my relationship with others?

The dental health team must remember to take care of and treat the whole person while concentrating on the physical dental difficulties that person is experiencing. Therefore, some overall knowledge of the body as a whole with its systems and their interrelationships is highly valuable for a dental assistant.

The Structure of the Body

The body is a structural unit, but it is composed of four kinds of smaller units: *cells, tissues, organs, and systems.* The organs are placed within body *cavities.* We locate the organs by use of body *planes.*

Health requires normal composition and functioning of our cells, tissues, organs, and systems. If conditions are not normal, disease or malfunctioning results. In the mouth, the most common diseases are *caries* and *periodontal degeneration.*

Since the organs are composed of tissues which are made up of cells, we will begin by discussing cells and proceed through the basic structural units before discussing the systems of the body.

Cells

Cells are the smallest units, often called the simplest, but they are not simple. Cells have specialized parts to carry on what we call life processes. Usually we think of the entire body performing certain functions. Actually, these functions are the combined activities of the cells of the body. A living cell is in a constant state of activity. There are nine separate **life processes** in the life of a cell or in the life of a human body as a whole.

They are **absorption, digestion, synthesis (assimilation), respiration, excretion, secretion, motion, irritability,** and **reproduction.**

These activities often are interrelated—that is, the **absorption, digestion,** and **synthesis** (or **assimilation**) of essential nutrients by the body as a whole affects the life of the cells because the nutrients so received enable the cells to live. The digestive system of the body *absorbs, digests,* and *assimilates* the nutrients which are then passed on to the cells. The cells in turn *absorb* the end products of the body's digestive process, *digest* these products by breaking them down into simpler compounds, and *assimilate* them (the process of synthesis) by utilizing the amino acids to build more complex molecules, resulting in cell growth.

The reason for **respiration** of the body as a whole (inhalation and exhalation by the lungs) is to provide the cells with a continuous supply of oxygen—without which they could not live. Thus, the respiration function of the body and the cells are closely associated.

The **excretion** of waste products begins in the cells. They must rid themselves of waste products. These wastes are carried away by the blood to be removed from the body. The several ways the body rids itself of waste matter will be discussed later.

The body as a whole and the cells both form and give off substances; this process is called **secretion.**

The body as a whole moves, and the cell content flows through the cell in a **motion** called *streaming.*

Irritability (or **sensitivity**) is the ability to respond to stimuli. Both body and cells—particularly nerve cells—respond to stimuli.

Cells **reproduce**—often by dividing into two new cells. The body as a whole reproduces by producing eggs or sperm. Eventually an egg and sperm can unite to become a new body.

Thus, the nine life processes of the individual cells and of the body as a whole are closely interrelated.

Cells are not all alike. Early in the formation of an individual, cells become specialized for a certain purpose. Groups of these cells form tissues. Some examples are muscle, blood, nerve, bone, and skin. Each cell of a tissue lives as an individual unit and must therefore perform all nine of the processes of life. In addition, each cell is able to perform one or more functions with great skill. For example, a nerve cell responds to stimuli skillfully—it is the chief purpose of the cell. However, it also performs all the other life processes. Some cells specialize in one function, others in a different life process.

Each cell is different—specialized for a specific purpose. Groups of similar cells form body *tissue,* such as bone or muscle.

Plate 1

Major bones of the skeleton: a) anterior; and b) posterior views.

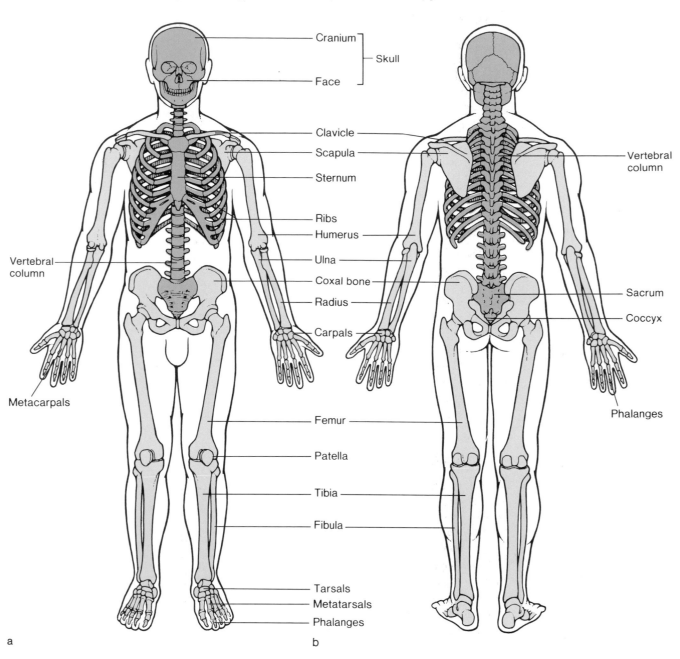

Cranium ⎤
           ⎬ Skull
Face   ⎦

Clavicle

Scapula

Sternum

Ribs

Humerus

Ulna

Coxal bone

Radius

Carpals

Vertebral column

Metacarpals

Femur

Patella

Tibia

Fibula

Tarsals

Metatarsals

Phalanges

Vertebral column

Sacrum

Coccyx

Phalanges

a

b

Plate 2

Superficial view of skeletal muscles: a) anterior; and b) posterior.

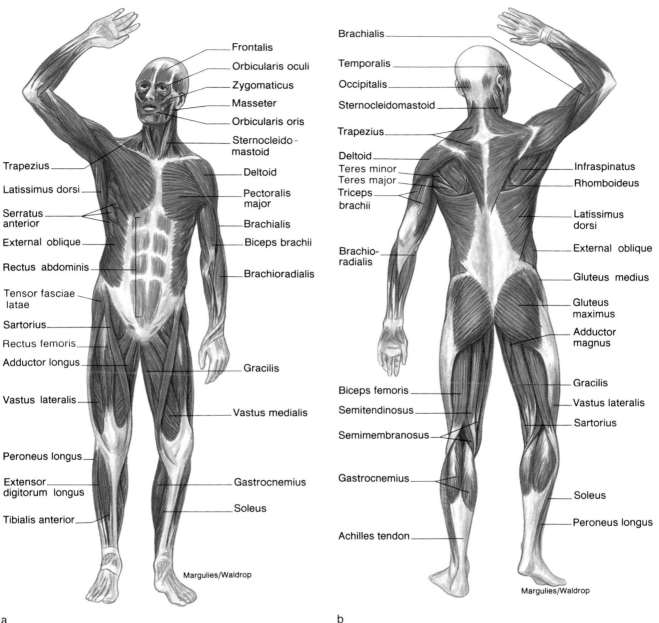

a — Anterior view

- Frontalis
- Orbicularis oculi
- Zygomaticus
- Masseter
- Orbicularis oris
- Sternocleido-mastoid
- Deltoid
- Pectoralis major
- Brachialis
- Biceps brachii
- Brachioradialis
- Gracilis
- Vastus medialis
- Gastrocnemius
- Soleus

- Trapezius
- Latissimus dorsi
- Serratus anterior
- External oblique
- Rectus abdominis
- Tensor fasciae latae
- Sartorius
- Rectus femoris
- Adductor longus
- Vastus lateralis
- Peroneus longus
- Extensor digitorum longus
- Tibialis anterior

Margulies/Waldrop

b — Posterior view

- Brachialis
- Temporalis
- Occipitalis
- Sternocleidomastoid
- Trapezius
- Deltoid
- Teres minor
- Teres major
- Triceps brachii
- Brachio-radialis
- Biceps femoris
- Semitendinosus
- Semimembranosus
- Gastrocnemius
- Achilles tendon

- Infraspinatus
- Rhomboideus
- Latissimus dorsi
- External oblique
- Gluteus medius
- Gluteus maximus
- Adductor magnus
- Gracilis
- Vastus lateralis
- Sartorius
- Soleus
- Peroneus longus

Margulies/Waldrop

Plate 3

Magnified cross section of the skin.

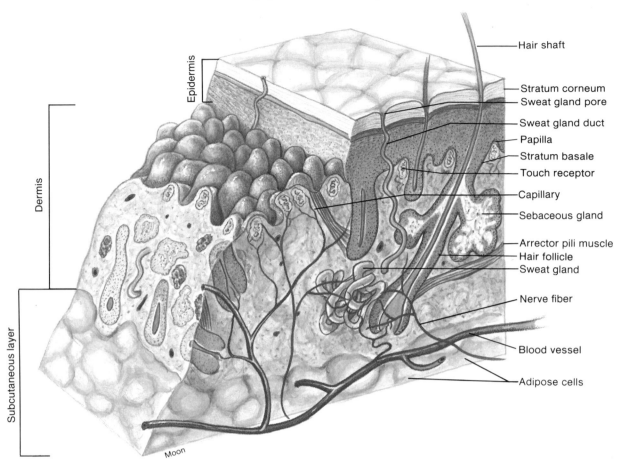

Epidermis

Dermis

Subcutaneous layer

Hair shaft

Stratum corneum
Sweat gland pore
Sweat gland duct
Papilla
Stratum basale
Touch receptor
Capillary
Sebaceous gland
Arrector pili muscle
Hair follicle
Sweat gland
Nerve fiber
Blood vessel
Adipose cells

Moon

Plate 4

The lungs, showing the bronchial tree and the capillary network.

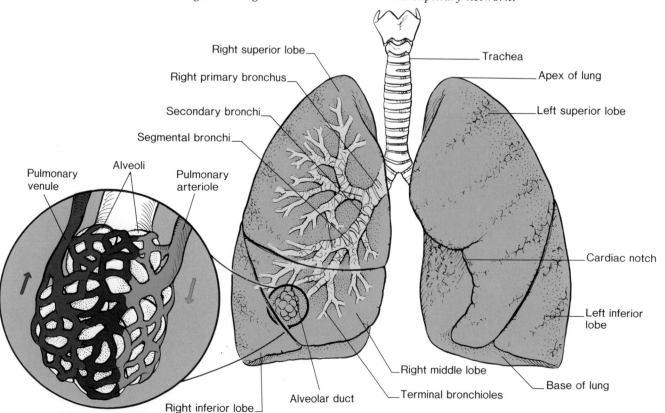

Right superior lobe
Right primary bronchus
Secondary bronchi
Segmental bronchi

Pulmonary venule
Alveoli
Pulmonary arteriole

Trachea
Apex of lung
Left superior lobe

Cardiac notch

Left inferior lobe

Right inferior lobe
Alveolar duct
Right middle lobe
Terminal bronchioles
Base of lung

Plate 5

The main veins of the head and neck.

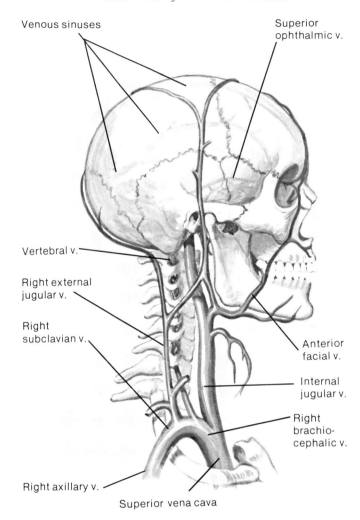

Venous sinuses

Superior
ophthalmic v.

Vertebral v.

Right external
jugular v.

Right
subclavian v.

Right axillary v.

Superior vena cava

Anterior
facial v.

Internal
jugular v.

Right
brachio-
cephalic v.

Plate 6

Schematic drawing of the circulatory system.

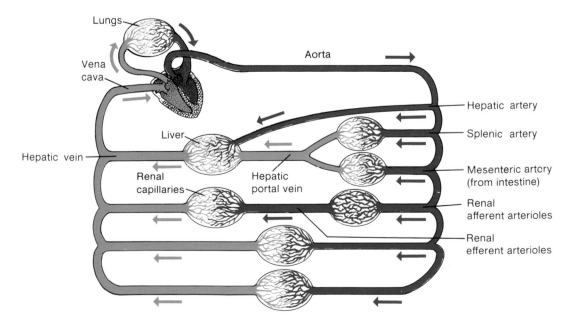

Lungs

Vena
cava

Aorta

Hepatic vein

Liver

Renal
capillaries

Hepatic
portal vein

Hepatic artery

Splenic artery

Mesenteric artery
(from intestine)

Renal
afferent arterioles

Renal
efferent arterioles

Plate 7

Major vessels of the venous system.

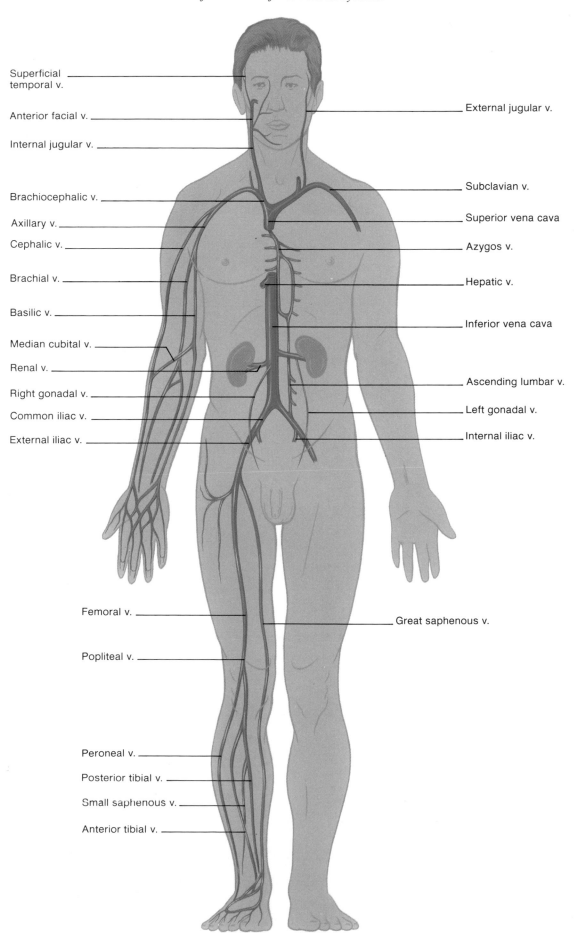

Superficial temporal v.

Anterior facial v.

Internal jugular v.

Brachiocephalic v.

Axillary v.

Cephalic v.

Brachial v.

Basilic v.

Median cubital v.

Renal v.

Right gonadal v.

Common iliac v.

External iliac v.

External jugular v.

Subclavian v.

Superior vena cava

Azygos v.

Hepatic v.

Inferior vena cava

Ascending lumbar v.

Left gonadal v.

Internal iliac v.

Femoral v.

Popliteal v.

Great saphenous v.

Peroneal v.

Posterior tibial v.

Small saphenous v.

Anterior tibial v.

Plate 8

Major vessels of the arterial system.

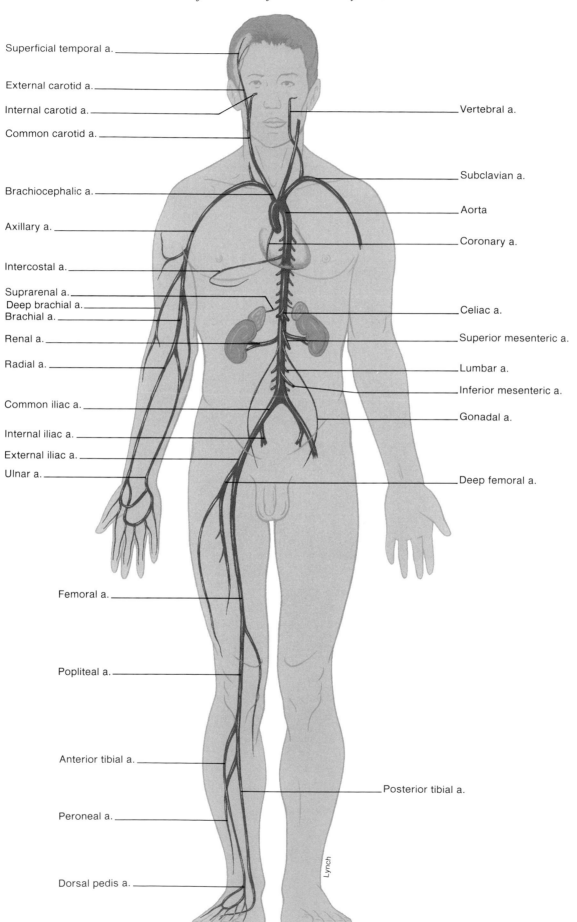

Superficial temporal a.

External carotid a.

Internal carotid a.

Common carotid a.

Brachiocephalic a.

Axillary a.

Intercostal a.

Suprarenal a.

Deep brachial a.

Brachial a.

Renal a.

Radial a.

Common iliac a.

Internal iliac a.

External iliac a.

Ulnar a.

Femoral a.

Popliteal a.

Anterior tibial a.

Peroneal a.

Dorsal pedis a.

Vertebral a.

Subclavian a.

Aorta

Coronary a.

Celiac a.

Superior mesenteric a.

Lumbar a.

Inferior mesenteric a.

Gonadal a.

Deep femoral a.

Posterior tibial a.

Lynch

Plate 9

These muscles help open and close the jaw (mandible).

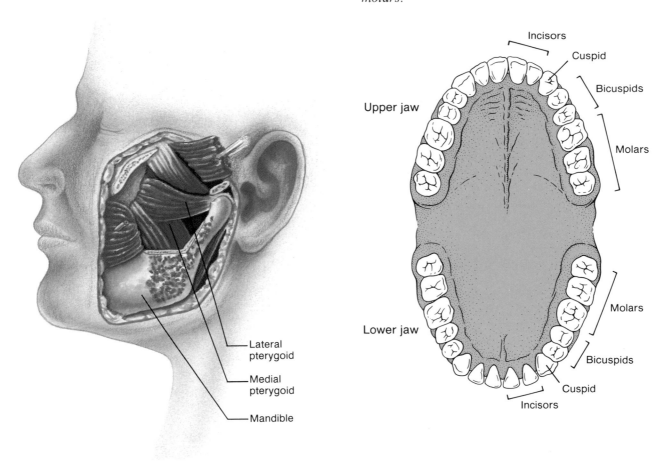

Lateral pterygoid

Medial pterygoid

Mandible

Plate 10

The permanent teeth of the upper and lower jaw, identifying the incisors, cuspids, bicuspids, and molars.

Incisors

Cuspid

Bicuspids

Upper jaw

Molars

Molars

Lower jaw

Bicuspids

Cuspid

Incisors

Plate 11

The articulation between the root of the tooth and the mandible.

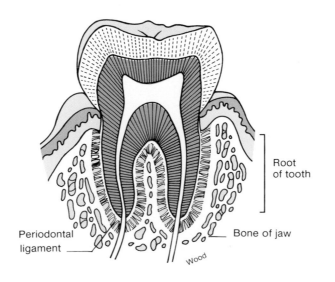

Root of tooth

Bone of jaw

Periodontal ligament

Wood

Plate 12

The hyoid bone supports the tongue and is an attachment for muscles that move the tongue and function in swallowing.

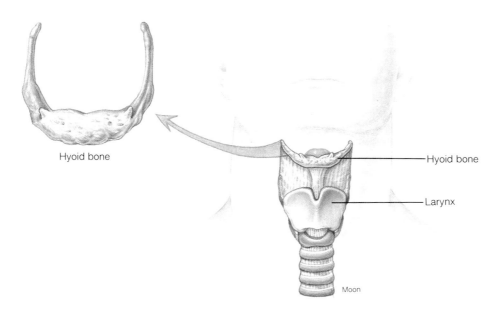

Hyoid bone

Hyoid bone

Larynx

Moon

Plate 13

A sagital section of the mouth, nasal cavity, and pharynx.

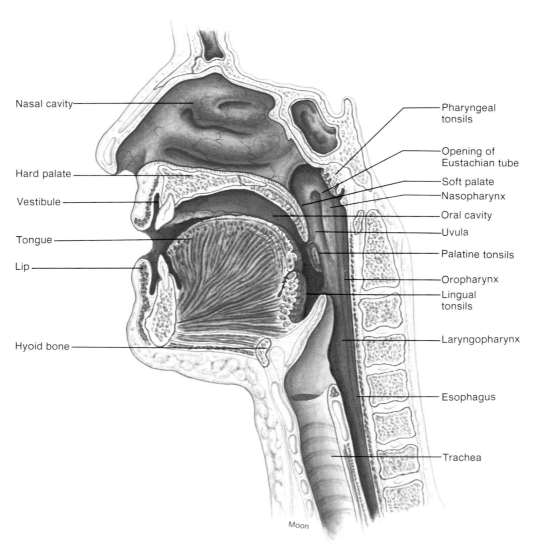

Nasal cavity

Hard palate

Vestibule

Tongue

Lip

Hyoid bone

Pharyngeal tonsils

Opening of Eustachian tube

Soft palate

Nasopharynx

Oral cavity

Uvula

Palatine tonsils

Oropharynx

Lingual tonsils

Laryngopharynx

Esophagus

Trachea

Moon

Tissues

The tissues of the body are divided into four groups.

1. **Epithelial tissues** are covering or lining tissues (mucous membranes). They form protective layers covering both inside and outside the body. Skin is an example of epithelial tissue. This tissue also lines the mouth, blood vessels, and the digestive tract through the entire body. There are three types of epithelial tissue: *simple squamous, stratified squamous,* and *simple columnar.*

2. **Muscle tissues** move body parts and are found everywhere in the body—in layers in the internal organs, in the walls of the internal organs, in the walls of the blood vessels, and in the heart. There are three types of muscle tissue:
   a. **Skeletal muscles** (also called striated, voluntary muscles) move bones, initiate the swallowing process, and cause extrinsic (outer) eye movements.
   b. **Visceral muscles** (also called nonstriated or smooth muscles) move substances through the digestive, respiratory, and genitourinary tracts, and through ducts; they also change the diameter of the blood vessels, the diameter of the pupils of the eyes, and the shape of the lens. Visceral muscles also cause the erection of hairs on the surface of the body.
   c. **Cardiac muscle** (also called striated, involuntary muscles) causes the contraction of the heart.

3. **Connective tissue** binds other tissues together and forms the framework to support the body. (For example, it connects bones to bones and muscle to bones.) It is the most widely distributed of all tissues. Types of connective tissues are:
   a. **Loose, ordinary connective tissue** connects other tissues and organs.
   b. **Cartilaginous connective tissue** consists of cartilage that is like bone, only softer and pliable. The end of the nose, which bends, is an example of cartilaginous tissue.
   c. **Fibrous tissue** consists of bundles of fibers in a fluid matrix. Ligaments and tendons are examples.
   d. **Bone** is rigid and the site for red blood cell production. It is also called osseous tissue.
   e. **Adipose tissue,** commonly called fat, is usually found in certain areas of the body called fat depots. It provides protection, insulation, and support.
   f. **Circulating tissue** is blood. It is different because the cells are not joined but float in plasma. It is sometimes called a fluid tissue because it is composed of a fluid portion (plasma) and a solid portion (blood cells).
   g. **Hemopoietic and reticuloendothelial tissues** are found in bone marrow space and the lymph system. These tissues are concerned with production of blood elements and lymph elements, and with the process of phagocytosis.

4. **Nerve tissue** is responsive to stimuli. It relates the individual to his or her environment and controls body activity. It is found in the brain, spinal cord, and nerves.

Organs

Cells are the basic structure that make up tissue. Tissue, in turn, is a group of structurally similar cells performing the same function. Several types of tissue may be found in an **organ,** each contributing its specialty to the satisfactory working of the whole organ. For example, the heart is an organ that has epithelial tissue as a covering, connective tissue binding other tissues together, muscle tissue, and nerve tissue throughout.

The organs of the body work better when they work in a system with other organs. For example, your stomach cannot digest a meal alone. Other organs that assist are: teeth, mouth, esophagus, small intestine, liver, gallbladder, and pancreas. These organs assist digestion by grinding food into small particles, and by manufacturing secretions such as ptyalin, insulin, pepsin, kinase, amylase, renin, and hydrochloric acid. Each vital process of the body is performed by a system. Each system is essential for good health. The systems are interdependent. A disturbance in one system will disturb the other systems and affect the general health of the individual.

Before we study the systems of the body, we should understand body cavities and body planes.

Body Cavities

The organs of the human body are housed in several **cavities**—actually two large cavities that are subdivided. The two large cavities are called the **dorsal cavity** (containing the cranial and spinal cavities) and the **ventral cavity** (containing the thoracic and abdomino-pelvic cavities).

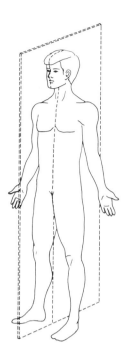

Figure 20.1
The sagittal plane.

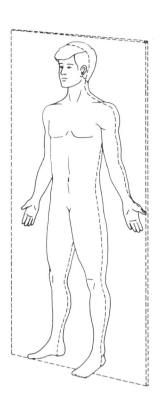

Figure 20.2
The frontal plane and the posterior plane.

The **cranial** (skull) **cavity** contains the brain and the facial organs of sight, smell, taste, hearing, and eating.

The **spinal cavity** holds the part of the central nervous system known as the spinal cord.

The **thoracic cavity** (also referred to as the chest cavity) contains the heart, lungs, large blood vessels, trachea, esophagus, thymus, and lymph nodes. It has three subdivisions separated by partitions of pleura. The lungs are in the part known as the **pleural cavity;** the space between the lungs that contains the esophagus, trachea, large blood vessels, etc., is called the **mediastinum.** The heart is protected in an envelope of connective tissue which is called the **pericardial sac.** All the viscera in the chest lie in the separate sections of the **thoracic cavity** between the lungs. The thoracic cavity varies in size during the act of respiration, enlarging on inspiration and decreasing on expiration. The **diaphragm** separates the thoracic cavity from the abdominopelvic cavity.

Below the thoracic cavity is the **abdominopelvic cavity,** within which are the organs of digestion, reproduction, and excretion. The upper portion is the **abdominal cavity,** containing the organs of digestion. Below is the **pelvic cavity,** containing the organs of excretion and reproduction.

Body Planes

Body planes are very important for the dental assistant to understand because they will be referred to in terminology.

Anatomists in all parts of the world have agreed to describe the human body with standard reference terms in relation to the *anatomical position,* which portrays the position of the living body standing erect, feet together, with the head, eyes, and toes directed forward, with the arms by the sides and the palms facing forward.

Sagittal Plane (Figure 20.1)

Divide the body into a right and left half vertically. The cut surface is the **sagittal plane** or section. If this cut is directly in the middle, it is the midsagittal section. However, it is possible to cut to the right or left of the middle and, providing the cut is still dividing right from left, the cut surface is still a sagittal plane or section.

Frontal Plane and Posterior Plane (Figure 20.2)

If the front half of the body is cut from the back of the body, the two sections thus discovered are called the **frontal plane** (for front) and **posterior plane** (for back).

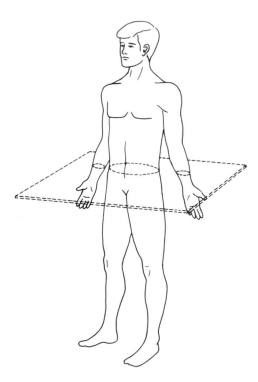

Figure 20.3
The transverse plane.

Transverse Plane (Figure 20.3)

If the cut were to divide the body into an upper and lower part, the exposed part is called the **transverse plane.** The term **superior** is used in referring to the upper part and **inferior** when referring to the lower part.

Body Surfaces

The front surface of the body is called the **anterior surface.** It includes the face, chest, abdomen, and front of the legs. The back surface is called the **posterior surface.**

Two other terms are used in referring to the anterior and posterior surfaces of the human body. **Dorsal** means back, and can be used interchangeably with posterior. **Ventral** is a French word that means "belly." The *ventral surface* is forward and can be used interchangeably with *anterior* in the human. In animals, it is the surface which faces downward.

Review of Certain Body Structures

Cells Have Specialized Parts to Carry on Life Processes
Absorption
Digestion
Synthesis
Respiration
Excretion
Secretion
Motion
Irritability
Reproduction

Body Cavities
Dorsal **containing**
Cranial
Spinal
Ventral **containing**
Thoracic
Abdominopelvic

Body Planes
Sagittal: right and left halves
Frontal and Posterior: front and back halves
Transverse: upper and lower halves

Body Surfaces
Anterior: front
Posterior: back
Dorsal: back (interchangeable with posterior)
Ventral: (French for "belly") underside; can be forward as anterior in humans, or downward surface in animals.

Review of Certain Body Structures— *Continued*

The Body is a Structural Unit Composed of
Cells
Tissues
Organs
Systems

Types of Tissues of the Body
Epithelial (covering or lining)
Muscle (attaches to bones and moves the body)
Connective (binds other tissues together)
Includes:
Loose, ordinary connective tissue
Cartilaginous connective tissue
Fibrous tissue
Bone
Adipose tissue
Circulating tissue
Hemopoietic and reticuloendothelial tissues
Nerve tissue

The Systems of the Body

Just as the cells work together to make better tissue, and the tissues are more efficient when they form an organ, and the organs when they form a system, the **systems** of the body also work together. The skeletal, muscular, and integumentary systems form the framework and covering of the body. Each system also has its separate function.

The Skeletal System

The **skeleton** of the body is usually referred to as the framework and protector of the vital living organs which make up the human body. The skeleton also accomplishes locomotion by action of attached muscles. Actually the bones are also living organs, supplied with blood, requiring oxygen and sustenance (nourishment), capable of growth and of self-repair. (Plate 1) The **skeletal system** includes these organs: *bones, cartilaginous structures,* and *ligaments of the framework of the body.*

Over 200 bones of many sizes and shapes are found in the human body. There are five functions bones perform.

1. They support the framework of the body (similar to a beam).
2. They help move the body by providing muscle attachment places (similar to a lever).
3. They protect vital organs from injury (similar to a shield).
4. They help to form red and certain white blood cells (similar to a factory).
5. They store the body's minerals (similar to a warehouse).

Three factors are necessary for bones to form and grow: the body must have an adequate supply of certain minerals, vitamins, and hormones. Should any of these elements be missing, the bones will either be weak and break easily or fail to grow. Since nature adapts bone to meet the needs of the body, a need must be present; that is, if one doesn't exercise and use one's bones, they are apt to become weak.

Table 20.1 gives the names of 206 of the bones.

The framework would be difficult to handle if it didn't have **joints** which make the framework movable. The ends of two bones meet (articulate) and a joint occurs. There are seven types of joints. **Cartilage** cushions the bone ends in the joint. Membranes cover the joint and secrete **synovial fluid** (sih-*nō*-vē-al) which lubricates the joint. **Ligaments** are similar to ropes. They bind the bones together and are tough and pliable. The seven types of joints have specific jobs to do, depending on the kind of movement needed for the joint. Table 20.2 summarizes the types of joints and their names, location, and use. Figure 20.4 shows the seven kinds of joints.

Review of Skeletal System

Organs of the Skeletal System
Bones
Cartilaginous structures
Ligaments

Table 20.1
Bones of the Skeleton

Part of Body and Number of Bones		Subdivision and Number of Bones		Description
Skull	(28)			
		Cranium	(8)	Houses the brain
		Face	(14)	
		Ear	(6)	
Hyoid	(1)			*U*-shaped bone in the neck between the jaw and larynx; the only bone not forming a joint with some other bone.
Vertebral column	(26)			The spine
		Cervical vertebrae	(7)	Upper seven vertebrae
		Thoracic vertebrae	(12)	Next twelve vertebrae (twelve pair of ribs are attached)
		Lumbar vertebrae	(5)	Next five vertebrae
		Sacrum	(1)	Wedge-shaped bone
		Coccyx	(1)	Tailbone
Sternum and ribs	(25)	Sternum	(1)	Breastbone
		True ribs (pair)	(7)	Upper seven pair—fastened to sternum
		False ribs (pair)	(5)	Lower five pair—not fastened to sternum directly
Shoulder girdle	(4)	Clavicle	(2)	Collarbones
		Scapula	(2)	Shoulder blades
Arms and hands	(60)	Humerus	(2)	Upper arm bone—long bone
		Radius	(2)	Forearm bone (on thumb side of forearm)—long bone
		Ulna	(2)	Forearm bone (on other side of forearm)—long bone
		Carpals	(16)	Wrist bones
		Metacarpals	(10)	Long bones in the hand (they form the palm)
		Phalanges	(28)	Finger and thumb bones
Pelvic bones	(2)		(2)	Large hip bones
Legs and feet	(60)	Femur	(2)	Thigh bone
		Patella	(2)	Knee cap
		Tibia	(2)	Shin bone
		Fibula	(2)	Slender bone to the outside of the lower leg
		Tarsals	(14)	Ankle and heel bones
		Metatarsals	(10)	Long bones of the feet
		Phalanges	(28)	Toe bones
Total bones in body	(206)			

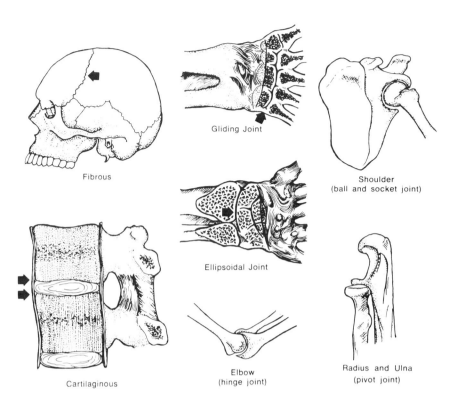

Figure 20.4
Seven kinds of joints illustrated.

Table 20.2
Summary of Joints of the Skeletal System and Their Use

Kind of Joint	Description	Example	Use or Movement Patterns
Ball and socket	One bone has a ball-shaped head which fits into the concave socket of the other bone	Shoulder and hip joints	Widest range of movement
Hinge	Spool-shaped bone end fits into concave end of other bone	Ankle, knee, elbow	Like a hinged door—one direction only (flexor and extensor action)
Pivot	One bone has rounded or peg-like end; other bone which is arch-shaped rotates around the peg-like end	Radius and ulna	Rotates
Ellipsoidal or condyloid	Oval surface of one bone fits into the concave surface of the other	Wrist	Up and down, side to side, flexor and extensor action, adduction—abduction
Gliding	Two almost flat surfaces glide across each other	Vertebrae	Gliding, limited movement with strong support
Cartilaginous	Cartilage grows between two bones and allows slight movement	Discs between vertebrae	Slight compression and bending to side or twisting movements
Fibrous	Connects bones which articulate; eventually becomes immovable	Skull	No movement; the fibrous joints actually become the places where the bones of the skull join

Review of Skeletal System—*Continued*

Functions of Bones

Support framework of body

Help move body by providing muscle attachments

Protect vital organs from injury

Help to form red and certain white blood cells

Store body's minerals

Types of Joints

1. Ball and socket: shoulder and hip joints
2. Hinge: elbow, finger, knee
3. Pivot: radius and ulna
4. Ellipsoidal or condyloid: wrist
5. Gliding: vertebrae
6. Cartilaginous: discs between vertebrae
7. Fibrous: skull

The Muscular System

We have learned that the skeletal system of bones forms a framework for our bodies; the joints of the bones allow us to bend and move. Muscles are attached to the bony framework to cause the bending when the muscle contracts, pulling the bone with it.

Muscle is one of the forms of tissue that, when stimulated, contracts or relaxes, and by so doing produces the movements of other connective tissues. Muscles are able to shorten, and this is called **contraction.** Skeletal muscles contract voluntarily in response to the wishes of the owner of the muscle. However, cardiac (heart) muscle contracts or relaxes in response to involuntary nerve impulses. That is, the contractions occur without conscious control by the person.

Muscular Action

Tone is important to muscles. **Tone** means that the muscle contains a certain amount of tension which keeps it ready to operate.

Muscles of the skeleton usually work in pairs. There is a **flexor** and an **extensor.** The flexor bends the joint and the extensor straightens it. This pair of muscles *oppose* each other. They cannot both work successfully at the same time. For example, the biceps muscle, which is in the arm, is a flexor. This muscle is attached to the shoulder, which is called the point of **origin** (immovable segment of muscle). The other end

fastens to the radius bone at the point of **insertion** (movable segment of muscle). (The radius bone is one of the two bones in the forearm just below the elbow. It is movable.) When the biceps contracts, it pulls the forearm up. It is a flexor muscle. If you wish to put your arm out straight again, another muscle is used. This muscle is called the triceps muscle. It is on the posterior side of the upper arm and has its origin in the shoulder. It is attached to the ulna at the point of insertion in the forearm. (The ulna is the other bone in the forearm.) This muscle works in opposition to the biceps. When it contracts, it straightens the elbow. It is called the extensor. All skeletal muscles function similarly.

The muscle **contracts** because a motor nerve tells it to do so. The individual has conscious control over most of the skeletal muscles. We call muscles we can control *voluntary* muscles. You can tell your voluntary muscles what to do.

Similar action occurs with muscles that have different functions. Abduction and adduction are terms you will hear. **Abduction** is the drawing away from the axis (or median line) of the body or of an extremity. An abductor muscle, on contraction, draws the part away from the axis of the body. The **adductor** muscle, on contraction, draws the part to the median axis. A good example of these opposing groups of muscles is the fact that the abductor muscles will move the legs apart and the adductor muscles will move the legs together.

The skeletal framework of bones, moved by the muscles, is held together and covered by another system: the *integumentary system*.

Review of Muscular System

Muscle contracts or relaxes to move body

Tone means certain amount of tension

Muscles work in pairs: flexor and extensor oppose each other

Muscles are attached at point of origin and point of insertion

Muscle control is voluntary and involuntary

Abduction is drawing away from the axis

Adduction is drawing toward the axis

The Integumentary System (Pertaining to or Composed of Skin)

The **integumentary system** includes *skin, hair,* and *fingernails*. The skin is more than just a smooth covering for the body. (Plate 3) If you look at it through a magnifying glass, you see a very coarse-looking covering with irregular ridges and valleys. The raised areas are called papillae (pa-*pill*-ee). The microscope reveals three different parts: the epidermis, the dermis, and the subcutaneous layer (sub-kyou-*tay*-nee-us).

The outer layer of the skin is the **epidermis** and is made of many layers of cells. The lower part of the epidermis contains pigment, which gives the skin color.

The **dermis,** which lies under the epidermis, is thicker. It makes the skin strong and elastic. The dermis contains two kinds of glands: sebaceous (seh-*bay*-shuhs) glands which produce an oil secretion that oils and protects the epidermis, making it soft and pliable; and sweat glands which lie deep within the dermis and even into the sebaceous layer. The sweat glands are controlled by the sympathetic nervous system and collect fluid from the blood which is called perspiration.

The innermost layer of skin, the **subcutaneous** layer, is fatty tissue and is a cushion against shock and an insulator against heat and cold.

Nails and hair are a modification of the epidermis, and hair extends beyond the surface of the skin. Hair roots are formed by cells that line a pocket called a follicle.

Review of Integumentary System

Three layers of skin:

Epidermis: outer layer

Dermis: makes skin strong, contains two kinds of glands

Subcutaneous: cushion against shock, insulation against heat and cold

Glands found in dermis:

Sweat glands

Sebaceous glands: produce oil to lubricate epidermis

The Circulatory System

The **circulatory system** is frequently compared to a transportation system. It is designed to deliver blood to and from the capillaries. The exchange of respiratory gases and metabolic substances occurs in the capillaries. Some of the fluid portion of the blood enters the tissues and drains back to large veins.

The circulatory system includes *the heart, the arteries, the arterioles, the capillaries, the venules, the veins,* and *the lymphatics.*

The Heart

The **heart** is the chief part of the circulatory system. It is a very muscular pump that weighs about three-fourths of a pound. It is the strongest muscle in the body and pumps between 4,000 and 5,000 gallons of blood a day. The rate of heartbeat varies, but between fifty and ninety beats per minute is considered normal.

The heart is usually located in the left thoracic cavity close to the lungs.

The heart has four sections or **chambers.** The upper chambers are called *atria* or *auricles.* There is a left atrium and a right atrium. The lower chambers are called *ventricles.* There is a left ventricle and a right ventricle. The atria receive blood from veins and pass it to the ventricles. The ventricles pump the blood out of the heart into the arteries.

The blood moves through the heart by use of what we might call one-way valves. When the **atrium** (or **auricle**) contracts, it forces the blood through valves into the ventricle, which is relaxed. The **ventricle** then contracts and forces the blood into the arteries. During the period when the ventricle is contracting, the atrium is relaxing and filling with blood for the next cycle.

The **right atrium** receives blood from all over the body. This blood has collected waste matter on its trip through the veins. When the atrium contracts, this waste-filled (deoxygenated) blood is forced into the **right ventricle.** When the ventricle is filled, it contracts, forcing the blood into the pulmonary artery, which conducts the blood to the lungs. When the blood reaches the lungs, carbon dioxide and water are discharged into the lungs, and the blood absorbs oxygen to be returned to the heart.

The blood then flows through the capillaries to the pulmonary veins and into the **left atrium** of the heart. The heart contracts, and the blood passes through the one-way valve (called the mitral valve) to the **left ventricle,** emptying the atrium and filling the ventricle. The heart contracts again, and the blood empties from the ventricle into the aorta to carry food and oxygen to all parts of the body.

Figure 20.5 shows the chambers of the heart and the direction in which the blood enters or leaves the heart chambers. Note that the openings for the flow of blood from the left ventricle are at the top of the ventricle. Note that there are four pulmonary veins opening into the left atrium. Also, the inferior and superior vena cava empty into the right atrium.

The Course of the Blood

The differences between veins and arteries are *the direction of the flow of blood* as well as structural differences. **Arteries** carry blood *away from* the heart. **Veins** carry blood *to* the heart.

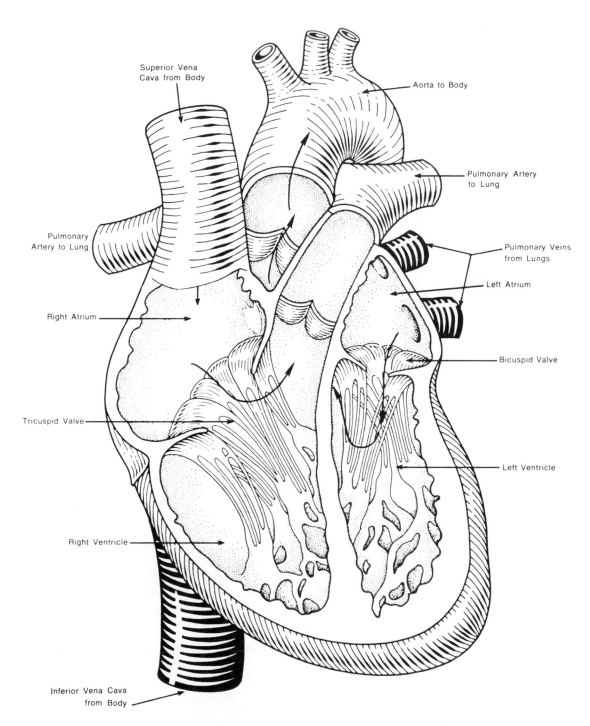

Superior Vena
Cava from Body

Aorta to Body

Pulmonary Artery
to Lung

Pulmonary
Artery to Lung

Pulmonary Veins
from Lungs

Left Atrium

Right Atrium

Bicuspid Valve

Tricuspid Valve

Left Ventricle

Right Ventricle

Inferior Vena Cava
from Body

Figure 20.5

The course of the blood through the heart.

The **aorta** is the main artery. Smaller arteries branch off from the aorta. These arteries branch into smaller units called **arterioles,** which carry blood into the **capillaries** (smaller units still). The exchange of nourishment and oxygen for waste matter from the tissues occurs in the capillaries and in spaces around the capillaries called tissue sinuses. (The process is called *internal respiration.*) The blood then flows from the capillaries into **venules,** then to veins, and finally into the **vena cava** (the largest vein). The process is from the largest artery to smaller arteries, to smaller arte-

rioles, to yet smaller capillaries, to small venules, to larger veins to the largest vein—and back to the heart. (Plate 6)

Arteries have thick walls, while veins have thinner walls.

The nerves to the vessels are of two kinds: vasodilators and vasoconstrictors. They cause contraction and dilation.

When the blood surges from the heart, the walls of the arteries are so elastic that they bulge. Arterial blood pressure is greatest now. We call it **systolic pressure.** Between the surges the wall springs back and clamps down on the blood. The pressure is lowest now. It is called **diastolic pressure.** The heart rests in diastole while the ventricle fills up again to be discharged into the circulation at systole. The arteries continue the pumping action by squeezing the blood while the heart is resting. When you feel a pulse, you are feeling the bulge in the artery wall caused by systolic pressure which is the rhythmical contraction of the heart.

Arteries branch freely through the body and lungs. They become smaller as they get farther from the heart. The veins follow the course of the arteries.

The blood carries nutrients and vital substances. The nutrients and vital substances pass into the tissues through the walls of the arterial capillaries. Waste products leave the tissue and pass through the thin walls of the venous capillaries where the blood picks them up. This exchange of nutrients and waste products occurs *only* in the capillaries.

Blood Circulating Systems

The heart is a double pump—with the two sides working together. The heart, with its pumping action, causes the blood to circulate through the arteries and veins of the circulatory system. It is a complex system, and there are several *circulations* within the blood circulation system. (See plates 5, 7, 8)

1. The **systemic circulation** is the one of which we are most aware. The aorta (largest artery in the body) leaves the left ventricle of the heart and sends branches to the neck, shoulders, arms, and downward along the spine. It then branches into an upside-down "Y" to feed both legs. The *veins* of the system then return to the right atrium of the heart. (The name of the important vein is the vena cava. *Inferior* and *superior* are two terms used with vena cava (meaning *below* and *above*) thus, the inferior vena cava services the lower part of the body—below the heart—while the superior vena cava services the upper part of the body—that which lies above the heart. Therefore, the teeth and head are served by the superior vena cava.)

    Within the systemic circulation are smaller circulations, each performing one function vitally necessary to the entire system.
    a. The **coronary circulation** supplies blood to the heart itself. It circles the top of the heart like a crown–thus, the name coronary, meaning crown.
    b. The kidneys also need blood, not only to nourish the cells of the kidneys, but to bring the waste matter that the kidneys eliminate. Thus, the **renal** (ree-nal) **circulation** is the branch of the systemic circulation that carries blood from the aorta to the kidneys and through them. The blood is then returned through the inferior vena cava. Since the blood "dumps" wastes into the kidneys for elimination, the blood returning to the heart from the kidneys contains the least waste of any of the blood in the vena cava (the returning circuit of the transportation system.)
    c. The **portal circulation** is the system that reaches the spleen, pancreas, stomach, small intestine, and colon. After the blood has transported oxygen to the portal system organs, it picks up digested food and water, which it carries to the liver. In the liver the blood picks up food to be delivered to the tissues.
    d. The veins carrying blood from the liver back to the inferior vena cava are called the hepatic veins, sometimes called the **hepatic circulation.**

2. When the blood leaves the left ventricle of the heart it moves through all these circulations to the right atrium and thence to the right ventricle where it enters the **pulmonary circulation** at the exit of the right ventricle. It travels to the lungs and back to the left atrium. During this trip the wastes are exchanged for oxygen in the lungs so that the blood now has fresh oxygen to carry into the rest of the body. Thus, the respiratory requirements of the body are met.

The circulatory system is closely allied with two other systems which utilize the circulatory system to deliver their products to the tissues of the body. They are the *lymphatic system* and the *hemic* or *blood system.* These two systems are discussed next.

Review of the Circulatory System

Four Chambers of the Heart
Right auricle
Right ventricle
Left auricle
Left ventricle

Blood Circulatory Systems
Pulmonary circulation
Systemic circulation
Coronary circulation
Renal circulation
Portal circulation
Hepatic circulation

Three Systems That Work Together
Circulatory system
Lymphatic system
Hemic or blood system

Course of the Blood Flow Is:
From left ventricle through aorta into arterioles; through arterioles into capillaries where the exchange of nourishment and waste from tissues occurs. Now the blood is ready to return to the heart. It flows from capillaries into venules; from venules into veins; from veins into vena cava to right auricle, thence to right ventricle; thence to pulmonary artery to lungs; thence to left auricle and back to left ventricle. Now blood begins its trip all over again.

The Lymphatic System (Figure 20.6)

The **lymphatic system** is closely linked with the circulatory system. In fact, blood carries lymph which it has obtained from the lymphatic system. (Lymph is a clear fluid.) The lymphatic system is composed of very *delicate capillaries, lymph nodes,* and the *thoracic duct.* Vessels called lymphatics carry the lymph from the capillaries to the great thoracic (thor-*as*-ik) duct. This duct is the largest of the lymph vessels and enters the subclavian (sub-*kla*-vee-an) vein at the junction of the subclavian vein and the internal left jugular vein. (The subclavian vein and the internal left jugular vein are part of the blood circulatory system.) Thus, lymph is poured into the bloodstream as it leaves the thoracic duct of the lymphatic system.

Lymph glands (also known as *lymph nodes*) are scattered throughout the pathways of the lymphatic system of vessels. They are relatively small bean-shaped or oval bodies. The glands act as filters to the lymph, screening out bacteria. They make one type of white blood cells, **lymphocytes,** and are an important part of the body's defense against infection.

Lymph, the liquid which flows through the lymphatic system and into the bloodstream, has almost the same composition as blood plasma. It contains many lymphocytes and sometimes red blood corpuscles. It is described as slightly yellow to colorless, watery fluid found in the lymphatic vessels. It is different from tissue fluid that is found outside the lymphatic vessels in tissue spaces.

Review of the Lymph System

Lymph glands (also called lymph nodes) manufacture
Lymphocytes (white blood cells, which are defense against infection) which flow in
Lymph (a liquid flowing through the lymph system and into the bloodstream). Lymph is almost the same composition as blood plasma.

The Hemic or Blood System

Hemic means pertaining to or developed by the blood: thus, the hemic system is the **blood system.** If we were to compare the heart and its vessels to a railroad system, the vessels would be the railroad tracks. The blood would be the railroad cars, transporting the vital life substances to all parts of the body. The food you eat and the air you breathe are converted to substances your body needs. These substances enter the bloodstream (or hemic system) and are carried to all cells of the body. The return trip from the cells is the way the railroad cars dispose of the wastes that have accumulated. Blood also picks up heat and distributes it through the body (which is the reason that running warm water over your hands or feet will soon make your body warm all over). Should your body develop excess heat, the blood carries it to the body surfaces and respiratory passages. Other blood cells help your body fight infection. Thus, blood is a **circulating tissue.** It is the delivery system that keeps the body alive by providing the correct environment (picks up wastes, delivers nutrients, equalizes temperature, and guards against infection).

What is blood? It is often described as a liquid tissue or as cells suspended in a liquid called **plasma.** It is a fluid tissue with live blood cells, both red and white, floating in the fluid. About twelve pints of blood are found in the average human body. This supply is maintained throughout life by the body process of discarding worn-out cells and manufacturing new ones.

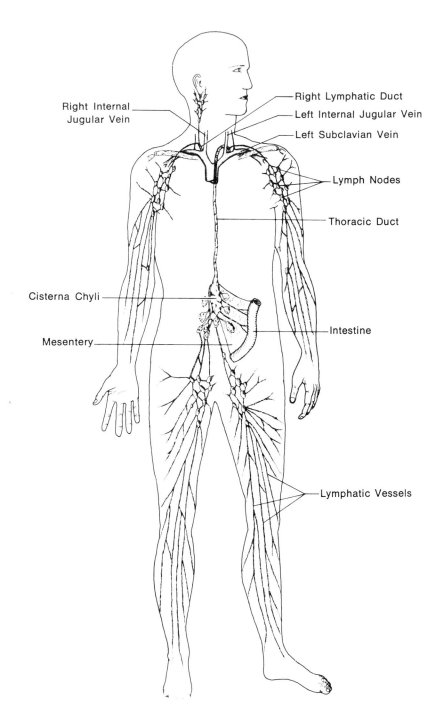

Right Internal Jugular Vein

Right Lymphatic Duct

Left Internal Jugular Vein

Left Subclavian Vein

Lymph Nodes

Thoracic Duct

Cisterna Chyli

Mesentery

Intestine

Lymphatic Vessels

Figure 20.6
The lymph system drawing.

Erythrocytes (or red blood cells) are the most numerous—between twenty-five and thirty trillion cells in total. A red cell count is used to determine certain health factors. (A person with a very low red count might have anemia.)

Red blood cells carry oxygen, and are shaped like two saucers placed face to face. This hollowed out shape allows them to absorb more oxygen because the shape increases their surface area.

A red pigment containing iron combined with a protein substance is called **hemoglobin** (hee'-moh-*gloh*-bin). It is this substance in blood that provides the red color. Hemoglobin turns bright scarlet when combined with oxygen. As blood delivers the oxygen to the tissues of the body, the cells turn dark red.

Red cells last about 120 days. They are destroyed by the liver, spleen, and regions within bone marrow. The iron that was in the worn-out cells is sent to the bone marrow and new cells are formed there. In addition, new iron is necessary to add to the reclaimed iron; thus, we must eat iron-containing foods. (The iron must be in a form that can be assimilated by the body, however.)

Leukocytes (white corpuscles), also found in the blood plasma, are the body's defense against infection. There are different kinds of white cells. Some are produced in the bone marrow while others are produced by the lymph nodes (from the lymphatic system).

The white corpuscles are capable of squeezing through the intercellular spaces of the capillary walls, and thus enter the tissue fluid. They travel to the center of an infection and dispose of the infectious bacteria. They may poison the bacteria with chemicals or consume the bacteria. Should the infection prove more powerful, the bone marrow simply produces more white cells. The white cell count rises dramatically during a serious infection.

Another formed blood element found in smaller numbers is called **platelets** (or thrombocytes). Platelets initiate the blood clotting process. A platelet lives only three to four days. The spleen, liver, and lymph nodes clear the bloodstream of the dead platelets.

The pale yellow liquid of the blood is **plasma.** It is about 55 percent of whole blood. By far the largest part of plasma (about 92 percent) is water in which will be found dissolved nutrients, mineral salts, and waste products. Three types of protein make up the rest of the plasma. **Albumin** (al-*byou*-min) regulates the amount of water in the plasma, thus regulating blood pressure.

Fibrinogen (fih-*brin*-oh-jen) assists platelets in clotting blood.

Globulin (*glob*-you-lin) is the vehicle for antibodies. Antibodies are chemicals that fight certain specific diseases. For example, one may have acquired antibodies against the mumps.

Serum is a part of plasma. Actually, serum is the combination of albumin and globulin.

Plasma delivers food to the tissues of the body and carries waste and heat away from the tissues. Another important fact is that plasma creates enough volume in blood to maintain blood pressure. If transfusions are to be given, the blood types must be carefully checked because the wrong type of blood can cause the death of a patient.

Blood is typed with the use of a microscope. The types are A, AB, B, and O. If type A or AB is added to type B, **agglutination** (uh-glue-tin-*nay*-shun) can occur. Agglutination means that the blood cells of one type settle out of the plasma in clumps.

If patients have blood type A, they cannot receive AB or B. They can receive A or O.

If patients have blood type B, they cannot receive A or AB. They can receive B or O.

However, type O may be added to any of the other types. Thus, type O is called a **universal donor** because it can be added to any of the other types.

Review of the Hemic System

Blood is a circulating tissue containing:

Red corpuscles: most numerous, carry oxygen

Hemoglobin: provides red color and carries iron

White corpuscles: body's defense against infection, manufactured in bone marrow and lymph nodes

Platelets: necessary for clotting, live three or four days.

Plasma: delivers food to tissues

  55 percent of whole blood

  92 percent of plasma = water with dissolved nutrients, mineral salts, and waste products

   8 percent of plasma = three proteins: albumin, fibrinogen, and globulin.

Serum = albumin and globulin combined

Similarly type AB may receive blood from any of the other groups, and type AB is, therefore, a **universal recipient.**

The Respiratory System

Respiration is the act of breathing wherein the exchange of gases takes place. The acquisition of oxygen by the cells of the body is absolutely vital to the life of the cell. Should a cell be deprived of oxygen, cell life ceases immediately. The cell receives oxygen from the tissue fluid around it. The tissue fluid has received the oxygen from the bloodstream. Within the cell the oxygen combines with glucose to make energy, and the waste products of this action are carbon dioxide and water. The process is called **oxidation.** The bloodstream carries the carbon dioxide and water away from the cells to the lungs where the exchange of carbon dioxide and water for oxygen occurs. **Internal respiration** is the term used to indicate the absorption of oxygen, oxidation of glucose, and giving off of carbon dioxide and water *by the cells*. **External respiration** is the name of the process by which the entire bloodstream is supplied with oxygen and relieved of the carbon dioxide and water. We breathe air by use of the respiratory system; and the blood system is the transportation mechanism to complete the cycle.

We inhale air through the **nostrils** or **mouth.** Both are part of the respiratory system—the openings through which air can reach the lungs. Normally we inhale about sixteen to twenty-four times per minute.

It is more desirable to breathe through the nose because nostrils contain hairs which catch dust and other particles of foreign matter. It is protection for the respiratory system. The nostrils are divided by the **nasal septum,** a cartilage and bone divider between the two nostrils. The **turbinates** (protrusions of bone and mucous membrane) within the nasal passages warm and moisten the air, and the sticky surface of the mucous membrane of the turbinates catches dust and dirt that may have evaded the nostril hairs. The air is then conducted from the back of the nasal cavities to the throat through two openings called the **internal nares** (*nair*-eez). The throat cavity is called the **pharynx** (*fair*-inks).

When we cannot get enough air through the nasal passages, we resort to mouth breathing. However, mouth breathing means our bodies are deprived of the advantages of the moistening and warming of the air that occurs in the turbinates.

The **sinuses,** which are found in the head, are also part of the respiratory system and help to warm and moisten the air. (They are also resonating chambers to assist with speech.)

The pharynx is the center where seven tubes converge:

1. The **internal nares** channel air into the pharynx.
2. The **eustachian tubes** are openings into the ears.
3. The **mouth cavity** permits food, beverage, and air to enter the pharynx.
4. The **esophagus** (for food) begins at the bottom of the pharynx, as does
5. The **glottis** (windpipe opening).

Automatically the **epiglottis** (a leaflike plate of cartilage that acts as a cover for the glottis) closes over the glottis when food and water descend into the esophagus. Automatically the epiglottis opens when air passes in and out of the lungs. On rare occasions the automatic signals become mixed, and the individual chokes as food or beverage attempts to enter the lungs.

The glottis contains the **larynx** (*lair*-inks), commonly called the voice box. The windpipe, actually the **trachea** (*tray*-kee-ah), is a tube about an inch in diameter and four and one-half inches long. It starts at the bottom of the larynx and ends at about the level of the fifth rib. At this point it divides into two tubes—the **bronchi** (*brong*-kee). The walls of the bronchi are lined with **cilia** (*sill*-ee-uh), hairlike processes (projections). These cilia fan upward toward the throat, moving dust particles that have been caught in the sticky membrane. Their purpose is to prevent any dirt from reaching the lungs.

The **lungs** (Plate 4) are cone shaped, curving outward on the sides where they press against the ribs. The lower surface is concave (curves upward) to make room for the **diaphragm,** which curves upward in the thoracic (chest) cavity. The lungs are covered by a double membrane. The **visceral membrane** covers the lungs; the **pleural** (*plur*-al) **membrane** (the pleura) lines the chest cavity. A thin layer of pleural fluid separates these two membranes to keep them from rubbing during breathing. If the pleura becomes inflamed, the condition is called *pleurisy,* which results in painful breathing.

Each **bronchus** (*brong*-kus) divides and subdivides within the lung so that there is a network of tubes a little like the branches of a tree. These divisions of the bronchi are called **bronchioles** (*brong*-kee-ohlz). The smaller the bronchioles, the thinner their walls so that as the bronchi divide and subdivide the ends become tiny chambers. Each tiny chamber is surrounded by a cluster of little air sacs which resemble a bunch of grapes. The air sacs are called **alveoli** (al-*vee*-oh-lie). Tiny capillaries of the blood system are in contact with the tiny alveoli. The thin walls of the capillaries and the thin walls of the alveoli, lying side by side, permit the exchange of gases between the blood and air sacs.

Review of the Respiratory System

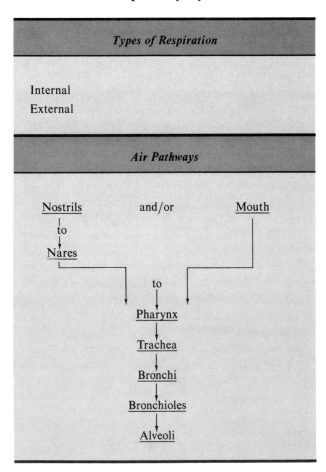

Protector	
Protectors:	**Protection:**
Turbinates:	Warm air
Cilia:	Move dirt out
Nasal hairs:	Keep dirt out
Epiglottis:	Keeps food out of trachea

Openings into Pharynx	
Channel:	**From:**
Internal nares:	Nostrils
Eustachian tubes:	Ears
Mouth cavity:	Mouth
Esophagus:	To stomach
Glottis: (windpipe opening)	Trachea

The Nervous System (Figures 20.7, 20.8, 20.9)

We said that muscles contract and move the skeleton voluntarily because the individual desires to move. If you decide to pick up an apple, your nervous system masterminds the action. It sends messages to your arm and hand to reach for the apple, pick it up, and carry it to your mouth. Actually, any voluntary desire and all involuntary actions are controlled by the **nervous system.**

A present-day computer with channels for incoming and outgoing coded messages is probably a good analogy for the nervous system.

The nervous system has two major parts:

1. **Central nervous system,** consisting of the brain and spinal cord.
2. **Peripheral nervous system,** consisting of the cranial nerves, the spinal nerves, and the autonomic nervous system.

The function of the nerves is to carry a message from the sense organ (for example, in your fingertip) to the central nervous system, and also from the central nervous system back to muscles or glands that in turn translate the return message into action. The nerves conduct an impulse, or message.

The Central Nervous System

The brain fills the **cranial** (*kray*-nee-al) **cavity,** which is the hollow space inside the skull. Three membranes cover the brain and spinal cord. There is fluid between the two inner membranes that cushions the brain and spinal cord from shock.

The brain is divided into regions. Bodily functions are controlled by specific regions within the brain. The **cerebrum** (*sair*-uh-brum) is the largest part of the brain. The **cerebellum** (sair-uh-*bel*-um), below the cerebrum, is smaller and in the back.

The enlargement of the upper end of the spinal cord is called the **medulla oblongata** (meh-*dool*-uh ahb-lon-*gah*-tah) and contains nerve centers which regulate the vital centers of breathing and heart actions. Nerve fibers form the spinal cord and branch out to all parts of the body. Just before the nerve fibers enter the spinal cord, they cross over. This is why the right half of the brain controls the left half of the body and vice versa.

The surface of the brain is the **cortex** and is gray in color, thus the term *gray matter* meaning "brain" or "intelligence."

The Peripheral Nervous System

The **peripheral nervous system** is composed of the cranial nerves and end organs and the spinal nerves and end organs.

The cranial nerves may be thought of as telephone wires. If you were to think of them as telephone wires between two computers, the analogy might be more correct, because the nerves carry impulses rather than conversation. In general those nerves that tell a muscle what to do are called **motor nerves.** Those nerves that carry a message back to the brain from an outlying area or organ are called **sensory nerves.**

There are twelve **cranial nerves** which, as the name implies, branch off from the brain (within the cranium). As with many other structures of the body, remember that we are again speaking of something in the singular sense, when actually the structures occur as a symmetrical pair, usually a left and a right.

The spinal nerves, thirty-one pairs of them, branch off the cord between the vertebrae of the spine. They are *pairs* because one nerve goes to each side of the body to perform the same function. Each cable contains both sensory and motor fibers so it is possible for the sensory nerve to send a message to the brain and the brain to return a command via the motor nerve.

The Autonomic Nervous System

The **autonomic nervous system** innervates three tissues in the body: glands, smooth muscle, and cardiac muscle. It is the system that automatically regulates the body, without the conscious control of the individual.

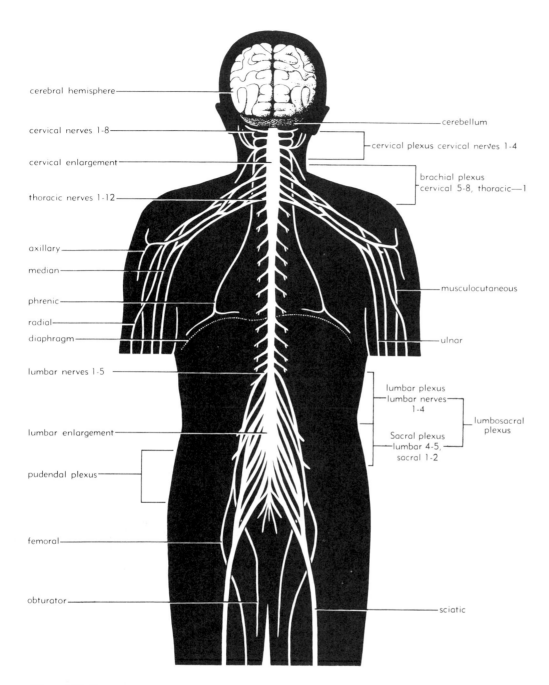

Figure 20.7
Nervous system of man, dorsal view.

Breathing and heartbeat go on or stop regardless of whether the individual wishes to stop or start these functions. The involuntary nervous system has two parts: the **sympathetic** and **parasympathetic.** They oppose each other, thus creating a proper balance. As an example, fear causes the sympathetic nervous system to increase the heartbeat. The parasympathetic system decreases the heartbeat. The eyes dilate in fear due to the action of the sympathetic system. When the fear reaction calms, the parasympathetic constricts the pupils.

The autonomic nervous system regulates the functions of the body that do not require voluntary reaction.

The Sense Organs
The nervous system is designed to permit us: (1) to perceive our environment and changes that occur in it, and (2) to adapt maximally to this environment.

Some highly developed special functions of the nervous system are: sight or **vision,** hearing or **audition,** smell or **olfaction,** taste or **gustation,** and touch or **taction.**

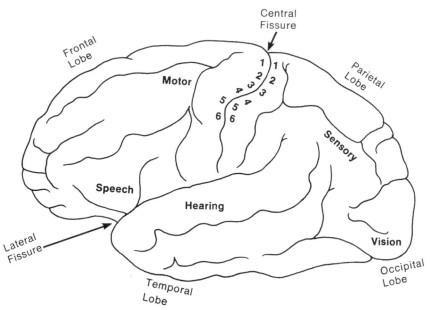

The sensory and motor areas of the frontal and parietal lobes are opposite each other. For example, the motor and sensory areas which control the leg are adjacent to each other.

1 = leg
2 = trunk
3 = arm
4 = neck
5 = face
6 = tongue

Figure 20.8
Control areas of the brain.

Kinesthetic (kin-es-*thet*-ik) sense is also important. This permits you to be aware of the position of your body: whether your leg is bent or straight is one example.

In addition, the body has millions of sense organs. The body's receptors sense change internally and externally and thus activate the body to react appropriately. They tell the individual what is happening in his or her body or to his or her body.

Review of Nervous System

Central Nervous System
Consists of
Brain
Spinal cord

Peripheral Nervous System
Consists of
Cranial nerves
Spinal nerves
Autonomic nervous system

Autonomic Nervous System
Innervates
Glands
Smooth muscle
Cardiac muscle

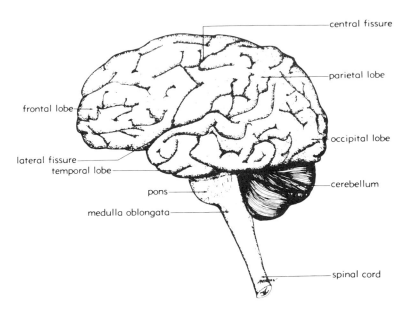

Figure A. Lateral View

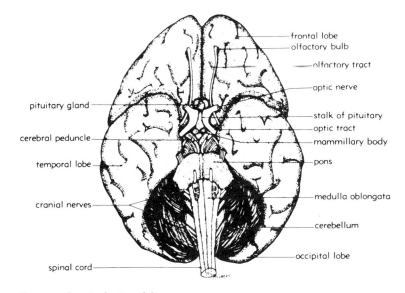

Figure B. Inferior View

Figure 20.9
Two views of the human brain.

Review of Nervous System—*Continued*

Autonomic Nervous System
Composed of Sympathetic System Parasympathetic System

Sense Organs
Vision—eye Audition—ear Olfaction—nostrils Gustation—taste buds Taction—body surface Kinesthesia—body position

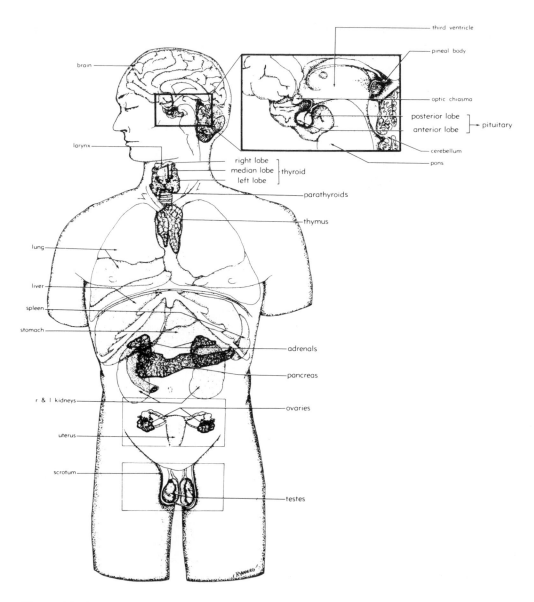

Figure 20.10
The endocrine system.

The Endocrine System (Figure 20.10)

Some glands scattered throughout the body are *ductless;* that is, their secretions are poured directly into the bloodstream. All the glands that are ductless are called **endocrine glands.** Because the endocrine secretions are poured directly into the bloodstream, they affect organs throughout the body.

Endocrine glands excrete a chemical exciter called a **hormone.** A hormone may have a strong effect on certain organs and tissues of the body. Either overactivity or underactivity of an endocrine gland produces abnormality.

Some of the endocrine glands influence other endocrine glands and there seems to be a delicate check-and-balance system among these glands. It is called the dynamic balance. **Hyperactivity** (overactivity) and **hypoactivity** (underactivity) of a gland may influence all the others to either speed up or slow down their production.

These glands work with the nervous system, responding to emotions to change the activity of the glands. The individual has no conscious control over the endocrine glands. When an individual's emotions of fear or anger become powerful, the emotions affect the autonomic nervous system, which in turn affects the endocrine glands.

The endocrine glands known to produce hormones are:

1. The **pituitary** and the **pineal,** located in the brain

2. The **thyroid** and the **parathyroids,** located over the larynx
3. The **thymus,** located in the chest
4. The **adrenals,** located in the retroperitoneum above the kidney
5. The **islet cells of Langerhans** within the pancreas, located in the abdominal cavity
6. Certain cells of the **gonads,** located in the testes and ovaries

Each endocrine gland has a function in the maintenance of the body.

Review of Endocrine System

Endocrine Glands

Gland:	Location:
Pituitary:	Brain
Pineal:	Brain
Thyroid:	Throat
Parathyroids:	Throat
Thymus:	Chest
Adrenals:	Retroperitoneum above kidney
Islet cells of Langerhans:	Pancreas in abdominal cavity

The Digestive System (Figure 20.11)

The **digestive system** is also called the alimentary system and related organs. Alimentation includes:

1. **Ingestion** (introduction of food into the alimentary system).
2. **Digestion** (the breakdown of foods into compounds that can be utilized by the body).
3. **Absorption** (the transfer of the completely digested products to the bloodstream for transfer to the tissues of the body).
4. **Utilization** (use of the products in the blood by the tissue for growth or energy).

As you can see, alimentation is a very complicated process involving the alimentary canal and related organs, such as salivary glands, teeth, liver, gallbladder, and pancreas. The **alimentary canal** starts at the mouth and ends at the rectum and anus. It is about thirty feet long. It includes the mouth, pharynx, esophagus, stomach, small intestines, and large intestines. The alimentation of food *begins* in the mouth where food is chewed and mixed with saliva.

A full set of teeth, or proper prosthetic substitute, is essential to good health. The teeth prepare the food for the stomach by chewing, grinding, tearing it into small pieces, and mixing the salivary secretions to start digestion.

After the food is chewed, it is swallowed, and the food is forced into the open **esophagus** where two sets of muscles help force it into the stomach.

The **stomach** is a digestive organ and a reservoir for food. When the food enters the stomach, there are three layers of muscles that contract at the same time causing the food to be churned and mixed with the digestive juices, including acid that is produced in the stomach for digestive purposes. When the work of the stomach is complete, the food is like thick syrup and is called **chyme** (kime). The valve at the lower end of the stomach is called the **pylorus.** It holds the chyme in the stomach, and opens when the mixture reaches the proper pH by relaxing the muscle and allowing the food to pass into the first part of the small bowel or **duodenum** (dew-oh-*dee*-num).

The duodenum is about ten inches long. In the mid-part of the duodenum, digestive juices from the pancreas and bile from the liver enter and mix with the chyme, which then passes into and through the other two sections of the **small intestine:** the **jejunum** (jeh-*joo*-num), which is about seven and one-half feet long and the **ileum** (*ill*-ee-um), which is about fifteen feet long. The small intestine is most important in digestion. The stomach only partially digests food and the greater amount of work is left for the small intestine. The digested food is also absorbed through the walls of the small intestine.

The intestinal juice, known as **enzymes,** causes further digestion of the chyme.

In the intestines the secretions of the liver, the pancreas, and the intestinal glands also help digest the chyme.

The **pancreas** secretes its fluid through a short pancreatic duct into the duodenum. It is responsible for the production of insulin.

The **liver** has many functions and is the largest gland of the body. It is just below the diaphragm. It is a storehouse for glycogen, fat, amino acids, iron, and many vitamins, as well as a producer of vitamin A and a reservoir for blood. It regulates metabolism for carbohydrate, protein, and fat. It also serves a protective function as a filter and produces clotting factors.

In addition to these functions the liver is also a digestive organ. It secretes about a quart of **bile** each day. It flows from the liver into the **gallbladder** where

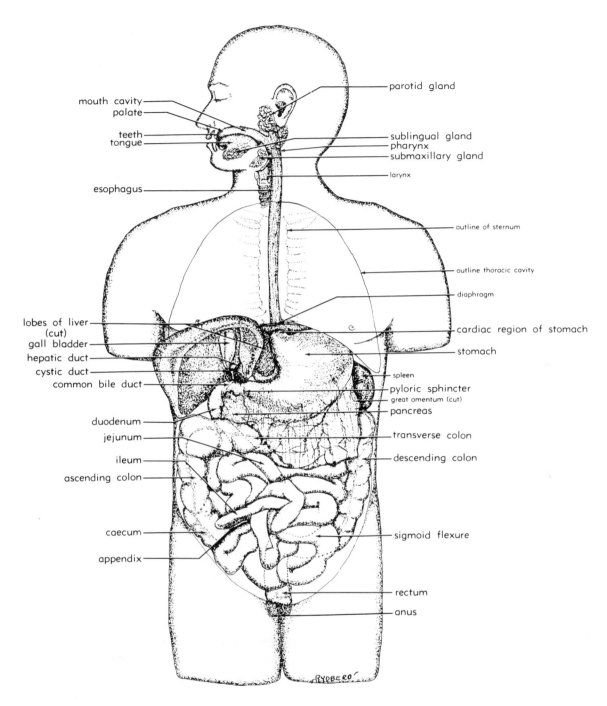

Figure 20.11
The digestive system.

it is stored until needed. The gallbladder releases the bile into the duodenum during digestion. Bile alters fats to form an emulsion so that they can be further digested. The bile is also weakly bacteriostatic (it helps to inhibit the action of the bacteria).

Peristalsis is a wavelike movement of the intestine which aids the passage of food. This movement is controlled by the autonomic nervous system. It takes about two to four hours for the food to move through the small intestine.

The **large intestine,** or colon, is the next section of the alimentary canal. It is divided into several parts. The junction of the small and large intestines is in the lower right corner of the abdomen. The junction leaves a blind end of the large colon. This blind end is called the **cecum** (*see*-kum). The **appendix** (a vestigial remnant) is an outgrowth from the end of the cecum.

The colon measures about five feet in length. It is about three inches in diameter. The residue of foodstuff leaving the small intestine enters the colon and travels up the **ascending colon** on the right side of the abdomen, then through the **transverse colon** across the top of the abdominal cavity just below the diaphragm, down the **descending colon** on the left side of the abdominal cavity to become the **sigmoid colon** lying in the pelvis, where it connects with the **rectum,** which is about six inches long and about one inch in diameter when empty. The rectum is very muscular and holds waste material until it can be discharged through the **anus.** The anus, or opening, is also very muscular and controlled by two sphincter muscles.

Excretion

Toxic substances cannot be allowed to build up significant concentrations in the body; therefore, waste products are eliminated from the body. (The elimination of waste products from the body is called **excretion.**) These substances (called excrement) include: **nitrogenous wastes** such as urea, uric acid, creatinine, and ammonia; **bacteria; excess water and mineral salts; undigested food;** and **carbon dioxide.**

Body processes are responsible for the presence of these toxic substances. For example, protein metabolism, the body's utilization of protein, produces nitrogenous wastes. Each cell's utilization of oxygen produces carbon dioxide, and so on.

Four organs are responsible for excretion: the **kidneys,** the **skin** (sweat glands), the **lungs,** and the **intestine.** Table 20.3 charts the various organs and excrement.

Review of Digestive System

Processes of Alimentation
Ingestion
Digestion
Absorption
Utilization

Digestive Tract
Mouth
Esophagus
Stomach
Duodenum ⎫
Jejunum ⎬ *Small Intestine*
Ileum ⎭
Pancreas
Liver
Ascending colon ⎫
Transverse colon ⎬
Descending colon ⎬ *Large Intestine*
Sigmoid colon ⎭
Rectum
Anus

Table 20.3
The Excretory Process

Excretory Organ	Name of Excrement	Excrement Composed of	Excrement Produced by
Skin (sweat glands)	Perspiration	Excess water	Ingestion, digestion
		Excess mineral salts	Ingestion, body metabolism
		Nitrogenous wastes	Protein metabolism
Lungs	Exhaled air	Water	Ingestion, digestion
		Carbon dioxide	Internal respiration
Intestine	Feces	Undigested food	Digestion
		Some salts	Body metabolism
Kidneys	Urine	Nitrogenous wastes	Protein metabolism
		Toxins	Bacteria in the body
		Excess water	Ingestion, digestion
		Mineral salts	Ingestion, body metabolism

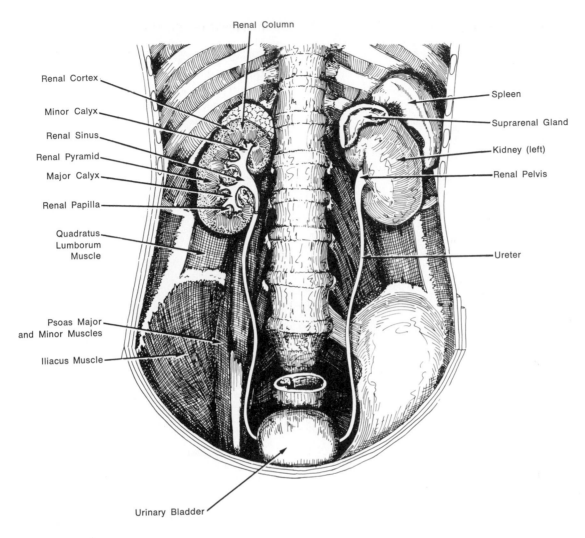

Renal Column

Renal Cortex

Minor Calyx

Renal Sinus

Renal Pyramid

Major Calyx

Renal Papilla

Quadratus Lumborum Muscle

Psoas Major and Minor Muscles

Iliacus Muscle

Spleen

Suprarenal Gland

Kidney (left)

Renal Pelvis

Ureter

Urinary Bladder

Figure 20.12
The urinary system.

The Genitourinary System

The function of the **genitourinary system** is two-fold: it is a filtration plant to expel body wastes, and it is also a reproductive system. These two systems (urinary and reproductive) are closely related developmentally and functionally, and so are sometimes discussed as one system.

The Urinary System

We will first consider the filtration plant function. The circulatory system transports the waste products to the kidneys, where these waste products are separated from the blood. These waste products are collected in the kidneys and emptied, via the ureters, into the bladder. During urination, the bladder contracts and urine is expelled from the body through the urethra. The urinary system, then, is comprised of **two kidneys, two ureters, the bladder,** and **the urethra** (fig. 20.12).

The Kidneys   The **kidneys** are two organs placed high in the retroperitoneal cavity, on either side of the lumbar vertebrae. An average-sized kidney is four and one-half inches long, one inch thick, and shaped like a lima bean. Usually the left kidney is slightly larger and higher than the right.

The kidneys are embedded in thick pads of fat that protect them and hold them in place.

Each kidney is encased in a tough white fibrous capsule. A cross section of a kidney exposes two layers of tissue (fig. 20.13). The outer layer is called the **renal cortex** or **cortex renis** (*ree*-niss), while the inner layer is called the **medulla renis.**

Within the medulla are a dozen or more **renal pyramids** (collecting elements). These triangular-shaped wedges deposit urine in the **renal pelvis.** The renal pelvis is the collecting area in the center of the kidney. The renal pelvis empties into the ureter.

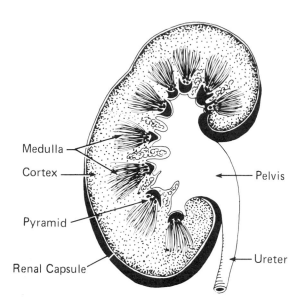

Figure 20.13
A cross section of the right kidney.

On a microscopic level, the kidney consists of about a million **tubules.** The individual tubule is the working unit of the kidney. Each tubule, consisting of a **glomerulus** and **Bowman's capsule,** is responsible for a small part of the daily urine output.

Urine Formation   The waste products are removed from the blood by a complicated process. These waste products are then collected in the renal pelvis, emptied into the ureter, carried by peristaltic waves to the urinary bladder, and expelled from the body via the urethra. As already noted, urine contains nitrogenous wastes such as urea, uric acid, creatinine, and ammonia; bacteria; excess water; and excess mineral salts.

Functions of the Kidneys   The kidneys regulate the composition and volume of blood in the body. They maintain a balance between the amount of electrolytes and water ingested and the amount excreted. For example, when a large volume of salty food has been eaten, a larger amount of salt must be excreted, or the chemical balance of the blood will be seriously disturbed.

The kidneys help regulate blood pressure by regulating the amount of body fluids excreted.

The two **ureters** connect the two kidneys to the urinary bladder. Each ureter is a muscular tube that carries the urine by peristalsis to the bladder.

The **urinary bladder** is a collapsible sac of muscle tissue lined with mucous membrane. It is low in the pelvic cavity, and its function is two-fold: the bladder collects the urine (from the ureters), and it expels the urine to the outside world. Both parasympathetic and sympathetic nerves innervate the bladder.

The **urethra** is a muscular tube lined with mucous membrane. The external opening of the urethra is called the **urinary meatus** (mee-*ate*-us). Urine is expelled from the body through the urethra.

In the male the urethra is much longer than in the female, and functions also in elimination of male reproductive fluid (*semen*).

Review of Urinary System

Urinary System Components
Two kidneys Two ureters One bladder One urethra
Kidney Function
Regulate composition and volume of blood
Urinary Bladder Function
Collects urine Expels urine from body

The Reproductive System

Reproduction is the name given the process by which organisms reproduce themselves. In humans, a single cell from each parent is all that is necessary to begin the reproduction.

In our discussion of cells we discovered that cells have a number of processes to perform, that some cells perform certain processes more efficiently than others, and that all cells perform all the processes to some degree or other. The chief function of the sex cells is to reproduce. The sex cells are called **gametes.** The male gametes are called **spermatozoa** and the female gametes are called **ova.** The organ that produces the gametes is called a **gonad.** The male gonads are called **testes,** and the female gonads are called **ovaries.**

The genital organs of the two sexes are structured for the production, transportation, protection, nourishment, and union of the gametes.

Review of Reproduction System

Sex Cells (Gametes)
Male: spermatozoa Female: ova

Gonads
(Organs which produce sex cells) Male: testes (produce sperm, secrete hormones) Female: ovaries (produce ova, secrete hormones)

Summary

The mouth involves the entire body, and dental treatment must consider the mental, emotional, and physical aspects of the patient as well as the moral values that affect his or her health.

The body is a structural unit composed of four kinds of smaller units: cells, tissues, organs, and systems.

These systems are housed in body cavities, and we look at them by the use of body planes.

Cells, the smallest units, carry on the nine life processes that occur in the life of a cell and also in the life of the body as a whole. They are *absorption, digestion, synthesis, respiration, excretion, secretion, motion, irritability,* and *reproduction.* Cells differ in structure and purpose. Similar cells form tissues. There are four groups of *tissues* in the body: *epithelial, connective* (including circulating), *muscle,* and *nerve.* Tissues form *organs.* Organs work best in a *system* with other organs.

The organs are housed in several *body cavities: cranial, spinal, thoracic,* and *abdominopelvic* are the major divisions.

The *body planes* with which the assistant should be familiar are: *sagittal, frontal, posterior,* and *transverse.*

The *body surfaces* also have names: *anterior, posterior, dorsal,* and *ventral* are some.

The systems of the body work together. The *skeletal system* is the framework and protector of the vital living organs. The skeleton also accomplishes locomotion. There are over 200 *bones* in the body. Bones have seven types of *joints* that make the framework movable.

The *muscular system* accomplishes the movement of the bony system. Muscles contract and thereby move a part of the body. The cardiac muscle contracts and relaxes involuntarily, but other muscles are controlled by the individual. Muscles work in pairs: *flexor* and *extensor* are two types of muscles that oppose each other and thereby can move the body. *Abductors* and *adductors* also work in pairs.

The skeletal framework of bones which can be moved by muscles is held together and covered by the *integumentary system.* The integumentary system includes the *hair,* the *fingernails,* and the *skin,* which is composed of three layers: *epidermis, dermis,* and *subcutaneous.*

The *circulatory system* is designed to deliver blood to and from the capillaries. It includes the *heart, arteries, arterioles, capillaries, venules, veins,* and *lymphatics.*

The heart is the chief organ of the circulatory system. From fifty to ninety heartbeats per minute is considered normal. The heart has four sections or *chambers.*

One difference between veins and arteries is the *direction of flow.* Arteries carry blood away from the heart, veins carry blood to the heart.

The *vena cava* is the important vein. The *aorta* is the important artery. The words *inferior* and *superior* are often used with vena cava to indicate the upper and lower sections.

The five blood circulatory systems include: the *pulmonary,* the *systemic,* the *coronary,* the *renal,* the *portal,* and the *hepatic.*

The *lymphatic* system is closely linked with the circulatory system, depositing lymph into the blood stream. The *hemic* system is actually the blood system. It carries nourishment to and waste from all parts of the body.

Respiration is the act of breathing wherein the exchange of gases occurs. The process of oxygen combining with glucose to make energy and giving off carbon dioxide and water is called *oxidation.*

Internal respiration is the absorption of oxygen, oxidation of glucose, and giving off of carbon dioxide and water by the cells.

External respiration is the process by which the entire bloodstream is supplied with oxygen and relieved of carbon dioxide and water.

Normally we inhale about sixteen to twenty-four times per minute.

The *nasal septum* is cartilage and bone between the two *nostrils. Turbinates* warm the air and catch dirt. The *internal nares* are the two openings through which the air passes into the *pharynx* where seven tubes converge. The *eustachian tubes* are openings into the ears. The *mouth cavity* permits food, beverage, and air to enter the pharynx. The *esophagus* begins at the bottom of the pharynx, as does the *glottis* (windpipe opening).

The *epiglottis* controls whether the esophagus or the *trachea* is open. The *larynx* is at the upper end of the trachea. The *bronchi* are below the trachea. *Cilia* tend to keep dirt from reaching the lungs.

The bronchi divide into *bronchioles,* which are surrounded by air sacs called *alveoli.*

The lungs are covered by two membranes: *visceral* and *pleural.* Fluid separates them.

The *nervous system* has two major parts: the *central nervous system* and the *peripheral nervous system.* The function of a *nerve* is to carry an impulse to and from the brain. The *brain* fills the cranial cavity. Some parts of the brain are the *cerebrum,* the *cerebellum,* and the *medulla oblongata.* The peripheral nervous system innervates glands, smooth muscles, and cardiac muscle. It is an involuntary system composed of *parasympathetic* and *sympathetic systems,* which oppose each other. The nervous system is designed to permit us to perceive our environment and the changes that occur in it; and to react to this environment. Some highly developed special functions of the nervous system are *vision, audition, olfaction, gustation, taction,* and *kinesthesia.* Two kinds of nerves are *motor* and *sensory.*

The *endocrine system* consists of numerous *glands* scattered throughout the body. These glands are ductless, and their secretions enter the bloodstream directly. The chemical exciter that an endocrine gland secretes is called a *hormone.* Different endocrine glands secrete different hormones, but each one has a strong effect on certain organs and tissues of the body. Abnormality occurs when a gland is either overactive or underactive. The delicate check-and-balance system among these glands is called the *dynamic balance.* There are eight types of endocrine glands.

The *digestive system* is that system which provides for the nourishment of the body. Another name for the digestive system is the *alimentary system.*

Alimentation includes *ingestion, digestion, absorption,* and *utilization.* The *alimentary canal* is about thirty feet long. The alimentation of food begins in the *mouth,* passes through the *esophagus* into the *stomach,* where the food is converted to *chyme.* The chyme moves into the *duodenum,* where digestion is continued. Chyme moves into the *jejunum,* and eventually the *ileum,* where the added secretions of the digestive organs continue to reduce the chyme to nutrients that are absorbed through the walls of the *intestines.* The *pancreas* secretes three enzymes which act on carbohydrates, proteins, and fats. The *liver* stores nutrients, produces vitamin A, and regulates metabolism.

Peristalsis is the wavelike movement of the intestines that helps move the chyme along to the large intestine, or *colon,* and down the descending colon to the *rectum.*

The *genitourinary system* has a two-fold function. It is a filtration plant to expel body wastes, and it is also a reproductive system. The circulatory system transports the waste products to the *kidneys,* where these waste products are separated from the blood. The waste products are collected in the kidneys and emptied, via the *ureters,* into the *bladder.* During urination, the bladder contracts and urine is expelled from the body through the *urethra.*

The working unit of the kidney is the *tubule.*

The kidneys regulate the composition and volume of blood in the body.

The *reproductive system* in humans requires a single cell from each parent to create a new human being. The organs that produce these cells are called *gonads.* The male gonad is the *testis,* the female gonad is the *ovary.* The cells these organs produce are called *gametes.* The male gamete is the *spermatozoa,* and the female gamete is the *ova.*

Study Questions

1. What are the four kinds of units of which the body is composed?
2. Describe the nine life processes carried on by cells.
3. Relate cells to tissues, tissues to organs, and organs to systems.
4. Describe the sagittal plane.
5. What is the work of the skeletal system? the muscular system? the integumentary system?
6. How many bones are there in the body?
7. What kinds of glands are in the integumentary system?
8. Describe the circulatory system.
9. Explain how the circulatory, lymphatic, and hemic systems work together.
10. How does the respiratory system relate to the circulatory system?
11. Discuss the two divisions of the nervous system.
12. How do the parasympathetic and sympathetic systems work?
13. List the regions of the brain.
14. How may cranial nerves are there?
15. What does the autonomic nervous system do?
16. Name the senses that are part of the nervous system.
17. What are the parts of the peripheral nervous system? the central nervous system?
18. What is another name for endocrine glands?
19. What do they secrete?
20. Explain their importance.
21. Describe the process of alimentation.
22. Describe the importance and contribution of the liver, pancreas, and gallbladder in the process of digestion.

23. What is chyme? peristalsis?
24. What is the two-fold function of the genitourinary system?

Vocabulary

anterior   front
articulations   joints
cranial   skull
endocrine glands   ductless glands
erythrocytes   red blood cells
esophagus   opening to stomach
eustachian tubes   openings into ears from pharynx
external respiration   respiration by the body as a whole
glottis   windpipe opening
hemic   blood
inferior   under or below
internal respiration   respiration by the cells
lateral   beside, on the side of
leukocytes   white blood cells
pharynx   throat cavity
posterior   back
superior   above
thoracic cavity   chest
ventral   belly

Word Elements	
Word Element	*Example*
dys combining form meaning: bad, improper	*dysfunction* malfunction of any part of the body
mal combining form meaning: bad, abnormal	*malocclusion* poor positioning of the teeth
necr combining form meaning: death	*necrosis* deadness of a certain portion of the body (dental necrosis is decay of a tooth)
oma suffix meaning: tumor	*odontoma* a tumor that is toothlike in structure
osis suffix meaning: abnormal increase in a process	*leukocytosis* an increase in the leukocytes in the blood
pathy suffix meaning: disease	*adenopathy* any disease of a gland, especially a lymph gland
path combining form meaning: disease, feeling	*psychopathic* a mental illness creating antisocial behavior
patho combining form meaning: relationship to disease	*pathology* the science that studies the nature of disease, its causes, effects, and the changes produced by disease
py, pyo combining form meaning: pus formation	*pyogenic* pus producing
tropism suffix meaning: a growth response in a motile organism elicited either toward or away from the stimulus	*neurotropism* having a special affinity for nerve fibers

Anatomy of the Head, and Anesthesia

Part One: Anatomy of the Head
Osteology (The Study of Bones)
    The Mandible
    The Maxilla
    Other Bones of the Skull
    The Temporomandibular Joint
    The Hyoid Bone
Myology (The Study of Muscles)
    Muscles of Mastication
    Suprahyoid Muscles
    Infrahyoid Muscles
    Facial Muscles
The Salivary Glands
    Sublingual Glands
    Submandibular Glands
    Parotid Glands
Exploration of Anatomical Landmarks
Teeth and Their Supporting Structures
    Teeth
        Primary Teeth
        Permanent Dentition
    Anatomy of Teeth
    Functions of Teeth
The Blood Supply to the Dental Area
The Nerve Supply in the Dental Area
Part Two: Anesthesia
Motor and Sensory Nerves
    How We Sense Pain
Prevention of Pain
    General Anesthesia
    Analgesia
    Local Anesthesia
    Topical Anesthesia

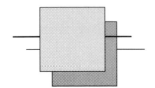

Part One: Anatomy of the Head

Anatomy is the science of form, structure, and inter-relationships of the parts of an animal body. A study of the anatomy of the human head and neck has an obvious and direct relationship with the practice of dentistry.

Although the dental assistant is not required to possess the same in-depth knowledge of anatomy as the dentist, the assistant should have a certain basic knowledge for responsibilities as a member of the oral health care team. The study of anatomy is complicated, but the basic essentials for beginning dental assisting included in this text are quite easily learned. If you wish further enrichment in this field, there are several excellent textbooks devoted specifically to the anatomy of the head and neck.

The illustrations in this chapter are planned to improve the student's visualization of the anatomy of the head. Please look at the illustrations and find the appropriate bones, muscles, and anatomical landmarks as you study the paragraphs describing each one. (Also see Plate 13)

Osteology (The Study of Bones)

The **skull** is composed of twenty-eight different bones: six auditory ossicles (forming the ear), fourteen facial bones, and eight bones of the cranium, which lodge and protect the brain. Although not considered a part of the skull, the hyoid bone is so important for the function of the mouth that it is, therefore, included in this discussion.

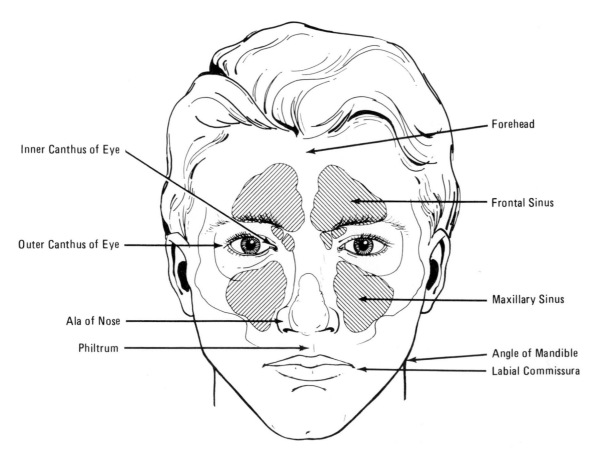

Figure 21.1
Facial landmarks.

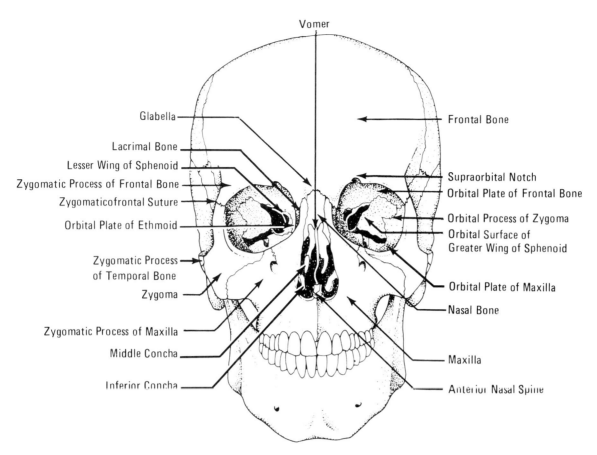

Figure 21.2
Anterior (front) view of the skull.

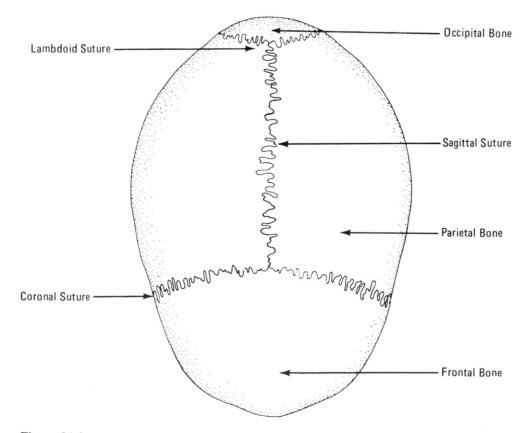

Figure 21.3
View of skull from above.

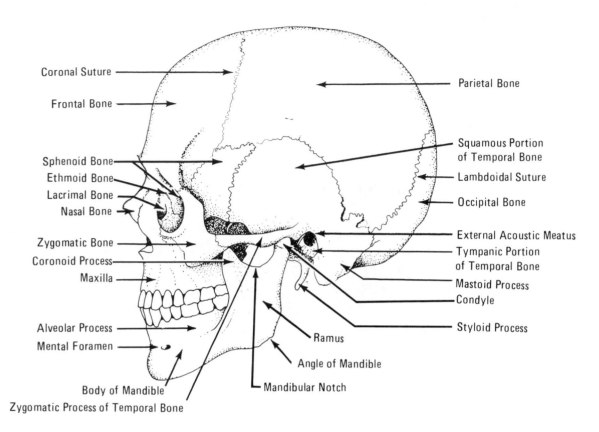

Figure 21.4
Lateral view of the skull.

Coronal Suture
Frontal Bone
Sphenoid Bone
Ethmoid Bone
Lacrimal Bone
Nasal Bone
Zygomatic Bone
Coronoid Process
Maxilla
Alveolar Process
Mental Foramen
Body of Mandible
Zygomatic Process of Temporal Bone

Parietal Bone
Squamous Portion of Temporal Bone
Lambdoidal Suture
Occipital Bone
External Acoustic Meatus
Tympanic Portion of Temporal Bone
Mastoid Process
Condyle
Styloid Process
Ramus
Angle of Mandible
Mandibular Notch

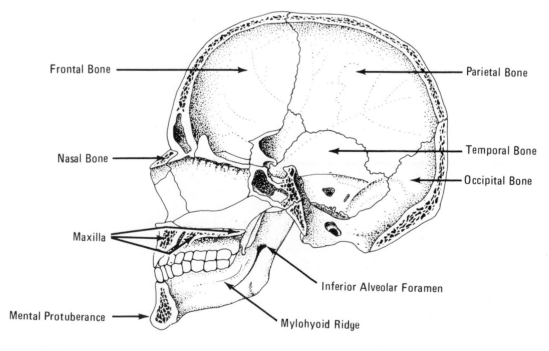

Figure 21.5
Cross section of interior of skull.

Frontal Bone
Nasal Bone
Maxilla
Mental Protuberance

Parietal Bone
Temporal Bone
Occipital Bone
Inferior Alveolar Foramen
Mylohyoid Ridge

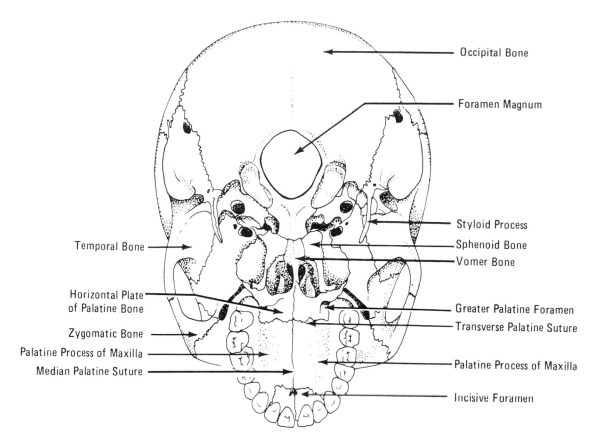

Figure 21.6
Inferior (from underneath) view of the skull.

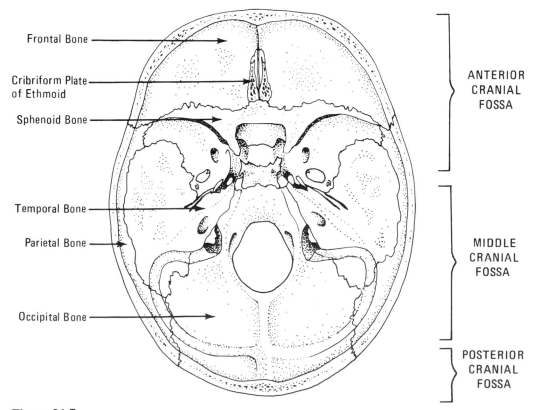

Figure 21.7
Inferior view of base of skull.

The fourteen facial bones and the eight bones of the cranium are connected by fibrous joints or **sutures** (immobile bony unions). The six ossicles of the ear are somewhat different: the **auditory ossicles** (the malleus, the incus, and the stapes) form a jointed column of bone. They are within the tympanic cavity and connect the tympanic membrane with the vestibular window. The outermost bone is the malleus, which is attached to the tympanic membrane. The innermost is the stapes, which is fixed to the vestibular window.

The mandible and the hyoid are connected to the rest of the head by muscles, tendons, and ligaments. There is only one mandible and one hyoid.

Most of the bones of the skull are paired; that is, there are identical bones on either side of the midline of the skull, each with the same name. These include the incus, malleus, and stapes (auditory ossicles); the maxillae; the palatines; the inferior, the middle, and the superior nasal conchae; the nasals; the lacrimals; the zygomatics; the temporals; and the parietals.

The single bones of the skull are the mandible, the vomer, the frontal bone, the sphenoid, the occipital bone, and the ethmoid bone.

The Mandible (Figure 21.8)

Run your finger downward from just behind the ear on one side of your head and follow the shape of the bone you will feel as it turns forward, around the point of the chin, then backward, until it turns upward again and seems to disappear just behind the other ear. The bone that you have followed forms the lower jaw and is called the **mandible.** It is a bone with a horseshoe-shaped body with certain extensions that are called **processes.** The curved alveolar process extends upward and surrounds the roots of the mandibular teeth, providing their support. It also provides places for the attachment of the various muscles that make it possible for us to chew. That portion of the mandible which extends on each side from near the ear downward to the angle is called the **ramus** (pronounced *ray*–muss). That portion which runs from one angle around the point of the chin to the other angle is called the **body** of the mandible. Each ramus has two processes, the anterior, or **coronoid process,** and the posterior, or **condylar process.** They are separated by a notch called the **mandibular notch.**

The condylar process **articulates** (joins) with the temporal bone to form the **temporomandibular joint.** Contraction and relaxation of the muscles of mastication cause movement of the mandible at the temporomandibular joint and thus permit speech and mastication of food.

There are four openings in the mandible. (The openings are called *foramen,* singular, and *foramina,*

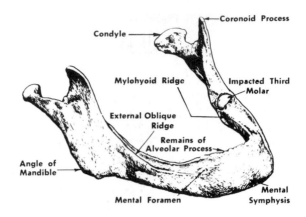

Figure 21.8
An edentulous mandible.

plural.) The two mandibular foramina are located on the inner *aspect* of the mandible, and the two mental foramina are on the outer *aspect.* (Aspect, in this usage, means the side or position from which the object is viewed.) The nerves and blood supply for the teeth and surrounding tissues pass through these foramina.

The Maxilla

Only the mandible moves as you open and close your mouth. The upper jaw is continuous with the rest of the skull and does not move. That portion of the upper jaw which corresponds to the mandible in providing the support for the upper teeth is made up of two bones joined in a suture at the midline (the **median palatine suture**) called the **maxillae.** By pressing firmly with your fingers, starting under the nose and following backward just under the cheekbones, you can feel the maxillae. The maxilla consists of a central body and four **processes,** or extensions. The frontal process extends upward to connect with the frontal bone. The **zygomatic process** (cheekbone) begins just in front of the ear, arches slightly outward, forward, and then curves slightly inward to an area just below the outer corner of the eye. The **arch** portion of this bone is just above the ramus of the mandible. You can't get your fingers under the **arch** because it is blocked by muscles. The **hard palate** is formed by the **horizontal palatine process** and the process from the other maxillary bone. The curved **alveolar process,** extending downward, surrounds and supports the roots of the maxillary teeth.

The central body of the maxilla has a hollow area called the **maxillary sinus.** The maxillary sinus has a direct connection with the nasal passage, and infections of the area commonly cause maxillary teeth to ache.

There are several **foramina** in the maxilla through which blood vessels and nerves pass. The **infraorbital foramina** are located below the eye socket.

Table 21.1
A Summary of the Bones of the Head

Facial bones	
Mandible	1
Maxilla	2
Palatine	2
Vomer	1
Conchae (inferior, middle, and superior)	2
Nasal	2
Lacrimal	2
Zygomatic	2
	14
Cranium	
Frontal	2
Parietal	2
Temporal	1
Sphenoid	1
Ethmoid	1
Occipital	1
	8
Ear	
Malleus	2
Incus	2
Stapes	2
	6
Total bones of the head: 28	
Of extreme importance to dentistry:	
The **Hyoid bone** (in the neck)	1
Total bones to recognize: 29	

Other Bones of the Skull

The **palatine bones** join the posterior border of the palatine process of the maxillary bones, completing the hard palate. The palatine bones also contain the anterior and posterior palatine foramina. These foramina provide an exit for the neurovascular bundles which supply both the hard palate anteriorly and the tissues of the soft palate posteriorly. The palatine bones and the maxillary bones together form the floor of the nose.

The **vomer** is a single bone attached to the maxillary and palatine bones in the midline and forms the lower and posterior part of the nasal septum.

The **inferior, middle,** and **superior conchae** are curved bones that project downward along the sides of the nose. The area beneath each conchae is known as a **meatus.** The middle nasal meatus has an opening that communicates with the maxillary sinus. This opening accounts for cross infections from the sinus to the nose and vice versa.

The **nasal bones** are small bones forming the bridge of the nose and are joined at the midline by a suture. Laterally, they are attached by the maxilla.

The **lacrimal bones** are very small bones between the ethmoid and maxilla and form a part of the medial wall of the **orbit.** (The orbit is the bony cavity that contains the eye.) The lacrimal bones together with the maxillary bones form the lacrimal fossae which contain the lacrimal sacs. The sacs provide the lubricating fluid, or tears, for the eyes.

The **zygomatic bones** are very prominent and are known as the cheekbones. The anterior processes of the zygomatic bones are attached to the maxillary bones. They also form a part of the lateral wall of the orbit.

The **frontal bone,** or the forehead, joins the zygomatic bone on its lateral surface and the nasal maxilla and lacrimal bones on the medial side. The frontal bone borders on the sphenoid and parietal bones posteriorly. The parietal bones form the major portion of the top and sides of the cranial vault. By sutures the parietal bones join the frontal bone anteriorly, the temporal and sphenoid bone laterally, and the occipital bone posteriorly.

The **temporal bone** is attached by sutures anteriorly with the zygomatic bone, and together they form the zygomatic arch. The temporal bone joins the sphenoid bone medially. The temporal bone contains the socket or the **mandibular fossa** (sometimes called the **glenoid fossa**) where the condyle of the mandible joins the skull. The temporal bone also contains the external auditory meatus, which houses the mechanism for hearing. Just below this meatus is the styloid process, a pencil-shaped bone that provides attachment for a strong ligament extending to the mandible.

The **sphenoid bone** is a biwinged bone in the center of the skull that forms part of the orbit wall as well as part of the nasal septum. This bone is in contact with all other bones of the cranium as well as some of the facial bones. In the body of the sphenoid bone is a depression known as the **cella turcica,** which houses the pituitary gland. The pituitary gland is a major part of the endocrine system, which we discussed in chapter 20.

The **ethmoid bone** contacts the vomer anteriorly and moves posteriorly and superiorly to form a part of the floor of the cranial fossa. (A **fossa** is a longitudinal depression.) The ethmoid bone thus forms part of the nasal septum as well as the passageway from the nose to the brain for the nerves that control smell. The ethmoid bone is also in contact with the nasal conchae.

The **occipital bone** forms the back of the head and joins the parietal bones anteriorly by sutures. It contains the largest foramen in the skull, the foramen magnum, through which passes the spinal cord from the brain to the vertebrae.

The Temporomandibular Joint

While you face a good light source, examine your own mouth very carefully, using a large, clear hand mirror. As you open and close your mouth, you will notice that the lower jaw swings on two joints, one just ahead of each ear. These two joints are called the **temporomandibular joints,** which are the connections of the mandible and temporal bones. They are considered as one joint because they function together.

The rounded condyle of the mandible fits in a depression of the temporal bone called the **mandibular fossa** (glenoid fossa). The joint is surrounded by a **fibrous capsule** and is separated by a **fibrous articular disc.** The disc divides the joint space into an upper and a lower compartment. The disc allows the mandibular condyle to both rotate and slide during jaw movements.

The operation of the temporomandibular joint can be felt. Put your little fingers in your ears. Now open and close your mouth. The movement you feel in the ear is caused by the operation of the temporomandibular joint. Now place your forefingers with firm pressure just in front of your ears, open and close your mouth, and move the lower jaw to both sides. You are feeling condyles functioning in the maxillary (glenoid) fossa.

The Hyoid Bone (Plate 12)

The **hyoid bone** is a horseshoe-shaped bone lying in the anterior part of the neck below the mandible. It is suspended from the styloid processes by the **stylohyoid ligaments,** and serves as an attachment for many muscles. The interaction of these muscles is important in the opening of the jaw and movement of the tongue.

Myology (The Study of Muscles)

We will review here some of the information already presented concerning myology in chapter 20.

The muscles of primary concern to the dental assistant are those involved in the functioning of the mouth and jaws. These are striated (voluntary) muscles and are composed of groups of individual muscle fibers bound together. The entire mass is covered with a tough, smooth skin to facilitate movement over body parts (nearby muscles, organs, and so on). Each muscle is attached at both ends; the end remaining relatively fixed during contraction is called the point of **origin,** while the end that moves is called the point of **insertion,** and the bulge in between is called the **belly.**

If the origin and insertion of a muscle are known, its action becomes obvious. For example, the origin of the biceps is at the shoulder and the insertion is at the elbow. When the bellies of the biceps contract, the elbow bends and the shoulder remains fixed.

Muscles are only capable of contracting (pulling); they cannot push. Therefore, muscles are most often found in pairs, or groups of muscles, with opposing actions. For example, the opening and closing of the mandible is accomplished by contracting one set of muscles, the lateral pterygoid, which opens the jaw; and the masseter, temporalis, and medial pterygoid which close the jaw. The opening and closing of the mandible, then, is produced by the coordinated contraction of opposing muscles. The more complicated motion of mastication is produced by a similar cooperation of several sets of muscles that generate not only the simple opening and closing movements, but a variety of anterior-posterior and lateral movements of the mandible as well.

The muscles of the mouth and jaws may be generally grouped into five areas:

1. **Mastication:** temporalis, masseter, medial pterygoid, and lateral pterygoid
2. **Suprahyoids:** geniohyoid, mylohyoid, digastric, and stylohyoid
3. **Infrahyoids:** sternohyoid, and thyrohyoid
4. **Muscles of the face:** orbicularis oris, mentalis, incicivus labii superioris and inferioris, quadratus labii superioris and inferioris, zygomatic, levator angula oris, depressor anguli oris, risorius, buccinator, and platysma
5. **Muscles of the tongue:** genioglossus; hyoglossus, and styloglossus

Muscles of Mastication

The **temporalis** is a fan-shaped muscle that originates on the side of the skull and extends under the zygomatic arch to insert on the coronoid process and the anterior border of the ramus of the mandible. You can visualize the action of this muscle pulling the mandible up by the coronoid process and ramus as it constricts.

The **masseter** is a muscle originating on the zygomatic arch and inserting on the outer surface of the mandible. If you place your fingers just below the zygomatic arch and clench your teeth, you can feel the masseter muscle in action. It is a powerful muscle that is used to close the jaw or move it forward.

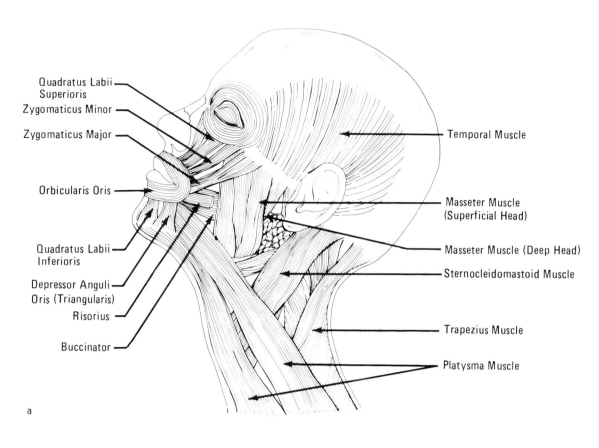

Quadratus Labii Superioris

Zygomaticus Minor

Zygomaticus Major

Orbicularis Oris

Quadratus Labii Inferioris

Depressor Anguli Oris (Triangularis)

Risorius

Buccinator

Temporal Muscle

Masseter Muscle (Superficial Head)

Masseter Muscle (Deep Head)

Sternocleidomastoid Muscle

Trapezius Muscle

Platysma Muscle

a

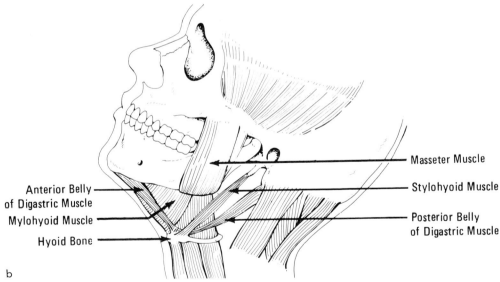

Anterior Belly of Digastric Muscle

Mylohyoid Muscle

Hyoid Bone

Masseter Muscle

Stylohyoid Muscle

Posterior Belly of Digastric Muscle

b

Figure 21.9

Muscles of the head and neck a–f (continued on next page).

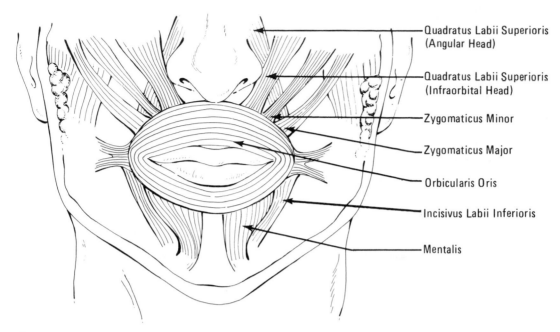

Quadratus Labii Superioris (Angular Head)

Quadratus Labii Superioris (Infraorbital Head)

Zygomaticus Minor

Zygomaticus Major

Orbicularis Oris

Incisivus Labii Inferioris

Mentalis

c

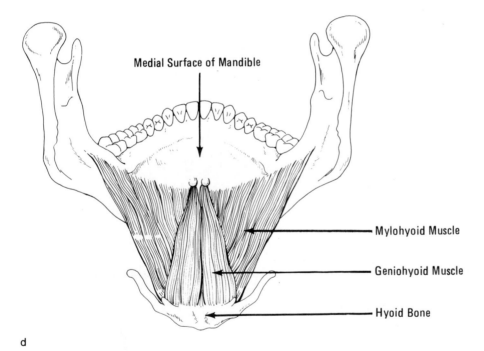

Medial Surface of Mandible

Mylohyoid Muscle

Geniohyoid Muscle

Hyoid Bone

d

Figure 21.9
(continued)

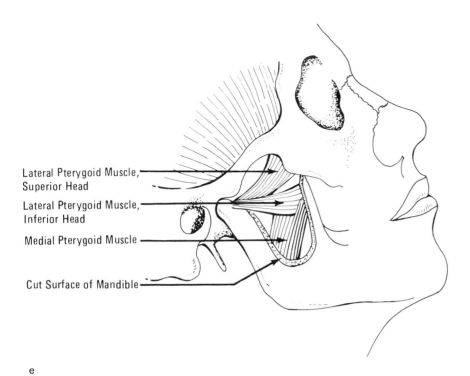

Lateral Pterygoid Muscle, Superior Head

Lateral Pterygoid Muscle, Inferior Head

Medial Pterygoid Muscle

Cut Surface of Mandible

e

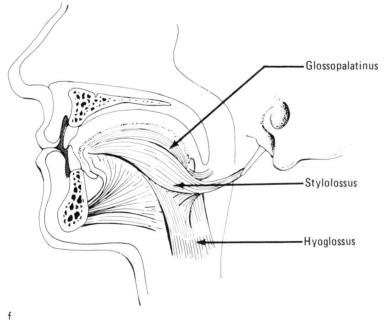

Glossopalatinus

Stylolossus

Hyoglossus

f

Figure 21.9
(continued)

The **medial pterygoid** is similar to the masseter but is located on the inner surface of the mandible. It originates on the lateral pterygoid plate and the tuberosity of the maxilla. Its point of insertion is on the inside of the ramus at the angle of the mandible. The medial pterygoid produces closing, side to side movements, and thrusting (protrusive) movements of the jaw.

The **lateral pterygoid** muscle has its origin on the greater wing of the sphenoid bone and on the infratemporal crest. It inserts on the neck of the condyle and the capsule of the temperomandibular joint. When these muscles act alternately, they move the jaw from side to side. When they act together, they assist in opening the mouth by pulling downward and forward.

Suprahyoid Muscles

The interaction of the muscles that attach to the hyoid bone are important in opening the jaw and moving the tongue. Note that the two groups of muscles, the suprahyoid muscles and the infrahyoid muscles, achieve functional significance due to their attachment to the hyoid bone.

The **geniohyoid muscle** originates from the genial tubercles (small bumps of bone on the inside of the front of the mandible) and inserts on the anterior surface of the body of the hyoid bone. Its action helps open the jaw.

The **mylohyoid muscle** originates on the mylohyoid line on each side of the inner mandible and inserts on the body of the hyoid. It forms the floor of the mouth. When this muscle constricts, it raises the tongue to the palate. It also assists in opening the mouth.

The **digastric muscle** is a muscle with two bellies that are connected by a tendon. The posterior belly originates on the temporal bone, while the anterior belly originates on the lower border of the mandible in the region of the symphysis (natural junction). The connecting tendon passes through a fascial loop attached to the hyoid bone. Constriction of this muscle can move the hyoid bone and open the jaw (the movement produced depends on which belly contracts, or if both bellies contract simultaneously).

The **stylohyoid muscle** originates from the styloid process of the temporal bone and inserts on the hyoid bone. It helps stabilize the hyoid when interacting with other muscles moving the jaw and tongue.

Infrahyoid Muscles

The **sternohyoid muscle,** originating on the sternum (breast bone), and the **thyrohyoid muscle,** originating on the thyroid cartilage, both insert on the hyoid bone and exert a downward pull on the hyoid when contracting. They can thereby assist in opening the mouth by depressing the mandible.

Facial Muscles

The **orbicularis oris** is a complex muscle forming the lips. The multifibered circular muscle isn't attached to bone, but to other muscles. It is responsible for the various lip actions.

The **mentalis muscles** originate in the mental area on either side of the mandible and insert in the orbicularis oris muscle, at the corners of the mouth. These muscles can extend the lower lip and pull the chin up.

The **incicivus labii** muscles (both inferior and superior) originate on the alveolar bone in the areas of the cuspid teeth and insert in the orbicularis oris muscle. They assist in closing the lips.

The **quadratus labii** (both inferior and superior) originate from the base of the nose, the zygoma and the infraorbital region, and are responsible for raising the upper lip and dilating the nostrils. The **zygomatic muscle** also originates from the zygoma and inserts in the orbicularis oris, and functions by pulling the corners of the mouth up and back.

The **levator anguli oris** originates in the canine fossa of the maxilla and inserts at the corner of the mouth. It can pull the corner of the mouth upward and a bit to the side.

Its counterpart on the mandible is the **depressor anguli oris,** originating in the mandible from the cuspid to the first molar and inserting at the angle of the mouth. This muscle pulls the corner of the mouth down and in.

The **risorius muscle** completes the angle of the mouth action with its origin in the anterior part of the masseter and its insertion at the corner of the mouth between the levator and depressor anguli oris muscles. When contracting, this muscle pulls the corner of the mouth laterally.

The **buccinator** or **cheek muscle** originates from the maxilla and mandible, inserts in the orbicularis, and functions in the varied movements of the cheek (especially in the mastication of food), as well as assisting the other muscles in pulling the corners of the mouth back.

The **genioglossus, hyoglossus,** and **styloglossus** muscles originate from the genial tubercle, the hyoid bone, and the styloid process, respectively; all inserting in the tongue. They are principally responsible for the functions of the tongue.

The Salivary Glands

Saliva has several functions: (1) it moistens and **lubricates** food we eat; (2) it contains enzymes that aid in the **digestion** of food; and (3) it acts to **cleanse** the oral cavity of food particles that contribute to caries and periodontal disease.

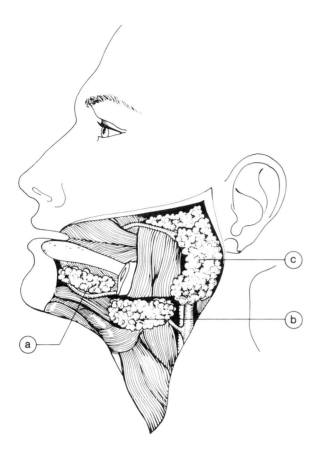

Figure 21.10
The salivary glands: (a) sublingual; (b) submandibular (submaxillary); and (c) parotid.

There are three major salivary glands: (1) **sublingual,** (2) **submandibular** (or submaxillary), and (3) **parotid.** There are also smaller glands that are close to the surface and open with numerous narrow ducts on the surface of the oral mucosa.

Sublingual Glands

The **sublingual gland** is also located in the floor of the mouth near the mandible, and its secretion, primarily mucus, enters the mouth through Bartholin's duct, which also opens on the sublingual caruncle. Bartholin's and Wharton's ducts may enter the mouth together, rather than individually.

Some patients have such an excessive flow of saliva (**sialorrhea**) that certain dental procedures are very difficult to perform. Sialorrhea may be involved in several physical disorders. The amount of secretions of all kinds in the body can be reduced by the use of one of the drugs classed as an *anti-sialogogue.* A substance that increases the flow of saliva is a **sialogogue.** Salivary glands or ducts can become blocked by calcareous deposits, one of the diagnostic symptoms being the

swelling of the gland at mealtimes. The removal of such deposits is a surgical procedure known as a **sialolithotomy.**

Submandibular Glands

The **submandibular gland** is located on the inner surface of the mandible and extends downward toward the hyoid bone. It is also called the *submaxillary* gland, which you can explain from your knowledge of dental terminology. This gland opens into the mouth through Wharton's duct, in a prominence called the **submaxillary caruncle,** which is located on the forward midline of the floor of the mouth near the lingual frenum. The submandibular gland produces both serous and mucous secretions and therefore is called a **mixed gland.**

Parotid Glands

The **parotid glands** are located in front and a little below the ear. The opening into the mouth is Stensen's duct, easily visible in the cheek just about opposite the upper second molar, as mentioned before. The parotid gland produces mostly a serous secretion (clear, almost watery), which is ptyalin. It is this gland that is involved in the disease you know as mumps—properly called parotitis.

Exploration of Anatomical Landmarks

Now examine your lips. They are composed of muscles and glands and are covered by skin on the outside and by *mucous membrane* on the inside. The area between these two, the **vermilion border,** is found only in human beings. The thin connecting fold at the corners of the lips is called the **labial commissure,** an area that is quite tender. During dental operations, it is wise to protect this area with a very light coating of Vaseline to prevent soreness.

You will notice a groove that runs from the **ala** or **wing** of the nose (the nostril) downward and outward beyond the corners of the mouth. This is the **nasolabial groove,** the deepening of which occurs with advancing age. When artificial dentures are constructed for a patient, the depth of this groove can be controlled to a great degree, and thus the appearance of aging can be influenced.

The little shallow, vertical groove that runs from the area between the nostrils of the nose down to the vermilion border of the lip is called the **philtrum.** Running parallel to the lower lip, and slightly below it, is the **labiomental groove.**

You will notice when you barely part your lips that the edges of the upper front teeth are just visible below your upper lip. This is true in the large majority

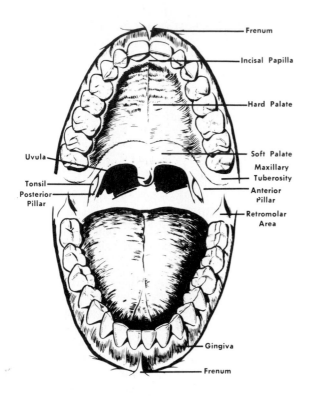

Figure 21.11
The mouth.

of people and is often used as a guide in making artificial dentures when no previous record of the natural teeth is available.

Look inside your mouth. The **oral cavity** is the space that is enclosed by the lips in front, the cheeks on either side, the **palate** above, and the floor of the mouth below. In a more restricted sense, the *oral cavity* might also refer to the space enclosed by the teeth, when closed together, with the palate above and the floor of the mouth below.

Place your finger on the outer (toward the cheek) surface of the last lower tooth in your mouth, moving it downward as far as it will go. Your finger is in a trough between the **gingivae,** or **gums,** and the inner surface of the cheek. As you slide your finger forward toward the front teeth, it is sliding along the **oral vestibule** or **mucobuccal fold.** If you pull your lower lip strongly forward and outward with your other hand as your finger follows the vestibule around, you will feel your fingers bump across a weblike structure almost exactly in the midline. This is the **frenum** of the lower lip. The upper lip has its *frenum* on the midline also, and it is usually more prominent, or larger, than the lower frenum. The *frena* contain no muscle tissue.

As your finger continues around the lower vestibule, this time follow around behind the last tooth (assuming that you have a full complement of teeth). Just behind and in line with the last tooth you will feel a

little rounded hump. This is called the **retromolar pad** or **area.** There will be one on each side. The same area, behind the *upper* tooth on each side, is called the **maxillary tuberosity.** These areas will be of importance to you when pouring casts in impressions that the dentist has taken for any reason. They should be included in the cast and not lost.

The pale pink tissue you see lining the mouth is called the **mucous membrane.** It is so named because it contains many tiny glands that secrete **mucus,** a viscid, watery secretion. That part of the **mucous** membrane which is located between the vestibule and the necks of the teeth is divided into two areas, that closer to the teeth being called the **gingiva** or **gum** (as in sugarless chewing *gum*). The area toward the vestibule is called the **alveolar mucosa.** That portion lining the cheeks is called the **buccal mucosa.**

The gum, or gingiva, is a pale pink color when in healthy condition and, when wiped dry, appears to be finely stippled, somewhat like a very fine sandpaper. The mucosa lining the cheeks, lips, vestibule, and up to the area of the gums is usually a deeper pink color with a smooth surface.

Around the base of each tooth the gum is not attached, forming a very shallow groove, actually, much like the cuff on a shirt sleeve except that the **free gum margin** is very snug around the tooth. The free portion, or the depth of the groove in that area alongside the base of the tooth, is very shallow. The depth normally does not exceed approximately one-sixteenth of an inch. The broad, thin end of a toothpick placed against a tooth, then gently moved downward into this groove, will demonstrate the free gum margin to you.

Now place the pad of your index finger on the palate just behind your upper front teeth. In the area exactly centered between the two *central incisors,* the two largest front teeth, you will feel a small hump. This is the **incisal papilla** or **palatine papilla.** Applying a firm pressure with your index finger, slide slowly from the incisal papilla backward toward the throat. You first feel a very firm section of the palate which extends as far back as the last teeth, if you have them all. This is called the **hard palate,** an area that has bony support and also forms the floor of the nasal passages.

At the end of the hard palate, the firm pressure will cause a slight amount of pain. Beyond this you will feel a soft area. This is the **soft palate,** also called the **palatine velum.** As you look at this area with the mirror say, *ah-h-h-h-h-h,* and repeat it several times. You will notice the rise and fall of the soft palate. That little finger-like projection hanging downward from the center rear edge of the soft palate is called the **uvula.** The soft palate and uvula close off the nasal passages when swallowing and are also used in speech. The soft palate and uvula are very muscular.

Looking at the area on either side of the uvula, you will notice two arched folds on each side, arching from the soft palate and disappearing beyond the edges of the tongue. Another heavier arch appears to run from behind the last upper tooth to the retromolar pad behind the last lower tooth. This latter archlike fold is called the **pterygomandibular fold.** The foremost of the next two arches is called the **palatoglossal arch** or **anterior pillar,** and the farthest back is the **palatopharyngeal arch** or **posterior pillar.** The **palatine tonsils** lie between the palatoglossal arch and the palatopharyngeal arch. These tonsils, if you still have them, are softly rounded, irregular masses of tissue appearing on either side between the aforementioned arches.

While examining this area, slightly close your mouth and with your free hand pull the cheek firmly away from the sides of the last upper teeth. If you look carefully, and think of eating something that you like very much, you may notice a small point jutting out from the inside surface of the cheek, just about opposite the next to the last tooth. This is the opening of the *parotid duct,* also called *Stensen's duct.*

Now look underneath the tongue. As you hold the tip of your tongue up behind the upper front teeth, with your mouth open wide, you will notice two little humps, one on either side of the *lingual frenum,* just behind the lower front teeth. These are the openings of the salivary ducts, called the *submaxillary caruncle.* The lingual frenum extends from the undersurface of the tongue to the floor of the mouth near the lower front teeth, along the midline. In some individuals it is more apparent than in others.

Now look at your lower teeth. Since they are arranged in a **U,** the entire group is often called the **lower arch;** the upper group is the **upper arch.** The teeth themselves are in pairs in each arch, starting at the midline. In the adult mouth having a full complement of teeth, thirty-two teeth are present. In the child, a complete **deciduous dentition** is twenty teeth. Very frequently the last tooth on each side in the adult mouth is not visible because it does not have room to come into the mouth and is **impacted.**

As you close your teeth together, they are **occluding,** and when closed are in **occlusion.** If you relax your muscles, you will notice that the teeth drop apart just a very small distance. This position of the lower jaw is called the **rest position.** When you close your teeth together (as though you are biting on the back teeth), your jaws are said to be in **centric occlusion.** Just what *centric* position is, with respect to the proper relationship of mandible to maxilla, and with respect to the proper relationship of the parts in the temporomandibular joints, is the subject of much discussion among dentists. The definition given is technically loose: "that position of the mandible in relation to the maxilla when the teeth are closed in the 'normal' position."

Teeth and Their Supporting Structures

Teeth

Every individual has two sets of teeth—primary and secondary. **Eruption** is the name given the process of a new tooth entering the mouth. It applies to the primary dentition as well as the permanent dentition.

Primary Teeth

There are twenty primary teeth, ten in the maxilla and ten in the mandible. These erupt at varying times from individual to individual, but generally between six months of age and two years. They are usually lost or "shed" between ages six and twelve and are replaced by the secondary teeth.

Permanent Dentition

The secondary teeth generally erupt between ages six and twelve with the exception of the third molars, or "wisdom" teeth, which erupt sometime around age eighteen. There is a total of thirty-two secondary teeth in most individuals. Table 21.2 shows the *approximate* ages when teeth erupt. Note that the mandibular teeth usually precede the maxillary teeth.

Anatomy of Teeth

A tooth is made of several kinds of material. That part which is visible in the mouth, under normal circumstances, is called the **crown.** The surface of the crown is **enamel,** the hardest material in the body. The enamel is in the form of a shell, covering the crown or **coronal** portion of the tooth. It varies in thickness, being heaviest on the chewing or biting surface of the tooth, and becoming thin toward that part of the crown that is farthest from the chewing or biting surface. The enamel consists of microscopic **rods,** which point generally in the same direction as the lines drawn across the enamel in figures 21.12, 21.13, and Plate 11.

Calcium and phosphorus make up approximately 90 percent of the enamel. The rest is made up of other minerals, plus a small amount of organic matter.

Inside the enamel shell, forming the main body of the tooth, is the **dentin.** The dentin has innumerable tiny canals and many nerve fibers that make the junction of the enamel with the dentin a very sensitive area. Dentin is slightly elastic, although not visibly so, and is very strong. It is approximately 67 percent calcium and phosphorus, about 5 percent other minerals, and about 28 percent organic matter.

In the central area of the tooth is a chamber that is filled with many different kinds of tissue: blood vessels, the main nerve supply of the tooth, connective tissue, and others. This central chamber **(pulp chamber)** has **canals** that form a passageway for the blood vessels

Table 21.2
Eruption Table for Primary and Permanent Dentition

Primary	Age in Months	Permanent	Age in Years
Lower central incisor	6	Upper and lower first molars	6–7
Upper central incisor	7½	Lower central incisor	6–7
Lower lateral incisor	7	Upper central incisor	7–8
Upper lateral incisor	9	Lower lateral incisor	7–8
Lower canine (cuspid)	16	Upper lateral incisor	8–9
Upper canine (cuspid)	18	Lower canine (cuspid)	9–10
Lower first molar	12	Upper canine (cuspid)	11–12
Upper first molar	14	Lower first premolar (bicuspid)	10–12
Lower second molar	20	Upper first premolar (bicuspid)	10–11
Upper second molar	24	Lower second premolar (bicuspid)	11–12
		Upper second premolar (bicuspid)	10–12
		Lower second molar	11–13
		Upper second molar	12–13
		Upper and lower third molars	17–70

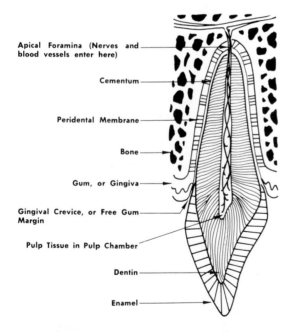

Figure 21.12
Schematic drawing of a tooth and its supporting tissues.

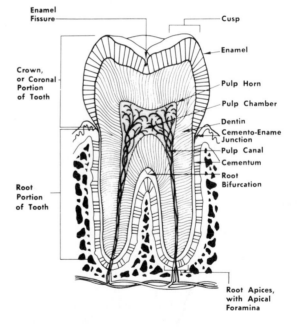

Figure 21.13
Schematic drawing of a cross section of a posterior tooth.

and nerve fibers to the tip of the root (the **apex**). These vessels and fibers pass through the apical foramen and thence to the circulatory and nerve structures of the rest of the body.

That portion of the dentin which lies beyond the enamel-covered coronal part of each tooth forms the **root.** The root, however, is covered by a thin, dense, sensitive material called **cementum.** The line at which

the cementum meets the enamel is called the **cemento-enamel junction** and locates the **cervical** portion of the tooth or the **gingival** portion, since the gingiva is attached to the tooth near this junction.

Thousands of tiny fibers run from the cementum to the tooth socket, the **peridental membrane,** supporting the tooth in the socket. Note that a tooth is not directly in touch with the bone of the jaw in which it is located. A slow, steady pressure on a tooth can move the tooth a noticeable amount in its socket. These supporting tissues of the teeth are extremely sensitive to pressure.

The words used here as the basic terminology the dental assistant should learn are not used by all schools and, therefore, are not used by all dentists. The differences, generally, are minor, but the dental assistant should be aware that differences do exist.

Functions of Teeth

The incisor teeth, four in the upper arch and four in the lower arch, are chisel-shaped. Their primary function is to "incise" food—to cut the food placed between them. When these teeth are recently erupted in a child's mouth, the biting edge has a lumpy appearance due to three small bulges or lobes. These teeth are formed in three sections, around three **centers of calcification** that fuse together as the tooth develops. This gives the biting edges the characteristic three-lobed appearance when they first erupt in the mouth. The biting edge wears to a more or less flat edge very quickly when the tooth begins to be used for incising food.

The incisor teeth normally erupt (at the proper time) just inside the mouth from the primary teeth, which often will still be in position in the child's mouth when the incisor of the permanent dentition erupts into view.

The next tooth distally in each quadrant of the adult mouth is the cuspid tooth. A cusp is a notably pointed or rounded eminence on or near the masticating surface of a tooth. The canine (cuspid) tooth is so named because it has a prominent, heavy cusp shaping the tooth to a relatively sharp point. Since the tooth also has a strong and very long root, it is ideal for its purpose—that of tearing food.

The premolars (bicuspids) are the next two teeth in each dental arch. As the name implies, the premolars have two cusps. Some premolars, particularly the lower first premolars, may not seem to comply with this description if they have a poorly developed cusp (the lingual cusp, in this case) or other minor variations in development. The upper first premolar generally has two roots; the others usually have one. The premolars begin the grinding or milling of food after the incisors and cuspids have performed their work. They cannot do the heavy-duty milling that is required of the group of teeth farthest back in the mouth.

The molars are the heavy-duty grinders of the dentition. With the advantage of position in relation to the temporomandibular joint, these teeth can be used to apply a tremendous pressure to food that the tongue and cheeks place on their masticating surfaces. To support these stresses, the lower molars generally have two broad, heavy roots—one under the mesial half of the crown, the other under the distal half of the crown. The upper molars generally have three roots—one longer heavy root toward the palate, and two somewhat shorter toward the buccal side of the tooth. The maxillary sinus can be seen (on a full-mouth X-ray series) dipping down between the lingual and buccal roots of the upper first and second molars.

The Blood Supply to the Dental Area

In order for tissues to survive, they must have a system that will bring food, nutrients, and oxygen and carry away waste products (carbon dioxide, urea, and so on). The circulatory system provides these necessities. Frequently compared to a transportation system, the circulatory system consists of the **heart** as the pumping station, the **blood** as the carrier, and the **blood vessels** as the transportation routes. The blood supply to the head and neck is an amazing network of large and small arteries (and corresponding large and small veins) that branch to every structure and area. The oxygenated blood leaves the left ventricle of the heart and passes into a large arched vessel, the **aorta,** from which many vessels branch off for all areas of the body. The first branch from the aorta is the **inominate artery,** from which the **right common carotid artery** branches. The second branch is the **left common carotid.** From this point, both right and left common carotid arteries are similar; that is, each gives off corresponding branches that supply corresponding areas on a particular side of the head and neck.

Each common carotid artery divides, forming an **internal carotid artery** and an **external carotid artery.** The external carotid arteries supply the lingual arteries (to the tongue) and the internal maxillary arteries.

From the **maxillary arteries** branch the **inferior alveolar arteries,** which supply the mandibular premolar (bicuspid) teeth and the molar teeth. The inferior alveolar arteries branch again into the **mental arteries,** which supply the chin area, and the **incisive arteries,** which supply the incisors and canines (cuspids) of the mandible.

The internal maxillary arteries also give rise to two other branches (on each side), the **posteriosuperior alveolar** (dental) **arteries,** which supply the premolars (bicuspids) and molars of the maxillae, and the **infraorbital arteries,** which supply the incisors and canines (cuspids) of the maxillae.

The Nerve Supply in the Dental Area

Specific nerves supply the dental area. There are twelve cranial nerves that, as the name implies, branch off from the brain (within the cranium). As with many other

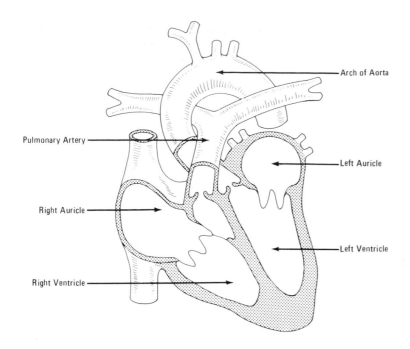

Figure 21.14

Schematic drawing of the heart.

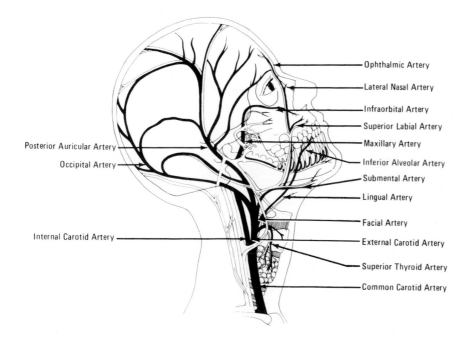

Figure 21.15

Arterial blood supply to the dental area.

structures of the body, remember that we are again speaking of something in the singular sense, when actually the structures occur as a symmetrical pair, usually a left and a right.

The first nerve to branch off the brain is the **olfactory,** a sensory nerve that provides our nasal mucosa with the sense of smell.

The second cranial nerve is the **optic,** again a sensory nerve, this time bringing impulses from the retina, giving us our vision.

The third cranial nerve is the **oculomotor,** a motor nerve involving control of many of the muscles that regulate the movement of the eye.

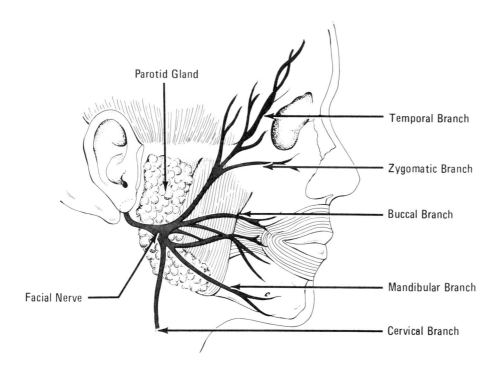

Figure 21.16
Facial nerve.

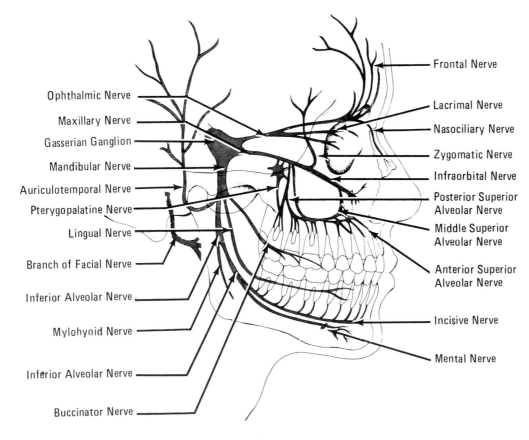

Figure 21.17
Trigeminal nerve pathway.

The fourth cranial nerve is the **trochlear,** again a motor nerve. Its function is the control of the muscle fibers that move the eyeball in an outward and downward rotation.

The fifth cranial nerve is the one most important dentally. It is both sensory and motor in its function— the motor root is the minor portion sometimes called the masticator nerve. The **trigeminal** (try-*gem*-in-al) nerve (a more common name for the fifth cranial nerve) is the largest of the cranial nerves with the exception of the optic.

As the fibers of the fifth cranial nerve approach the brainstem, there is found a kidney-like shape called the **Gasserian,** or **semilunar, ganglion.** From the convex portion, the root of the nerve enters the brainstem. From the concave portion (which is directed forward), three divisions of the trigeminal are given off. These branches are the **ophthalmic, maxillary,** and **mandibular.** Each of these is purely sensory, although the mandibular nerve is joined by the fibers of the masticator nerve (which is motor) and serves to innervate some of the muscles of mastication.

The ophthalmic nerve is the smallest of the three branches of the trigeminal. The ophthalmic again divides into three terminal branches that are involved with the cornea, iris, tear gland, eyelid, eyebrow, and skin of the forehead, among other areas, through further branches.

The maxillary nerve is the second division of the trigeminal and is also intermediate in size—larger than the ophthalmic but smaller than the mandibular nerve (the third division).

The branches of the maxillary nerve are many, but the first to be specifically involved in the innervation of teeth are the posterosuperior alveolar nerves, which are usually two in number. These give off branches to the gums and the posterior portion of the mouth, then pass on to enter the posterior alveolar canals and join with the other alveolar branches to form the superior dental plexus, through which they give innervation to the upper molar teeth.

The branches of the maxillary nerve given off in the infraorbital area are the middle-superior and anterosuperior alveolar nerves.

The middle-superior alveolar nerve gives off branches that again join with other alveolar branches to form the superior dental plexus, and through this it supplies the bicuspid teeth as well as the mucous membrane of the maxillary sinus and the gums.

The anterosuperior alveolar nerve is given off by the infraorbital nerve, unites with other alveolar nerves to form the superior dental plexus, and supplies the canine (cuspid) and incisor teeth, and again supplies

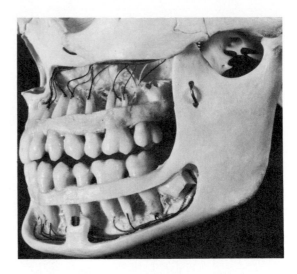

Figure 21.18
Skull reproduction, illustrating the nerve supply to the teeth.

an area of the mucous membrane of the maxillary sinus and the gums, plus another small branch to part of the nasal cavity.

As has been said, these branches are but part of the many divisions of the maxillary or second division of the trigeminal nerve.

The superior dental plexus is a network formed in the alveolar canals by the three superior alveolar nerves: the posterosuperior alveolar nerve, the middle-superior alveolar nerve, and the anterosuperior alveolar nerve. This network makes connection across the midline with the corresponding network on the other side. It is due to this that the dentist in anesthetizing a central incisor, lateral incisor, or canine (cuspid) on one side of the arch, will also add some anesthetic to an area over the apex of the opposite central incisor.

The third division of the trigeminal nerve is the mandibular nerve, the largest of the three divisions. It is commonly described as formed by the union of two distinct nerves: the entire masticator nerve (motor in function) and the large bundle of sensory fibers from the Gasserian ganglion that is actually the third division of the trigeminal. The single trunk divides into the anterior portion and the posterior portion.

The anterior portion is smaller than the posterior and is composed mainly of motor fibers of the masticator nerve, which supply the muscles of mastication (temporal, masseter, and external pterygoid). The balance of this anterior division is sensory and forms (mainly) the long buccal nerve, innervating the cheek as far forward as the angle of the mouth.

The posterior part of the mandibular nerve forms into three branches. Two, the lingual and the auriculotemporal, are sensory; the third contains some motor fibers from the masticator nerve for the innervation of the mylohyoid muscle.

This third branch of the posterior portion of the mandibular nerve is directly concerned with innervation of the mandibular teeth. It is the largest of the three branches and is called the inferior alveolar nerve. Shortly after its formation it enters the ramus of the mandible at the mandibular foramen.

The inferior alveolar nerve branches to form the inferior dental plexus and the mental nerve. (A bundle of motor fibers to the mylohyoid muscle is given off before the interior alveolar nerve enters the mandibular foramen.)

The inferior dental plexus is a series of fine branches intermingling within the bone, giving off two definite sets: the inferior dental branches, which go to the mandibular molars and premolars (entering through the single or multiple foramina at the tip of each root) and the inferior gingival branches, which supply the gums.

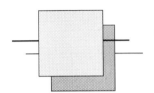

Part Two: Anesthesia

Motor and Sensory Nerves

There are two types of nerves: motor and sensory. The motor nerves control the function of muscle fibers; the sensory nerves carry messages to the brain from their sensory endings.

The message that cries "Pain!" to the brain must be received or perceived before the person is aware of pain. If the perception of this message is interfered with by some chemical means, the individual is **anesthetized.** If the message is not permitted to leave the area of origin, the anesthesia is **local.** If the message is sent but not perceived by the brain, the anesthesia is **general.**

How We Sense Pain

The function of the nerves is to carry a message from the sense organ (for example, in your fingertip) to the central nervous system, and also from the central nervous system back to muscles or glands that in turn translate the return message into action. The nerves act exactly like the telephone wire that connects your telephone to the central office—they conduct an impulse, or message. Nerves can be seen. They appear as long cords of whitish, translucent material. Large nerve "trunks" may be half an inch in width and at their terminal distribution have end branches so tiny as to be almost invisible. The messages, or impulses, that these nerves transmit or carry are actually tiny electrical impulses. On an "incoming" message these impulses are read in the spinal cord and brain. The brain and spinal cord again make up the answering message, or signal, and send it out along the nerve trunk to the proper place for action.

Let's take an example. Imagine that your finger is touching a hot stove. The sense organs in the deeper layers of the skin feel the excessive heat and are stimulated or excited, and electrical impulses leave the sense organ to travel along the nerve to the spinal cord and brain. There the message is interpreted to indicate that your finger has been placed in contact with a hot stove. Immediately another message is relayed from the brain and spinal cord as a series of impulses along a nerve trunk, finally reaching the muscles that move your finger, hand, and arm. The muscles accept the order and promptly remove your finger from the hot stove—and have most likely been told to take it to your mouth so that you could have another set of muscles squeeze air out of your lungs to blow on the hot finger!

Prevention of Pain

The word **pain** is derived from the Latin *poena,* meaning "penalty." Humans have been trying since the earliest of times to eliminate pain from their sensations, and perhaps thought of pain as a penalty for misbehavior in much the same way that disease or injury also was thought to be a penalty.

Pain is a very personal and individual experience. What one person considers pain may not be considered pain by another person. A pain that is intolerable to one person may be quite tolerable to someone else. Our response is conditioned by practice, by general health, by mental conditions, and by environment, and many of these can change from day to day or hour to hour.

Anesthesia, from the Greek *an + aisthēsia* meaning "not feeling," is the word given to the state or condition that exists when the sensation of pain has been eliminated. The word is used whether the entire body or only a part is involved. More correctly *anesthesia* is used to indicate a lack of sensibility to impressions of any kind that originate from outside the area concerned (again, whether it be the entire body or a part of the body).

An *anesthetic* is an agent that is capable of producing anesthesia.

General Anesthesia

In **general anesthesia,** the brain and spinal cord are no longer able to read messages or to send out messages, except for a few that are set on "automatic," such as breathing and heartbeat. While under general anesthesia, therefore, the patient will feel no pain since the general anesthesia produces unconsciousness, and as a result, the message or impulses cannot be "read" by the spinal cord and brain.

Ether was one of the earliest agents used to produce anesthesia, as was nitrous oxide. While the arguments about names and dates still do occur, it should be remembered that there have been instances when various people have actually made numerous discoveries but have not publicized them. Sometimes a later worker in the same field of research repeated the identical discovery and, because he made it known, became the one credited with the original discovery. This has been the case with early work with general anesthesia. Oxygen and nitrous oxide, the gases, were discovered by Joseph Priestley in 1772, but their use as an anesthetic agent was not known. It wasn't until December 1844 that Horace Wells, a dentist, had nitrous oxide used as an anesthetic on himself for the removal of a tooth. William T. G. Morton first demonstrated in public in October 1846 the use of ether to stop pain in surgery.

The use of nitrous oxide requires a "gas machine," a mechanism for mixing nitrous oxide gas with oxygen in the proper proportion to produce and maintain anesthesia. The mechanism provides a support for cylinders of gases that are attached to mixing valves, pressure gauges, hoses, mask, and breathing bag for the patient.

While nitrous oxide with oxygen continues to be administered as an inhalant anesthetic, there are also other combinations and other inhalant anesthetics. The oral surgeon will select the combination of anesthesia and tranquilizers that he or she prefers.

Analgesia

Analgesia is the loss of the ability to feel pain without loss of consciousness. This insensibility to pain is "general" as it is in general anesthesia. Often the same anesthetic agent is used to produce analgesia when inhaled

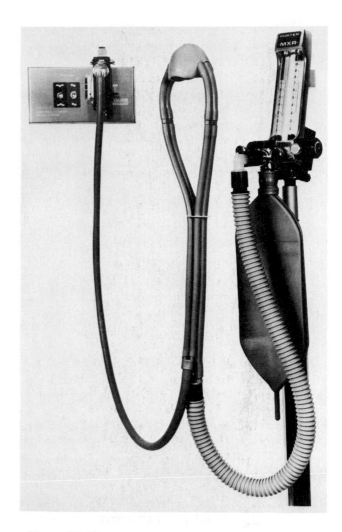

Figure 21.19
Wall mount unit by Porter for the administration of nitrous oxide and oxygen.

in smaller quantity as is used to produce anesthesia when higher concentrations or greater quantities are inhaled. This is true of nitrous oxide and oxygen.

Generally, the patient controls the amount of the gas inhaled for analgesia. If the patient begins to pass from analgesia into anesthesia, he or she also loses control of the equipment, which is generally made to automatically reduce or completely stop providing anesthetic gas if the patient is unable to squeeze a bulb or hold a slide against the pressure of a spring.

As a dental assistant, you will not be required to give general anesthesia. It is given by a person thoroughly trained in anesthesia, under conditions that provide the patient with every safeguard possible. While there are dental offices that are able to meet these requirements, they are not common.

If analgesia is used in the office in which you are employed, you will be expected to learn the proper use and care of the equipment concerned. This should be

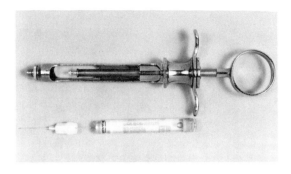

Figure 21.20
Local anesthetic syringe, disposable needle, and carpule.

carefully and thoroughly studied, because there are dangers present whenever an anesthetic agent is used, whether for analgesia or for anesthesia, whether it is a local or a general anesthetic.

Local Anesthesia

In **local anesthesia,** the manner in which the patient is relieved of the sensation of pain is somewhat different from the manner in which general anesthesia relieves pain.

Local anesthesia is by far the most common form of anesthesia for dentistry and is produced by using a syringe to inject the anesthetic agent into an area that is as close as possible to the nerve the dentist desires to anesthetize.

The local anesthetic agent is particularly attracted to the actual nerve fibers that make up the "telephone line." When a quantity of this agent is placed where it will infiltrate (soak into) the area through which a nerve passes, it especially seems to soak into the nerve fibers and incapacitates the nerve. Impulses or messages will no longer be able to pass the point at which the local anesthetic agent has been absorbed by the nerve until the agent has been carried away by the blood circulation in the area.

There is an additional peculiarity in this situation. The feeling of numbness that occurs when a local anesthetic is blocking a nerve at a given spot seems to extend from the spot at which it actually is soaking into the nerve all the way to the end of the nerve at the sensory organs. If, for example, all the nerve trunks at your elbow were penetrated with local anesthetic solution, your arm from the elbow to the fingertips would feel numb, or "asleep."

To help maintain this condition of local anesthesia, the anesthetic agents are commonly used with another chemical that acts as a **vasoconstrictor,** a chemical or drug that shrinks or constricts the blood vessels in the injected area to retard or slow down the rate at which the blood stream can circulate so that

it cannot carry away the local anesthetic solution as rapidly.

The original local anesthetic was **procaine hydrochloride,** which was made in a laboratory by Einhorn in 1905. It was introduced as **Novocaine,** a product of the Noval Chemical Company, and this name is used by the public today for all local anesthetic agents, whether or not they are procaine hydrochloride. Others used are metycaine, nupercaine, pontocaine, and lidocaine hydrochloride; almost all have trade names by which they are known and sold by dental supply houses.

Local anesthetic solutions as discussed above are designed to produce anesthesia when injected close to a nerve or nerve trunk. Few of these solutions will produce any anesthetic action when applied on the surface of the mucous membrane (the lining of the mouth) or on the surface of the skin.

Topical Anesthesia

There are anesthetic agents, however, that are designed to work when applied to the surface of the mucous membrane. They are called **topical anesthetics** and can be found as liquids or as pastes. Many dentists use a topical anesthetic on the mucous membrane before injecting a local anesthetic solution, since most of the discomfort of an injection is caused at the surface of the mucous membrane by the act of puncture with the hypodermic syringe.

Summary

Anatomy is the science of form, structure, and interrelationships of the parts of an animal body. The study of anatomy of the head and neck is important to dentistry.

Osteology of the skull includes the recognition of twenty-eight bones of the skull and the hyoid bone, on which important functions of the mouth depend.

Of importance to dentistry are the *mandible* (lower jaw) and the *maxillae* (two bones forming the upper jaw). The two *temporomandibular joints* permit the mandible to move.

The *hyoid bone* is a horseshoe-shaped bone lying in the anterior part of the neck below the mandible. It serves as an attachment for many muscles that interact to open the jaw and move the tongue.

The muscles with which dentistry is concerned are striated muscles (voluntary muscles). There are five areas of muscle involved in the use of the mouth and jaws: *mastication, suprahyoids, infrahyoids, muscles of the face,* and *muscles of the tongue.*

Saliva is manufactured in the salivary glands, of which there are three major glands: the *sublingual,* the *submandibular,* and the *parotid.*

Anatomical landmarks can be utilized in learning the necessary anatomy of the head and neck.

Teeth are *occluding* when the mouth is closing and are *in occlusion* when the mouth is closed and the upper and lower arches are touching. Each individual has two sets of teeth: *primary* and *permanent* or *secondary*. The approximate ages when teeth first appear in the mouth are indicated.

A tooth is composed of *enamel, dentin, pulp chamber,* and *cementum. Incisors* incise (cut) food, *canines* tear food, *premolars* grind food, and *molars* mill food.

A *blood supply* is directed to each area of the mouth.

Nerves may be compared to wires between two telephones. The *fifth cranial nerve* supplies the dental area. *Motor nerves* control the function of muscle fibers. *Sensory nerves* carry the messages to the brain.

Anesthetics are capable of blocking feeling. *General anesthesia* makes it impossible for the brain and spinal cord to recall or send messages. *Analgesia* is loss of ability to feel pain without loss of consciousness. *Local anesthesia* temporarily blocks the ability of a particular nerve to transmit messages. *Topical anesthetic* temporarily blocks the nerves in the surface of the mucous membranes.

Study Questions

1. Describe the bones of the skull that are important to dentistry.
2. Explain the function of the temporomandibular joint.
3. Why is the hyoid bone important?
4. Discuss the muscles of mastication.
5. Explain the function of the suprahyoid and infrahyoid muscles.
6. What are the three major salivary glands, and where are they located?
7. Discuss the anatomical landmarks that are important to dentistry.
8. How many primary teeth are there and how do they differ from permanent dentition?
9. Describe the structure of a tooth.
10. What is meant by *erupt?* When do teeth erupt?
11. Detail the functions of the various types of teeth.
12. Describe the blood supply to the teeth.
13. Describe the nerve supply to the teeth.
14. Differentiate between sensory and motor nerves.
15. Explain how we sense pain.
16. Differentiate between general anesthesia and analgesia.
17. Explain local anesthesia.
18. Discuss topical anesthetics.

Vocabulary

The student is expected to find and memorize definitions within the chapter of the anatomical names of parts of the skull and neck that are important to the study of dentistry, particularly the names of the parts of teeth. The vocabulary drill given here is limited, then, to additional words that might be omitted from the drill on the many definitions within the chapter of anatomical parts.

anatomy   science of form, structure, and interrelationships of the parts of an animal body
articulates   joins
aspect   side or position from which object is viewed
auditory canals   ears
deciduous dentition   primary dentition
foramen   opening in bone
fossa   depressed channel
mandible   lower jaw
maxilla   upper jaw
myology   study of muscles
osteology   study of bones
processes   extensions on bone
sialogogue   substance that increases flow of saliva
striated muscle   voluntary muscle
sutures   immobile bony unions
zygomatic process   cheekbone

Word Elements	
Word Element	*Example*
emesis suffix meaning: vomit	*hematemesis* vomiting blood
emia suffix meaning: blood	*cholemia* excess bile in the blood
hystero combining form meaning: relationship to hysteria (also to uterus)	*hysterical* lack of control over acts and emotions
itis suffix meaning: inflammation of	*gingivitis* inflammation of the gingivae (gums)
myx prefix meaning: mucus	*myxedema* mucinous edema
phage suffix meaning: to eat, devour	*lipophage* a cell that has devoured lipid
plasia suffix meaning: to form	*hyperplasia* excessive formation of normal cells
rhea, rrhea suffix meaning: abnormal or excessive flow	*sialorrhea* excessive flow of saliva
septi prefix meaning: disease produced by microorganisms and their poisonous products	*septicemia* a disease condition caused by microorganisms and their poisons in the blood
toxi prefix meaning: poison	*toxicity* kind and amount of poison produced by a given organism

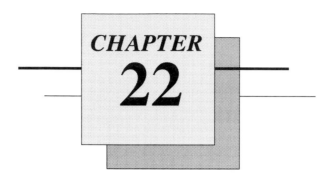

CHAPTER 22

Identification of Teeth and Cavity Classification

Names for Teeth
Written Identification
Tooth Terminology
Identification of Children's Teeth
Cavity Classification for Restoration
Charting

Names for Teeth

Individual teeth have been given specific names (for verbal) and specific systems of annotation (for written) identification in order that we can discuss them intelligently. These names are important to know so that you can recognize the specific tooth and area involved in a planned dental operation, and with this knowledge can be better prepared to assist the dentist.

Assuming we are discussing a mouth that has a complete set of teeth, we have an upper and a lower arch of teeth. Each arch we can imagine as being divided into two halves—the left half and the right half. Since each half-arch is one-quarter of the full set of teeth, we call each half-arch a quadrant. Thus, four quadrants make a complete set of teeth.

Left and *right* are always noted from the patient's point of view. That is, the teeth on the patient's left are annotated as *left* in referring to position. The four quadrants are called the upper left quadrant, the lower left quadrant, the upper right quadrant, and the lower right quadrant (fig. 22.1).

A complete adult dentition contains thirty-two teeth—eight teeth in each quadrant. (Plate 10) The teeth in *each* quadrant, starting from front to back, have the same names, in the same sequence, as the teeth in any other quadrant:

> central incisor
> lateral incisor
> canine (cuspid)
> first premolar (first bicuspid)
> second premolar (second bicuspid)
> first molar
> second molar
> third molar ("wisdom" tooth)

Since this means that in a complete set of teeth we have four teeth with the same name (one in each quadrant), we also add to the name of each tooth the location of the quadrant (fig. 22.1).

The teeth in the upper left quadrant, for example, are labeled as follows:

> upper left central incisor
> upper left lateral incisor
> upper left canine (cuspid)
> upper left first premolar (bicuspid)
> upper left second premolar (bicuspid)

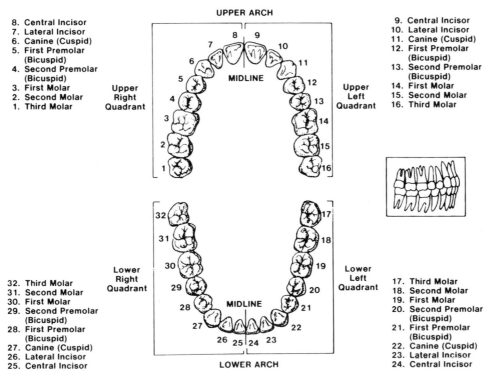

PERMANENT TEETH

UPPER ARCH

8. Central Incisor
7. Lateral Incisor
6. Canine (Cuspid)
5. First Premolar (Bicuspid)
4. Second Premolar (Bicuspid)
3. First Molar
2. Second Molar
1. Third Molar

Upper Right Quadrant

MIDLINE

Upper Left Quadrant

9. Central Incisor
10. Lateral Incisor
11. Canine (Cuspid)
12. First Premolar (Bicuspid)
13. Second Premolar (Bicuspid)
14. First Molar
15. Second Molar
16. Third Molar

32. Third Molar
31. Second Molar
30. First Molar
29. Second Premolar (Bicuspid)
28. First Premolar (Bicuspid)
27. Canine (Cuspid)
26. Lateral Incisor
25. Central Incisor

Lower Right Quadrant

MIDLINE

Lower Left Quadrant

17. Third Molar
18. Second Molar
19. First Molar
20. Second Premolar (Bicuspid)
21. First Premolar (Bicuspid)
22. Canine (Cuspid)
23. Lateral Incisor
24. Central Incisor

LOWER ARCH

Figure 22.1

Schematic drawing showing quadrants, names, and numbers of teeth in both upper and lower arches as you face the patient's mouth.

upper left first molar
upper left second molar
upper left third molar

Each quadrant is similarly labeled—upper right incisor, lower left incisor, and lower right incisor—throughout the entire quadrant.

Written Identification

If we wished to quickly write a list of various teeth, this would be a cumbersome way to write an identification of each tooth; therefore, various shortcuts have been devised to make it easier to write such an indication of a particular tooth. Several methods are used, but each dentist uses only one method routinely in his or her office.

The **universal numbering system** (adopted by the American Dental Association in 1968) is the most commonly used method. The teeth are numbered from one to thirty-two as follows: the upper teeth are numbered in sequence from right to left and the lower teeth in a continuing sequence from left to right. Thus, the upper right third molar is tooth number one; the upper left third molar is tooth number sixteen; the lower left third molar is tooth number seventeen; and the lower right third molar is tooth number thirty-two. This is the most widely used method of tooth identification.

An **alternate method** numbers the teeth in the upper quadrants from one to eight, beginning with the front tooth in each quadrant, as follows:

1. central incisor
2. lateral incisor
3. canine (cuspid)
4. first premolar (bicuspid)
5. second premolar (bicuspid)
6. first molar
7. second molar
8. third molar

In the lower arch, number the teeth in each quadrant from nine to sixteen, beginning with the front tooth in each quadrant, as follows:

9. central incisor
10. lateral incisor
11. canine (cuspid)
12. first premolar (bicuspid)
13. second premolar (bicuspid)
14. first molar
15. second molar
16. third molar

In this method we can tell by the number alone whether the tooth is an upper or a lower tooth. To indicate which side the particular tooth is on, all we need to add is the letter *L* for left side or *R* for right side. Thus, an upper left first molar would be written as "L6," a lower left cuspid as "L11," or a lower right second molar as "R15."

Ask your dentist which method he or she uses. Practice until you can write the correct identification for any tooth easily and quickly.

To help yourself learn this more quickly, first make up a list of the teeth in each quadrant as they are listed in figure 22.1. After each tooth indicate the number and position by the method your dentist uses. Follow this with a fully written list of all thirty-two teeth in a mixed-up order and do the same. Show this listing to your dentist to be checked for error.

Tooth Terminology

Each tooth has five sides (called **surfaces**) that have names for identification either in speech or in writing. The six upper front teeth and six lower front teeth actually have four surfaces and a biting edge, while the back teeth have four sides and the chewing surface. On the six upper and six lower front teeth, these five surfaces are named as follows:

incisal	biting edge
labial (or facial)	surface toward the lip
lingual	surface toward the tongue
mesial	side toward the midline of the arch
distal	side away from the midline of the arch

As a group, the six upper and six lower front teeth are referred to as the *anterior* teeth, **upper anteriors** and **lower anteriors.**

For the back or **posterior** teeth, the five surfaces are named as follows:

occlusal	chewing surface
buccal	surface toward the cheek
lingual	surface toward the tongue
mesial	surface toward the midline of the arch
distal	surface away from the midline of the arch

A tooth touches its neighbor toward the front with its *mesial* surface and its neighbor toward the back with its *distal* surface. Of course the last tooth in each quadrant has no tooth behind it, so its distal surface does not touch another tooth. The two central incisors in each arch are the first teeth in their respective quadrants, and their two mesial surfaces touch each other. Their mesial surfaces both touch the imaginary midline of the dental arches. The portion of a tooth that touches the tooth next to it is called the **contact area.**

You will notice that only the first two surface names differ for anterior and posterior teeth, as listed. The *incisal* edge of the anterior teeth becomes the *occlusal* surface of the posterior teeth, and the *labial* surface of the anterior teeth becomes the *buccal* surface of the posterior teeth. All teeth have a lingual, mesial, and distal surface.

You may be required to write the location of surfaces named by the dentist during an oral examination. There are abbreviations of the surface names. The abbreviations, when written as single surfaces, are:

incisal	Inc	distal	D
occlusal	Occ	lingual	Li
labial	La	mesial	M
buccal	Bu	facial	F

Frequently you will hear references to surfaces in groups of two or three. The surface names take on a uniform change when combined into such groups: mesial and occlusal become **mesio-occlusal;** distal and occlusal change to **disto-occlusal;** and mesial, occlusal, and distal become **mesio-occluso-distal.**

In writing *groups* of surfaces, the following abbreviations are used:

mesio-occlusal	MO
disto-occlusal	DO
mesio-occluso-distal	MOD
mesio-incisal	MI
occluso-lingual	OLi
disto-buccal	DB
mesio-buccal	MB
disto-lingual	DLi
mesio-lingual	MLi
disto-labial	DLa
mesio-labial	MLa

This same pattern is used with all the group abbreviations.

Identification of Children's Teeth

The **primary teeth** are the first set of teeth. They are also properly called the **deciduous teeth,** although this term is not often used. You will hear parents refer to them as *milk teeth* or *baby teeth.*

The child has a complete set of twenty teeth in his or her mouth at approximately two years of age. Their replacement by the permanent teeth begins at about six years of age and is completed at about twelve to thirteen years of age. From the age of six to the age of twelve or thirteen, both primary and permanent teeth usually will be found in the mouth—not all the primary teeth have been shed, and not all the permanent teeth have come into position. This period is referred to as the period of **mixed dentition.**

There are five primary teeth—central incisor, lateral incisor, canine, first molar, and second molar—in each quadrant. The first three are eventually replaced with their identically named permanent teeth, while the last two are replaced by the first and second permanent premolars.

The American Dental Association official method of annotating primary teeth uses the letters *A–T,* starting with the upper right second deciduous molar and following the same pattern as the permanent teeth (fig. 22.2). The upper left second deciduous molar would be *J* and the lower left second deciduous molar would be *K,* with the lower right second deciduous molar labeled *T.*

Another method of annotating these primary teeth uses the subletter *A* on the deciduous tooth that corresponds to the permanent tooth. Thus, the upper left central incisor in the permanent teeth annotation is 9 and in the primary dentition is 9_A. (Compare figures 22.1 and 22.2.)

Cavity Classification for Restoration

Your dentist may indicate the cavity classification for the carious lesion he or she has discovered in examining the patient's mouth as it relates to the preparation necessary for the restoration.

Class I.   Pit and fissure cavities
   a. In the occlusal surfaces of bicuspids and molars
   b. In the occlusal two-thirds of the buccal surfaces of lower molars
   c. In lingual surfaces of upper incisors
   d. In the occlusal one-third of the lingual surfaces of upper molars

Class II.   Cavities that occur in the proximal surfaces of bicuspids and molars and necessitate the involvement of the occlusal surface for restoration

Class III.   Cavities that occur in the proximal surfaces of incisors and cuspids and *do not* involve the removal and restoration of the incisal angles

Class IV.   Cavities that occur in the proximal surfaces of incisors and cuspids and *do* involve the removal and restoration of the incisal angles

Class V.   Cavities that occur in the gingival third of labial, buccal, or lingual surfaces of any teeth

Class VI.   Incisal edges of anterior teeth

In addition, a cavity may be referred to as a simple cavity or a compound cavity. A **simple cavity** involves but one surface of a given tooth; a **compound cavity** involves two or more surfaces of a given tooth.

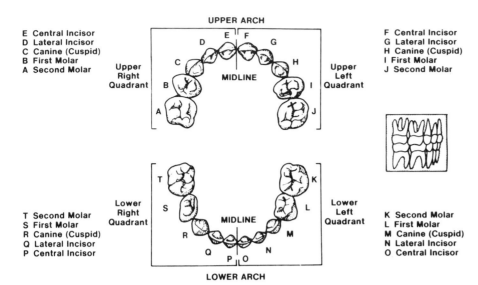

DECIDUOUS TEETH

UPPER ARCH

E Central Incisor
D Lateral Incisor
C Canine (Cuspid)
B First Molar
A Second Molar

Upper Right Quadrant

F Central Incisor
G Lateral Incisor
H Canine (Cuspid)
I First Molar
J Second Molar

Upper Left Quadrant

MIDLINE

Lower Right Quadrant

T Second Molar
S First Molar
R Canine (Cuspid)
Q Lateral Incisor
P Central Incisor

Lower Left Quadrant

K Second Molar
L First Molar
M Canine (Cuspid)
N Lateral Incisor
O Central Incisor

LOWER ARCH

Figure 22.2

Schematic drawing of upper and lower deciduous arches (children's teeth).

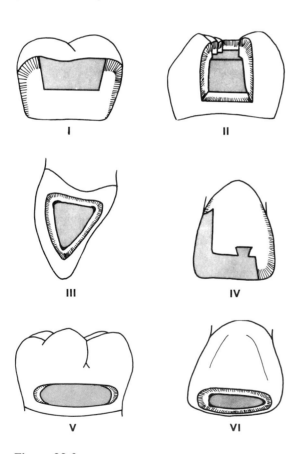

Figure 22.3

Cavity classification: I. pit and fissures; II. proximals of bicuspids and molars; III. proximals of incisors and cuspids not involving incisal angles; IV. proximals of incisors and cuspids involving incisal angles; V. gingival third of labial, buccal, or lingual surfaces of any teeth; and VI. incisal edges of anterior teeth.

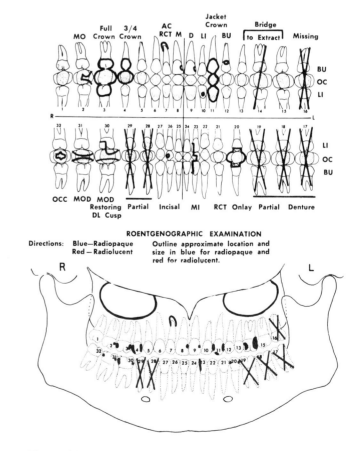

ROENTGENOGRAPHIC EXAMINATION

Directions: Blue—Radiopaque   Outline approximate location and
Red—Radiolucent   size in blue for radiopaque and
red for radiolucent.

Figure 22.4

One method of charting teeth.

Charting

Dentists vary in the type of information they wish recorded in an oral examination. If the patient is new to the dental office, it is well to record all previous work present in the patient's mouth (including the material used for each restoration), the areas that need restoration because of visible caries activity, the restorations that need replacement because they are no longer serviceable, missing teeth, drifting of teeth, information in detail on all oral structures, condition of the gums, presence and depth of periodontal pockets, teeth with questionable prognosis, marginal ridge discrepancies, overhangs, poor or open contacts, mobility, and perhaps other details. On recall examinations, only areas of new caries or new pathological conditions are generally noted.

Charting of the dental restorations already present in the patient's mouth, and the material of which they are constructed, is usually done in detail and must be done accurately if it is to be useful to the dentist. Colored pencils may be used to indicate different materials. On the tooth outlined in the patient's chart, color the restored area with the correct color for that type of restoration.

Regardless of the form or amount of detail required for examinations in your dental office, be very certain *to write legibly and accurately.* If for any reason you do not get one notation written before the next is given, immediately ask your dentist to slow down. Do not expect to remember. There may be so many items that you will be hopelessly confused, and the examination will have to be started over again. You will gradually develop speed in writing these notes as you become more familiar with them. Your dentist will be glad to dictate at a speed at which you can notate accurately if you will ask him or her to do so. The dentist does not usually realize how rapidly he or she gives these notes.

It is preferable to write out fully any terms with which you are not familiar. When you have learned the terms well, then proceed to use the proper abbreviations.

Summary

Identification of teeth requires a fundamental use of technical terms. The dental assistant must learn to use these terms with ease and facility because their use will save time through efficiency and will prevent error through accuracy. The basic technical terms provide the dental assistant with tools with which to work. Practice in their use is essential. Proficiency in their use is very desirable.

Study Questions
1. Name the teeth in each quadrant of the mouth.
2. Identify the teeth by the universal numbering method.
3. Name the five surfaces of the anterior teeth.
4. Name the five surfaces of the posterior teeth.
5. Write the abbreviations of the surface names.
6. Write the abbreviations for groups of surfaces.
7. Describe identification of children's teeth.
8. Describe the cavity classifications in terms of classes.
9. Distinguish between a simple cavity and a compound cavity.
10. Discuss charting of teeth and practice the methods.

Vocabulary
compound cavity   involving two or more surfaces of a given tooth

contact area   area where two teeth touch

deciduous teeth   first set of teeth in a baby

mixed dentition   both primary and permanent teeth are present

primary teeth   first set of teeth in a baby

simple cavity   involving only one surface of a tooth

Tooth Surfaces of Anterior Teeth
incisal   biting edge

labial   surface toward the lip

facial   surface toward the lip

lingual   surface toward the tongue

mesial   side toward the midline of the arch

distal   side away from the midline of the arch

Tooth Surfaces of Posterior Teeth
occlusal   chewing surface

facial   surface toward the cheek

buccal   surface toward the cheek

lingual   surface toward the tongue

mesial   surface toward the midline of the arch

distal   surface away from the midline of the arch

Word Elements	
Word Element	*Example*
cardio, card combining form meaning: heart	***cardiac*** pertaining to the heart, a patient with a heart disorder who may require special care
chole combining form meaning: bile	***acholic*** without bile
denti, dento combining form meaning: tooth	***dentifrice*** a product used to clean teeth
lip combining form meaning: fat	***lipedema*** an excess of liquid and fat in the subcutaneous tissues
osteo prefix meaning: bone	***osteomyelitis*** inflammation of bone
pnea suffix meaning: breath	***dyspnea*** labored or difficult breathing
psych combining form meaning: mind	***psychology*** study of the interactions of living organisms with their environment
stom combining form meaning: mouth, orifice	***stomatitis*** inflammation of the oral cavity
stomy suffix meaning: artificial mouth	***tracheostomy*** surgical creation of an opening in the trachea so air can enter lungs when normal passage is blocked
trophy suffix meaning: nourish	***dystrophy*** defective or faulty nutrition

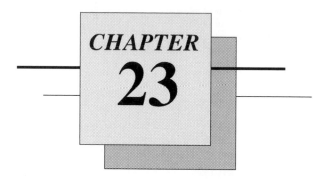

Diet and Nutrition

Food and You
Diet
Nutrition
    The Energy Foods—Proteins, Carbohydrates, and
        Fats
    Minerals
    Vitamins
        The Fat-soluble Vitamins
        The Water-soluble Vitamins
Recommended Dietary Allowances
Diet AND Nutrition
Diet and the Oral Cavity
    Diet for Control of Caries

Food and You

Did you have breakfast? Did you eat an egg? cereal? fruit? . . . or did you just have a cup of coffee?

What did you eat for lunch today? a pizza slice and pop? a hot dog? a doughnut? a gooey sundae?

What you eat determines your vitality, your enthusiasm, and your health—sometimes not immediately, but always eventually! It is a rare person who understands enough about diet and nutrition—or who uses the knowledge to establish the very best diet possible for excellent nutrition. Most of us are inclined to eat for reasons other than health.

We find that present-day psychiatrists are relating eating habits to events in the early stages of a baby's life—whether a baby received enough milk, whether he or she received it when needed, and whether he or she received enough love and cuddling. Many children learn to use food as a weapon in defying their parents. Parents often unwittingly, and sometimes consciously, use food as a reward or punishment. In some homes the parents refer to a food as "good" and to be eaten, yet they don't eat it themselves. Other foods or beverages are called "bad," yet parents indulge themselves in front of their children. Our eating habits are therefore developed emotionally, and we eat to satisfy emotional cravings more frequently than to satisfy our hunger or nourish our bodies.

Diet and nutrition are not one and the same thing. **Diet** refers to everything we eat as food or medication to satisfy a need or an appetite. **Nutrition** refers to how these foods and medications are used by our bodies after we put them in our mouths—their use after assimilation. (Assimilation is the process of the absorbing of food by the digestive organs and turning it into living tissue.)

Food serves three purposes:

1. It provides energy.
2. It regulates body functions.
3. It promotes growth.

A well-balanced diet includes foods that supply all the elements the body needs. If an adequate amount of any one of these elements is not included in the diet *regularly,* your health suffers. Your vitality is lowered, your resistance to fatigue and disease is lowered, your teeth may show more decay, and anemia may develop. Prolonged lack of certain food elements brings on the deficiency diseases: scurvy, rickets, pellagra, beriberi.

Your **appetite** is your pleasant emotional desire for food, and quite probably for specific foods, especially chocolate cake or coconut cream pie, whether or not they are nutritious.

A **nutrient** is a food element that provides material the body cells can use. The essential food elements that must be present in your diet are:

1. Carbohydrates
2. Fats
3. Proteins
4. Minerals
5. Vitamins
6. Water
7. Bulk or roughage

If you see to it that these essential food elements are in your diet, it really does make a difference in your health. Studies show that mental performance may be measurably inferior due to depleted energy, inability to concentrate, and fatigue.[1]

One study of teen-age boys with and without breakfast showed a need for an adequate breakfast if the boys were to be attentive and achieve scholastically in the latter morning hours.[2]

Nervous stability is also affected by malnutrition. Tests show undernourished humans are more irritable and restless.[3] The ability to work physically—strength, speed, endurance, and the amount of work accomplished—is adversely affected by poor nutrition. Illness, resulting in absenteeism from the job, is also found more frequently if an individual has a nutritionally poor diet.[4] It is also reported that resistance to infectious diseases is lowered by poor nutrition[5] and that the body (bony framework and soft tissue) is directly affected by nutrition.

Good nutrition produces larger, stronger bodies. During World War II the diet of children in Norway was changed due to food rationing. They received less sugar and refined carbohydrates and more whole grains and milk. There was a marked improvement in their teeth—less caries. Following the war, the Norwegians returned to a free choice of diet. The caries rate began to increase.[6]

Whether we wish to face up to the facts or not, it remains that nutrition determines the health of our bodies, and eating can no longer be considered just our pleasure. We must feed our bodies for their own good if we wish to live long and feel enthusiastic about doing so.

Diet

We must consume the aforementioned seven essential food elements to meet the nutritional demands of our bodies.

Foods have been grouped into the **Basic Four.** If you see that your diet includes the proper number of foods from each of these four groups every day, you can be *reasonably* certain that your diet is providing the nutrients you need. Beyond that it is important to realize that other foods—those snack or treat foods not included in the Basic Four—usually are actually harmful for you to eat if you are considering your longevity and health.

The foundation food groups, then, are:

1. **Dairy foods.** Milk, including cheese, ice cream, and other milk products. Milk supplies proteins, calcium, minerals, vitamins, and fat. Sometimes it is called nature's most nearly perfect food. Vitamin A is already in the cream, and vitamin D can be added to milk since milk is considered one of the most suitable carriers for vitamin D. Milk provides energy and promotes growth. Drink one to two glasses daily as the minimum requirement for an adult. There are differences of opinion about the quantity of milk needed in the diet. A pint is recommended for everyone, and for some people a larger quantity. Some pediatricians have shown that more than a pint per day may increase the caries rate in the teeth of some children. When this is discovered to be true for a child, his or her milk intake should be restricted to no more than a pint per day.

2. **Meat, poultry, fish, and eggs.** This group may be called the protein group—the tissue-building and tissue-repairing foods. Some of these foods contain iron and other minerals as well as protein. Two or more servings are needed. The servings should be approximately three ounces of cooked meat. At least three eggs per week are recommended for health.

3. **Vegetable-fruit foods.** Four or more servings are needed per day. A dark green or deep yellow vegetable is to be eaten at least every other day and citrus fruit or other rich vitamin C source used daily. Other fruits and vegetables are added to make up the four servings.

    Green and yellow vegetables have a high vitamin A value. They contain carotenes which our bodies are capable of using to form vitamin A. Certain of the leafy vegetables also have iron and calcium in a form that can be used by the body. Some leafy vegetables contain riboflavin and ascorbic acid. Careful preparation is

necessary to keep these food values. This group provides vitamins, minerals (iron and calcium), some proteins, and roughage.

Citrus fruits and tomatoes provide vitamin C or ascorbic acid as well as vitamin A and minerals. The vitamin C is so important that one should always have his or her orange juice or *equivalent* each day.

Potatoes are included each day for their high energy value as well as for the thiamine and iron they add to the diet. Primarily they are a carbohydrate. Other vegetables help the mechanical action of the digestive tract.

4. **Bread or cereal foods.** Four or more servings are suggested, with one slice of bread, two-thirds cup of cooked cereal, or one cup of ready-to-eat cereal constituting a serving. These, of course, should be the enriched, whole grain, or "restored" foods.

    Some of our energy foods (carbohydrates) are found in this group. There are vitamins in whole grain foods also, especially the B complex. Of course, if you are overweight, your physician may reduce your carbohydrate intake.

    Other foods that are to be added to increase the calorie limit to the required amount per day include fats, sweets, unenriched cereals, and flavorings.

Your daily diet, then, should include:

4 servings of vegetables and fruit, including
  2 leafy green or yellow vegetables
  1 orange, or grapefruit or tomato equivalent of the C content of an orange
  1 serving of other vegetables or fruit
  2 servings of meat, fish, or poultry (3-ounce servings)
  2 glasses of milk
  1 egg or a minimum of 3 per week
  4 servings of bread or cereal
  8 glasses of water per day

Coffee and tea do not count as water intake because they contain caffeine, which has a strong diuretic action and causes the elimination of the same quantity of liquid as the coffee or tea you drink.

The other foods that are not listed in the Basic Group should be eaten only after you have had the proper amounts of food from each group of the Basic Four.

Nutrition

Now that you understand the Basic Four, you should learn something about nutrients. Most commonly mentioned as nutrients are foods that can be classified as carbohydrates, fats, proteins, minerals, and vitamins. Some nutritionists mention water as a nutrient; others mention it only as essential to life.

Nutrients are taken into the body in the foods you eat. Then they must be sorted, separated, and simplified so that your body can put them to work. The processes that make these foods part of you are *digestion, absorption,* and *assimilation.* You cannot expect to have a well-nourished body unless the nutrients your body needs are present in adequate amounts in the foods you eat.

Metabolism is the chemical process that releases energy or builds tissue in the body. If the nutrients are lacking, the energy or tissue-building process is affected.

The Energy Foods—Proteins, Carbohydrates, and Fats

We are concerned first with the energy foods. **Energy** is the power for doing work. Our bodies need energy for two kinds of work—that which goes on inside us twenty-four hours a day, the action of the heart, lungs, digestion, etc., and that which we do ourselves externally, like working, playing, swimming, etc.

The amount of energy required varies with the activity of the individual and with his or her age. The energy that the body uses is largely in the form of heat. In nutrition, therefore, we use the heat unit—the Calorie—to measure the energy our bodies use.

A **Calorie** is the amount of heat necessary to raise the temperature of one kilogram of water 1° centigrade.

The body's daily requirement for energy is met by three types of nutrients: carbohydrates, fats, and proteins. These nutrients are found in varying amounts in different foods. Some foods are primarily composed of one of these nutrients and will be so listed in any table of foods.

Carbohydrates: Chemically, carbohydrates are made up of carbon, hydrogen, and oxygen. They contain twice as much hydrogen as oxygen.

Sugars and starches are carbohydrates. Sugar is found dissolved in fruits and vegetables as well as in a package of cane or beet sugar. Starch must be changed to sugar before the body can make use of this nutrient.

One gram of carbohydrate contains four Calories. (Twenty-eight grams is roughly an ounce.)

The body changes carbohydrates to glucose, which then passes to the liver and is used by the body as needed. The glucose not needed immediately is changed to glycogen and is stored in the liver and in the muscles. If more carbohydrates are consumed than the body can use and store as glycogen, they are stored as *fat.*

Fats: Chemically, fats are made up of carbon, hydrogen, and oxygen. They are arranged in different proportions from carbohydrates. Fats are low in oxygen and, therefore, can absorb oxygen in large quantities. Fat burns quickly and gives more than twice as many Calories as carbohydrates or proteins. One gram of fat contains nine Calories; thus, small amounts of fats have high Caloric value.

Fats stay with us because they require more time to digest, which is the reason that a slice of bacon with breakfast makes us feel satiated much longer. Four of the important jobs fats do for our bodies are: (1) carry phosphorus, (2) carry fat-soluble vitamins, (3) conserve body heat, and (4) spare protein since the body will not use protein for energy if there is fat or carbohydrate present in the body.

For digestion, absorption, and assimilation, fat must be broken down into glycerol and fatty acids. Essential fatty acids cannot be synthesized by the body; they must be eaten. However, any excess fat (that which is not utilized by some part of the body during absorption) is stored in the body as *fat.* Since only a small quantity of fat is needed each day, it follows that only a very small amount should be eaten by anyone. People who are overweight can completely eliminate fat from their diets, because the essential fatty acids will be provided by the tiny amount of fat that is inseparable from meat and some other foods. This lack of fat intake will cause the body to draw on its reserve fatty tissue. Since protein foods and carbohydrates also become fat when eaten in excess, overfed Americans need to watch their food intake most carefully.

Proteins: Proteins are the nutrients that build the body, repair worn parts, and supply heat and energy. The word *protein* comes from the Greek *prōteios,* which means "primary or holding first place." Protein is essential to all living plant and animal tissue. Milk, milk products, meat, and eggs are protein foods.

Chemically, the same three elements of carbon, hydrogen, and oxygen are present in protein as in carbohydrates and fats. There are also the elements nitrogen, sulphur, and sometimes phosphorus and iron. Proteins are made of amino acids, the materials with which our body can build or rebuild tissue. Amino acids are the final products of digestion of protein. In a watery solution, the amino acids are absorbed through the walls of the small intestine into the bloodstream. They are carried to the liver and then to the tissues and organs of the body. The tissues and organs select the amino acids they need. What acids are not used by the body are returned to the liver. The nitrogen in them is removed and excreted. Then the remaining carbon, hydrogen, and oxygen can be used for energy—or if not needed immediately, stored as fat.

One of the important points to remember about the differences between amino acids and the final products of carbohydrate and fat digestion is that amino acids provide nitrogen in addition to carbon, hydrogen, and oxygen. Nitrogen is essential to every cell of the body and thus to life itself. But if you eat more protein than you need for building, repairing, and maintaining the cells of your body, the excess is stored as fat, just like the carbohydrate and fat excesses you may eat as cookies or sweets.

Minerals

The body is made up of cells, tissues, and organs. They in turn are composed of different chemical elements. Chemical elements are the building blocks of the body. Carbon, oxygen, and hydrogen are the chief elements of the body. Nitrogen is a fourth important element. These four elements make up 96 percent of the body weight and are supplied by carbohydrates, fats, and proteins in our food. These, the energy foods, we have just discussed. Let us turn our attention to the other elements.

Four percent of the total body weight is composed of mineral elements. They are small but exceedingly important to life. Other minerals present in trace amounts, considered to be essential to health, are cobalt, fluorine, molybdenum, silicon, and zinc.

Although they may only be needed in minute amounts, mineral elements are essential and must be present in the diet to maintain life. It is not possible to say that because calcium and phosphorus are required in larger quantities, they are therefore more important to the body. Iron is one of the most vital elements for the well-being of the body. However, only a few thousandths of a gram is needed daily. (**Iron** is needed for making hemoglobin. **Copper** is necessary to the making of hemoglobin, but it is not present in hemoglobin.)

Most of the metallic elements needed in trace amounts seem to be useful as part of the enzymes, hormones, or vitamins necessary to create some essential chemical reaction in the tissues. **Cobalt** is known to be an essential component in vitamin B_{12} (the vitamin that helps form new red blood corpuscles). **Iodine** is a necessary part of the hormone *thyroxine,* made by the thyroid gland. **Zinc** is used as part of the pancreatic hormone *insulin.* **Magnesium** has been linked to some enzymes that are necessary to body oxidation.

Table 23.1
Percent of Body Weight Composed of Mineral Elements

Elements	Percentage of Total Body Weight
Calcium and phosphorus	2.3–3.4%
Potassium, sulfur, chlorine, sodium, and magnesium	0.95%
Iron	0.004%
Manganese	0.0003%
Copper	0.00015%
Iodine	0.00004%

Most of the trace elements are found in so many foods that they are usually provided by a normal diet. One exception is iodine. There are sections of the country where a lack of iodine in the water causes a greater incidence of thyroid problems.

Fluorine is not considered an essential nutrient, but it is an element that is very important to dental health. Water containing one part fluorine per million parts water is considered safe. Large amounts of fluorine have caused stiffening of the backbone and mottling of teeth. Test studies have shown that dental caries is reduced or arrested in young children when they drink water that has up to one part per million of fluorine.

The need for mineral elements is summarized in table 23.2. Bones and teeth need **calcium** and **phosphorus.** There are two to three times as much calcium and phosphorus in the body as the other elements, most of it in the bones and teeth. However, calcium is present in blood plasma, also. Calcium is needed for blood clotting. It is also needed for muscle tone, for proper regulation of the heart (with **sodium, potassium,** and **magnesium**). The *parathyroid gland* regulates the blood calcium level through its hormone. *Vitamin D* is required for the utilization of calcium.

Phosphorus has more uses in the body than any other element: tooth development; skeletal growth; carbohydrate, fat, and protein metabolism; brain and nerve metabolism—all are affected by phosphorus. It is vital to the functions of the cells of the body's soft tissues as well as the bones and teeth. Whole blood contains phosphorus.

Iron is concentrated in the blood, specifically in the red corpuscles. It is also found in the liver, spleen, and bone marrow. Iron has a special ability to be alternately oxidized and reduced; that is, to take on oxygen and later give it up. It is precious to the body, but it is difficult for the body to absorb it from food. However, the body stores this element and uses it over and over again. The best sources for humans are liver,

Table 23.2
Body's Need for Minerals

Minerals Needed	Purpose	Penalty If Lacking
Calcium	Build bones and teeth; regulate body processes, especially clotting of blood	Rickets Malformed teeth Caries
Phosphorus		Stunted growth Soft or weak bones

All salts
  potassium
  sulfur
  chlorine
  phosphorus
	Build soft tissues including muscles	

Phosphorus and all salts	Nervous tissue	
Iron, calcium, phosphorus, sodium, and chlorine	Blood	Nutritional anemia
Sulfur	Skin, nails, hair	
Iodine	Thyroid secretion needs iodine	Enlargement of thyroid gland
Iron and iodine	Allow oxidation in digestion	
All salts	Maintain normal exchange of body fluids	

eggs, lean meats, legumes, nuts, dried fruits, whole grains, and all green, leafy vegetables. Milk is poor in iron value.

Copper is necessary for the production of red corpuscles, although copper will not be found in the blood.

Iodine is most essential to the body. Each cell has traces of iodine in it. About three-fifths of the iodine in the body is in the thyroid gland, located in the neck. This gland selects iodine from the blood, stores it, and uses it to make thyroxine, the hormone so necessary for metabolism. The thyroid gland mixes iodine and an amino acid called tyrosine to obtain thyroxine. *Thyroxine* regulates the rate of body metabolism. Physical changes go on in the body whereby the chemical energy in food is changed to heat that the body can use for its work.

Minerals are equally important with energy foods and proteins as nutrients. Minerals are tissue builders, repairers, and aids to digestion. Calcium, iron, and iodine are very important. Calcium and phosphorus (usually considered together) build strong bones, sound teeth, and regulate the body processes. Calcium and phosphorus are found in large quantities in milk and milk products. Some nutrients our bodies need are found in food in a form our bodies cannot use—cannot assimilate. The calcium and phosphorus must be in a usable form. Iron builds rich, red blood and is needed for carrying oxygen to all parts of the body. Iodine is usually

found in saltwater fish and shellfish. It is also found in water, but certain parts of the country (around the Great Lakes) have a low iodine content in the soil and water. In these parts of the country, people should use salt that has been iodized.

Mineral elements are not used up nor do they provide energy. When they are no longer needed, they are discarded. A regular supply is needed to keep up with the body's process of using and discarding them.

Most mineral salts are water-soluble.

Vitamins

Vitamins are body regulators. They are defined as organic compounds different from any food materials, needed only in small amounts, but necessary for normal growth, regulation of the body functions, and the protection and maintenance of health. Vitamins must be supplied in food. They are either fat-soluble or water-soluble. They have been named and numbered. The **fat-soluble vitamins** are A, D, E, K; the **water-soluble vitamins** are the B complexes and vitamin C. Fat-soluble means "stored in fats in the bloodstream." Water-soluble means "carried by water," and water-soluble vitamins are much harder to control because they can escape from a leafy vegetable into the water in which it is cooked.

Vitamins promote growth, the ability to produce healthy offspring, normal functioning of the digestive tract, good nutrition, and central nervous system stability. They also regulate health of the body tissues and resistance to bacterial infections.

Vitamin deficiency causes illnesses. A multiple vitamin deficiency refers to a lack of several vitamins in the body.

The Fat-soluble Vitamins

Vitamin A: This vitamin may either be present in the body as vitamin A or be formed in the body from carotene. When vitamin A is present in foods as vitamin A, it is called *preformed vitamin A*. Some of the carotene in foods is converted into vitamin A in the intestines during digestion. Carotene is called *provitamin A*. Carotene is found in both animal and vegetable foods, but preformed vitamin A is present only in animal foods.

Vitamin A is essential to growth, is important for resistance to infection, is necessary for vision (functional night blindness is due to an insufficient supply of vitamin A), prevents certain eye diseases, increases longevity, delays senility, and aids bodily functions.

Sources of vitamin A are liver, spinach, carrots, and sweet potatoes. (A two-ounce serving of liver provides three times as much vitamin A as the next most important source. Liver is the body organ that stores vitamin A, thus its high content.)

The most important sources of vitamin A and the number of international units of vitamin A these foods contain are shown in table 23.3.

Table 23.3
Sources and International Units of Vitamin A

Food	Measure	International Units of Vitamin A
Liver, beef	2 oz.	30,330
Spinach	½ cup	10,600
Carrots	½ cup	9,000
Sweet potato	one, medium	9,000
Cantaloupe	½ melon	6,600
Squash, winter yellow	½ cup	6,350
Broccoli	½ cup	2,550
Apricots, dried, cooked	½ cup	2,290
Tomato juice, canned	½ cup	1,270

It is possible to have too much vitamin A in your diet. The Council on Foods and Nutrition of the American Medical Association has warned that taking vitamin A in excess of 50,000 international units over a prolonged period of time can result in loss of appetite, irritability, and bone and joint pains.

Vitamin D: There are two forms of this vitamin found in the body: preformed and provitamin. Vitamin D is needed for the utilization of calcium and phosphorus in the normal nourishment of bones and teeth. It helps make and keep a satisfactory balance between calcium and phosphorus in the body. A serious shortage of this vitamin produces a disease called rickets. Bones bend easily and sometimes are malformed. Teeth erupt early and decay readily.

Vitamin D is found in its most concentrated form in an oil that contains ergosterol. The ergosterol (from yeast) is irradiated and then dissolved in the oil. It is used by the *drop* because it is so powerful. It is regularly added to milk. Other sources are butter, egg yolk, beef liver, salmon, sardines, cod liver oil, and halibut liver oil. Another excellent source is sunlight. The recommended dietary allowance for vitamin D is 400 international units per day for all ages.

Vitamin D is stored in the liver. It is stable and does not disappear with normal cooking temperatures. Excesses of this vitamin can cause toxicity, illness, nausea, diarrhea, and loss of appetite. Usually an overdose is unintentional. No figure is given for an overdose since this varies with individuals and how much sunlight they receive.

Vitamin E: This vitamin is important because it can unite with oxygen and protect red blood cells from being destroyed by such substances as hydrogen peroxide. It also prevents the destruction of vitamin A and carotene by oxidation in the body and in foods. It is stored in the body in muscles and fat deposits. It is not affected by ordinary cooking temperatures. Since it is fat-soluble, it is not dissolved in cooking water. It isn't likely that anyone will be short of vitamin E. It is present in wheat germ, leafy vegetables, legumes, whole grains, vegetables, oils, liver, butter, milk, and eggs.

Vitamin K: Vitamin K is essential to normal clotting of the blood and normal functioning of the liver. It has not been possible to determine a dietary allowance since the natural sources of vitamin K vary with the individual human. Vitamin K_1 is found in common foods: green, leafy vegetables, egg yolk, and organ meats. Vitamin K_2 is produced by intestinal bacteria and varies from individual to individual.

The Water-soluble Vitamins

The water-soluble vitamins are the larger group. All of the B vitamins and vitamin C, or ascorbic acid, are water-soluble. They generally are not stored in the body.

This means that the possibility of toxicity from an overdose is not possible as with the fat-soluble vitamins.

Three of the B complex are better known vitamins, and dietary allowances have been established for them. We will consider them first.

Thiamine or B₁: Thiamine is one of the first three B vitamins that function together to make it possible for carbohydrate to "burn" at body temperature. It is known as the appetite vitamin. In addition, its uses include helping the nervous system to function normally and helping carbohydrate metabolism. Deficiency in thiamine hydrochloride or B₁ results in beriberi.

Some of its best sources are whole grains, enriched flours and breads, lean pork, peas, liver, milk, vegetables, and fruits. It is difficult to find a very rich source. One must eat several foods to maintain the minimum daily requirement.

Riboflavin B₂: Also known as G, vitamin B₂ is necessary for growth of all tissues of the body and for maintenance of healthy skin. Deficiency in this vitamin produces cheilosis. Lesions are present on the lips, the tongue is sore and purplish, and the skin of the nose is rough and scaly.

The major sources of riboflavin are in three groups: milk, meats, and grains.

Riboflavin can be lost in discarded cooking water and meat drippings. It is unstable when exposed to direct sunlight, daylight, or artificial light. It is best to store milk in paper or dark-brown glass containers.

Niacin: The third vitamin of the B complex, niacin is concerned with the problems of translating sources of energy into energy that the body can burn and is also helpful in cellular respiration. Lack of niacin (or nicotinic acid) produces a disease called pellagra. It is known as the disease of the three *d's*—dermatitis, diarrhea, and dementia. If the disease is not treated, dementia eventually occurs and death follows.

Niacin is available to the body in two forms, niacin and proniacin. Proniacin is tryptophan—one of the amino acids. The human body can make 1 mg. of niacin from 50 to 60 mg. of tryptophan.

The other water-soluble vitamins: Other water-soluble B vitamins that are nutritionally important include: folacin, B₆, B₁₂, pantothenic acid, biotin, and choline.

Vitamin C, ascorbic acid: Ascorbic acid, or vitamin C, is very important in our diet. It prevents scurvy. It is used to help make a substance that binds cells together. If this material is weak, the walls of small blood vessels will hemorrhage. Hemorrhage commonly occurs in the gums. Ascorbic acid also helps build body resistance to bacterial infection and helps heal wounds. It is an unstable vitamin and must be supplied daily.

Health can be poor if the intake of C is low, even though it is high enough to prevent scurvy. People can be irritable, have minor illnesses, and be generally listless.

Ascorbic acid is found in greatest concentration in citrus fruits, especially oranges. Since ascorbic acid is unstable and can be destroyed by oxidation, care must be used in handling foods high in ascorbic acid. The recommended dietary allowance for ascorbic acid is 70 mg. daily. To be safe, for daily use it is advisable to choose a very rich source of vitamin C, such as an orange.

Recommended Dietary Allowances

Opinions about diet have changed. It has been decided Americans need fewer Calories per day because we are not as active as the day laborer of years ago, or our life is more sedentary. Each individual's daily Calorie intake is determined by his or her height, ideal weight, size of build, age, and physical activity. It is recognized now that the weight reached by twenty-five to thirty years of age should be maintained throughout life.

It becomes increasingly evident that in planning meals and re-forming one's eating habits, it is necessary to recognize that certain foods must be eaten for adequate body nourishment. After the food plan has included all the necessary items for nutrition, it is possible to build to the total Caloric consumption allowed for that day with foods that you eat strictly for pleasure. Not only is it necessary to eat the foods recommended for daily diet each day, but also to select the type of meat, the individual vegetables, fruits, and other foods that together provide you with the correct amount of vitamins, minerals, carbohydrates, proteins, and fats needed for complete nourishment of your body. Emphasis was formerly on providing *enough* food elements, with no thought of harm from overproviding. We must now face the recognition that it may be just as harmful to overeat, to provide too many nutrients. It isn't enough to say that you will eat two servings of meat, four of vegetables and fruits, two servings of milk, and four servings of breadstuffs. It is necessary to check these food items for their nutrient content as well as for their Caloric content.

Eating to keep our bodies healthy rather than satisfying emotional needs may take severe self-discipline. Habits formed even beginning in early childhood influence our reaction to food subconsciously. Food becomes a symbol of many different things as we grow up. It may become a reward or a punishment symbol with some families. It may have been used by the child to control his or her parents (by eating, refusing to eat, creating a scene). In some homes the food is not nutritious, and food habits are built around a poor diet and habit sets in. Many adults eat as they do because they acquired the habit of eating in such a fashion from long exposure to certain foods. A "finicky" eater (one who doesn't like certain foods and makes his or her dislikes known to everyone) conditions little children to such eating patterns. A child learns to eat by example, and parents need to eat well-balanced, nutritionally excellent meals if they expect their children to do likewise.

It is wise to remember that appetite is our desire for food and the pleasure we remember from eating. Hunger is our need for food. Few of us are ever really hungry. The sensations we experience that we think of as hunger are often the result of emotional problems.

It can be a very satisfying experience to learn about good nutrition and change our eating habits to give us the opportunity to have better health, disposition, and longevity.

Diet AND Nutrition

We have said that food serves three purposes: to provide energy, to regulate body functions, and to promote growth.

The essential food elements that serve the first purpose are carbohydrates, fats, and proteins. They are high in calories. They furnish heat and energy. If you eat more carbohydrates and fat than you need, the excess is stored in your body as fat. If you have a tendency to overweight, avoid that cinnamon roll or candy bar!

The essential food elements that serve the second purpose, regulating body functions, are the following:

Proteins	Build and repair body tissue (except body fat).
Some Minerals	Regulate body functions. Example, iodine regulates the rate at which the body uses other energy foods.
Water	Aids in regulation of body functions, such as digestion and elimination of body waste. Controls temperature.
Vitamins	Promote growth and help the body remain healthy and vigorous.
Roughage	Aids in the elimination of body waste.

The third purpose of food, promoting growth, is accomplished by these elements:

Proteins	Build and rebuild tissue.
Minerals	For calcification. They build teeth, build and repair bones, and build blood.
Water	The structure of all body tissue is composed of cells. Cells need water to maintain life.

It is possible to plan an adequate diet to satisfy all these nutritional needs of the body. The best way for the average person to be certain that he or she is nourishing his or her body as well as satisfying the appetite for food is to use the Basic Four as a daily plan of diet, checking carefully, at least for a time, to be certain that the menus so planned do include the necessary daily food nutrients.

A brief summary of the important functions of vitamins will help clarify the deficiency diseases that can be encountered in the dental office from insufficient nutrients. **Vitamin A** is necessary for: (1) growth, (2) vision, and (3) structure and function of the epithelial tissue. Lack of vitamin A may cause night blindness and xerophthalmia (dry eye), retarded growth, defective tooth formation, changes in the epithelial tissue, and increased susceptibility to infection.

Vitamin B is important to cellular processes concerned with internal respiration, so the functioning of the circulatory system is affected. It is important to prevent a breakdown of the capillary wall and to provide for absorption of food elements through the alimentary system. Deficiencies of B or B complex vitamins 1, 2 through 6, and 12 lead to some symptoms such as beriberi, blurred vision, burning and soreness of the eyes, inflammation of the tongue, premature aging, and fissuring at the corners of the mouth, pellagra and upset of the functioning of the nervous and digestive systems, dermatitis, and pernicious anemia.

Vitamin C is important for maintaining blood vessels, tooth development, and health of the gums. Scurvy, bleeding gums, hemorrhages around bones, and tendency to bruise easily are results of low vitamin C intake.

Vitamin D is necessary for the regulation of metabolism and building and maintaining bones and teeth. Rickets, soft bones, dental decay, and poor development of teeth are results of vitamin D deficiency.

Vitamin E is considered the reproductive vitamin and seems to show some relationship to the normal reproduction function.

Vitamin K is important to normal blood clotting. Hemorrhages result if there is a lack of vitamin K.

Diet and the Oral Cavity

Certain diseases and mouth conditions result from insufficient nutrients. (See "Oral Pathology" for further discussion of this topic.)

The supporting tissue of the teeth will not be healthy without an adequate vitamin C intake. Sometimes the deficiency shows in bleeding gums. If the deficiency continues over a long period of time, scurvy results.

Vitamin B is important in preventing a breakdown of the capillary wall. Milk in proper quantities will prevent this breakdown.

The effect of carbohydrate (especially the refined carbohydrates—sugar, candy, gum) on the oral cavity is particularly important. The use of too much sugar, especially in children, is responsible for much dental caries. The time of day that sugar is used is also important. Snacks should not be of high sugar content and should be followed by careful cleansing. Use raw apples, celery, or carrot sticks to cleanse teeth at the close of a meal or snack, if brushing is impossible.

Diet for Control of Caries

Some individuals have an unusually high degree of susceptibility to dental decay. These people should adhere strictly to a special diet for the reduction of decay. If the problem is less serious, they may follow the diet less strictly, remembering that its extreme form is intended for individuals with a very high rate of decay.

Food habits in general warrant a careful scrutiny to improve general nutrition as well as to limit or eliminate foods that are high in refined starches and sugars. Sumter S. Arnim, D.D.S., Ph.D., of the University of Texas, Dental Branch, has suggested a dietary regime for caries control, which is given in table 23.4. The patient's physician should be consulted before the dietary change is made in case any item should be restricted or omitted. In the list of foods to be included each day, the amount indicated is a minimum; the patient may use as much as he or she wishes.

Some general suggestions should be stressed in conversing with the patient about the dietary regime. They include:

1. Finish a meal with a piece of raw fruit or a raw vegetable, such as celery, carrot, apple, or orange. These foods act as a cleanser, removing some of the deposits of soft foods left from eating the meal.
2. Sugar-free gums following a meal may be helpful, but avoid the use of sugar-sweetened chewing gum. Each stick contain one-half teaspoonful of sugar.

Table 23.4
Diet Suggestions for Control of Caries

Include Daily
1 pint of milk: whole, skim, or buttermilk
1 egg
vegetables, especially leafy green and yellow, preferably 1 raw each day
potato, cooked in the skin is best
butter or substitutes, enriched margarine
cream, cheese, other fats
lean meats, poultry, fish, liver
fresh fruits, unsweetened fruit juice, canned or fresh citrus fruits

Limit
bread to 1 or 2 slices a meal; at least half should be whole wheat
biscuits to 1 a day
cereals to 1 serving a day, cooked preferred
hot breads to 1 piece if made without sugar

Omit or Greatly Restrict
sugar, syrups, molasses, jam, jellies, preserves, honey, candy, soft drinks, sundaes, ice cream, sherbet, milk shakes, sodas, cookies, crackers, cakes, pastries
fruits canned or prepared with sugar
salad dressings prepared with sugar or starch
sweet pickles, ketchup, chili sauce
chewing gum that is sweetened with sugar

---

3. Substitute oranges, apples, and other fresh fruits or vegetables for the in-between meal snack. Avoid the snacks of candy, sweet carbonated beverage, cake, peanut butter and jelly sandwich, and processed cheeses. Many processed cheeses contain sugar. Use the natural cheeses instead because they contain minerals and vitamins and are a valuable addition to the diet.

The most successful method of stopping carious lesions is the use of restorations. Restorations have served for many years as effective agents for controlling the ravages of this disease. When the diseased portion of the tooth is surgically removed by the dentist and the remaining tooth substance correctly prepared to receive a restoration, and that restoration is placed, one may safely assume that the carious process has been stopped. Unfortunately, that portion of the tooth which has not been protected with a restoration is still susceptible to dental caries.

Careful mouth examinations, with X rays, at regular intervals are necessary for early diagnosis. It is especially important that we instruct our patients (and follow our own advice) to have all carious lesions treated as soon as we detect them. It is the dentist's responsibility to prevent the ravages of this universal disease by using all means at his or her disposal:

> *early diagnosis*
> *preventive measures, and*
> *restorations properly made.*

An important factor to remember about sugar and sweets in connection with diet for caries control is that it isn't the quantity. It is the fact that caries-producing materials are in the mouth. If sweets are used, follow them with a thorough cleansing, including brushing *immediately.* The sooner the residue is removed from the teeth and oral tissues, the less damage will occur.

It has also been suggested that if one insists on eating sticky rolls, he or she should eat them at a meal with other foods that will help remove the gummy caramel from the teeth as the food is eaten. As a separate snack, they create a caries-inviting environment.

Nutrition is important, then, for your teeth and mouth because what you eat as a child influences largely the calcification of your permanent dentition. The prenatal diet of the mother influences largely the calcification of the deciduous teeth of the baby.

There is no way to separate the health of one part of the body from the rest of the body. All the parts are interdependent, and a good, well-balanced diet with sufficient nutrients in a form that can be utilized by the body is the best way to preserve the health of the dental organs—or any other organ.

The diet of the late teen-age period is usually poor, unbalanced—overloaded with refined carbohydrates. The nutritionists believe that the diet during these years directly affects the ability of the young woman to carry a baby effectively during the young adult years. What you eat as a late teen-ager affects your health and the health of any children you may have in the early adult years!

Diet, health, and longevity have been associated in a strikingly clear statement by a well-known authority in nutrition and public health, H. W. Sebrell. He says, "Diet is one of the most important factors in determining how long an individual lives. . . . Even though you never suffer from acute malnutrition, years and years of improper eating will add up to various kinds of damages to your body that will eventually shorten your life. . . . While a good diet can't guarantee that you will be in good health, you can't be in the best of health unless you live on a good diet."

Now to return to your lunch.

What will you have tomorrow? a coke? a caramel roll? a malt?

. . . or a meat sandwich, milk, and carrot straws?

How about breakfast? The milk, fruit, egg, and toast or cereal that you need? . . . or a cup of coffee?

Summary

Diet refers to everything we eat to satisfy a need or an appetite. *Nutrition* refers to how the foods and medications are used after assimilation.

Food serves three purposes: provides energy, regulates body functions, and promotes growth. The essential elements needed in the diet are carbohydrates, fats, proteins, minerals, vitamins, water, and bulk or roughage.

Nutrients must be changed into simplified forms for absorption by the cells. *Energy foods* are proteins, carbohydrates, and fats. We measure energy by the Calorie, a unit of heat.

Chemical elements form the tissues of the body. *Vitamins* are body regulators. The recommended dietary allowances are based on research findings and should be used as a guide in planning the food intake of each individual.

Eating is closely related to emotions. *Appetite* is the desire for food. *Hunger* is the need for food. Most of us eat to satisfy emotional needs. We need to consider nutrition in planning our diets to properly nourish our bodies so we can enjoy a healthier and longer life.

Diet also affects oral health. Certain diseases and mouth conditions result from insufficient nutrients. *When* snacks are eaten, as well as *what* food is used for the snack, is important when considering the effect of snacks on teeth. *Adequate care of the oral cavity after eating is essential.*

Study Questions

1. Differentiate between diet and nutrition.
2. Name the energy foods.
3. What are the three purposes of food?
4. Why should we limit our fat intake?
5. Discuss the Basic Four food groups.
6. Discuss vitamins.
7. Discuss essential elements for nutrition.
8. Why do we have a conflict between diet and proper nutrition?
9. Discuss the effect of diet on the oral cavity.
10. Discuss proper care of the oral cavity following eating.

Vocabulary

appetite   desire for food
Calorie   the amount of heat necessary to raise the temperature of one kilogram of water one degree centigrade
diet   what we eat
energy   the power for doing work
fat-soluble vitamins   A, D, E, K
hunger   the need for food
metabolism   chemical process which releases energy or builds tissue in the body

nutrition   how our diets are utilized after assimilation by the body
water-soluble vitamins   C, B complex

Word Elements	
Word Element	*Example*
bronch, broncho root word meaning: windpipe	***bronchitis*** inflammation of the bronchi
cerebro root word meaning: brain	***cerebrum*** main portion of the brain
cerv root word meaning: neck	***cervical line*** line at which cementum meets enamel on a tooth
cheilo, cheil root word meaning: lip	***cheilosis*** fissuring at the corners of the mouth
chondr, chondro, chondri, chondrio combining form meaning: relationship to cartilage	***chondroseptum*** the cartilaginous part of the nasal septum
gastr root word meaning: stomach	***digastric muscle*** a muscle with two bellies. (The muscle that assists in the opening of the mouth is digastric.)
hem, hema, hemo, hemat root word meaning: blood	***hemorrhage*** copious bleeding
nephr root word meaning: kidney	***nephritis*** inflammation of the kidney
os, osteo root word meaning: bone	***osteoblast*** bone forming cells
pneum, pnea, pnoe root word meaning: lung, air	***pneumatic*** operated by air pressure

Microbiology and Sterilization

Part One: Microbiology
Understanding Microbiology
Bacteriology
    Protozoa
    Fungi
    Rickettsiae
    Viruses
Part Two: Sterilization and Related Processes
Practical Applications
Cleanliness
    Scrubbing procedure
    Cleansing the Environment
Preparation of Materials for Disinfecting and
        Sterilizing
Sanitizing and Disinfecting
    Chemical Agents
    Sanitizing by Boiling in Water
Sterilization
    Purposes in Sterilizing
    Autoclave
    Dry Heat
    Ethylene Oxide Sterilizers
Cleanliness and Sterilization Routine Reviewed

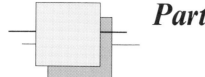

Part One: Microbiology

Understanding Microbiology

Microbiology is the science of the nature, life, and actions of microorganisms—those organisms visible only through a microscope. These microscopic organisms are either animal or plant. Bacteria, protozoa, algae, fungi, rickettsiae, and viruses make up the microorganisms (although some viruses differ from true microorganisms in some respects).

While each group has some members that are pathogenic (cause disease) in man, not all are by any means harmful to man. This is a common misconception of the importance of microorganisms in everyday life. The truth is that without bacteria there could be no other living thing in the world. All plant and animal life is dependent upon the fertility of the soil. Soil fertility depends, in turn, upon the activity of the microorganisms that inhabit the soil in inconceivable numbers.

Knowledge of the existence of a world of small creatures was noted in the early part of the seventeenth century. The major advancements came at a much later date and were the product of the labors of many persons, but notably of the three mentioned here.

Louis Pasteur (1822–1895) was a French chemist. His earliest work in the field of bacteriology was concerned with beer and wine, the process of fermentation, then diseases of silkworms. His later work was concerned with isolating the causative bacteria in other diseases, some affecting man. You may be familiar with his name as used in the "pasteurization" of milk.

Joseph Lister (1827–1912) was an English surgeon, considered to be the founder of antiseptic surgery but whose work involved many other aspects of surgical procedures.

Robert Koch (1843–1910), a German bacteriologist, was awarded the Nobel prize for medicine in 1905. Koch developed the conditions that he felt must be met to prove a given bacterium was the cause of a given disease. Known as Koch's law, the conditions are these: the microorganism must be present in every case of the disease; it must be capable of cultivation in pure culture; it must, when inoculated in pure culture, produce the disease in susceptible animals. To these has been added a fourth condition: the organism must be recovered and again grown in pure culture.

Bacteriology

Bacteriology is the science and study of bacteria, a very large group of one-celled microorganisms. They do not contain chlorophyll. In structure and form (morphologically) these microorganisms exist as oval or spherical cells called **cocci,** or they exist as cylindrically shaped rods called **bacilli.**

The two general morphologic types of bacteria—bacilli (rod-shaped), and cocci (spherical)—also have many variations. Some bacilli are slender with parallel sides, others are short and fat with rounded sides, some have pointed or tapered ends, others are flat-ended. Some bacilli occur singly, others lie end to end in pairs or chains, or they may be stacked. Those bacilli that are curved are called **spirilla** (spiral-shaped) or **vibrios** (comma-shaped). Spirilla also may occur in many forms. They may have a single curve, may be coiled, may have many curves, or may be coiled and curved at the same time.

Cocci are named by size and arrangement, rather than by variations in shape. Occurring singly after division, they are called **micrococci;** if they remain in pairs, **diplococci;** in chains, **streptococci;** in sheets or grape-like clusters, **staphylococci;** in cubes or packets of eight, **sarcinae.**

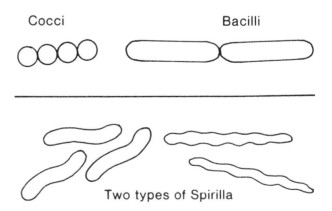

Cocci   Bacilli

Two types of Spirilla

Figure 24.1
Representative cell shapes of bacteria.

Bacteria are **aerobic,** requiring free oxygen in order to survive, or **anaerobic,** able to live without oxygen. Some can live under either condition and are called **facultative** aerobes or anaerobes. The cells are either **motile,** able to move under their own power, or **nonmotile,** unable to move by themselves. If they exist on living hosts, they are **parasites;** if they exist on dead hosts, **saprophytes.** Again, some bacteria can do either and are called facultative parasites, while others are true parasites.

In cell structure, it is evident that the bacterial cell is extremely complex. It is known that a definite cell wall exists, surrounding the **protoplasm** of the cell. In addition to the cell wall, many bacteria have a **slime layer** that, when enlarged or thickened, is called a capsule. The **capsule** is a defensive structure for the protection of the bacteria and is usually present on a pathogenic organism. The capsule is one type of cell structure.

Bacteria may also have organs of locomotion, called **flagella.** If the organism is flagellated, it is motile; otherwise it is nonmotile. Special stains are required to make the flagella visible under the microscope. Flagella are a second type of cell structure.

Bacterial cells reproduce by division. The material of the cell itself increases in volume; spherical forms become oval, and rod forms become nearly double their original length. The cell becomes constricted at the middle, and eventually the cell contents are held in two compartments separated by a wall formed at the place of constriction. Soon the separation is complete—two new individuals, or daughter cells, have been formed that are exactly the same as the mother cell and identical to each other.

Some species of bacteria also are capable of a third morphology (form) called a **spore,** and considered a form of hibernation. Spores generally are formed when conditions for reproducing by division have become unsatisfactory for any reason, such as dryness, heat, cold, or through the presence of a chemical substance that is poisonous. In some cases, spores are formed in the normal life cycle of the bacteria. The spore form of the organism is most difficult to destroy. Some sporulating organisms have been known to remain alive for more than ten years (the organisms capable of multiplication only by cell division usually are dead in twelve months or less). Later, when conditions are right for the sporulating organism, the spore becomes a cell again. Either the spore wall softens, thins, and the cell assumes its typical form (called **vegetative**), or the wall of the spore thins and breaks down either at one end or the middle of the cell, permitting the cell

contents to emerge and assume the typical form, leaving the empty spore shell behind. The spore form is a third type of cell structure.

Spores are by nature of their structure extremely resistant to the usual types of sterilization. They will survive hours of boiling and dry heat of more than 100°. No method of sterilization can be considered satisfactory and entirely safe if it ignores the sporogenic types of bacteria.

Microorganisms are so tiny that a small dot could cover as many as 250,000 bacteria of average size. The unit of measurement used for such tiny sizes is the micron μ, which is 1/1000 of a millimeter, or roughly 1/25,000 of an inch. An average bacillus may measure about 2 microns in length and ½ micron in width; but there is a considerable variation in size. Lengths of 40 microns may occur; others are as short as 0.4 of a micron. The cocci, or round forms, may be between 0.8 and 1.3 of a micron in diameter.

Bacteria are identified in various ways. In cultivating growths or colonies of the unknown bacteria in a laboratory, the addition of certain chemicals to the **media,** or material on which the bacteria can grow, might stimulate certain species to grow more rapidly, while the growth of others might be slowed. The media may be either a broth (liquid) or agar-agar (a gel-like solid). When various dyes are placed in the media, some species will absorb the color, others will not. If blood is added to the media, some pathogens may destroy the red blood cells, others will not. All these tests give a basis for determining the particular bacteria under examination.

One of the most common staining techniques used in identifying bacteria is called the **Gram stain,** named for the man who developed the technique. Some bacteria will withstand decolorizing agents such as alcohol and acetone, while others will not. In applying this test, a prepared sample of the organism (usually on a glass slide) is first washed with a purple stain, then decolorized; then a red counterstain is applied. The organisms that resist the decolorization remain purple in color and are said to be **gram positive.** Those that do not resist the decolorization lose the purple dye and take on the red color of the counterstain. These organisms are called **gram negative.** This test is widely used to tell the difference between organisms that frequently appear identical.

Many types of stain tests are used in bacteriology, but it is not necessary to investigate further. If the office in which you are employed has special reason to use tests of this nature, the required techniques will be taught to you.

Protozoa

The **protozoa** are the simplest form of animal life, because they are essentially one-celled animals. Each single protozoan must perform all the life processes we have described for humans. Yet humans have a multiplicity of cells and systems with which to achieve these functions. Therefore, the one-celled protozoan is indeed a highly complex organism.

Protozoa generally require a fluid environment for active life. They are found in pools and puddles, oceans, lakes, in bodies of higher animals and plants, as well as in soil—wherever moisture is present. In a dormant state, they may exist in dry conditions.

At times no definite line can be drawn at this primitive level between animal and plant kingdoms. For example, some of the flagellated protozoa contain chlorophyll. Under certain conditions they may synthesize food as do green plants; under other conditions they are able to engulf and digest solid food. The majority of protozoa are aerobic.

Protozoa reproduce mainly by binary fission, budding, and sporulation. Sporulation is especially characteristic of the parasitic forms that have been most intensively studied because they produce diseases in humans. Of these, the most well known are the malarial organisms.

Fungi

The **fungi** are a low form of plant life. They are, however, without chlorophyll. The four classes are Phycomycetes, Ascomycetes, Basidiomycetes, and Fungi Imperfecti. Most of the pathogenic fungi belong to the Fungi Imperfecti.

Fungi reproduce by spores, which may consist of one or many cells.

Since fungi do not have chlorophyll, they are dependent on other plants or animals for food. When the food is obtained from living organisms, the fungi are parasitic; when (as is more common) it is obtained from dead remains, the fungi are termed saprophytes. The number of species is probably in excess of 100,000.

The **yeasts** and **molds** are fungi. The drug penicillin is a product of the fungus *Penicillium notatum*. Another fungus, the common mushroom, *Psalliota campestris*, is a wholesome food. *Candida albicans* is the fungi responsible for the disease we know as thrush. Thus, fungi provide humans with medicine, food, and disease.

Rickettsiae

These microorganisms are smaller than bacteria but larger than most viruses. **Rickettsiae** are pathogenic parasites, which can survive only briefly outside their host. The natural hosts of these microbes include a variety of small animals, arthropods, and humans. Humans become infected by rickettsiae only through the bites of infected arthropods (lice, fleas, ticks, mites, and so on). Rickettsiae are difficult to grow under laboratory conditions.

Rickettsia rickettsi is that species which is the causative agent of Rocky Mountain spotted fever. Other diseases found in man are: Q fever (caused by *Coxiella burneti*), trench fever (*Rochalimaea quintana*), epidemic typhus (*Rickettsia prowazeki*), and Boutonneuse fever (*R. conori*).

Viruses

The **virus** (Latin: poison) organism is even smaller than the rickettsiae. In fact, most viruses are impossible to see in an ordinary microscope. They usually will pass through a filter that catches bacterial forms.

A virus is a bundle of genetic material surrounded by a tough protein coat that protects it from the environment. Viruses cannot be grown on inanimate (non-living) media, such as the broth that can be used to cultivate bacteria. Rather, they must be grown in cell tissue cultures (a group of living animal cells) or in proliferating embryonic cells.

Since viruses are made up only of genetic material, they are incapable of reproduction unless attached to an animal cell. Strangely enough, the virus uses this cell's reproductive apparatus to reproduce the virus's own genetic material.

The ultraviruses, those of the smallest particle size, are about 10 millimicrons. The larger sizes range up to 200 millimicrons.

The better-known viral diseases are rabies, encephalitis lethargica, poliomyelitis, herpes facialis, herpes zoster, smallpox, chickenpox, the common cold, yellow fever, influenza of various types, mumps, and infectious and serum hepatitis.

In the case of the two types of hepatitis and other diseases caused by the viruses, the low "dosage" required to produce infection is amazing. As little as 0.0004 ml of contaminated blood or serum will produce infection.[1]

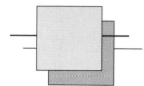

Part Two: Sterilization and Related Processes

Practical Applications

Procedures in the dental office must protect patients from the pathogenic organisms that flourish. The average adult mouth contains a total of 160,000,000,000,000,000,000,000,000,000,000 microorganisms.[2] The organisms may include hepatitis, syphilis, or tuberculosis in addition to such common annoyances as colds. The spread of these microorganisms from one patient to another (called **cross-infection**) must be prevented by using proper techniques of cleanliness, disinfection, and sterilization.

Always prepare instruments and equipment as you would prepare them for use in your own mouth.

Proper sterilization of instruments, materials, and equipment in the dental office is one of the greatest responsibilities of the dental assistant toward the patients who come for treatment.

Unless you have had training in hospital surgical procedures, be assured that you will confuse cleanliness with sterility. You can care for instruments, for example, with a high degree of cleanliness, and yet not have sterile instruments. Conversely, you will not have sterile instruments without a habit of cleanliness in their care and handling. In many cases, in the dental office particularly, it is not always possible to sterilize everything in the true sense of the word. The effort should be made, however, to approach sterility as much as possible.

We have discussed the general groups of microorganisms that concern us: bacteria, protozoa, fungi, rickettsiae, and viruses. To do our best to properly prepare instruments, materials, and equipment for the dental patient, *we must proceed as though the most difficult organisms, the bacterial spore forms and certain of the viruses, were to be constantly encountered in routine preparations.*

For example, how resistant are the causative viruses of hepatitis? Experiments have established that they will withstand an *indefinite exposure* to 0.25 percent phenol, 2 percent tricresol, 1:2000 merthiolate, 70 percent alcohol or ether USP. They will withstand for one month or longer exposure to any of the quaternary ammonium disinfectants in any commonly used concentration. The viruses are *not* destroyed by twenty minutes' boiling. Autoclaving, the use of ethylene oxide gas, or exposure to dry heat at 160° C. (320° F.) or higher for one hour are the best methods of destroying them.

How resistant are bacterial spores in some cases? They have been known to withstand boiling water for sixteen hours. It has been suggested that disease-producing spore-forming types of bacteria are rarely encountered in dental practice, which is irrelevant, if true.

As long as infectious and serum hepatitis maintain their present high incidence, in addition to the fact that an individual, though apparently healthy, may have hepatitis and be a carrier, there can be no acceptance of a sterilization procedure that does not adequately consider the destruction of the viruses.

Proper preparation of syringes is so easily accomplished in a modern dental office with modern equipment that no question of their sterility need arise. A presterilized disposable needle is a tremendous aid in the elimination of one source of infection, although the needle does not eliminate the entire problem.

In order to better understand the various methods of preparation and what each can accomplish, it is desirable to define the commonly used terms.

Sterilization is the removal or destruction of all forms of life. Therefore, an object is either sterile or it is not sterile. All forms of life, including spores and viruses, must be destroyed for an object to be considered sterile.

A **germicide** is an agent that kills pathogenic organisms. Many agents that are labeled germicide are not capable of killing *all* pathogenic organisms. Therefore, you must know the capabilities of the agent you are using. (For example, zepheran chloride is not reliable.)

A **disinfectant** is an agent, usually a chemical substance, that destroys or inhibits the microorganisms causing disease. Ordinarily, spores are not destroyed. Usually this refers to an agent that is used, for example, in cleaning a hospital room.

An **antiseptic,** one of a large group of compounds, stops or inhibits the growth of bacteria without necessarily killing them. Alcohol, mercuric chloride, and phenol are examples.

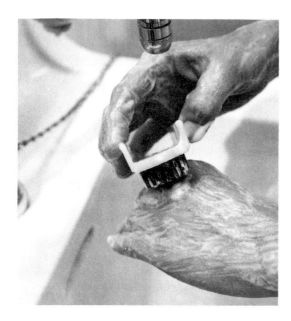

Figure 24.2
Scrubbing the hands.

Various methods of disinfection or sterilization are available to the modern dental office. The choice of method is determined largely by the instruments, equipment, or surgical materials; by their ability to withstand various methods of preparation; and by the necessity to sterilize or merely to disinfect.

Cleanliness

Before anything can be disinfected or sterilized it must be clean. Cleanliness *begins* with the individual staff member.

Foremost in importance is self-cleanliness, or personal hygiene. You cannot possibly have clean instruments and equipment if your own hands and clothing are not clean. Uniforms or other clothing worn in the office must be clean at all times. Hands and arms should be washed thoroughly with a good soap and scrubbed with a hand brush before touching instruments and before assisting with each patient.

A special process known as **scrubbing** is important to practice regularly.

Scrubbing Procedure

1. Turn on the water and adjust the temperature to be warm enough to clean well, but not so hot as to be uncomfortable. If you have a foot or knee control on the faucet, scrubbing will be easier than with hand-operated faucets.

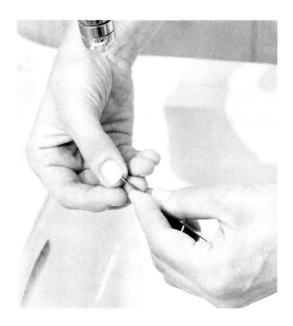

Figure 24.3
Cleaning the fingernails.

2. Wet your hands thoroughly.
3. Apply a generous amount of soap or detergent, either by rubbing the wet bar of soap between your hands or dispensing the proper amount of liquid, powder or leaves from your dispenser.
4. Rub your hands together briskly and work up a good lather. This first soaping is to remove the gross contaminants and dirt.
5. Rinse well under running water until all lather is removed.
6. Add soap or detergent again.
7. Work up a good lather. Rub each side of each finger, massaging the lather between the thumb and fingers of your other hand.
8. Rub between the fingers where they join the hand.
9. Rub well around the fingernails.
10. Use an orangewood stick to clean under each nail if you wish.
11. Use a nail brush to scrub the nail and cuticle of each finger.
12. Scrub the knuckles well.
13. Scrub the palms thoroughly.
14. Scrub the backs of the hands thoroughly.
15. Be sure to wash well above your wrists.
16. Rinse well with lots of running water. Be sure all the soap or detergent residue is removed from arms and hands and from under nails.

17. Dry thoroughly with a clean towel. Be sure to dry under your fingernails, too. Take time to do a good job.
18. Shut the water off. If faucets are hand-operated use your towel over your hand.
19. Set out a fresh towel.

You will notice that this is a thorough process—a time-consuming but necessary step. During the rest of the day it may not be necessary to wash your hands as thoroughly as you should at the beginning of the workday.

In between patients, when you touch your hair, face, or person, you usually do not deposit grime underneath nails or in the crevices of the cuticle. If you have soiled some part of your hands and do need to disinfect them or cleanse them with a bacteria-destroying soap, a good sudsing, brisk rubbing, and thorough rinsing should suffice for almost all necessary washing after the first hospital scrubbing procedure in the morning and again after lunch.

Some of the preparations on the market today actually remove bacteria from the skin and prevent recontamination by bacteria for a few hours. The routine use of these products is better than ordinary soap.

When it is time to disinfect or sterilize instruments, be sure to clean your hands first. They can be washed with detergents containing three-fourths of 1 percent, or less, hexachlorophene, which will reduce the natural skin flora and eliminate the contaminating organisms.

Cleansing the Environment

Next the area must be clean in which sterilization and sanitizing occur.

The residue from bar soap left in a soap dish or the gummy deposits left around the opening on a liquid soap dispenser foster the growth of microorganisms. Be careful to remove these deposits frequently.

Be certain that you have cleaned the laboratory bench and sink where you will sanitize or sterilize.

Now hospitals find that five major sources of bacteria are important causes of cross-infection. These same sources may apply in the dental office:

1. *Dust and dirt on floors* are major sources. Floors should be carpeted or smooth-surfaced and easy to clean. Wet spots of blood, pus, or debris should be wiped up before they can dry and be carried into the air.
2. *Ventilated air.* Fans are taboo in operating rooms. Air conditioners should be mounted five feet above the floor to prevent stirring up of floor bacteria. Humidified air (about

50 percent relative humidity) helps settle airborne bacteria. Aerosols can be used effectively to settle air, but they are not effective if humidity is less than 50 percent.
3. *Respiratory passages* of personnel are a major source of cross-infection both for the individual and for others in the office.
4. *Dirty linen and towels* are a menace to all who handle them.
5. *Dandruff and hair clippings* from a fresh haircut are sources of cross-infection.

With cleanliness of the personnel and area accomplished, the preparation of instruments for sanitizing or sterilizing occurs.

Preparation of Materials for Disinfecting and Sterilizing

Cleaning dirty instruments is a major menace to anyone working with them. It is extremely easy to prick a finger or hand. The dangers of cross-infection for patient, doctor, and staff exist in every operatory. Be careful as you handle these dirty instruments.

Regardless of the method of disinfecting or sterilizing used in your office, the first step is to start with instruments cleaned of all debris, blood, grease, and oil. Bulk-rinse the instruments in a commercial cleaning solvent to remove any possible grease or oil. After this rinsing, the instruments should be individually scrubbed with a brush and a very warm non-ionizing detergent solution. Soaps are quite alkaline and not compatible with germicides; soap residues will prevent disinfection. *Thoroughly* rinse the detergent off the instruments and remove the excess moisture by rolling the group of instruments in a towel.

Pay attention to serrated edges. Be sure they are clean and rinsed. Check movable instruments to see that they are workable. Then wrap them for sterilization.

An alternative method for preparation of instruments for sterilization is to use an **ultrasonic cleaner** which can eliminate much of the danger of infection from working with dirty instruments and will insure thorough removal of the loosened dirt and cleaning solutions. The ultrasonic tank should be cleaned at periodic intervals; rubber gloves should be worn when removing any scum.

There are alternative methods for disinfecting instruments having a sharp or cutting edge. Your office may use chemical solutions, a dry heat oven, or the autoclave.

Several methods for sterilizing and disinfecting are acceptable in dental practice. Some offices use only the one method; others use several. Learn the methods your dentist prefers. With these methods in mind, group the prepared instruments according to the type of sterilizing technique to be used with each group.

With instruments *cleaned,* the next step will be to **sanitize** or **sterilize.**

Sanitizing and Disinfecting

Disinfecting and sanitizing are processes used in the dental office for certain objects. *Do not confuse sanitizing and disinfecting with sterilizing!*

Rubber goods, such as the rubber tip on the saliva ejector hose into which the saliva ejector is placed, can be kept new-looking by wiping with a gauze moistened with benzene. This process merely refreshes the surface of the rubber and does not take the place of disinfection.

All operating levers on the chair, unit, lights, and any other item in the operating room that is touched in the course of treating a patient should be washed frequently with soap and water. Between patients they may be wiped with a gauze moistened with 70 percent isopropyl alcohol or sprayed with a disinfecting spray.

The low-speed handpieces and contra-angles are preferably disinfected and lubricated after each use according to the manufacturer's directions.

Examining lamps may be wiped with 70 percent isopropyl alcohol, but the removable mirrors may be treated by other more effective methods, preferably autoclaving.

Chemical Agents

There are many preparations available to the dental office that are used to make up a disinfecting solution by the addition of water. Many of these chemical disinfectants will not destroy the causative agent of viral hepatitis.

The germicidal solution concentration is critical. Mix it exactly as directed; or use ready-to-use solution or premeasured concentrates.

The quaternary ammonium compounds, such as benzalkonium chloride (zephiran) have soaplike properties and kill ordinary vegetative bacteria. They are used most widely as cold disinfecting solutions. While they have the same limitations of effectiveness as other types of solutions, they have achieved wider use through their nonirritating qualities.

Chemical disinfectants kill microorganisms by coagulating their protein. Dirty instruments, coated with blood and tissue fluids, placed in a chemical disinfectant would result in the coagulation of the surface protein and prevent further penetration of the chemical, thus protecting the microorganisms below the surface. *All instruments going into disinfectants must be*

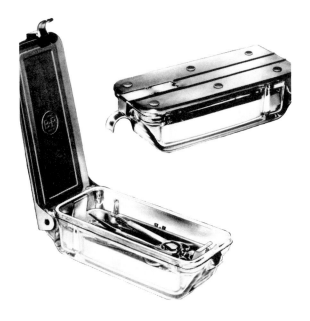

Figure 24.4
An instrument container for use with chemical agents.

clean and free from grease and soap. They must also be dry. Even an autoclave cannot sterilize dirty instruments.

Learn the proper minimum time of immersion for the solution used in your office, as well as the number of days or weeks the solution remains effective for use. Write the date of change on tape that is applied to the container. You will be reminded when it is time to change the solution.

Sanitizing by Boiling in Water

Boiling-water sanitizers are not highly effective. Instruments disinfected in this manner must be boiled for a minimum of ten minutes, completely immersed, and timed after the water is boiling vigorously. Check the water level frequently during the day. Use anti-rust tablets in the water. Dry instruments thoroughly with a sterile towel immediately after removal from the water. Deposits of lime in the boiler itself should be removed regularly, daily if necessary, by draining all the water and scrubbing the boiler with a stiff brush and cleanser. If you have a particularly difficult problem with deposits, you may find it worthwhile to use distilled water instead of tap water.

Many spores will survive hours of boiling water, but most vegetative forms of bacteria are destroyed in ten minutes. Boiling is not recommended for instruments that come into contact with blood or otherwise penetrate the oral mucosa.

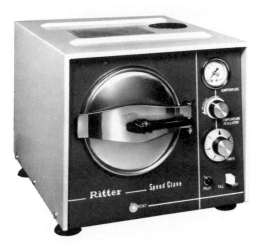

Figure 24.5
An autoclave.

Sterilization

Sterilization is the most exacting process in the entire routine of avoiding cross-infection. The accepted methods of sterilization include:

1. Steam under pressure (autoclave)
2. Ethylene oxide gas
3. Dry heat, prolonged

Be aware of sterilization—what it means and how it is accomplished. *Never substitute a lesser process where sterilization is required.* Be certain that you have sterilized.

Purposes in Sterilizing

The two reasons for sterilizing instruments must be understood by the person who cares for the sterilization. *Instruments are sterilized after use* to prevent cross-infection. These instruments are cleaned and replaced carefully to keep them clean. *Instruments are sterilized before use,* and must be kept sterile for use. They must remain in sterile wrappings or be placed on sterile towels in a sterile cabinet, using sterile tongs so that the instruments are not touched by the person transferring the instruments from the sterilizer to the sterile cabinet.

Instruments should not be touched with hands when removed from the sterilizer. Use transfer forceps or instruments forceps (fig. 24.6). If transfer forceps are not available, the instruments can sometimes be tipped from the sterilizer tray into a sterile towel, the towel folded over the instruments and used to dry them, then used to place the instruments in storage. The instruments that are sterilized after use can be as free from contamination as possible if this toweling process is used.

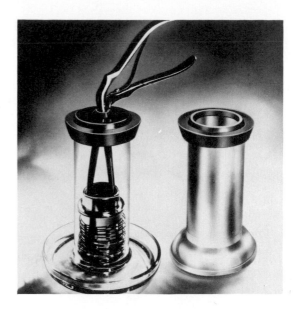

Figure 24.6
Transfer forceps.

Always be certain that your hands are clean when you handle instruments. Even instruments that are sterilized *after* use must be clean for the next use.

Autoclave

Autoclaving is the preferred method of office instrument sterilization. Steam under pressure rises in temperature. It is this rise in temperature, together with the moisture necessarily present, that makes autoclaving so desirable. Less corrosion of sharp-edged instruments occurs. Packaging and loading must be done correctly, and you should regularly test your method of loading the autoclave. Packaging envelopes and tape for sealing wrapped autoclave loads indicate whether sterilization has been achieved. (The envelope or tape changes color.)

An autoclave may be operated correctly to achieve its purpose. No living thing can survive ten minutes of direct exposure to saturated steam at 121° C (249.8° F). When an autoclave is operated correctly (fifteen pounds' pressure at sea level elevation), it achieves these conditions. It is the moist heat that is lethal.

Air must be completely removed from the sterilizing chamber. In most autoclaves this is accomplished automatically, if the operator correctly positions items that can entrap air. Cannisters or open jars wrapped in muslin must be placed on their sides so that air can be "poured" out by displacement with steam. Think of air, in this case, as behaving like water; that is, always place items in such a way that if they contained water instead of air, the water would be able to run out of them. Space items out as much as possible.

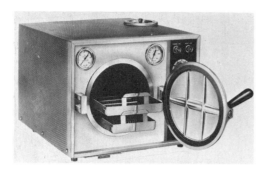

Figure 24.7
Omniclave sterilizer for both heat and steam sterilizing.

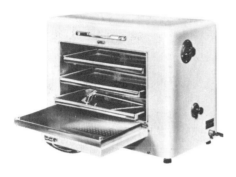

Figure 24.8
Dri-Clave sterilizer for dry heat sterilizing.

Hinged instruments, such as forceps, should be placed in the autoclave in an open or unlocked position so that steam can reach all of the surfaces.

It is possible to autoclave instruments that have sharp cutting edges without damaging them by using one of the products prepared for this purpose. Coating the cutting edge or hinges of scissors and forceps protects them from the steam. Follow the directions for use supplied with the product. An autoclave is shown in figure 24.5.

Dry Heat

Dry heat sterilizers are available in very satisfactory designs for dental office use. A dry heat sterilizer is essentially an oven. Care in loading in order to aid proper circulation of air is important. Dry heat is especially satisfactory for cutting instruments, since corrosion is eliminated.

Instruments must be thoroughly cleaned. Instruments or other materials to be sterilized should be spread out well either on gauze in racks or should be wrapped in aluminum foil. Unusually large loads should be avoided.

Temperature recommended for dry heat sterilizers ranges from 160° to 180° C (320° to 355° F) for at least one hour. When the load in the oven has

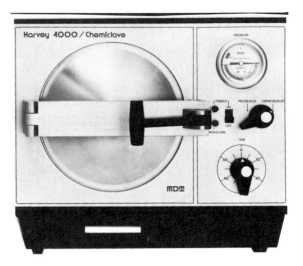

Figure 24.9
The Harvey sterilizer: a vapor-type sterilizer using a special alcohol-base solution called Vapo-steril.

reached this range, the temperature should be maintained for at least one hour—preferably longer.

The factor that is important in dry heat sterilization is to remember that both time and temperature are to be considered in sterilizing. Bacteria in the dry state are more resistant to heat than in the moist state. The time and temperature should be checked very carefully according to the directions with the dry heat sterilizer found in your office.

Dry heat sterilization can be used to sterilize materials that might be affected adversely by steam. Dry heat penetrates organic films on metal, glass, enamel, and anhydrous materials (chemicals, powders, vaseline, oil). It also prevents chemical reactions between medications and glass.

Too high a temperature will shorten the life of materials so sterilized. Some of them may be destroyed by dry heat. It is important to remember this because dry heat penetrates slowly and the inclination of the operator is to hurry the process by increasing the heat. Remember to *take time* when you dry sterilize.

Figure 24.7 shows a combination autoclave-dry heat sterilizer. Figure 24.8 shows a dry heat sterilizer.

Ethylene Oxide Sterilizers

Another method of sterilizing is the use of ethylene oxide gas, used mainly in large institutions such as hospitals and dental school clinics. A moderately heated mixture of ethylene oxide gas is used for some types of sterilization. The temperature is low so that heat-sensitive materials can be sterilized. The directions that are provided with the gas sterilizer should be followed. Figure 24.10 shows an ethylene oxide gas sterilizer.

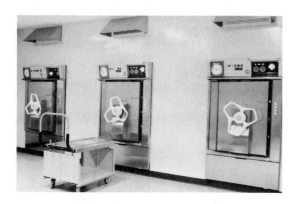

Figure 24.10
An ethylene oxide gas sterilizer.

Cleanliness and Sterilization Routine Reviewed

Clean yourself.

Clean the area in which sterilization is to occur.

Clean the instruments and materials to be sterilized.

Sterilize.

Put away. Be certain that those materials which must remain sterile do remain sterile and that no contamination occurs of the clean instruments which are sterilized after use.

Whatever is done to achieve asepsis in your office, be aware of the need to be constantly on your guard against habits or procedures which prevent the achievement of your primary responsibility: *the protection of your patient, the protection of your doctor, and the protection of yourself.*

Summary

Microbiology is the science of the nature, life, and actions of microorganisms which are either animal or plant. Bacteria, protozoa, algae, fungi, rickettsiae, and viruses make up the microorganisms.

Protection of all persons in the dental office from *cross-infection* requires cleanliness, disinfection, and sterilization procedures. Hospitals suggest five major sources of bacteria that are important causes of cross-infection. These five sources also apply to the dental office problems in cross-infection.

Sterilization is the removal or destruction of all forms of life. A *germicide* is an agent that kills pathogenic organisms. A *disinfectant* is an agent that destroys or inhibits the growth of bacteria without necessarily killing them.

Careful cleansing of all instruments and materials is necessary prior to either disinfecting or sterilizing them.

Disinfectants can be *chemical agents* and *boiling water.*

The approved methods of sterilization are: *steam under pressure (autoclaving), dry heat,* or *ethylene oxide gas.*

Instruments that are sterilized are either sterilized after use to decontaminate them or sterilized before use to prepare them for use on the patient.

Be aware of the procedures that protect the patient, the dentist, and the assistant, and establish them as your routines.

Study Questions
1. Discuss the general morphologic types of bacteria.
2. Why is it important to understand spores?
3. Explain the differences between protozoa, fungi, rickettsiae, and viruses.
4. Why do we sterilize?
5. Discuss the need for cleanliness.
6. What five major sources of bacteria are important causes of cross-infection?
7. Explain scrubbing procedure and its value.
8. Explain the use of chemical agents in the dental office.
9. Describe the three best methods of sterilization.
10. How do you prepare a syringe for sterilization?
11. How do you remove instruments from the sterilizer?
12. How should you prepare instruments for use on patients?

Vocabulary
aerobic bacteria   require free oxygen to survive
anaerobic bacteria   able to live without oxygen
antiseptic   a substance that stops or inhibits the growth of bacteria without necessarily killing them
bacilli   rod-shaped bacteria
bacteria   a large group of one-celled microorganisms, not containing chlorophyll
bacteriology   the science and study of bacteria
capsule   defense structure for protection of bacteria, present usually in pathogenic organisms
cocci   oval or spherically shaped bacteria

cross-infection   transferring infection from one person to another by means of contamination

diplococci   paired cocci after division

disinfectant   an agent that destroys or inhibits microorganisms causing disease

facultative   bacteria able to live either with or without oxygen

flagella   organs of locomotion found on some bacteria

germicide   an agent that kills pathogenic organisms

Gram stain   technique for identifying bacteria

media   material on which bacteria can grow

microbiology   the science of the nature, life, and actions of microorganisms

micrococci   single cocci after division

motile   bacteria able to move under their own power

nonmotile   bacteria unable to move under their own power

parasites   bacteria that live on living hosts

pathogenic   causing disease

protoplasm   the physical basis of all life, found in all cells

saprophytes   bacteria that live on dead hosts

sarcinae   cocci in cubes or packets of eight after division

spirilla   spiral-shaped bacilli

spores   a form of bacteria that can remain alive under difficult conditions; most difficult to destroy

staphylococci   a type of cocci commonly found in grape-like clusters or sheets

sterilization   removal or destruction of all forms of life

streptococci   a type of cocci, commonly found in chains

vibrios   comma-shaped bacilli

Word Elements	
Word Element	*Example*
acro prefix meaning: extremity	*acromegaly* a disease characterized by large extremities
aur combining form meaning: ear	*auricle* part of ear not contained within the head
oto combining form meaning: relationship to ear	*otogenous* originating within the ear
cranio combining form meaning: relationship to the skull	*craniofacial* pertaining to the upper part of the head and the face
derm root word meaning: skin	*dermatosis* any disease of the skin
encephal combining form meaning: brain	*encephalic* within the skull
gingiva root word meaning: gums	*gingivitis* inflammation of the gingiva
glosso root word meaning: tongue	*glossitis* inflammation of the tongue
gnatho root word meaning: jaw	*gnathodynamometer* an instrument used for measuring biting pressure
hepato root word meaning: liver	*hepatitis* inflammation of the liver

CHAPTER 25

Oral Pathology and Dental Caries

Oral Pathology
  Inflammation
  Other Tissue Changes
Dental Caries
  Pulp Reaction
  Periapical Abscess
  Granuloma
  Periodontitis
Control of Dental Caries

Oral Pathology

Pathology (from the Greek *pathos,* meaning disease, and *log,* meaning science of) is that branch of biological science which deals with the nature of disease through a study of its causes, how it proceeds, and its effects, including changes in function and changes in structure. Pathologic changes in the tissues of the body may be caused by microorganisms, wounds or injuries, chemicals, cold or heat, or pressure. These may act individually or several may act together to produce pathologic results.

Oral pathology (diseases of the mouth) concerns the area of immediate interest to the dentist but also includes diseases that affect that area indirectly. Many systemic diseases (diseases of the body as a whole) produce visible effects in the mouth or cause accompanying changes that are apparent in the mouth. Many diseases of the mouth are not related to the teeth.

When we speak of diseases of the teeth themselves, such as **dental caries** (a localized, progressive disintegration of tooth structure) and the abnormal conditions that may follow dental caries, we use the general term **dental pathology,** which means diseases pertaining to or relating to the teeth.

The discussion of oral pathology in this volume will be limited to those diseases which are most frequently of interest to the dental assistant, either as observations in the course of her or his normal duties or as diseases that require certain preparations on the part of the dental assistant in their treatment. (Books are available for the advanced student of oral pathology.)

Inflammation

The response of the tissues of the body to pathologic changes is called **inflammation** (from the Latin *inflammare,* to set on fire). It is the body's defense against injury and disease. Inflammation is indicated in terminology by the suffix *itis.* If we say *gingivitis,* we indicate that the gingival tissues have an inflammatory reaction present. If we say *pulpitis,* we indicate that the pulp of the tooth is undergoing an inflammatory reaction.

The characteristics of inflammation are such basic responses that it is something every person who works in the health profession should know. For the dental assistant, knowledge of the inflammatory process is applied to conditions that commonly occur in the oral cavity.

If you should scratch the skin of your hand with a pin, you would notice a reaction to this injury within minutes. The skin around the scratch would be reddened due to increased blood flow in the area. If you ran your finger across the scratched area, you would feel an elevation of the tissue, indicating that the reddened area is also swollen. This is due to excess fluids

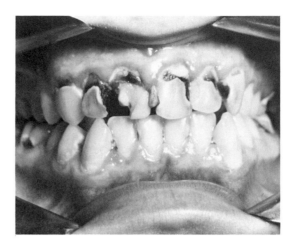

Figure 25.1
Dental disease caused by oral neglect (caries, gingivitis).

from the bloodstream in the tissue, diluting and attacking any toxins that may be present. You would also note increased sensitivity or pain when anything comes in contact with the scratch, causing you to favor the area and avoid further irritation. If you had a delicate thermal-sensitive instrument, you would be able to detect an increase in temperature in the area of the wound due to the increased blood flow. The **cardinal symptoms of inflammation** are *redness, swelling, heat, pain,* and *impairment of function.* If the area were to continue to show a more severe reaction, you would note an increased degree of these cardinal symptoms and, perhaps, the formation of pus.

In the inflammatory reaction, the increase in blood supply (*hyperemia*) brings additional white blood cells (*leukocytes*) and fluids to the damaged area in an effort to fight invading bacteria and toxins. The cells phagocytize the bacteria by engulfing them and destroying them. The leukocytes die in the process, forming what you know as pus.

Immediately after the injury there is an initial constriction of the vessels, followed very closely by a dilation of the vessels, which results in hyperemia. The total current of the blood through the area is slower due to the dilation of the vessels, which permits the blood cells and fluid to penetrate the vessel wall and migrate into the injured or diseased area.

Inflammation of the tissue may be produced by microorganisms, wounds or injuries, chemicals, cold, heat, or pressure. One factor may act alone or several may act together. Some authorities, in discussing inflammation, also include the process of repair, which encompasses new capillary formation, the formation of granulation tissue, organization of the wound, and finally, cicatrization (formation of scar tissue).

Inflammation is a form of body resistance to injury and disease. *Inflammation is a helpful process.*

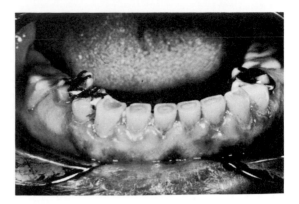

Figure 25.3
Attrition-abrasion (anterior teeth worn down, posterior teeth missing).

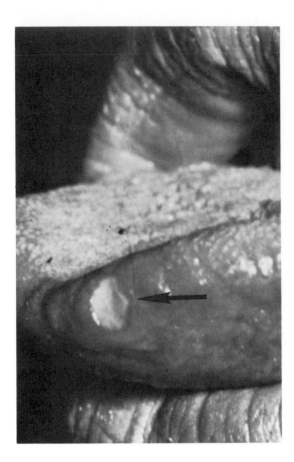

Figure 25.2
Aphthous ulcer.

Other Tissue Changes

If you were to look through a textbook of pathology, you would most likely think, "There are so many disorders and diseases how can anyone be healthy?" Even with reference to those diseases which most directly affect the oral cavity, the number seems overwhelming. In actual practice, however, most dentists will contact but a few pathologic conditions that are not directly associated with gingival, pulpal, or periapical changes in teeth. In dental schools the number will be greatly increased because practicing dentists tend to refer anything unusual for diagnosis and treatment to faculty in these areas.

The diagnosis of oral pathology is not always simple. A **diagnosis** may be made from recognition of the clinical symptoms of the disease alone; this is known as a **clinical diagnosis.** A **differential diagnosis** involves distinguishing between two or more diseases of similar character by comparing symptoms and any other known factors. A diagnosis can only be made after considering all the manifestations of the disease, visualizing the disorder in terms of its physiology and histochemistry, examining a biopsy of the lesion if indicated, conducting clinical tests, and finally, reasoning about the collected data.

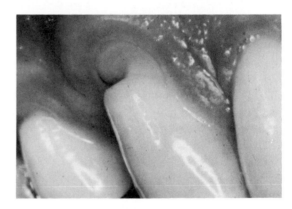

Figure 25.4
Erosion.

Here is a brief list of the conditions that are most commonly observed in the dental office:

Abscess: An abscess is a localized area of pus. In the mouth this may be caused by infection: (1) inside the tooth, resulting in a periapical abscess; (2) alongside the root, resulting in a lateral or periodontal abscess (a periodontal pocket); or (3) around the crown of a partially erupted tooth, resulting in a pericoronal abscess.

Aphthous ulcer (aphthastomatitis): This lesion is commonly called a canker sore. It is an ulcer of unknown origin that appears on the mucous membrane. It is similar to the herpes simplex lesion that occurs on the skin, but the aphthous ulcer is definitely not of viral origin whereas the herpes lesion is.

Attrition, erosion, and abrasion: Pathologic wear from attrition, erosion, or abrasion can lead to pulpal injury (or even exposure) if secondary dentin does not deposit rapidly enough to protect the pulp.

Burns: On occasion, patients may attempt self-medication and place such drugs as aspirin directly on gingival tissues at the site of pain, producing a serious burn lesion.

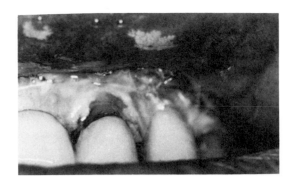

Figure 25.5
Aspirin burn.

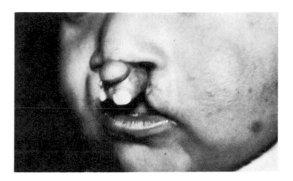

Figure 25.7
Cleft lip and/or palate.

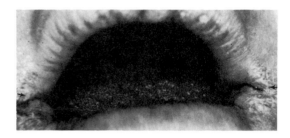

Figure 25.6
Cheilosis.

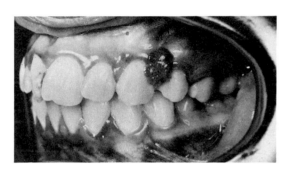

Figure 25.8
Epulis.

Cheilitis: Inflammation of the lip. The lower lip is more often involved. Persons who are outdoors a great deal may have cheilitis occur as a swelling of the lip with a white, leathery covering sprinkled with red areas where erosion has occurred.

Cheilosis: A fissuring at the corners of the mouth due to vitamin B complex deficiency; or in the case of the patient who wears dentures, it may also develop because the vertical dimension (distance of the chin from the nose) is not great enough, resulting in a constant wetness of the corners of the mouth with cracks and fissures eventually forming.

Cleft palate: A condition probably originating early in uterine life (congenital) characterized by the failure of the soft and hard tissues of the palate to join along the midline. When this condition extends through the lip, it is along the lines of the premaxillary region, so that the cleft (or harelip) is visible below the ala of the nose on one side (unilateral) or both sides (bilateral). The premaxillary region is a pie-shaped segment extending its point back to the midline of the hard palate approximately in the region of a line drawn across the palate from first premolar to first premolar. While cleft palate is a failure of two halves to join properly during development, harelip is a failure of one side to join properly with the premaxillary segment on one or both sides.

Diabetes mellitus: A disorder of carbohydrate metabolism. Dental involvement is characterized by multiple periodontal abscesses (which also can be recurrent), changes in alveolar bone, lowered resistance to infection, and slow healing following any oral surgery.

Epulis: Any benign neoplasm of the gingiva, usually pedunculated and raised like a small toadstool.

Exostosis: Overgrowth of bone projecting outward from the usual surface; the most common are the *tori,* bony protuberances occurring along the midline of the hard palate in about 20 percent of the population. (This protuberance is called a *torus palatinus.*) The bilateral or unilateral protuberances occur on the lingual surface of the mandible in the premolar region in about 7 percent of the population (*torus mandibularis*).

Fibroma: A benign neoplasm of fibrous connective tissue.

Fistula: An oral fistula is usually an abnormal passage or communication from an abscess to the outer surface. It may be at the gingival tissue or may drain to the outer skin on the cheek or chin. This is a symptom of trouble that indicates that the body's defenses are unable to cope with some infection, such as that caused by infection within root canals and some periodontal pockets.

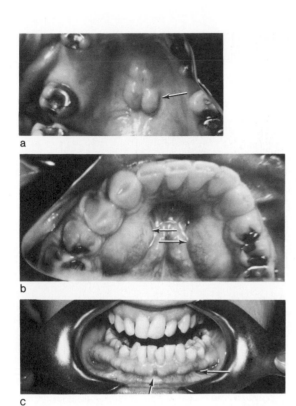

Figure 25.9
Exostosis: (a) palatal; (b) lingual; and (c) labial.

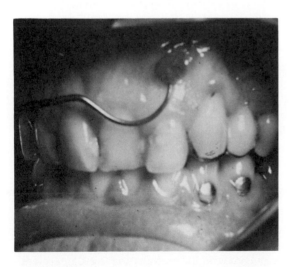

Figure 25.10
Fistula.

Fordyce's spots: Harmless, brownish, slightly raised spots on the oral mucosa or lips, found in more than 70 percent of the population. Erroneously called Fordyce's disease.

Herpes simplex: An infection caused by a virus of the same name. It usually occurs on the skin and rarely on the mucous membrane.

Hyperplasia: The abnormal increase in *number* of normal cells of a tissue, resulting in an enlargement

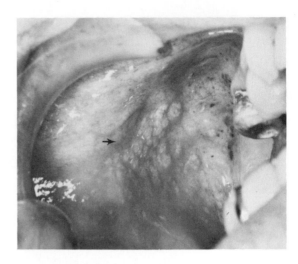

Figure 25.11
Fordyce's spots inside of cheek.

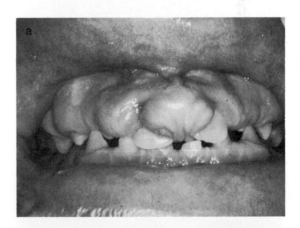

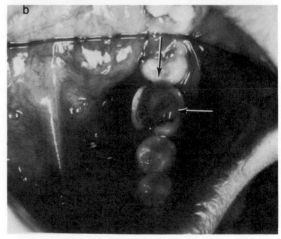

Figure 25.12
(a) Dilantin hyperplasia; and (b) pulpal hyperplasia (soft tissue growing out of pulp).

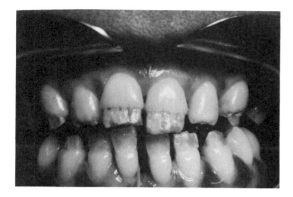

Figure 25.13
Hypoplasia.

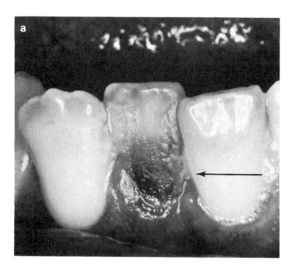

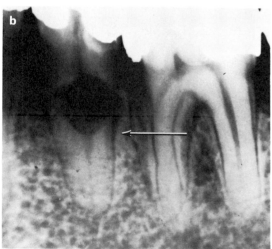

Figure 25.14
(a) Clinical photograph of lower lateral incisor; and (b) radiograph of lower bicuspid; both showing internal resorption.

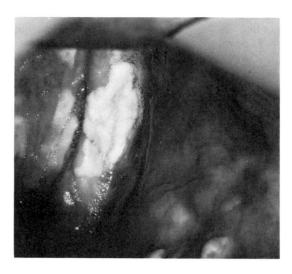

Figure 25.15
Leukoplakia.

or thickening of the tissue. One of the possible reactions of tissue to irritation, injury, or drugs. For example, continued long-term intake of Dilantin to control epileptic seizure may cause the formation of hyperplastic gingival tissue (Dilantin enlargement).

Hypertrophy: The abnormal increase in the *size* of the cells of a tissue, resulting in an enlargement or thickening of the tissue. True or physiologic hypertrophy results from excessive activity of muscle; for example, exercise makes a muscle larger.

Hypoplasia: Defective or incomplete development of any tissue; in dentistry, mostly associated with enamel hypoplasia: pits or ringlike grooves left in enamel due to interference with the function of the ameloblasts (enamel-forming cells) at the particular time this area was being formed. Hypoplasia is often associated with a highly infectious illness with high temperature. The age at which this occurred can be estimated quite accurately by the position of the defect.

Internal resorption: When the resorptive process involves the crown of a tooth and sufficient dentin is destroyed, the translucent enamel shows the pinkness of the vascular tissue underneath. This condition is verified by roentgenographic examination (fig. 25.14, a and b).

Leukoplakia: A white, opaque, leathery plaque formed upon the oral mucous membrane. Considered premalignant. Resembles lichen planus in appearance; differentiated by *biopsy* (the removal of a small tissue sample from the suspect area for the purpose of microscopic examination).

Lichen planus: A disease of unknown etiology affecting either skin or oral mucous membranes, sometimes both together. The oral lesion appears on the buccal mucous membrane most commonly, a lacy pattern of raised bluish-white or white porcelainlike fine lines or dots. Painless and harmless. Distinguished from leukoplakia by biopsy.

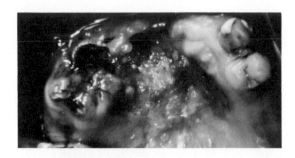

Figure 25.16
Malignancy.

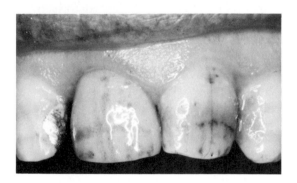

Figure 25.17
Mottled enamel.

Malignant neoplasms (cancer): Can occur in the mouth. Lesions suspected of being malignant are biopsied by the dentist and sent to a pathologist for microscopic examination.

Mottled enamel: Due to excessive intake of fluoride during tooth development. See *fluorosis* in Glossary.

Mucocele: A dilated gland or duct filled with mucous secretion.

Necrotizing ulcerative gingivitis: (Vincent's *gingivitis*): A periodontal disease. The gingival tissues are puffy, red, very painful, and bleed easily. The interdental papillae are gray, necrotic, and contribute to a very foul breath. The patient usually has an elevated temperature and feels sick.

Nevus: A congenital malformation seen occasionally on the oral mucosa; can be vascular (similar to a birthmark) or nonvascular with pigmentation. Some types can develop into malignancies.

Papuloma: A benign neoplasm made up of epithelial cells, warty in appearance.

Periodontitis: Inflammation of the tissues that surround and support the teeth—the gingivae, the cementum of the tooth, the periodontal membrane, and the alveolar and supporting bone.

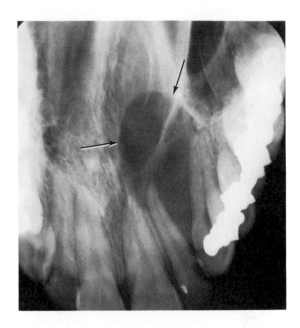

Figure 25.18
Periapical (Root-end) cyst of maxilla.

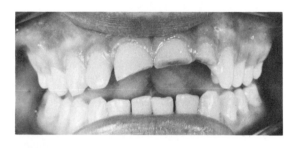

Figure 25.19
Traumatic injury.

Periodontosis (diffuse alveolar atrophy): A noninflammatory condition, affecting the tissues listed under periodontitis, in which the fibers of the periodontal membranes degenerate, alveolar bone is resorbed, and the epithelial attachment is proliferated along the root surfaces. The end result of the process is the loosening and moving of teeth.

Radiation necrosis: Death of the tissue caused by radiation. If treatment of carcinoma (cancer) of the throat, mouth, or lip is undertaken by means of X rays or cobalt, heavy destruction of bone and teeth with formation of a sequestrum (piece of dead bone, usually being expelled from the body) is generally one result. The destruction is apparently more easily controlled when teeth, if present in the area of treatment, are removed prior to exposure.

Residual cyst: An odontogenic cyst that remains within the jaw after the tooth with which it was associated has been removed.

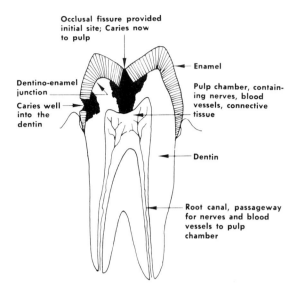

Figure 25.20
Schematic illustration of the progress of dental caries.

Sialolithiasis: The formation of salivary calculi within the ducts of the salivary glands, or the condition or infection caused by such formation.

Stomatitis: A general term for inflammation of the oral cavity, which may occur from bacterial, viral, mechanical, chemical, electrical, thermal, or radiation injury, from allergens, and as secondary (in sequence of time or development) manifestation of a systemic disease. May also occur as a reaction to medications or irritants, or systemic changes such as pregnancy. In the case of pregnancy it is often referred to as *pregnancy stomatitis,* and at this time a patient may also exhibit a gingivitis with hypertrophy of the gums, and occasionally develop a "pregnancy tumor" on the gingiva. Such pregnancy tumors are easily removed.

Thrush (moniliasis): A disease caused by the yeastlike *Candida albicans,* characterized by white, curdy, raised patches which can be scraped off, leaving a base that bleeds.

Trauma: Trauma to the oral cavity is manifested in a variety of ways, from lacerated, swollen, soft tissue damage through fractures of the teeth and supporting structures.

Dental Caries

Dental caries, which you may have called decay until now, is a disease that is present in almost everyone's teeth at some time or other. It can begin at a very early age—as soon as the primary teeth begin to appear in the mouth. In some cases of an extremely active degree of dental caries, called *rampant caries,* the primary teeth have been destroyed by three or four years of age.

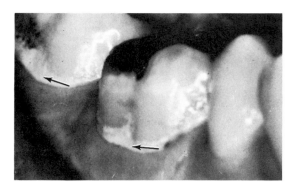

Figure 25.21
Decalcification (whiteness) of enamel (creating a chalky appearance).

What is dental caries? It is a disease process that attacks the hard tissues of the teeth, demineralizing and eventually destroying these hard tissues through loss of both organic and inorganic elements. Its exact cause is not known.

In the process of eating we deposit a considerable amount of food debris in the nooks and crannies around our teeth, as well as over some of the flatter surfaces in certain areas. We also know that we do have bacteria in our mouths in considerable numbers. These bacteria cover various areas of the teeth in what is called a **bacterial plaque,** a filmlike covering that is often very difficult to see in a well-kept mouth. However, if we should paint the teeth with a dye, such as a 5 percent basic fuchsin or a 1 percent Mercurochrome solution, then rinse the mouth well with water, the bacterial plaques will become stained with dye and be easily visible. An area of the tooth that is really clean and not covered with a bacterial plaque will not retain the dye. In the average well-kept mouth, even one that is scrupulously clean to all appearances, these bacterial plaques will be made visible most commonly in that area of each tooth which is close to the gum, tending to encircle the tooth and broadening in the area toward a neighboring tooth.

Most authorities think that the enzymes produced by the bacteria that provide the plaque cause an action on fermentable carbohydrate foods, forming relatively weak acids in the process, during and following eating. This production of acid proceeds rather quickly. Experimentally, it is apparent within ninety seconds after placing a 10 percent solution of glucose (a simple sugar) in the mouth. It can reach its maximum formation within thirty minutes and may be hard to detect again after an hour.

When a certain level of acidity is reached, the acids are thought to cause a demineralization of the enamel, which produces an opaque white spot in the enamel substance. This acid-forming cycle is repeated

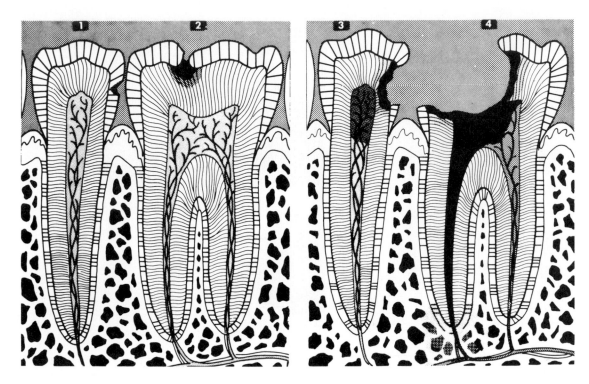

Figure 25.22
Four stages of dental caries.

whenever more fermentable material is brought into the plaque. The process is indicated first by this opaque white area, then by a loss in hardness of the enamel, then by the indication that everyone recognizes— cavitation, or the formation of a cavity in the tooth. This, if allowed to proceed farther, causes a discoloration of the surrounding area and eventually, although not always, results in pain.

Pain may occur when the advance of caries first reaches the dentino-enamel junction, where it usually is not severe, or when the advancing caries has affected the pulpal tissues, at which time the pain is often most severe.

The *Atlas of the Mouth* groups ten stages in the progress of dental caries into four larger classifications: (1) the formation of a small cavity in the enamel of the tooth, frequently detected by X ray; (2) the enlarged cavity beginning to make inroads in the dentin, usually with discoloration present; (3) penetration of the caries process into the pulp chamber, resulting in infection of the pulp; and (4) the formation of a periapical lesion, with the death of the pulp.[1] (See fig. 25.22.)

Pulp Reaction

If dental caries has penetrated a tooth to any degree, the pulp responds to the irritation so produced by showing certain inflammatory reactions similar to those described in soft tissue. However, within the tooth, secondary dentin forms to protect the pulp. As the caries

progresses into the dentin, a mild hyperemia exists as white blood cells are carried to the area. If the caries is allowed to proceed without interruption, the inflammatory reactions become more severe.

There is one essential difference between the skin on your forearm and the pulp of the tooth in their inflammatory responses. In the case of your forearm, swelling can occur freely. The pulp of the tooth, however, is contained in a definite hard-walled chamber. The effort to swell merely produces pressure on nerves and blood vessels.

The pressure may cause certain reactions: mild toothache (if any toothache is mild to the person who is experiencing it); severe toothache; mild toothache progressing to severe toothache; or an intense toothache, followed by sudden cessation of the pain. First, the capillaries are contained within the hard walls of the canal and pulp chamber. A surge of increased blood pressure in the capillaries occurs. When the pressure created by the hyperemia and edema of the pulpal tissues has made the tooth more sensitive than normal, the pressure of the hyperemia (increase in blood supply) is sometimes sufficient to cause quite severe pain. This is **pulpitis** (toothache).

If the hyperemia proceeds slowly, the pain is usually less severe, often intermittent, as the invasion of bacteria progresses toward the pulp. If the invasion of bacteria and toxins is rapid, an intrapulpal abscess occurs before secondary dentin can form. Death of the pulp tissue progresses to the apex of the root(s). The

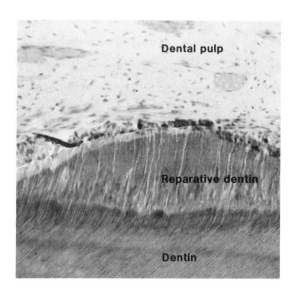

Figure 25.23
Histological section of reparative dentin.

patient will often give a history of a severe throbbing or pulsating pain that suddenly stopped (upon the death of the pulp). The severe stage is referred to as **acute pulpitis,** which is an advanced inflammatory involvement of the pulp of the tooth. Bacteria have invaded the pulp chambers in numbers. The battle with the white blood cells can extend to an area around the apex of the root, where the early stages of **periapical abscess** formation are now evident.

Periapical Abscess

As the pulpal infection proceeds through the apical foramen into the periapical area, the body defenses through the inflammatory process are usually more capable of containing the bacteria and preventing the spread of the disease.

A root canal containing necrotic, perhaps infected material, acts as a reservoir for toxins that may escape into the periapical area. In this situation, the inflammatory process (the body's resistance to disease) is not capable of entering the minute apical foramen into the root canal to remove the toxic products and probable bacteria present. The best it can do is attempt to prevent the dissemination of the toxins by walling off the apical foramen with granulation tissue. This tissue will convert to normal periapical tissue or scar tissue when the source of irritation is removed from the root canal.

If the host's defenses are inadequate to counter the virulence of the invading microorganisms, the pressure of pus and gas will cause increased redness, swelling, heat, and pain. The tooth will be extremely tender, and obviously its function will be impaired. An **acute abscess** exists. The patient seeks immediate relief from the dentist, who will open into the pulp chamber

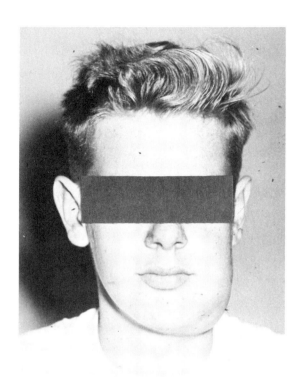

Figure 25.24
Periapical infection with acute swelling.

and root canal to release the pressure and concomitantly the reason for the pain. On occasion, the swollen area is localized enough as evidenced by a palpable fluid mass in the gum, and relief may be obtained by lancing (fig. 25.25).

The dentist may decide to assist the patient in fighting the infection by prescribing systemic antibiotics and may also prescribe a medication, such as Darvon or aspirin with codeine, to relieve the intense pain during the early stages of gaining control of the infection.

When infection invades the periapical area, bone is destroyed. Calcified bone is removed during the walling-off process by the inflammation. A definite area of bone loss appears on the X ray as a radiolucency, which means the area is darker because the X rays have less bone to travel through than where the bone is complete from outer to inner surface of the alveolar process as seen in figure 25.18.

If the body's defenses are fairly evenly balanced with the invading infection, the severe inflammatory reaction does not occur, and an abscess may form without too much concern by the patient. Sometimes a **fistula** forms, providing drainage of the pus to the outside. While the fistula keeps the tooth comfortable, it does not eliminate the infection. Patients recognize the outer opening of the fistula as a "gum boil" (fig. 25.10).

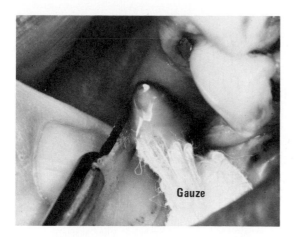

Figure 25.25
Lancing acute abscess (scalpel penetrates gum to release pus from abscess, gauze collects pus as it is released).

At times it is necessary to trace the course of the fistulous tract to its source in order to determine which tooth is causing the problem. The dentist inserts a gutta-percha point or wire probe into the tract, and X-rays it in position (fig. 25.26).

Granuloma

The walling off of the periapical infection is usually accomplished by granulation tissue, and consequently, such lesions are called **granulomas.** If the wall of the sac is lined with epithelium, the lesion is called a **cyst.** If a tooth bearing a cyst is extracted and the cyst remains in the jaw, it is called a **residual cyst.**

With few exceptions, the chronic periapical conditions discovered during routine radiographic examination are granulomas. The patient may give a history of toothache of short duration that he or she thought did not require dental attention; or the death of the pulp and its extension periapically may have been so gradual that the patient was unaware of any serious trouble.

Since most of the lesions that wall off root ends with infected pulp canals are granulomas, a more detailed description of their microscopic structure is important for the dental assistant to more fully understand the problem involved and the dentist's treatment of the problem.

Fish presented an excellent means of describing the periapical granuloma by dividing the area into four zones.[2]

1. Infection
2. Contamination
3. Irritation
4. Stimulation

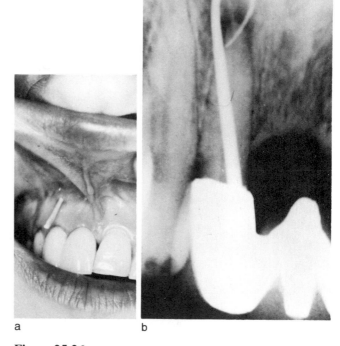

a   b

Figure 25.26
a) Gutta-percha marker in fistulous tract; and b) X ray of marker in place.

Figure 25.27 shows a diagram of a root canal that contains necrotic and probably infected tissue. The necrotic area may be infected with organisms that gained entrance to the canal through a carious lesion, a pulp exposure caused by trauma, or perhaps through a transient bacteremia that may have allowed bacteria to have access to an area of low resistance within the pulp tissue. On the other hand, the tooth may have been traumatized without fracture but with subsequent death of the pulp. In such cases, the pulp may not demonstrate microorganisms by routine culturing methods. Whether the toxins are produced by bacteria or break-down products of decomposed tissue, they have an irritating effect on periapical tissues.

1. The **zone of infection** is the area adjacent to the apical foramen. It represents an area in which the toxins exuding from the root canal are in their most concentrated state. Microorganisms may also be present. The microscopic picture is that of acute inflammation, with PMNs (a type of leukocyte) and macrophages dominating the scene. The function of the PMNs is to devour any bacteria present. The macrophages reinforce the PMNs in attacking bacteria and removing the debris from the area.

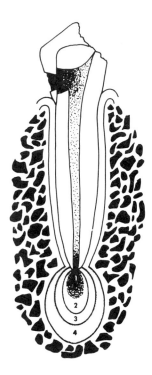

Figure 25.27
Four zones of periapical granuloma as described by Fish:
(1) infection; (2) contamination; (3) irritation; and
(4) stimulation.

2. In the **zone of contamination,** the toxins are becoming diluted by the exudate from the blood. (*Exudate* means fluid oozing out.) Microscopically, this area presents a picture of chronic inflammation with lymphocytes and plasma cells predominating.
3. The **zone of irritation** is still farther from the source, and the toxins become more dilute. Their effectiveness may be reduced to that of a mild irritant. Osteoclasts may be found attacking the bone. (An *osteoclast* absorbs and removes bone.)
4. In the fourth zone, the **zone of stimulation,** the toxins are so dilute that they act as a stimulant to osteoblasts and fibroblasts, whose respective functions are to build new bone and tissue. Thus, there is present an active core of inflammation that gradually changes to an area of healing at the periphery as the toxins become diluted and lose their destructive effectiveness.

When a granuloma is well organized, an area of healing exists. If the source of irritation within the root canal is removed, there will be **complete regeneration** of periapical bone and periodontal membrane. This statement is the premise on which the principle of intracanal therapy for periapically involved teeth is based.

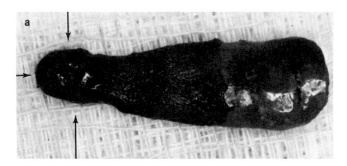

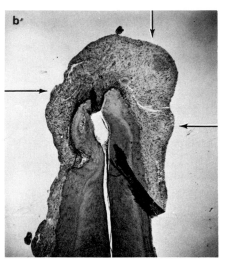

Figure 25.28
Cross section of tooth with sac on apex (arrows indicate sac).

However, the virulence of the toxins in the granuloma may be so strong that the body's defense mechanisms may be barely holding the infection in check. (Remember, the body's defense mechanism is the inflammatory process, but the inflammatory process cannot always reach the purulent material.) The histologic picture may show a thin peripheral sac of granulation tissue filled with purulent material. Although proper intracanal therapy should remove the irritant inaccessible to the inflammatory process and allow periapical regeneration, this purulent mass may be self-sustaining and require intervention. Such residual infections have been observed following intracanal therapy, or following extraction of teeth where such periapical areas have not been properly curetted at the same time as tooth removal. Unfortunately, it is impossible to diagnose the histologic condition without viewing prepared sections of the tissue under a microscope.

If toxins exuding from the root canal are highly virulent (extremely poisonous) and maintain or increase their strength, the area will become larger. However, if the virulence is reduced, the condition will become static, and granulation tissue will make up the bulk of the lesion.

An acute apical abscess is entirely made up of the zone of infection, while the disease is actively spreading. When the inflammatory process becomes effective in counteracting the infection, the zones of irritation and stimulation become established.

Periodontitis

Periodontitis is an advanced stage of gingivitis, affecting the tissue supporting the teeth. As the disease progresses, the periodontal membrane is destroyed and alveolar bone is resorbed forming a **pocket.** If not treated with success, the teeth or tooth involved will lose so much support that a periodontal abscess may form or removal of the tooth may eventually become necessary. This disease is commonly referred to as **pyorrhea.** It is preventable if attention is given to the first signs of poor oral health. If the causative factors are treated first, periodontitis is treatable providing there is sufficient tissue to support the tooth.

Periodontosis, or diffuse alveolar atrophy, is a degenerative disease, the end result of which is similar to that of periodontitis. Simplifying their differences to some extent, we might say that periodontosis is similar to periodontitis except for the lack of inflammatory reactions.

Control of Dental Caries

In any disease, many people are inclined to look for assistance or cure in a tube of this, a bottle of that, or a shot of some wonder drug to banish the difficulty. This is true in respect to dental caries as well.

Dental caries can only be corrected by the use of dental restorations. Teeth that have been damaged by dental caries cannot repair themselves. Caries *activity,* however, can be strongly influenced by personal habits. A correction of dietary habits combined with an improvement in oral hygiene can and does work wonders with the majority of individuals. This does not have particularly wide appeal because it does not consist of a tube, a bottle, or a shot—just the application of time and effort. This application often falls victim to the lethargy of which we are all guilty to some degree.

Fluoride in community drinking water has proved its usefulness in reducing the incidence of dental caries. The direct application of stannous fluoride to teeth has also proved dramatically effective. These methods are only helpful, however, if we exercise control of other areas of strong influence such as oral hygiene and diet at the same time.

With a better understanding of the significance of the attachment of dental plaque in relatively thick, large masses, and the rapidity with which these organisms with their enzymes can produce acid within the plaque, oral hygiene can be made more effective than before. *First, the plaque must be removed at least daily.* This involves proper toothbrush technique and the proper use of dental floss. The use of both must be carefully taught the patient. *Second, food must be removed from the mouth as soon as possible after eating,* remembering the time element in the production of acid within the plaque. The removal of food can be accomplished by eating coarser foods last, rather than finishing with a dessert. Thorough rinsing and the use of toothbrush and dental floss are also helpful. The chewing of a small piece of paraffin wax or sugar-free gum immediately after eating is a good detergent, aiding in cleansing the teeth and in stimulating flow of saliva, which dilutes and washes away food residue from tooth surfaces.

Some individuals have an unusually high degree of susceptibility to dental decay. These people should adhere rigidly to a special diet for the reduction of decay. If the problem is less serious, they may follow the diet less strictly, remembering that its extreme form is intended for individuals with a very high rate of decay. (See chap. 23.)

The most successful method of stopping carious lesions is the use of restorations. Restorations have served for many years as effective agents for controlling the ravages of this disease. When the diseased portion of the tooth is surgically removed by the dentist and the remaining tooth substance correctly prepared to receive a restoration, and that restoration is placed, one may safely assume that the carious process has been stopped. Unfortunately, that portion of the tooth which has not been protected with a restoration is still susceptible to dental caries.

Careful mouth examinations, with X rays, at regular intervals are necessary for early diagnosis. It is especially important that we instruct our patients (and follow our own advice) to have all carious lesions treated as soon as we detect them. It is the dentist's responsibility to prevent the ravages of this universal disease by using all means at his or her disposal:

1. **Early diagnosis**
2. **Preventive measures**
3. **Restorations properly made**

Summary

Oral pathology is a study of the diseases of the mouth.

Inflammation is the body's defense against injury and disease. The cardinal symptoms of inflammation are redness, swelling, heat, pain, and impairment of function.

Diagnosis of oral pathology is not simple. There are clinical and differential diagnoses. A number of conditions that are pathological are commonly observed in the dental office. Learn them from your text.

Dental caries is decay. The four stages of progress of dental caries are: (1) formation of a small cavity in the enamel of the tooth; (2) enlarged cavity beginning to make inroads in the dentin; (3) penetration of the caries process into the pulp chamber, resulting in infection of the pulp; and (4) formation of a periapical lesion with the death of the pulp.

The pulp responds to irritation of caries and if neglected can result in periapical abscess and granuloma.

Periapical granuloma is described by dividing the area into four zones: (1) infection, (2) contamination, (3) irritation, and (4) stimulation.

Periodontitis is an advanced stage of gingivitis.

Dental caries can be controlled by daily removal of plaque, removal of food from the mouth as soon as possible after eating, eating proper foods, and having careful examinations at regular intervals, followed by adequate care of any diseased areas.

The dentist's responsibility is to prevent the ravages of caries by means of early diagnosis, preventive measures, and restorations properly made.

Study Questions

1. Name five causes of pathologic changes in the body.
2. Differentiate between oral pathology and dental pathology.
3. Describe inflammation.
4. Familiarize yourself with the definition of oral pathologic conditions described in this chapter.
5. Describe caries and explain how and why it occurs.
6. Describe pulp reaction to dental caries.
7. Describe a periapical granuloma, dividing the area into Fish's four zones. Clarify each zone.
8. What is periodontitis?
9. What is the most successful method of stopping carious lesions?
10. What means for preventing caries does the dentist use?

Vocabulary

abscess   localized area of pus

aphthous ulcer   canker sore

cheilitis   inflammation of the lip

cheilosis   fissuring at corners of mouth due to vitamin B complex deficiency

clinical diagnosis   one made by considering the clinical symptoms

dental caries   a localized progressive disintegration of tooth structure

dental pathology   diseases pertaining to or relating to the teeth

differential diagnosis   distinguishes between two or more diseases of similar character

exudate   fluid oozing out

gingivitis   inflammation of the gingival tissues

hyperemia   increase in blood supply

inflammation   response of tissues of body to pathologic changes

leukocytes   white blood cells

oral pathology   diseases of the mouth

osteoclast   a large multinucleate cell, associated with the dissolution of unwanted bone

pathology   branch of biological science that deals with nature of disease through a study of its causes, how it proceeds, and its effects

pulpitis   inflammation of the pulp of the tooth

stomatitis   inflammation of the oral cavity

systemic   body as a whole

Word Elements	
Word Element	*Example*
ad prefix meaning: to, toward, addition to, intensification	*adhesion* molecular binding
ad suffix meaning: to, toward	*cephalad* directed toward the head
cephalo, cephal combining form meaning: relationship to the head	*cephalalgia* headache
aden combining form meaning: relationship to gland	*adenopathy* enlargement in size of glandular organs
blast combining form meaning: root, germ cell	*odontoblast* a dentin-forming cell
cyt combining form meaning: relationship to cell	*cytology* study of cells
ana prefix meaning: again, back, up, excessive	*anaphylaxis* excessive allergic reaction to a foreign protein, drug, or infection; hypersensitivity
anim prefix meaning: life, mind	*animation* the state of being alive
ics suffix meaning: characteristic qualities	*numeric file* a file using numbers for identification of the contents

CHAPTER

26

Drugs, First Aid and Emergency Care

Part One: Drugs
Drug: From Poison to Panacea
   Incompatible Drugs
   Food-Drug Reactions
Dispensing or Administering Drugs to Patients
     Dispensing Drugs to Patients
     Administering Drugs to Patients
Drug Terminology
   Drugs as Liquids (Solutions)
   Drugs as Solids
   Generic and Proprietary Drugs
Types of Drugs
Controlled Drugs
The Use of Drugs in the Dental Office
Part Two: First Aid and Emergency Care
Preparation for Emergency Action
The Emergencies Encountered in a Dental Office
   Allergies
   Chest Pain
     Hypertension
   Circulatory Reactions
     Mouth-to-Mouth Resuscitation
   Convulsions (Adult and Child)
   Death
   Fainting (Syncopé)
   Hermorrhage (Bleeding)
   Insulin Shock
   Psychosis
   Respiratory Reaction
   Shock

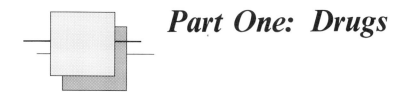

Part One: Drugs

Drug: From Poison to Panacea

"A **drug** is any chemical compound that may be used on, or administered as, an aid in diagnosis, treatment, or prevention of disease or other abnormal condition;" further it may be used "for the relief of pain or suffering, or to control or improve any physiologic or pathologic condition."[1] While many people tend to associate the word *drug* with drug addicts and drug dependency, it is also used to label those substances which help humans fight disease.

It is true, however, that many drugs are helpful when used in prescribed quantity but act as poisons if used in an excessive quantity.

Learn to exercise care in all procedures in which you use or dispense drugs upon the order or instruction of your dentist.

Your dentist has received training in **pharmacology**—the science that deals with the nature, properties, and use of drugs. This training is required by law for anyone who is to prescribe drugs. Your dentist, therefore, is the one person in the dental office who is qualified and licensed to prescribe drugs for use by your patients. It is your obligation to follow his or her instructions exactly and carefully.

Should you discover that you cannot remember how much premedication you are to give a patient, *do not guess.* If you find that you do not know for certain what is used to refill the topical anesthetic bottle in the instrument cabinet, *do not guess.* Ask your dentist. Be certain.

Further, remember that drugs or medications can be dangerous. Verify every medicine when you remove it from its container or when adding to it in the storage area. If it is necessary to refill a container, double check both the large container and the smaller one you plan to refill. Do not remove a container and replenish a smaller one without looking at the labels simply because that is the place in the cupboard where that drug is always kept. Someone may have moved the containers. *Keep labels in good condition at all times.* Be certain that you can clearly read the label—and then do so.

If you wish to broaden your knowledge of pharmacology as it applies to the practice of dentistry, one of the books most commonly available in any dental office is *Accepted Dental Therapeutics,* which is published annually by the American Dental Association.

It lists commercial products that are currently accepted by the Council on Dental Therapeutics and describes nearly all the official and nonofficial therapeutic items that are of demonstrated usefulness in dental practice. It deserves your study because of its specific and thorough application to dental practice.

Incompatible Drugs

One difficulty with prescribing medications is that certain drugs cannot be mixed because the two substances may cause undesirable or dangerous side effects. (A **side effect** is a consequence other than the one for which the medication was used. Thus, if a particular medication to relieve pain also gives the individual hives, the hives are a side effect.)

Through usage and research some drug interactions have been determined to be incompatible—to cause dangerous reactions and even death. For example, the tranquilizers potentiate (magnify the effects of) alcohol, anesthetics, hypnotics, and narcotics. Thus, if a patient is using a drug from the phenothiazine group (tranquilizers), he or she should not mix alcohol with the medicine. The use of phenothiazine medication should be carefully considered prior to the use of anesthetics, hypnotics, or narcotics because there may be a synergistic effect.

Food-Drug Reactions

In addition to the possibility that a patient may be given two drugs that are incompatible, it is possible that a food and drug combination may cause mild or severe reactions.

Thus, drugs can be poison or panacea. It is imperative that the correct drug in the correct amount be given the patient.

Dispensing or Administering Drugs to Patients

Sometimes the dental assistant is instructed to give the patient a medication to be taken either right then at the office or to be taken home and used. Accuracy in the performance of this task is imperative. Follow the directions given in this section. Also, remember that whenever any drug is administered, dispensed, or prescribed, it must be recorded on the patient's record. The

```
┌─────────────────────────────────────────┐
│  School of Dentistry      Department of Oral and  │
│  University of Minnesota   Maxillofacial Surgery   │
│                           Telephone: 373-3276      │
│ ───────────────────────────────────────── │
│                                           │
│     This envelope contains tablets to be taken │
│  for pain. If more tablets are required, ordinary │
│  5-grain aspirin tablets may be used in the same │
│  manner.                                   │
│                                           │
│                                           │
│     Dosage:                                │
│                                           │
│        Adults—Two tablets every 4 hours.  │
│                                           │
│                                           │
│  If care is necessary after clinic hours, please │
│  call 373-8484.                            │
│                                           │
└─────────────────────────────────────────┘
```

Figure 26.1
Envelope (with printed instructions for use of contents) which is given to patient to take home.

notations about the medication, quantity, exact description, and date (with year) must be entered on the patient's record.

Dispensing Drugs to Patients

If you are instructed to give a patient a medication to be taken at home before the next appointment:

1. Place the medication in a small drug envelope with instructions clearly written on the envelope stating the time at which the medication is to be taken.
2. Hand this envelope to the patient and orally state the instructions.
3. If the medication is in capsule form, mention that the capsule is to be swallowed with water. Occasionally you will find individuals whose experience with medications is limited and they will not be quite sure whether the capsule is to be taken apart to make the powder available, or whether the capsule itself is safe to swallow.
4. Be sure the patient completely understands all instructions concerning the medication.
5. Note the medication on the patient's record.

Administering Drugs to Patients

If you are instructed to give a patient a medication in the office:

1. Verify that the medicine you are about to give the patient is the one the dentist has prescribed. Double check it.
2. Place that medication in a disposable paper cup.

3. In a second disposable cup bring water for the patient's use in swallowing the tablet. Hold the cup near the bottom rather than at the upper edge where the patient's lips will be during drinking.
4. Say to the patient, "I am going to give you a pill. Will you hold out your hand, please?"
5. You then "pour" the tablet from the paper cup into the palm of the patient's hand, and at the same time extend your hand with the cup of water so that the patient may take the cup easily with his or her free hand.
6. Stand by the patient to be sure that the medication is taken as requested. Occasionally the patient will question the purpose or kind of medication given. Refer the question to the dentist.

Drug Terminology

A crude drug is unrefined, containing its entire ingredients from which the active parts are taken. When it has been refined, we have a pure drug. The pure drug is any powder, crystal, liquid, or gum used in its highest concentration and purity as a medicine.

Drugs as Liquids (Solutions)

Drugs can be in **solution.** A solution is **saturated** when it is holding all of the substance that can be dissolved and still remain in solution. For example, when you mix water and sugar together until the water can dissolve and hold absolutely no more sugar, the solution is *saturated* with sugar. Certain drugs follow this principle. When the largest amount of the drug that the liquid can hold is dissolved, we have a saturation.

A **stock solution** is a concentrated form of the drug. It may not be saturated, but it is close to its saturation point. It is used to make up weaker solutions of the medicine according to prescriptions.

A **suspension** is different from a solution in that the particles of the drug remain in their solid form and are just suspended in the liquid. A drug that is in suspension has a label that reads, "Shake well."

A **diluent** is added to reduce the strength of the solution or mixture.

A **tincture** is an alcoholic solution of a soluble drug or chemical. (For example, tincture of iodine.)

An **extract** is obtained by dissolving the drug in alcohol or water and evaporating it to a certain prescribed consistency.

A **mixture** is a combination of two or more drugs. These drugs do not unite. They retain their individual properties. The mixture can be either liquid or dry ingredients.

Aerosol is a drug in solution that can be atomized finely and inhaled to alleviate respiratory or systemic problems, or it can be sprayed topically.

Parenteral is a sterile solution or suspension of a drug that is prepared for injection.

A **vehicle** is something that is used to administer a medicine. Some vehicles are:

1. An **elixir,** which is a sweetened, aromatic, alcoholic preparation used to administer an active medicine such as elixir of phenobarbital.
2. A **syrup,** which is a sugar solution used to administer a drug.
3. An **ointment,** which is a semisolid preparation of a drug in a base used externally.
4. An **emulsion,** which is an oily or resinous drug held in suspension in some liquid which makes it possible for the patient to swallow it.

Drugs as Solids

Drugs can also be in a solid state, or some form that makes it possible to swallow without being in solution. The following are four examples.

1. A **pill** is a small globular or oval molded, medicated dosage intended to be swallowed.
2. A **tablet** is a solid dosage form of varying weight, size, and shape which may be molded or compressed, containing a medicinal substance in pure or diluted form.[2]
3. A **capsule** is usually rod-shaped, made of soluble material such as gelatin. It contains powders or liquids that can be swallowed without being tasted. The capsule dissolves in the stomach, and the medicine is thus delivered to the system.
4. A **suppository** is usually made of a material that will melt when it reaches body temperature. Whatever the vehicle, the medicine is embedded in it; and as the vehicle melts the medicine is distributed and absorbed. The suppository is designed to be inserted into an opening in the body, such as the anus.

Generic and Proprietary Drugs

Generic names are family names of drugs. The generic name comes from the source or compound used to make the particular drug. The name refers to a certain chemical entity. Pharmacists will use generic name chemicals to prepare prescriptions if the prescription does not specify a proprietary drug.

Proprietary names are names given to drugs by the manufacturer. Each firm may package a particular drug under its own brand name. Thus, a drug called by a generic name might have two or three proprietary names given by different manufacturers. For example, *Pentids* is a brand name of penicillin manufactured by one drug firm. Other firms have penicillin, but they do not call their penicillin *Pentids*. The use of a proprietary name for a drug means that the manufacturer guarantees that each tablet of that drug is exactly like the other tablets of that drug.

Types of Drugs

Drugs are grouped by type. Some of those with which you should be familiar are discussed in the following paragraphs.

Analgesics relieve pain.
Anesthetics produce loss of feeling.
Antibiotics are called the "wonder drugs."

Probably the best known antibiotic is penicillin. The antibiotics were prescribed first in the 1940s. The medicine is made from particular molds that destroy many disease-producing bacteria. The word was derived from two Latin words, *anti* (meaning "against") and *biotic* (meaning "relating to life"). A dentist usually inquires as to whether the patient has a known allergic reaction to any antibiotic. This reaction can be severe. It is also possible for the organism to build up resistance to a given antibiotic through too much use. A change to another antibiotic may be necessary. In this case the patient does not respond to the treatment because her or his system no longer is affected by the antibiotic. Thus, a patient can have a form of disease that has grown immune to a specific antibiotic. A complete dosage of antibiotic should be taken because failing to do so may give the bacteria an opportunity to become resistant to the antibiotic and make the individual ill again. Absolutely no antibiotics should be administered without the specific direction of the dentist or physician!

Amphetamines act as a stimulant on the central nervous system. They are prescribed as appetite depressants by some physicians.

Antidepressants relieve depression (often called "mood elevators").

Antidotes are medicines that neutralize or precipitate a poison. The administration of an antidote lessens the toxicity of the poison.

Antihistamines are medicines that are used to regulate and control the secretions in the body of a person suffering from allergies. They help reduce the swelling of mucous membranes with the discharge of fluids.

Antilaxatives are medicines that counteract diarrhea or loose stools.

Astringents are drugs that stop or retard bleeding or discharge. They are used topically and cause constriction of the tissue. *Alum* is one of the most commonly used.

Cathartics evacuate the bowels. There are laxatives which work mildly, such as mineral oil. There are purgatives which work more severely, such as castor oil. There are drastic purgatives, such as croton oil, which are rarely used.

Decongestants are drugs that decrease or reduce congestion or swelling.

Diuretics are medicines or beverages that increase the output of urine.

Emetics cause vomiting.

Expectorants cause the liquefaction of phlegm.

Hemostatic agents arrest the flow of blood by helping it to coagulate (harden and form a scab). They may be taken internally or applied locally as a solid. Vitamin K is a common hemostatic agent. Such an agent may be applied during oral surgery.

Hormones are the secretion produced by the endocrine glands which are used for patients whose own glands are malfunctioning.

Hypnotics are sleep-producing drugs.

Muscle relaxants are drugs that are used to relax a smooth muscle spasm. (They are called *antispasmodic* drugs.)

Narcotics are a class of drugs that produce stupor, complete insensibility to pain, or sleep. There are many forms. The opiates produce sleep. The use of this class of drugs is strictly regulated by federal law, and they may only be prescribed by a dentist or a physician who has a narcotic license.

Sedatives are drugs that quiet patients. They reduce nervous tension.

Stimulants are substances that stimulate the heart to beat faster and stronger. Adrenalin and caffeine are examples. The amphetamines are also considered stimulants.

Tranquilizers calm patients who are agitated.

Vasoconstrictors are substances that cause the blood vessels to constrict.

Vasodilators are drugs that dilate the blood vessels and help to reduce blood pressure by relaxing the muscles in the blood vessels.

Vitamins are necessary for the proper functioning of every human. They are produced synthetically now, although the primary source is still food products. Some vitamins are synthesized by the body itself. (See chapter 23 for further explanation.)

Controlled Drugs

Many medications for home remedies can be purchased without a prescription. These purchases are called over-the-counter sales. Permission to purchase these medications is not required.

Other drugs are considered dangerous if used in the wrong quantities or for the wrong purposes. For these drugs the patient must have a written prescription from a dentist or a physician: a person licensed to prescribe drugs.

In addition to this precaution about most drugs there is further restriction on drugs that are known to be **addictive.** (A person who uses an addictive drug over a period of time develops a physical and/or emotional dependency on the drug and cannot be without it.) Narcotics are known to be habit-forming, addictive drugs. Thus, narcotics, or medications containing narcotics, are carefully supervised by the federal government. Because all narcotics dispensed must be accurately reported to the federal government, complete records must be maintained.

Many dentists will prescribe narcotics, and thus possess prescription blanks with the dentist's federal registry number printed on them. These prescription blanks and any narcotics kept in the office must be guarded carefully. *The dental assistant must be aware of the necessity to keep accurate and complete narcotics records if the dentist prescribes or dispenses any drugs containing narcotics.*

At one time, only narcotics were thought to be addictive drugs. However, in recent years, we have discovered that some drugs that are not narcotics are addictive. These drugs are also carefully regulated. They are frequently referred to as **mood drugs.**

Amphetamine is one such drug classification. Amphetamines were quite freely prescribed for persons who wished to lose weight until their addictive capacities were discovered. Amphetamines are frequently called "uppers" because they raise a person's spirit and enthusiasm.

Another group of drugs, called "downers," are also addictive. They are more likely to contain narcotics. However, *all* these drugs are addictive and must be carefully controlled and prescribed.

Whatever the reasons a person uses drugs for personal or social satisfactions, those who work in the health professions must be aware that many people are trying to find sources to acquire their particular drug because an addict is unable legally to purchase the quantity he or she needs. To obtain any controlled drug without a prescription means purchasing on the black market, which is very costly. Often habits can cost $150 a day or more. To support such a habit usually means stealing. Often attempts are made to steal the drug or prescription blanks with a federal registry number on them.

If a pharmacist calls the office concerning a prescription that you discover has not been issued by your dentist, contact the nearest office of the Bureau of Narcotics. Whenever a pharmacist calls you about a prescription, double check by looking at the patient's record. Don't trust to memory, no matter how wonderful yours is!

The Use of Drugs in the Dental Office

Most drugs used by dental patients are prescribed by the dentist as a written order to the pharmacist who supplies the medication for the patient. However, drugs are also used in the office during the treatment of the patient. Many preparations must be carefully handled. They include: anesthetics, disinfectants, surgical dressings, medicated cements, irrigating solutions, cauterizing agents, topical drugs, and systemic drugs. Some solutions may be caustic if carelessly placed, or they may stain the skin and clothing if spilled. Learn to respect these drugs for what they can offer in the treatment of patients as well as for the problems they can create if misused. For further information concerning the specific use of drugs in the practice of dentistry, consult *Accepted Dental Therapeutics,* published by the American Dental Association. It is an excellent compendium of acceptable brands of drugs used in dentistry.

Parts of a prescription: If the dentist wishes to have the patient take a medication at home, either before or after treatment in the office, the dentist writes the prescription on a printed prescription blank. Certain information is imprinted on the blank including the dentist's name, address, telephone numbers and Federal Registry number. Usually there is designated space for the patient's name. The center section is blank, providing room for the dentist to write the desired medication and directions.

The written prescription contains:

1. The name of the patient
2. The name of the drug or medication, either proprietary or generic
3. The size of the dosage
4. The total quantity of the drug to be given the patient for this prescription
5. The directions (called the *Signa* or *Sig*)
6. The dentist's signature
7. The dentist's federal registry number, if the prescription contains drugs that are regulated by the narcotics acts
8. The number of times the prescription can be refilled (indicated at the bottom of the blank)

The second through fourth items are sometimes grouped under the expression, *Rx,* which means prescription.

Thus, a prescription for *penicillin V* could read either "penicillin V" (the generic name), or "PenVee" (Wyeth's proprietary name), or "V-Cillin-K" (Lilly's proprietary name), and so on. Also on the prescription blank would be listed: (1) the size of the tablet, such as *250 mg* or *500 mg;* (2) the number of tablets, such as *20* or *30;* and (3) the frequency with which they are to be taken (in abbreviated form), such as *q.i.d.*

Figure 26.2 is a properly written prescription.

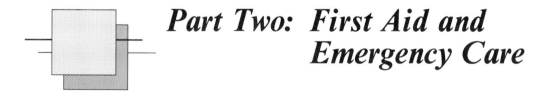

Part Two: First Aid and Emergency Care

Preparation for Emergency Action

Many patients who come to a dental office can develop medical emergencies. Perhaps your dentist will not be in the office area in which the emergency condition arises. You must be prepared to handle these situations. You should be able to recognize the person who needs emergency care, and you should know how to help your dentist in all office emergencies.

The dental assistant's association with a health profession makes it desirable to have formal training in first aid. The American Red Cross courses are most commonly available.

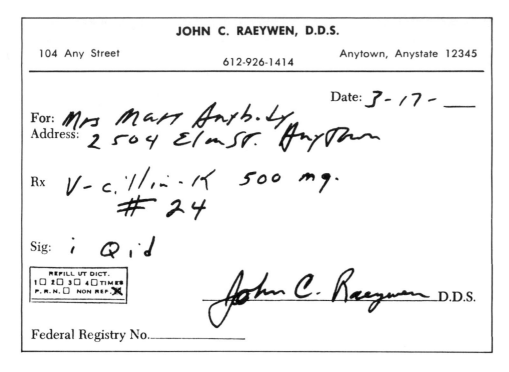

Figure 26.2

A properly written prescription.

An emergency in the dental office is described as an unanticipated combination of circumstances requiring immediate action in order to prevent serious injury or loss. Key words are *unanticipated, immediate action,* and *serious injury or loss.*

Certain types of emergencies are more common in a dental office. Recognition of these emergencies should be developed. For example, if a patient begins to faint, your dentist might have his or her back turned at the moment, and your quick attention may prevent the patient from losing consciousness.

What you are permitted to do for emergency care will depend on your dentist. For example, it is nice to know that a pressure pack in a tooth socket will help clotting and reduce hemorrhaging, but legally only the dentist or the patient can place that pack in the socket. The more likely emergencies that may be encountered in the dental office are syncopé (fainting), several forms of shock, procaine allergies, hypertension, hemorrhage, convulsions, and respiratory failure.

Dental procedures are the source of considerable tension and strain to some patients. If the patient is in good health, as are the majority of patients who come to the dental office, these stresses and strains may not bring on any unusual symptoms. However, every dental office will, at times, have a patient who suffers a reaction from one cause or another, which requires that the patient be handled properly and quickly to prevent serious consequences. It is most important that the type of disturbance and its cause be recognized as early as possible. This is necessary in order that difficulties which are not serious may be recognized as such, and difficulties which are serious may be handled with due regard for the responsibilities involved.

In any emergency **a primary attempt should be made to call the attention of the dentist to the problem.** If the dentist is not available, procure medical assistance as rapidly as possible after taking the necessary preliminary precautions required by the condition of the patient.

The fundamental rules for your conduct during an emergency are:

Rule number one: Anyone who needs emergency treatment is likely to be frightened. Your first responsibility is to remain calm, to reassure the patient, be interested, sympathetic, but do not show surprise or fear. Watch your comments.

For example, one assistant to a periodontist inadvertently upset a patient by opening her eyes wide as she changed a dressing and commented audibly to the patient, "I've never seen a hole *that* big." The poor patient, who was already wondering about her recovery, could only be more frightened about permanent damage. This same reaction of surprise in an emergency can panic the patient. Rule number one, then, is to be reassuring, calm, and sympathetic.

Rule number two: Call the attention of your dentist to the emergency if he or she is not aware of the situation.

Rule number three: Follow your dentist's instructions exactly, whether they are to call the patient's physician or bring a cold pack.

In an Emergency

Remain calm and reassuring

Call the attention of the dentist to the emergency if necessary

Follow the dentist's instructions quickly and efficiently

The Emergencies Encountered in a Dental Office

Some of the more common emergencies that may occur in the dental office, descriptions of symptoms, suggestions for care, and any pertinent information are given here in alphabetical order. The boxed summary of instructions for each emergency delineates the pertinent actions.

Allergies

Patients should be questioned regarding their possible allergic problems as part of the history when they register in the office. The most positive means of avoiding difficulties is to omit the use of drugs to which the patient reports a previously unfavorable reaction. *If they are not sure of their response to proposed drugs, their physician should be consulted.* Although allergists do not consider skin sensitivity an absolute indication of hypersensitivity, if the tests are positive, some other agent should be used. For example, sensitivity to a local anesthetic is occasionally encountered. With the variety of solutions available today, an alternative choice is no problem.

If a patient begins to show pallor, apprehension, tremor, or dyspnea (difficult or labored breathing), your dentist should be alerted if he or she is not observing the patient. Oxygen should be available.

Allergic Reaction

Call dentist to patient if not present

Ready oxygen

Assist in whatever way your dentist directs

Chest Pain

Chest pain can be dangerous. If the patient is sweating profusely, has an ashen appearance or looks gray, and perhaps clutches his or her chest, call your dentist at once. Time may be most important. Adjust the chair so that the patient is sitting upright, ready oxygen, and follow your dentist's directions, which may include calling the patient's physician.

Hypertension is one cause of chest pain.

Hypertension

The term *hypertension* is used three ways.

1. It means a disease called "essential hypertension."
2. It means a symptom associated with heart-blood vessel-kidney disease.
3. It means a symptom of arteriosclerosis (hardening of the arteries).

Hypertension is an increased blood pressure and is usually uncommon before thirty years of age. A systolic pressure of over 150 mm. of mercury is suggestive of hypertension, and in severe cases, systolic pressures of over 250 mm. of mercury are not unusual.

The treatment of essential hypertension is aimed more at relief of the symptoms than at curing the disease. Attempts are made to lower the blood pressure to a degree that will minimize the symptoms.

Anything that results in an elevation of blood pressure or causes nervousness should be avoided in hypertensive patients. Premedication will materially reduce nervousness but should be given only if your dentist has given the instructions to do so or has consulted with the physician acquainted with the patient's medical history. The physicians of all hypertensive patients are usually consulted by the dentist before proceeding with extractions or extensive oral surgery.

The usual local anesthetic is not used on these patients because no vasoconstrictive agent should be used. Most local anesthetic solutions are available without a vasoconstrictor and should be kept in stock in the office for use on such patients.

Chest Pain

Observe symptoms

Call dentist and follow his or her directions

Ask patient if he or she is short of breath

Ready oxygen for dentist

Stay with patient

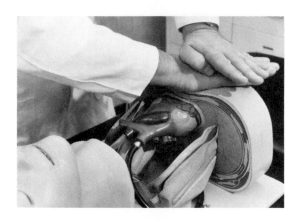

Figure 26.3
External cardiac massage demonstrated on model to show hand position and effect of compression on heart; the sternum should be depressed 1½" to 2" 80–100 times per minute.

Circulatory Reactions

The dental assistant should be certified in CPR (cardiopulmonary resuscitation).

Syncopé may be involved in a mild circulatory reaction or in a severe circulatory reaction or collapse. If the reaction is mild, the total effect is usually self-limiting.

Severe circulatory reaction or collapse, however, is extremely serious and requires immediate attention. It may occur with no warning. Circulatory collapse involves cardiac arrest, or stoppage of the heart, and every effort must be made to reinstitute cardiac rhythm rather than to desert the patient and seek medical help.

Learn to feel for a carotid pulse, rather than the usual radial pulse. The radial pulse, if a pulse is present at all, will be too faint to be identifiable; the carotid pulse would be more easily felt. The carotid pulse is best felt just ahead of the sternocleidomastoid muscle in the neck area by depressing the tissues firmly with three fingers held together. If no pulse is detected, promptly feel the chest and, with the ear pressed to the rib cage, listen for a heartbeat. The pupils will not respond to light stimulus, as is also true in milder syncopé.

The dentist will generally have taken charge of the patient, leaving the assistant free to secure medical assistance if the dentist so instructs. If the dentist is not available, the assistant must not desert the patient but, rather, must be able to apply the necessary emergency measures. **Circulation must be reestablished within three minutes to avoid irreversible CNS damage.**

Oxygen inhalation or mouth-to-mouth resuscitation should be started at once. Closed chest resuscitation methods can be applied by the dentist while the assistant cares for the breathing.

If cardiac arrest is suspected, the chair should be adjusted so that the unconscious patient is lying horizontal, with the chest supported by the backrest. Begin external cardiac massage by placing the palm of the right hand over the sternum and the left hand on top of the right. The sternum is then depressed one and one-half to two inches 80–100 times a minute. If the patient is also suffering from pulmonary arrest, necessitating mouth-to-mouth resuscitation, and if you are alone with the patient, compress the sternum fifteen times and give two quick inflations of the lungs through mouth-to-mouth contact. If there are two people available for first aid, the lungs should be inflated after each fifth compression of the sternum. This process should be continued until spontaneous pulse returns.

Mouth-to-Mouth Resuscitation

When a patient suffers pulmonary arrest, the head should be tilted back and the mouth and throat explored with the fingers to remove any mechanical obstructions, such as loose dentures. The aspirator may be used to remove any accumulated fluids that may be obstructing the airway. *If the patient is breathing, administer oxygen.* Inhalation of aromatic ammonia may be used to support the oxygen administration.

If the patient is not breathing, close the nose with the thumb and forefinger of one hand. With the other hand take a firm grip on the mandible and hold the mouth open. The patient's head should be tilted back with the neck fully extended. Lift the lower jaw forcefully upward or lift the neck to accomplish the same purpose. Then cover the patient's mouth completely with your mouth, so that it is airtight, and blow air into the lungs until you visibly see the chest rise. Remove your mouth; let the patient exhale. Repeat the process approximately twelve times a minute for adults and twenty times a minute for children. When the patient has established his or her own breathing pattern, oxygen may be administered. Drugs for cardiac or pulmonary arrest should be administered by either the dentist or the physician. A **Resusitube** may be utilized effectively if someone is trained in its use.

A discussion of procedures and a rehearsal are desirable in the training of the entire staff. If plans are practiced for the various types of emergencies, competent action by the office staff is far more certain.

Circulatory Reactions

Alert dentist and follow his or her directions

Ready oxygen

Apply mouth-to-mouth resuscitation or closed chest resuscitation, depending on condition of patient

Assist dentist as necessary in these procedures

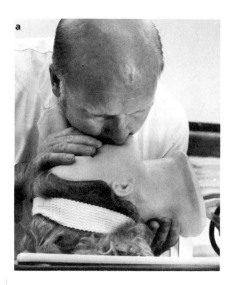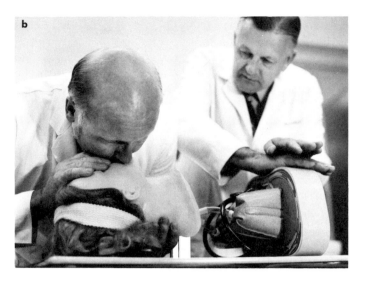

Figure 26.4
CPR on manikin: (a) Nasal openings closed by thumb and forefinger of the right hand; and (b) combined mouth-to-mouth resuscitation and external cardiac massage demonstrated on model.

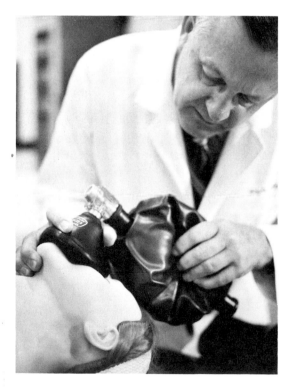

Figure 26.5
Artificial respiration with portable respirator demonstrated on model; chin is pulled upward and forward to pull the tongue forward and maintain an open airway.

Convulsions (Adult and Child)

Convulsions are irregular, intermittent, and variable muscular contractions involving large areas of the body. Generalized convulsions are usually accompanied by a loss of consciousness. Such seizures are much less common in adults than in children, but are generally much more serious in adults. Oxygen should be given for such seizures.

Convulsions may occur in a person who is subject to epileptic seizures. A history of taking Dilatin-sodium or a steady intake of barbiturates is indicative of susceptibility to such seizures. If Dilantin has been taken steadily over a period of time, the soft tissues of the mouth will show a marked hypertrophy (overgrowth), which should arouse suspicion of an epileptic history.

It is possible for some people to have a convulsion without being subject to epileptic seizures. Fever, indigestion, and nutritional deficiency can be causative factors.

A person experiencing such a seizure will frequently gnash his or her teeth violently and seriously lacerate the tongue and cheeks. A bite block, towel, or other soft object may be held between the jaws to prevent such damage. Never put your fingers or hands in the mouth of a person experiencing a seizure. The force of the jaw clenching is great enough to break bones.

The patient should be held in the chair to protect the patient from flailing his or her arms, falling, or bumping his or her head against the dental unit or cabinets, or otherwise harming himself or herself.

A child or an adult known to be subject to epileptic seizure should be premedicated as an aid in prevention.

Regardless of the type of convulsion, keep the patient warm and prevent the patient from harming himself or herself. No doubt your dentist will contact the patient's physician for whatever instructions the physician deems essential.

Convulsions
Make patient as comfortable as possible
Prevent patient from harming self
Assist your dentist as directed
Remove other patients or observers from area
Call patient's physician if dentist so requests

Death

Although the occurrence is rare, it is possible that a patient may die in the office (as is possible anywhere). Should this happen, it is necessary to notify the coroner or medical examiner in your community. The office personnel should know the requirements in case of sudden death and be prepared to make the necessary telephone calls immediately. Quite likely your dentist will ask you to call the patient's physician.

Death
Know the procedure required in your community
Alert the dentist if he or she is not in the same area of the office as the patient
Make necessary telephone calls
Follow dentist's instructions for relating to the family of the deceased person

Fainting (Syncopé)

The term *syncopé* refers to a sudden lack of circulation of blood to the brain. The most common conditions that are likely to cause syncopé (fainting) are fear, emotional disturbance, and pain. The lack of circulation is the result of a temporary lowering of the pulse pressure, which creates a shortage of blood supplied to the brain. A feeling of uneasiness and lightheadedness usually precedes the actual syncopé or faint.

The picture of syncopé is quite startling. The skin is pale, cool, and clammy. The pupils are dilated and do not become smaller when in a strong light. Pulse pressure is weak, and respiration is slow, feeble, and irregular.

Usually the patient will indicate when he or she feels faint. Where the patient is will determine your action. If the patient is already in the dental chair, lower the backrest to a horizontal position so that the head is level with, or lower than, the body. A cold, wet towel should be placed on the patient's forehead either to prevent loss of consciousness or to assist the patient to regain consciousness.

If the patient is in the beginning stages of syncopé and still conscious, place the head between the knees, with the arms hanging loose. Place your hand on the back of the patient's head and say, "Push against my hand with your head as if you are going to sit up." The patient's exertion will bring blood to the brain quickly and help avoid syncopé. Aromatic spirits of ammonia are furnished in small, cloth-packaged vials. A vial may be broken and briefly held under the patient's nose because the spirits act as a reflex stimulant. Be sure to use it sparingly, as the ammonia is quite strong and will be offensive to the patient.

If the patient happens to be standing and is likely to fall before he or she can be seated, do not hesitate to have the patient lie down quickly on the floor.

Tight clothing should be loosened in all cases of syncopé. A short period of oxygen inhalation will be very helpful.

After such recommended treatment for syncopé, the patient may appear to recover quite rapidly but should not be placed in an upright position too quickly,

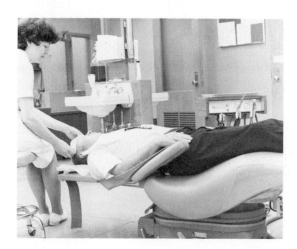

Figure 26.6
Patient in horizontal position.

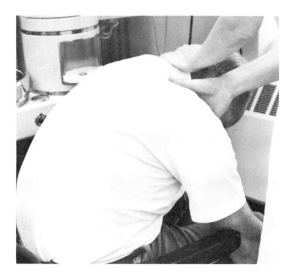

Figure 26.7
Patient applying upward pressure against dental assistant's hand.

nor should an effort be made to continue dental procedures immediately unless it is necessary. Give the patient sufficient time to readjust to the situation before proceeding—better overall progress will frequently result.

Fainting
If the patient is sitting: Have patient put head between knees Apply pressure to back of neck Ask patient to push against your hand Use spirits of ammonia briefly, if needed Loosen tight clothing **If patient is standing:** Have patient lie down Loosen tight clothing **If patient is in dental chair:** Lower back rest Apply cold cloth Loosen tight clothing **In all cases:** Do not leave patient alone Have patient remain quiet Do not allow patient up too soon

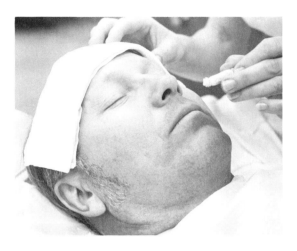

Figure 26.8
Ammonia being administered.

Hemorrhage (Bleeding)

The control of hemorrhage during and following dental surgery may be a problem. Extraction sockets or other surgical sites in the mouth may continue hemorrhaging due to improper clotting or partially severed vessels, either in the bone or soft tissue. Pressure packing by holding gauze over the wound for three to five minutes is the most reliable method of stopping hemorrhage in a patient with normal clotting time. Occasionally it is necessary for the dentist to place additional sutures where indicated at the wound site to tie off the bleeding vessels.

Clot formation and control of bleeding is the goal when hemorrhage occurs. A hemostatic agent is an agent that stops the flow of blood. Several hemostatic agents are being used to assist in the clot formation when it is necessary. Oxidized cellulose, a specially treated material that is capable of being gradually dissolved in relatively undamaged or normal tissue, may be placed in the wound and sutured in position. Therefore, when surgery is contemplated, it is very important to have materials for suturing available, as well as the hemostatic agents.

Epistaxis (nosebleed), should it occur to a patient, may be stopped with a large piece of cotton moistened with cold water and packed as high as possible in the nostril. Cold packs on the nose and lifting the head until the nose assumes a horizontal position (not low in relation to the rest of the body) are also helpful. An epinephrine pack might be used for a young person, but definitely not for an older patient, particularly one with any history of a cardiac disturbance.

Hemorrhage (Bleeding)
Pressure pack immediately Alert dentist if necessary Set out suture materials

Epistaxis (Nosebleed)
Prepare packs if needed While awaiting dentist, elevate patient's head until the nose is horizontal Apply pressure to base of nose

Insulin Shock

Diabetic patients can experience a condition known as insulin shock. It is imperative that you immediately call the physician of a patient who is experiencing insulin shock. Records of a diabetic patient should be marked with some arresting color to indicate that this patient is diabetic. The physician's telephone number should be written in bold digits where it can be easily seen in order to facilitate the telephone call that could be necessary to save a life.

Abnormal behavior in a diabetic patient may mean insulin reaction. The individual may be weak, sweat profusely, experience palpitation, sometimes becoming confused, unable to speak proficiently and unable to tell you that he or she is experiencing a problem. The patient may become unconscious. If a diabetic patient appears to be going into, or is already in, a state of shock, rush to phone the patient's physician.

Insulin Shock
Be certain diabetics' records are marked for recognition of these patients. Have telephone number of physician in conspicuous place. Diabetic patients should be continually observed for behavior that might indicate shock. Alert dentist Alert physician Follow instructions

Psychosis

Many persons are unstable emotionally. Some of them can be psychotic. The dental personnel must be aware that persons who have emotional problems do come for dental treatment. Most patients who are unstable emotionally cause no problem in behavior, but occasionally a patient will be a known psychotic or drug addict. Should such a patient be in your practice, be sure the dentist is scheduled to be in the room with the patient the entire time. Have two staff members present with the psychotic patient.

Psychotic Patient
Always have two staff members present in the room with a psychotic patient or drug addict.

Respiratory Reaction

Respiratory reaction is observed in many degrees of difficulty and for a number of reasons. It can be cardiac disease, reaction to a drug, inhalation of fumes, asthma, or other diseases of the lungs.

Allow a conscious patient to choose the position in which breathing is most comfortable. This may not be lying down. Clothing should be loosened. The patient may be or become unconscious.

Regardless of the cause of the respiratory reaction, oxygen must be given. If the patient is unconscious, artificial respiration may be necessary.

Of course, the dentist must be alerted at once and his or her directions followed. A Resusitube is a valuable emergency instrument to have available . . . and to know how to use. It may work more efficiently than mouth-to-mouth resuscitation.

Respiratory Reaction
Free airway (Remove any obstructions such as dentures, gum, and so on.) Alert dentist and follow instructions Help patient find position most comfortable for breathing Loosen tight clothing Ready oxygen and/or artificial respiration Call patient's physician

Shock

Shock covers a broad range of difficulty. It becomes a matter of degree. A very mild state of shock may produce nothing noticeable in the patient's physical appearance. Severe shock may leave the patient unconscious. Shock can result in symptoms of varying degrees of severity between these two extremes.

It is unusual to see more severe forms of shock than syncopé in the dental office. The rules for treating serious shock are similar to those for care of the person with syncopé. Keep the patient warm and loosen tight items of clothing, such as belts and collars, and call the patient's physician.

Shock May be Recognized by These Symptoms

Cool, moist skin

Pale or cyanotic lips

Increasingly weak pulse

Falling blood pressure

Thirst and restlessness

Collapsed peripheral veins

Suppression of urine formation

Emergency Actions for Shock

Stop hemorrhage

Maintain free airway

Elevate feet (unless head injury, pulmonary edema, or chest wounds—which are unlikely in a dental emergency)

Conserve body warmth

Relieve pain and anxiety

Summary

A *drug* is any substance that is used as a medicine. In the correct quantity drugs can be helpful, but excessive amounts may be poisonous. Certain drugs when taken together cause unfavorable reactions. Also, some drugs and foods cannot be mixed because the combination produces an unfavorable reaction.

Learn to exercise care in all procedures in which you use or dispense drugs. Do not guess. Be certain that you are accurate when you dispense or administer drugs for patients. Drugs are usually liquid or solid. Fourteen classifications are given for liquid drugs and four for solid drugs. *Generic* drug names are family names, deriving from the source or compound used to make the drug. *Proprietary* names are those given to a specific drug formula by the manufacturers of the specific formula.

Certain drugs are controlled by law. Care must be exercised so that such drugs are accounted for to the proper authorities. Mood drugs are controlled as well as drugs containing narcotics.

The dentist is the only member of the oral health care team who is qualified to prescribe medications. A written prescription must be given the patient for any medication requiring it. A prescription blank has eight items to be completed: the name of the patient, name of drug, size of dosage, total quantity to be dispensed, directions, signature of the dentist, the federal registry number, if necessary, and the number of times the prescription may be refilled.

An *emergency*—unanticipated combination of circumstances requiring immediate action to prevent serious injury or loss—may occur in the dental office. Anxiety may be the cause. The primary attempt of the dental assistant is to call the attention of the dentist to the emergency condition should it be necessary. Fundamental rules for the dental assistant's conduct include:

1. Be calm and reassuring for the patient.
2. Call attention of your dentist to the emergency.
3. Follow the dentist's instructions exactly.

For each emergency there is a summary of procedures listed alphabetically in this chapter. Refer to them as necessary.

Study Questions

1. Discuss the values and dangers of drugs.
2. Why must you keep labels in good condition so that you know what is in the containers?
3. What is meant by "From panacea to poison"?
4. Differentiate between a saturated solution and a stock solution.
5. Choose five types of drugs used in the dental office and explain their use.
6. Differentiate between generic and proprietary drug names.
7. Differentiate between "administer," "dispense," and "prescribe."
8. What is an emergency? How do you determine that you have an emergency?
9. Discuss what you would do with a person who is about to faint.

10. Describe the emergency and explain the dental assistant's role in meeting the following emergencies: syncopé, chest pain, hemorrhage, shock, allergic reaction.
11. What is hypertension?

Vocabulary

administer   give the medication to the patient and watch him or her take it

analgesics   relieve pain

anesthetics   produce loss of feeling

capsules   rod-shaped, soluble material such as gelatin, which forms a case containing powders or liquid to be swallowed without tasting the contents

coagulate   harden and form a scab

compendium   a summary of knowledge of a specific field, gathered together and presented in concise or outline form, presenting all the essential facts and details of a subject

dispense   give the patient the medication with instructions for use at home

drug   any substance that is used as a medicine

dyspnea   labored breathing

epistaxis   nosebleed

generic   family name of drug

hemostatic agent   something that arrests the flow of blood

narcotic   class of drugs that produce stupor, sleep, and/or complete insensibility to pain

pills   small, hard objects made of sugar and starch mixed with medicinal drugs

potentiate   magnify the effects

prescribe   designate by written order a medication and instructions for its use

proprietary   name given to drug by manufacturer; drug conforms to a specific formula, manufacturer guarantees each tablet is exactly like all other tablets packaged under that name

saturated solution   liquid containing largest amount of drug that will dissolve in that amount of liquid

sedative   drug that quiets a patient

side effect   a consequence other than the one for which the medication was used

stock solution   concentrated form of drug

tablets   disc-shaped mixtures of sugar of milk, and the drug

tincture   alcoholic solution of soluble drug or chemical

Word Elements	
Word Element	*Example*
ante prefix meaning: before, preceding, in front of	*anterior* front or forward part
cau prefix meaning: burn	*caustic* chemical that burns or eats away tissue
cret combining form meaning: distinguish, separate off	*discrete* made up of separate parts
ecto prefix meaning: outside	*ectoderm* the outer layer of the skin
er suffix meaning: one who belongs to or is connected with	*bookkeeper* one who maintains the business records of a firm or dental practice
exo prefix meaning: beyond, out of, without, from, off, outward, outside	*exodontics* art and science of the removal of teeth
form prefix meaning: shape	*formation* process of giving shape or form
gno combining form meaning: know	*diagnose* to recognize the nature of a disease
grad, gress, gred combining form meaning: go, step, walk, degree	*graduated* marked by a succession of degrees, lines, steps (a graduated measure)
leuk, leuc combining form meaning: white	*leukocyte* white blood cells

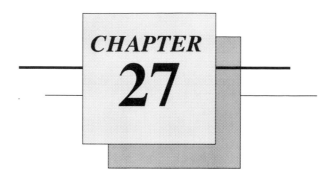

CHAPTER
27

Preventive Dentistry and Personal Oral Hygiene

Oral Hygiene
  Plaque
  Calculus
  Stains
  Dental Prophylaxis (Prevention Through
      Cleaning)
  Fluoride
  Dentifrice
Toothbrushes and Toothbrush Technique
  Electric Toothbrushes
Flossing
Water Jets
Other Aids

Oral Hygiene

For decades the dental profession has attempted to care for the oral health needs of patients with a treatment-oriented philosophy and practice. Treatment alone, however, cannot maintain teeth. Dental decay and periodontal disease destroy the teeth and their supporting structures faster than the nation's dentists can treat them.

Dental research has shown that sound preventive practices coupled with good restorative treatment is the only way adequate dental health care can be achieved. The goals of preventive dentistry are to prevent the occurrence or recurrence of dental disease. Preventive practice demands a commitment to the philosophy of prevention by all members of the oral health care delivery team; and they, in turn, must *motivate* their patients to provide the home care. Frequently, too little attention has been given to POH (personal oral hygiene) education: teaching the patient how to give his or her mouth the correct daily care that is so important in maintaining good oral health. Further, on each prophylaxis appointment the patients must be evaluated on the results of their personal oral hygiene performance. Only with this supervision can individual patients intelligently accept their responsibility for the maintenance of a healthy mouth.

The dental assistant should be prepared to explain to patients the objectives of a good preventive program and be able to instruct the patients in proper oral hygiene, proper diet, correct toothbrush technique, and correct flossing. These measures form the foundation of sound preventive practices. The assistant must also present this instruction without scolding or degrading the patient for poor techniques or failure to perform the necessary tasks in personal oral hygiene. A gentle, firm, continual reminder of the importance of these home duties will produce better results than causing the patient to lose face.

Some of the basic information necessary for teaching patients personal oral hygiene will be discussed here, but it must be emphasized that there are many ways to accomplish the same objective. Each dentist may have a somewhat different method he or she will wish to teach. The methods of brushing the teeth and the types of brush to use are subject to variation. The dental assistant should learn exactly what the dentist wants patients taught and then use every opportunity to *motivate* the patients to perform their home care routines well.

Plaque

The salivary glands (the parotids, the submaxillary, and the sublingual glands) produce a clear, alkaline, and usually viscid (to a greater or lesser degree) fluid called

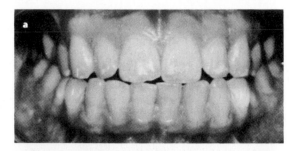
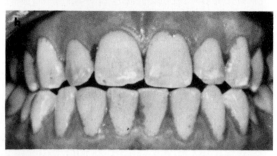
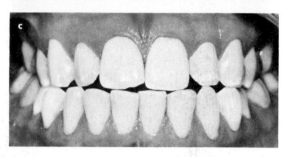

Figure 27.1

Plaque staining: (a) Patient has brushed teeth, apparently clean. The patient is now instructed to chew and dissolve a disclosing tablet thoroughly, swish the liquid throughout the mouth for sixty seconds, spit it out, then rinse with a mouthful of water; (b) results of the staining; and (c) mouth after the second brushing.

saliva. The saliva enters the mouth in three general areas: one in each cheek approximately opposite the buccal surface of the upper first or second molars and another in the floor of the mouth nearest the lower anterior teeth. Mucous glands, which are present wherever there is a mucous membrane, like the lining of the mouth, add their mucous secretion. Saliva contains the enzyme called ptyalin, which begins the conversion of starches in food to maltose (a sugar). Saliva also contains serum-albumin, globulin, and cell debris.

A yellow-white sticky substance, *mucin,* is a precipitate of saliva that combines with bacteria, food, and cell debris in the mouth to form a gelatinlike layer on those surfaces of the teeth that are somewhat sheltered. The surfaces that are constantly rubbed by the tongue, lips, or cheeks, or are cleaned in the process of chewing food, do not accumulate this gelatinous layer which is called *bacterial plaque.*

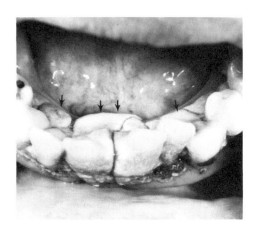

Figure 27.2
Calculus.

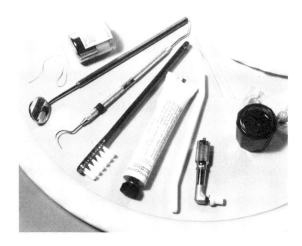

Figure 27.3
Armamentarium for POH.

Plaque is the principal cause of dental caries and periodontal disease. If you can teach your patients to eliminate this slippery mass of microorganisms from the surfaces of the teeth through meticulous brushing and flossing techniques, their dental diseases will be all but eliminated. The maintenance of a healthy dentition is dependent on a plaque-free mouth.

Calculus

Various salts, such as the salts of calcium and phosphorus, are also precipitated from saliva. The gelatinous matrix of the bacterial plaque provides a base for the accumulation of these salts, and eventually a hard cementlike substance evolves that is impossible to remove with a toothbrush. The substance is calculus. This particular type of calculus is *salivary calculus*. When calculus forms on the teeth, it must be removed with scaling instruments as the first stage of the dental prophylaxis. If allowed to accumulate, it collects progressively into the subgingival area as well and compounds the periodontal problems. Loss of supporting bone occurs, and pockets of infection are created.

Stains

A commonly seen stain is that caused by smoking. The brown or blackish stains are tobacco tars precipitated on the tooth surface and are extremely difficult to remove. Once the teeth are thoroughly cleaned, the patient can often retain a nice appearance, in spite of smoking, by doing a very thorough brushing job, and especially if the patient smokes cigarettes not more than halfway through.

Green stains on the gingival third of the tooth is sometimes seen in children. Less commonly, a red or red-brown stain is seen. These stains are caused by chromogenic bacteria attached to the remains of *Nasmyth's membrane,* a covering present over the unerupted enamel crown of the tooth. The stains are extremely disfiguring but can usually be removed by the dentist.

Dental Prophylaxis (Prevention Through Cleaning)

Dental prophylaxis is an operation for which scaling instruments and polishing pastes are used to remove the hard and soft accretions and stains from the tooth surfaces and the gingival crevices.

Scalers are necessary to plane the surfaces of the teeth and free them from all calculus deposits. The prophylaxis paste is used to remove all soft accretions and leave a smooth, polished surface.

Flour of pumice, a powdered grit made from lava rock, was formerly the powder of choice for prophylaxis. Today, however, less harsh cleaning agents containing zirconium not only clean the tooth surfaces well, but leave them highly polished and less susceptible to plaque formation. These commercially prepared powders also contain fluoride for its topical effect against caries.

The paste is used with brushes, rubber cups, and dental floss to eliminate all plaque and debris from pits, fissures, and interproximal surfaces.

The prophylaxis contra-angle is an instrument made specifically for use with rubber cups. A regular contra-angle is used to hold the prophylaxis brushes. The grit in the cleaning pastes can gain access to the interior gears of the contra-angles, and consequently these instruments must be meticulously cleaned after each use to keep the gears functioning properly and to

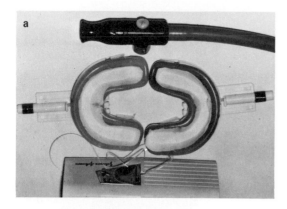

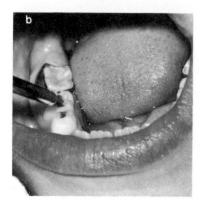

Figure 27.4
*Flouride treatment (a) trays for flouride application,
(b) drying prior to fluoride application.*

effect sterilization between patients. Care on your part will greatly increase the service your office can expect from these contra-angles (or right angles).

Stains and calculus can also be removed with the ultrasonic instrument that gently and quickly removes attached debris with an instrument tip that vibrates or oscillates 25,000 cycles per second.

Fluoride

Dental research has confirmed that flouride in the drinking water during the years of tooth development drastically reduces the incidence of dental caries. The effectiveness of fluoride is directly related to the concentration of fluoride ion in the water, up to 1.5 parts per million (ppm). There is also sufficient evidence to support the ingestion of fluoride tablets to provide the necessary caries-preventing flouride where drinking water does not contain sufficient fluoride naturally, or where the community water supply is not fluoridated. These tablets would be prescribed by the dentist when indicated.

In the dental office, further protection can be given by the topical application of a concentrated fluoride solution or gel. This application is generally performed by the dental hygienist, or where permitted by law and with proper training, by the dental assistant. The teeth are first thoroughly cleansed to remove all debris and plaque so that the fluoride will have maximum access to the enamel surface. Some prophylaxis pastes contain fluoride (usually stannous fluoride) to increase anticariogenic effectiveness.

Three types of fluoride are currently used for topical application: sodium fluoride (2 percent), stannous fluoride (8 percent for children, 10 percent for adults), and acidulated phosphate-fluoride (1.23 percent). All produce essentially the same protective reaction on the enamel surface. Sodium and stannous fluoride applications are made as a solution painted on the teeth. Acidulated phosphate-fluoride may be applied either as a solution or in the form of a gel held in place by a tray.

Following a prophylaxis, the teeth are rinsed, isolated with cotton rolls, and dried with warm air. The exposed surfaces of the teeth are then covered with the fluoride solution or gel. Solutions are painted on with cotton swabs, keeping the teeth wet with the solution for four minutes. Although there is some evidence that shorter periods of time are effective, the consensus is that the four-minute application offers the maximum benefit. The same timing applies to the tray application of the gel. The patient is advised not to eat, drink, or rinse the mouth for at least half an hour following the application.

Topical applications are repeated at intervals prescribed by the dentist, based on the needs of the patient. This is usually every six to twelve months from the age of two years to fifteen years. Applications are made at less frequent intervals after that time.

None of these methods of fluoridating teeth is completely effective in controlling dental caries. Consequently, the maximum effectiveness is obtained by using a combination of fluoride prophylactic paste and topical fluoride application in the dental office, followed by the use of a toothpaste containing fluoride for home care, supplemented with the use of fluoridated drinking water. Brushing teeth with fluoridated toothpaste for as long as one lives is considered most important in preventive dentistry.

Fluoride mouth rinse may be used at a concentration of 0.2 percent sodium fluoride for the weekly rinse or at a concentration of 0.05 percent sodium fluoride for the daily rinse.

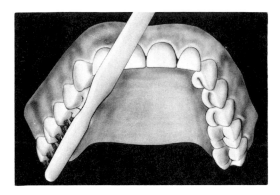

Figure 27.5

Start on the right side and brush the occlusal surfaces of the upper teeth; next, the lower teeth. The ends of the bristles reach into the fissures and pits of the teeth to dislodge food debris. Use short, horizontal strokes with reasonable pressure.

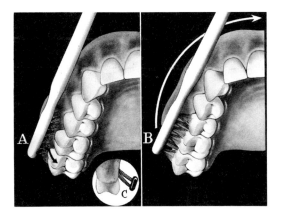

Figure 27.6

With handle horizontal, place brush on gums above the buccal surfaces on three posterior teeth, upper right side (figure A). The bristles are directed toward the roots of teeth with their sides touching the gums. With sweeping strokes, move brush downward to the occlusal surfaces. As the bristles enter the spaces between the teeth (figure B), with a gentle vibratory motion cleanse these areas and stimulate the soft tissue. Figure C shows sides of bristles with downward sweeping stroke over the gums. After brushing the three posterior upper teeth, move on around the arch, using the same strokes.

Dentifrice

Actually, for the adult patient, the energy expenditure and proper action in using the toothbrush is more important than the dentifrice placed on the bristles.

The formation of calculus begins with the accumulation of food deposits and the retention of bacterial plaques for a period of time. If plaque is removed as thoroughly as possible on a daily basis, the dentist or hygienist can easily complete the cleansing of those

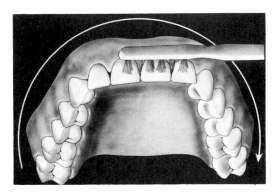

Figure 27.7

This picture shows the brush moved around to the upper anterior teeth. Use the same downward sweeping stroke as shown in figure 27.6. Care is taken so that the ends of the bristles do not pierce or otherwise injure the gums. Continue brushing until you have brushed all the upper teeth.

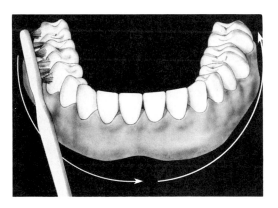

Figure 27.8

Next, brush the facial surfaces of the lower teeth, beginning with the posterior teeth on the right side and continuing around the arch until you have brushed every lower facial surface. Note that on the lower teeth the sweeping stroke is upward.

areas the patient misses or cannot readily reach. The daily removal of as much as possible of these soft accumulations reduces the irritation and inflammation and provides exercise for the gums.

Fluorides and other additives purported to be anticariogenic are incorporated into many commercial toothpastes for patient use. Fluoride is the only additive that has been proved effective against caries.

The Council on Dental Therapeutics of the American Dental Association has approved certain stannous fluoride dentifrices as aids in reducing the incidence of dental decay, along with the usual programs of dental care.

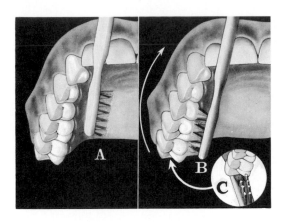

Figure 27.9
Now brush the lingual surfaces of the three posterior upper teeth on the right. Place the sides of the bristles (figure A) toward the center of the palate; use a sweeping stroke and move the brush to the lingual surfaces of the teeth until it is in figure B. Use a gentle rotary motion; the ends of the bristles work into the spaces between the teeth. Figure C shows how the distal surfaces of the last molar teeth, both upper and lower, are cleaned with a few short strokes. The toe or end of the brush is used.

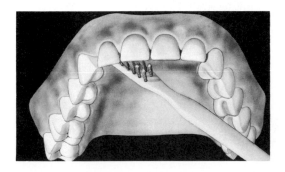

Figure 27.10
Now clean the lingual surfaces of the upper anterior teeth. The brush handle is in a more vertical position. The stroke is downward toward the occlusal surfaces with a gentle vibratory motion. Use the same method for the lingual surface of the lower anterior teeth.

Toothbrushes and Toothbrush Technique

A variety of toothbrushes are available for patients to buy. The patients should be instructed to purchase a brush with soft bristles that will not injure the delicate gingival tissues and yet will be stiff enough to adequately reach and clean the gingival areas and interproximal spaces as well as the easier-to-brush occlusal surfaces.

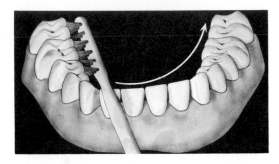

Figure 27.11
To clean lingual surfaces of lower posterior teeth, the toe or end of the brushhead is used with controlled rotary motion. The tufts work into the spaces between the teeth. The brush is moved around the arch until no lingual surface is neglected.

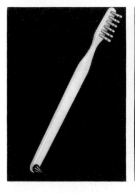
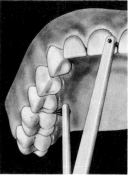

Figure 27.12
Effective stimulation of the gum tissue and cleaning of spaces between the teeth with the rubber stimulator tip. Reasonable pressure with the tip is exerted against gum tissue. Intermittent action forces stagnant blood from the capillaries, allowing fresh blood to replace the supply. In addition to the use of the rubber tip, flossing is necessary to clean the interproximal areas.

The method of brushing you teach your patients is the decision of your dentist. The objective is to de-plaque all surfaces of the teeth. Although method is important, there are many ways to brush teeth and successfully accomplish the objective. Whatever the method, it should be specific and should be mastered by your patients under your instruction. One method, a modified Charters-Stillman method, is illustrated in figures 27.5 through 27.12.[1]

Another widely accepted and popular brushing technique, the Bass technique, utilizing short back-and-forth strokes of the bristles pointed into the gingival and interproximal areas.

Electric Toothbrushes

Many brands of electrically powered toothbrushes have been introduced in recent years. They have varied widely in their construction, cost, and operating methods. The Council on Dental Therapeutics included powered toothbrushes in its evaluation program in order to provide authoritative information to dentists and the public, as well as to encourage manufacturers to establish adequate testing of their products.

Regardless of the manner of movement of the head of the particular electric toothbrush, it is possible to alter to a considerable degree the direction of the brush movement on the teeth and gums by holding the brush handle in various positions.

The electric toothbrush can be an invaluable aid for persons with limited function of the hands and arms, such as persons with arthritis and patients in hospitals and nursing homes.

Flossing

Flossing is a process of cleaning the areas between the teeth with pieces of dental floss. Flossing may be accomplished by holding the dental floss firmly between the fingers and inserting it gently between the contact areas of the teeth. Care must be taken not to "snap" the floss through the contact and damage the interdental papilla. The proper procedure is to pass the floss through the contact at a forty-five-degree angle to the occlusal plane, moving it slightly back and forth (fig. 27.14).

Cleaning with the floss is accomplished with an up-and-down motion, drawing the floss subgingivally as comfort permits. Floss in an organized pattern, making sure to polish the interproximal surfaces of all contacting teeth.

Water Jets

Another device marketed as an aid for oral hygiene delivers a stream of water to flush debris from hard-to-reach areas. One popular device is the water pik (fig. 27.15). This instrument projects a jet of water at adjustable pressures to wash out debris. Although this instrument cannot accomplish complete cleansing and plaque removal, it can remove debris from under fixed bridgework and around orthodontic appliances. It can also be used following brushing and flossing to rinse interproximal spaces where gingival recession exists. Care must be taken not to use too forceful a jet stream, which may harm the gingival attachment.

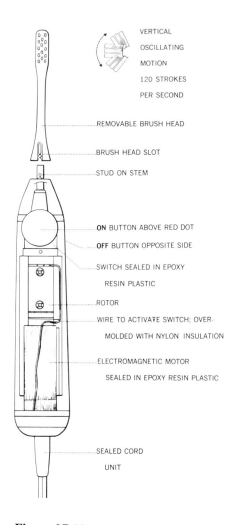

Figure 27.13
Broxident electric toothbrush.

Other Aids

Additional aids to remove plaque and maintain a healthy mouth include:

1. A perio-aid that uses a frayed toothpick as an additional brush for the free gum margin area
2. Rubber tips to stimulate the tissue between the teeth; and pipe cleaners or interproximal type brushes for reaching areas in which the bone loss has caused a deeper indentation

However, all of these aids must be used only with instruction from the dentist who prescribes them.

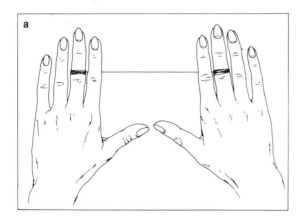

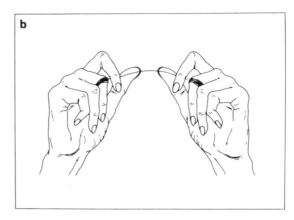

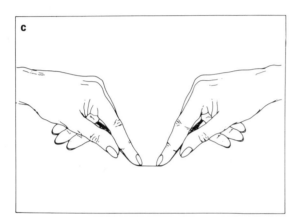

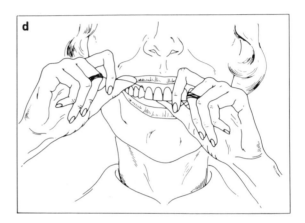

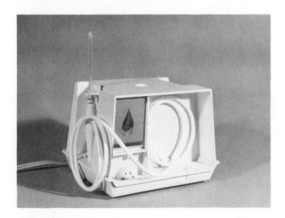

Figure 27.14
Flossing: (a) stabilizing the floss; (b) thumb position for flossing upper teeth; (c) position for flossing lower teeth; and (d) flossing upper teeth.

Figure 27.15
Water pik.

Summary

Adequate dental health care can be achieved through a combination of good restorative treatment and sound preventive practices. Preventive dentistry means that the oral health care delivery team is committed to the philosophy of preventive dentistry, and the members attempt to motivate patients to practice good personal oral hygiene.

The dental assistant should be able to explain to patients the objectives of a good preventive program, to instruct them in proper oral hygiene, proper diet, correct toothbrush technique, and correct flossing. Patients must learn to meticulously cleanse the mouth of substances that cause dental disease.

Plaque forms and must be removed. Bacterial plaque is a gelatinlike layer caused by the mixing of food with mucin. *Mucin* is a yellow-white sticky substance precipitated by saliva.

Calculus must be removed with scalers since the toothbrush cannot remove the hardened salts.

Stains, such as those caused by smoking, can be removed by dental prophylaxis.

Dental prophylaxis is the process by which the hygienist or dentist removes all deposits from the teeth with scalers, rubber cups, prophylaxis contra-angles, or ultrasonic instruments.

Fluoride reduces the incidence of caries when properly administered. Both care in the dental office and at home are required.

Dentifrice is helpful. Toothpaste with flouride does assist in retarding and eliminating dental disease.

The *toothbrush* is used as an instrument of cleaning and exercise. The objective of brushing is to deplaque all surfaces of the teeth. The method taught and the type of brush used will be prescribed by the dentist. Electric toothbrushes are available and are particularly helpful for persons who have limited function of arm and hand movement.

Flossing is a process of cleansing areas between teeth with pieces of dental floss.

Water jets deliver a stream of water to flush debris from hard-to-reach areas.

Other aids are prescribed by the dentist for certain patients.

Study Questions

1. What forms the foundation for sound preventive practices for adequate health care?
2. What does POH mean?
3. Describe fluoride treatment and explain its advantages.
4. Who can benefit from the use of fluoride?
5. Describe plaque and explain its effect on teeth.
6. Describe dental prophylaxis.
7. For the adult patient, what is more important than the choice of toothpaste?
8. Describe a good method of toothbrushing.
9. Describe flossing.
10. Of what value is a water jet?

Word Elements

Word Element	Example
hyper combining form meaning: excessive	**hypersecretion** increased or excessive secretion
hypo combining form meaning: insufficient, defective, under, deficient	**hypodontia** fewer teeth than normal
iatr combining form meaning: heal, treatment	**pediatrics** medical specialty that treats only children
ject combining form meaning: throw, cast	**injection** introducing (forcing) a liquid into tissue
labi combining form meaning: lip	**labial** pertaining to the lips
lact combining form meaning: relationship to milk	**lactobacillus** bacteria that produce lactic acid
lith prefix or suffix meaning: stone	**lithotomy** removal of a stone
lysis suffix meaning: decomposition, destruction, dissolution	**autolysis** self-dissolution (some bacteria are autolytic)
myo prefix meaning: muscle	**myology** study of muscles
ob prefix meaning: over, to, against	**obesity** overweight

CHAPTER 28

Dental Specialties

Endodontics
Oral and Maxillofacial Surgery
    Definition
    The Role of the Assistant
    Preoperative Duties and Preparation
    Efficient Assisting in Oral Surgery
    Postoperative Duties
Orthodontics
    Angle's Classification
    Parts of the Orthodontic Appliance
    Duties of an Orthodontic Assistant
Pedodontics
Periodontics
    Duties of the Periodontal Assistant
Prosthodontics
    Duties of the Prosthodontic Assistant

A dental assistant for a specialist will have some duties that are peculiar to the practice of the specialty. In this chapter the brief descriptions give a general idea of the particular work of each specialty discussed.

Two of the specialties, *oral pathology* and *dental public health,* have been omitted since they do not commonly require assistants. The other specialties are discussed in alphabetical order.

Endodontics

Endodontics (*end,* "within" + *dont,* "tooth") is that specialty of dentistry which deals with the diagnosis and treatment of irritated or infected pulps of teeth and their periapical tissues. Its purpose is to retain such teeth as healthy functioning organs. To thoroughly understand the problems involved in the treatment of pulpal and periapical disorders, the dentist must have a sound knowledge of the origin and effect of the various irritants that may attack the tooth, the ability to utilize diagnostic aids to their best advantage, and the faculty to correlate subjective and objective symptoms to arrive at a correct diagnosis. The correct treatment is the goal. Correct diagnosis is the means to that goal.

As a dental assistant, you will record much of the patient's history and symptoms and assist in performing such tests as vitality testing to help the dentist arrive at the diagnosis (figs. 28.10, 28.11). Patients frequently come to the dental office with pain, and this pain is most often of pulpal origin. Such patients not only need immediate attention, but also more understanding and gentle care. Be supportive.

The following description explains the scope of endodontic therapy. The treatment of pulpal and periapical conditions may be divided according to various objectives.

1. **Desensitization of dentin** is the treatment of dentin exposed through normal gingival recession, periodontal disease, or surgical intervention on adjacent tissues (fig. 28.1, tooth 1).
2. **Pulp protection** refers to the placement of an insulating, protective, and perhaps analgesic cement or paste on the pulpal or axial wall of dentin when fractures of the tooth or the removal of deep caries approximates, but does not expose, vital pulp tissues (fig. 28.1, tooth 2).
3. **Pulp capping** is a superficial treatment of vital dental pulps exposed through trauma or during caries removal. This is an attempt to stimulate a hard tissue healing over the exposed area and to insure continued vitality of the remaining pulp tissue (fig. 28.1, tooth 3).

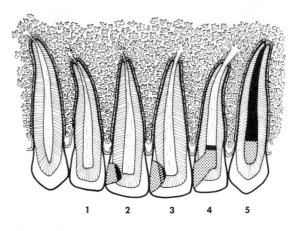

Figure 28.1
Conservative endodontic treatments.

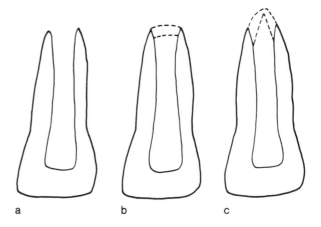

Figure 28.2
Apexification: (a) incompletely formed nonvital tooth; (b) apical closure; (c) apical development.

4. **Pulpotomy,** or partial pulpectomy, is the removal of part of the vital pulp tissue and the treatment of the remaining pulp stump or stumps in an attempt to stimulate hard tissue healing over the exposed wound(s) and maintain the vitality of the remaining pulp tissue. In principle, this latter operation is identical with pulp capping; however, the site of capping is selected at a more favorable position in this procedure (fig. 28.1, tooth 4).
5. **Root canal therapy,** or complete pulpectomy, is the removal of all pulpal tissue, followed by sterilization and filling of the root canal (fig. 28.1, tooth 5).
6. **Apexification** is a method of inducing apical closure or the continued apical development of the root(s) of an incompletely formed tooth in which the pulp is no longer vital. Usually the apex is formed by osteodentine or a similar hard tissue (fig. 28.2).

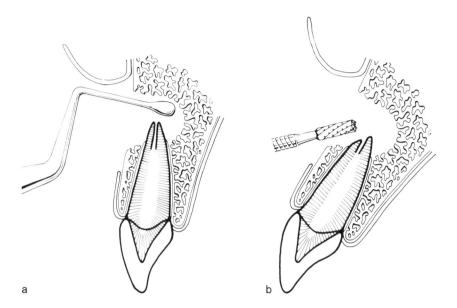

Figure 28.3
*(a) Root end exposed for retrofilling by curetting apex;
and (b) root resection for retrofilling.*

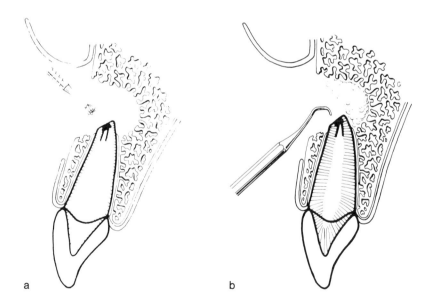

Figure 28.4
*(a) Retrofilling preparation; and (b) placement of
retrofilling.*

7. **Apical curettage** is the surgical removal of
   pathologic periapical tissues, which may be
   accomplished following root canal therapy
   or simultaneously with it.
8. **Apicoectomy** is the removal of a portion of
   the root apex, performed concurrently with
   apical curettage where indicated.

9. **Retrofilling** is a method of filling the root
   canal, particularly the apical portion, from
   the apex of the root following apical
   curretage and root resection (figs. 28.3–
   28.8).
10. **Hemisection** or **root amputation** must
    occasionally be performed. The root portion
    is sacrificed, but the remaining tooth
    structures are retained for restoration.

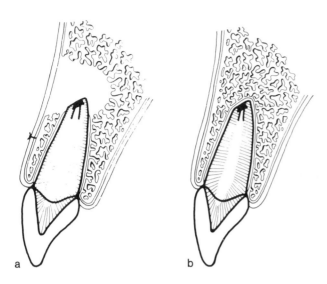

Figure 28.5
(a) Placement of suture; and (b) complete healing.

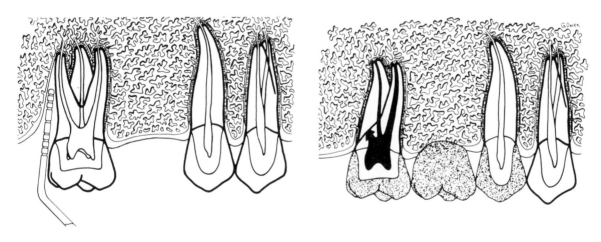

Figure 28.6
Root amputation.

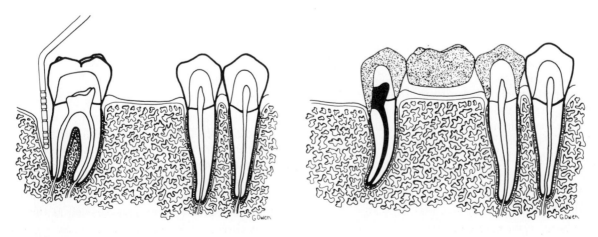

Figure 28.7
Hemisection.

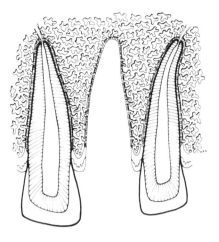
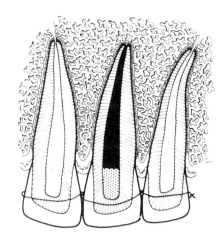

Figure 28.8
Replantation.

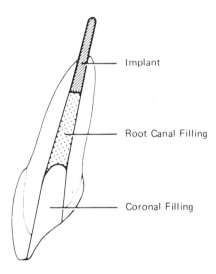

Implant

Root Canal Filling

Coronal Filling

Figure 28.9
Endodontic implant.

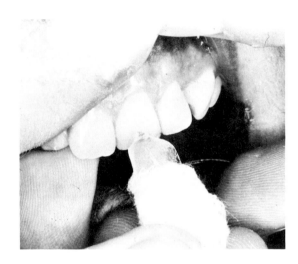

Figure 28.10
Pulp testing with ice.

Figures 28.6 and 28.7 diagram root amputation and hemisection. Root amputation is usually performed on upper teeth. The process removes the root portion and leaves the crown. Hemisection is usually performed on lower teeth. In this therapy, part of the crown is removed along with the root. The remaining part of the crown is then used for a restoration.

11. **Replantation** is the insertion of a totally luxated (accidental or intentional) tooth in its socket usually following endodontic therapy (fig. 28.8).

12. **Endodontic implant** is a method of stabilizing a tooth by lengthening the existing root with a metallic implant extended through the root canal into the periapical osseous tissue (fig. 28.9).

The problem in pulpal therapy is to determine through correct diagnosis which treatment is indicated for any given case. The endodontist has been trained to arrive at the correct diagnosis by studying all available data, including comments from the patient. Frequently this process of evaluating all the data is difficult. Therefore, it is important to carefully preserve all notes concerning the patient's comments as well as the endodontist's clinical observations.

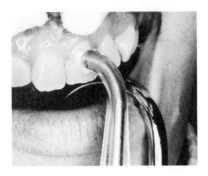

Figure 28.11
Pulp testing with electric pulp tester.

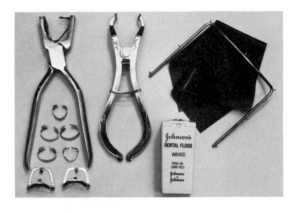

Figure 28.12
Rubber dam tray.

A thorough knowledge of microbiology and sterilization methods is paramount to the practice of endodontics. The assistant will frequently assist the endodontist on surgical cases as well as with the routine procedures performed under rubber-dam isolation.

Oral and Maxillofacial Surgery

(William P. Frantzich, D.D.S., M.S.D.)

Definition

Oral and maxillofacial surgery is that part of dental practice which deals with the diagnosis and the surgical and adjunctive treatment of diseases, injuries, and defects in the oral and maxillofacial region.

The most common procedure in oral surgery offices is the removal of impacted teeth. Other procedures common to the oral and maxillofacial surgeon are:

1. Diagnosis.
2. Radiographic interpretation.
3. Removal of cysts and tumors.
4. Biopsies of lesions.
5. Treatment of facial injuries and fractures of the jaws as a result of auto accidents or other trauma.
6. Correction of jaw deformities, such as protruding or recessive upper and lower jaws and correction of apertognathia (open bite). (This type of surgery is termed *orthognathic surgery* and is generally performed in conjunction with an orthodontic consultation and treatment.)
7. Diagnosis and treatment of diseases of the temporomandibular joint.
8. Surgical placement of osseo integrated implants.
9. Closure of clefts of the palate using bone grafts. Orthognathic surgical procedures may also be necessary to further correct the jaw relationships in cleft palate patients. The oral and maxillofacial surgeon becomes an important team member in the cleft palate clinic.

The oral and maxillofacial surgeon operates both in the office and the hospital and may expect the dental assistant to be competent and comfortable assisting him or her in either location.

The Role of the Assistant

An assistant working in an oral and maxillofacial surgery office will require specific knowledge associated with this specialty. This specific knowledge will include the use and maintenance of sophisticated equipment for monitoring, anesthesia, X ray, and others. It will also include application of the knowledge learned in anatomy, physiology, pharmacology, and other basic sciences. In addition, a successful oral surgery team member develops a very special attitude toward the patients who come for treatment and toward the other oral surgery team members. That attitude permits the team member to lead and be assertive when necessary and then to follow the lead of others in this very special blend of team membership. This unique attitude permits the placing of patient care above any individual needs. In other words, the team player's job description is "whatever it takes to get the job done." All team members must be sensitive to the patient's needs. Giving quality care and treating every patient with respect is of prime importance.

The job of the oral surgery team is to care for the patient in the most beneficial and efficient way. When doing surgery the assistant and the surgeon must be coordinated in their efforts so they can accomplish this goal.

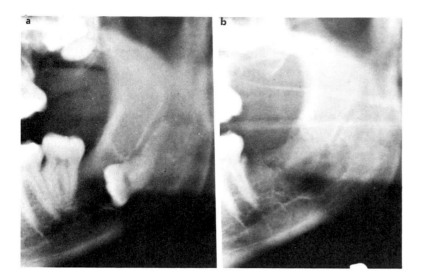

Figure 28.13
X rays: (a) before; and (b) after impaction removal.

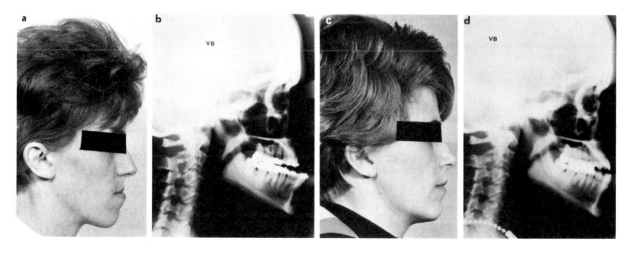

Figure 28.14
Mandibular prognathism: facial photo & skull X ray;
before treatment (a and b); and after treatment (c and d).

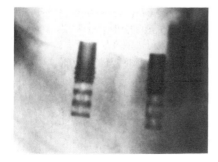

Figure 28.15
X ray of osseo integrated implants.

An assistant must be thoughtful, kind, and reassuring to the patient. Apprehension and anxiety are commonly experienced by oral surgery patients. The assistant must be able to instill in these patients a sense of confidence in the oral surgery team. In addition, the assistant must be able to anticipate the needs of the surgeon in order for the team to perform efficiently and effectively. A good oral surgery office cannot function without the services of such an assistant.

Preoperative Duties and Preparation

1. Patient registration must be complete and accurate (fig. 28.16a).
2. The patient must be thoroughly informed about the treatment options and also given a fair appraisal of the benefits and the risks involved. The patient is to sign an informed consent statement.

   If surgery is to be performed for a minor, the parent's consent form must be attached to the minor's chart, dated and signed by the parent or guardian.
3. A current medical history must be obtained about the patient. (Figure 28.16b is one such form. Questions similar to those in figure 28.16b may be included in the oral surgery medical history.)
4. Certain preoperative preparations are required for some surgeries. The dental assistant is expected to ascertain that these requirements have been met.
   a. The patient has had nothing to eat or drink for six hours.
   b. A responsible person is present to take the patient home.
   c. Removable dental appliances have been removed.
   d. The patient's bladder has just been emptied.
   e. You have checked the buck slip (fig. 28.17) to be sure you have accomplished all the appropriate items for which you are responsible.
   f. The patient with a history of rheumatic fever must have proper premedication with antibiotics prior to the appointment.
   g. Other stipulations concerning preoperative instructions may be routine in an oral surgery practice. Each surgeon will specify his or her requirements in this area.

      It is the duty of the assistant to verify that the patient has followed the preoperative preparation directions and/or taken the appropriate medication. The assistant should write a note on the chart stating whether the patient has complied with the instructions for preoperative preparation. The oral surgeon can then observe this notation prior to performing the surgery. (Figure 28.17 is a *buck slip* that can be passed from one team member to another to accomplish the necessary communications concerning each patient.)
5. If the procedure is more complicated, a consultation appointment may be made for the patient. At this time the patient will be informed about the surgery, possible complications, and likely postoperative course. A video visual aid film may be used to assist the patient in understanding the procedure. If hospitalization is necessary, additional preparation and information will be given.
6. The assistant is responsible for sterilization of instruments by use of an autoclave and cold sterilization. The assistant should know when to use each type of sterilization and be certain that sterilization has been accomplished. Many of the instruments used in oral surgery are individually packaged before placing in the autoclave for sterilization. The assistant is responsible for this task and to see that the packaged, sterilized instruments are placed in the proper storage drawers.
7. The assistant prepares the operatory and the patient for the surgical procedure. The following minimum essentials are necessary for the operating team, and the assistant must be responsible for having them available.[1]
   a. A clear, recent radiograph of the tooth and some of the surrounding structures
   b. A suitable anesthetic agent
   c. Appropriate forceps and elevators for the teeth to be removed
   d. A flap tray of instruments for performing flap operations, sterile and immediately available
   e. The oral surgeon's headlight or other brilliant light
   f. Suction aspiration
   g. An efficient assistant, necessary throughout the entire surgical procedure

---

ORAL AND MAXILLOFACIAL SURGERY SPECIALIST

PATIENT'S NAME (Mr/Mrs/Ms) _____ AGE _____

ADDRESS_____ CITY _____ ZIP _____

HOME PHONE ( )_____ BIRTHDATE _____ SOCIAL SECURITY # _____

OCCUPATION_____BUSINESS NAME_____

BUSINESS ADDRESS_____ CITY _____ ZIP _____

BUSINESS PHONE ( ) _____

MARITAL STATUS - M W S D SPOUSE NAME _____ SPOUSE BUSINESS PHONE _____

PERSON TO GUARANTEE ACCOUNT PAYMENT   ☐ SAME AS ABOVE

NAME _____ ADDRESS _____ CITY _____ ZIP _____

HOME PHONE ( )_____ BIRTHDATE _____ SOCIAL SECURITY # _____

OCCUPATION_____BUSINESS NAME_____

BUSINESS ADDRESS_____ CITY _____ ZIP _____

BUSINESS PHONE ( ) _____

INSURANCE

DENTAL INSURANCE _____ POLICY _____ GROUP _____

MEDICAL INSURANCE _____ POLICY _____ GROUP _____

MEDICAL ASSISTANCE_____VALID FROM_____TO_____

SECOND PARTY WITH INSURANCE

NAME (parent/spouse/self/other) _____

ADDRESS_____ CITY _____ ZIP _____

HOME PHONE ( )_____ BIRTHDATE _____ SOCIAL SECURITY # _____

OCCUPATION_____BUSINESS NAME_____

BUSINESS ADDRESS_____ CITY _____ ZIP _____

BUSINESS PHONE ( ) _____

DENTAL INSURANCE _____ POLICY _____ GROUP _____

MEDICAL INSURANCE _____ POLICY _____ GROUP _____

IS THIS VISIT DUE TO AN ACCIDENT (yes/no)

REFERRED BY: DENTIST_____ORTHODONTIST_____

              PHYSICIAN _____OTHER _____

Person to contact in case of emergency (other than above)_____

Address_____ City _____ Zip _____

Home Phone _____ Work Phone _____ Relationship _____

FINANCIAL ARRANGEMENTS:

  A FINANCE CHARGE of 1% per month (ANNUAL PERCENTAGE RATE of 12%) or $1.00, whichever
  is greater, will be applied to accounts not paid within 45 days after date of service.

_____ Receive a 5% savings—payment of service in full today—cash or check

_____ Payment by Visa or Master Card

_____ 20% down payment on the day of service—required on all insurance claims—balance of 80% due within 30 days.

I have read the above and understand I am financially responsible for the account. I authorize the release of information
and x-rays regarding examination or treatment related to this claim and authorize payment of any insurance benefits directly
to the oral surgeon.

_____Date_____

SIGNATURE

Figure 28.16a

Registration form used by an oral surgeon.

HEALTH HISTORY RECORD

GENERAL DENTIST _____

REFERRED BY _____

Your health is important to us. In order to provide excellent care with safety, it is necessary to become acquainted with vital information related to each patient. Thus, it is extremely important that you answer the following questions as accurately as possible. If you have any questions regarding the information requested, please feel free to ask the doctor or a member of the staff for assistance.

Birthdate: _____

Age: _____ Weight: _____

1. Have you been a patient in a hospital during the past 2 years? _____   YES   NO
2. Have you been under the care of a physician during the past 2 years? _____   YES   NO
3. Have you taken any kind of medicine or drugs during the past year? _____   YES   NO
   PLEASE LIST THIS MEDICATION:

   _____   _____

   _____   _____

4. Are you allergic to penicillin or any drugs or medicine? _____   YES   NO
5. Have you ever had any excessive bleeding requiring special treatment? _____   YES   NO
6. Circle any of the following which you have had:

Heart Trouble	Asthma	Arthritis	Alcoholism
Congenital Heart Lesions	Persistent Cough	Stroke	Emphysema
Heart Murmur	Diabetes	Epilepsy	Bronchitis
High or Low Blood Pressure	Tuberculosis	Psychiatric Treatment	Kidney Disease
Anemia	Venereal Disease	Ulcers	Liver Disease
Rheumatic Fever	Sinus Disease	Drug Dependency	Aids
Scarlet Fever	Porphyria	Cancer	Artificial Joints
Jaundice/Hepatitis	Allergies/Hayfever	Glaucoma	Other _____

7. Do you smoke? _____ How much _____   YES   NO
8. Women: Are you pregnant now? _____ How many months? _____   YES   NO
9. Do you wear contact lenses? _____   YES   NO
10. Have you had any other serious illnesses? _____   YES   NO
11. Do you have difficulty in opening your mouth wide? _____   YES   NO
    Jaws ever click or pop _____   YES   NO
12. Do you have pre-existing T.M.J. problems _____   YES   NO
13. Have you ever had any difficulty with past dental treatment? _____   YES   NO
    Please explain: _____

    _____

14. Have you or any member of family experienced any problems with
    general anesthetic or "twilight sleep"? _____   YES   NO
    Please explain: _____
15. Physician's Name, City, and Phone Number _____

    _____

    _____

    _____

The above medical history is accurate and current to the best of my knowledge.

Signature of Patient (Parent or Guardian, if minor) _____ Date: _____

- -

MEDICAL HISTORY / PHYSICAL EVALUATION UPDATE

Date   *Addition*

_____   _____

_____   _____

_____   _____

Figure 28.16b

A typical medical history form used by an oral surgeon.

```
Patient's Name: _____ Date:_____

Procedure to be performed:_____

_____Referral attached
_____Pre Op Preparation completed. Problems:_____
_____NPO (No food or drink for six hours)
_____Significant medical problems: _____
     _____
_____Return in ____days ____ weeks _____months
_____Check bleeding
_____Post Op X ray
_____Dr. to see before discharge.
_____Ice pack Jaw Support Bandage

_____
_____Analgesic Medication
_____Penicillin 250 mg., 500 mg.
_____Erythromycin 250 mg., 500 mg.
_____Other _____

_____Acute infection instructions
_____Sinus instructions
_____TMJ surgery information
_____Orthognathic surgery information

_____Driver available _____ call for ride, Phone:_____
```

Figure 28.17
The oral surgeon's buck slip.

Efficient Assisting in Oral Surgery

The oral surgeon should be kept occupied using his or her skill at peak efficiency. This goal can be achieved providing the oral surgeon has efficient assistants who are well trained in the specific functions and hand motions that will be required. These duties are:

1. Use the suction aspirator constantly to remove blood, saliva, and debris from the floor of the mouth, the dorsum of the tongue, the right and left retromolar triangles, and the wound itself. If this duty is faithfully performed, the patient should never have to use the cuspidor. The operation proceeds more rapidly and neatly. If the aspirator tip becomes plugged, the assistant must instantly clear the obstruction with a cleaning wire.

2. Use the water syringe in conjunction with the aspirator to cool the bur and to clear a film of blood from the surface of the bone. This task should be performed without a specific request from the oral surgeon.

3. Use the 3 × 3 inch gauze square in the left hand (a) to receive debris picked up by the aspirator tip and (b) to clean the beaks of instruments such as the rongeur forceps or side-cutting bone forceps. A fresh sponge is taken from the pile on the table as needed. If the aspirator becomes plugged, a gauze square should be firmly placed against the wound to keep the field dry. The obstruction in the aspirator can then be removed and the procedure resumed.

4. Use a retractor to hold back the lip or cheek at the moment when suture knots are to be tied.

5. Reassure the patient in a pleasant, affirmative manner.

6. When scrubbed for an operation, the assistant must remain at the chairside until the completion of the procedure. An additional circulating assistant who has not scrubbed is highly desirable to attend to the needs of the scrubbed assistant and to accomplish duties away from the chair.

7. Check airway, bleeding, patient's color, blood pressure, and pulse. Report any abnormal findings to the oral surgeon.

8. Have a knowledge of anesthesia and emergency drugs.

9. Be certified in cardiopulmonary resuscitation.

10. The oral surgery dental assistant may have to be competent in these areas: operation of blood pressure, oximeter, EKG, and defibrillating equipment.

Postoperative Duties

The assistant should continue to monitor the patient in the recovery room, reporting any unusual conditions to the oral surgeon.

Ice therapy is frequently started in the recovery room. A new, efficient way of applying ice after third molar surgery is with the ice-pack mandibular support bandage (fig. 28.18).

The assistant should discharge the patient from the office when the patient is ready. The bleeding should be stopped, and the patient should be awake and able to walk with ease. Any prescriptions should be dispensed at this time.

An appointment for follow-up care and/or suture removal is made before the patient leaves the office.

Discuss postoperative care and give the patient an information pamphlet. The following instructions are usually found in such a brochure. The patient is instructed to read it carefully at home.

Care of the Mouth Following Oral Surgery

1. BLEEDING: After your surgery a gauze compress usually is placed firmly against the surgical area, and you are to keep firm pressure against the area for 30 minutes or until you get home from the office. This is to allow the blood to clot in the tooth socket. If bleeding persists, repeat the procedure. The gauze may be discarded when the bleeding stops. Slight bleeding (blood in the saliva) may be present up to three more days. This is not unusual and is no cause for alarm.

   If EXCESSIVE BLEEDING occurs, the blood is usually bright red and may be pooling in the mouth. Eating and talking

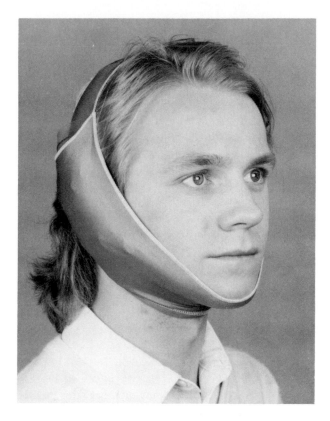

Figure 28.18
Ice-pack mandibular support bandage.

may be difficult, and large clots often form at the surgical site. If CLOTS FORM, rinse your mouth thoroughly and remove any large clots from the bleeding area. Locate the bleeding site and place a compress of folded gauze or facial tissue directly on the bleeding area and hold firm pressure for 30 minutes.

   If BLEEDING PERSISTS, moisten a tea bag and use it as a compress and repeat the above procedure. Tea contains tannic acid and promotes clotting. (EXERCISE AND SPORTS the first six days after surgery will increase bleeding and swelling.)

   IF THE ABOVE MEASURES DO NOT SUCCEED, CALL THE OFFICE FOR ADVICE.

2. DIET: Good nutrition is the key to good healing and rapid recovery. You will feel better, have more strength, less pain, and heal faster if you continue to eat. After surgery, it may be necessary to start by eating soft or liquid foods, such as soup, jello, cooked cereal, milk shakes, baby foods, or liquid diet preparations. As soon as possible return to a normal diet.

FLUIDS: It is important that your fluid intake be adequate. An adult should consume eight to twelve glasses of fluid each day, not counting diuretics, such as coffee and tea. Children should have a proportional amount. Avoid drinking with a straw. Also avoid alcoholic beverages and smoking after surgery.

3. RINSES: Do not rinse the mouth vigorously the first day of surgery. Beginning the next day, rinse the mouth gently, using a full glass of warm water in which a half teaspoon of table salt or mouthwash has been dissolved. This is important for healing and hygienic purposes. For extensive surgical procedures these rinses should be repeated every two to four hours, while awake, during the first week. A syringe may have been dispensed to you to irrigate food from the socket. Use it if food collects in the tooth socket. This irrigation should be performed after meals and at bedtime.

4. PAIN: If you are having more pain than can be controlled by the medication you received, it would be best to call the office.

5. SWELLING: To keep swelling to a minimum, ice packs should be applied as soon as possible. The ice packs should be applied to the jaw continuously the day of the surgery. It is also important to keep the head elevated the first day to reduce swelling and pain.

If swelling recurs after it has once subsided, you should call the office.

6. FEVER: A slight fever (100 degrees) is not unusual the first 48 hours even after a simple procedure. Fever may be caused by an inadequate fluid intake, so it is important to drink eight to twelve glasses of fluids a day after surgery not counting coffee, tea, or any other beverage that is a diuretic.

If the fever is excessive (above 101 degrees), call the office for advice.

7. SUTURES: When sutures have been placed, they should be removed one week after the surgery unless other arrangements have been made. You should arrange an appointment for this procedure.

8. COMPLICATIONS: DRY SOCKET—A dry socket is a breakdown of the normal healing process in the tooth socket of unknown cause. It is diagnosed by the onset of pain in the tooth socket approximately three days after the surgery. It generally occurs in lower molar tooth sockets and the pain is dull, constant, and radiates up to the ear. This problem can be treated easily by returning to the office to have a "dry socket" medicated dressing placed in the tooth socket.

INFECTION—Usually infection is diagnosed by a fever above 101 degrees and an increase in swelling after the swelling has subsided. It may occur from three days post surgery to eight weeks post surgery. If you have these symptoms, please call the office.

NAUSEA AND VOMITING—During the first 24 to 48 hours nausea and/or vomiting may occur, quite normally, due to the anesthesia, the procedure itself, swallowing blood, or the prescribed pain medications. Pain medications should be taken with some food or liquid in the stomach to reduce the possibility of nausea or vomiting. If you are troubled with nausea and it doesn't subside, call the office.

9. A. You should not drive the car or do any dangerous tasks the day that you have had general anesthesia or intravenous drugs.
B. You should not do any aerobics, physical exercise, or sports for six days after the surgery. These activities will increase bleeding, swelling, and pain. They actually slow down an athlete's early recovery.

Orthodontics

(Hugh R. Silkensen, D.D.S., M.S.D.)

Orthodontics (*ortho*, "straight" + *dont*, "tooth") is that science which has for its objective the prevention and correction of malocclusion of the teeth.

Have you worn braces on your teeth? This assorted group of wires and bands or bonded brackets applied to a person's teeth is correctly termed a **fixed orthodontic appliance. Removable orthodontic appliances** are also often used, particularly in the mixed dentition between ages six and twelve. The most obvious purposes of the appliance are to realign that person's teeth into a more pleasing appearance and to establish normal function.

The effect produced by a successful orthodontic treatment, however, extends much further than that simple statement. "More pleasing appearance" is made up of many more factors than alignment of the visible

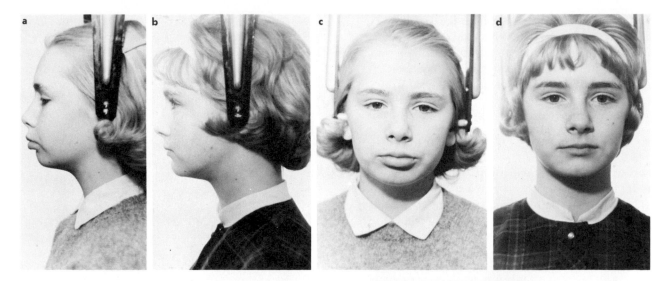

Figure 28.19

An orthodontic patient before and after treatment: a and c are side and front views before treatment; b and d are side and front views after treatment.

front teeth. Very commonly it includes a complete alteration of the relationship of *all* the teeth, for example:

1. An orthodontic treatment may involve changing within the same dental arch the original relationship of the teeth to each other.
2. An orthodontic treatment may involve changing the original relationship of the lower arch to the upper arch.
3. An orthodontic treatment may involve changing the original relationship of the anterior sections of both arches to the rest of the facial structures, such as lips, or to the upper lip and nose (seen in profile).

Orthodontic treatment is a complex specialty. Besides achieving the improvement in appearance, which is the chief interest of both the patient and the parents, the orthodontist must also restore normal function (ability to chew) to the complete mouth in order to achieve a correction that is stable and healthy for the individual. This normal function involves the temperomandibular joint complex as well as the teeth in each arch.

Malocclusions that occur have many variations, causing difficulty in classifying them. In order to achieve a common basis for analyzing various cases, however, it is essential that some form of classification be used. One of the most commonly used is the form developed by Dr. Edward H. Angle, who became a pioneer specialist in this field in 1892 while practicing in Minneapolis, Minnesota. Dr. Angle's classification

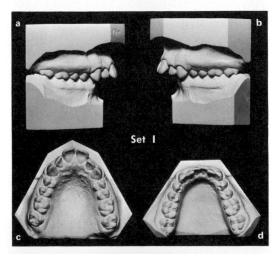

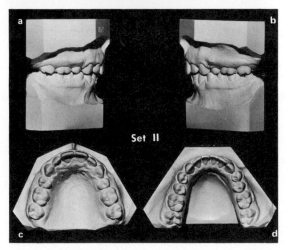

Figure 28.20

Casts of the orthodontic case shown in Fig. 28.19 before and after treatment. Set I is before treatment; Set II is the same mouth after treatment. Notice the alignment of the teeth in the arch: (a) right profile; (b) left profile; (c) upper arch; and (d) lower arch.

dates back to 1899. The assistant in the specialty of orthodontics would do well to memorize the classification and at the same time to match each class with a typical case from the collection of the dentist's orthodontic models made from cases before treatment.

Angle's Classification

Class I. All cases of malocclusion in which the lower dental arch and body of the mandible are in normal mesiodistal relationship to the anatomy of the skull.

Class II. Division 1. Cases in which the lower dental arch and body of the mandible are in bilateral, distal relationship to the maxillary arch and in which the upper incisor teeth show labial protrusion.

Subdivision. Cases in which the lower dental arch and body of the mandible are in unilateral, distal relationship to the maxilliary arch and in which the upper incisors manifest labial protrusion.

Division 2. Cases in which the lower dental arch and body of the mandible are in bilateral, distal relationship to the maxillary arch and in which the upper central incisors are tipped lingually.

Subdivision. Cases in which the lower dental arch and body of the mandible are in unilateral, distal relationship to the maxillary arch and in which the upper central incisors are tipped lingually.

Class III. Cases in which the lower dental arch and body of the mandible are in bilateral mesial relationship to the maxillary arch.

Subdivision. Cases in which the lower dental arch and body of the mandible are in unilateral, mesial relationship to the maxillary arch.

Parts of the Orthodontic Appliance

The orthodontic appliance is made up of several parts. That part which is fitted to an individual tooth and cemented to that tooth after it has been fitted is called a **band.** Many bands may be used as part of an individual orthodontic appliance.

Individual brackets are often cemented or "bonded" directly to the surface of a tooth and can be used instead of a band with a welded bracket. Clear or tooth-colored ceramic brackets are also used, especially for adult patients.

Another part of the orthodontic appliance appears to be a wire, usually following the shape of the dental arch around the outside (buccal and labial surfaces) of the teeth but at times placed on the inside (lingual) surfaces of the teeth. The wire is correctly called an **arch wire.**

The arch wire is used to apply gentle, steady pressures to the teeth that the orthodontist wishes to move. The arch wire applies pressure to the bracket, which is cemented solidly to the tooth. At times **rubber**

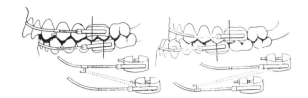

Figure 28.21
Intermaxillary rubber elastics.

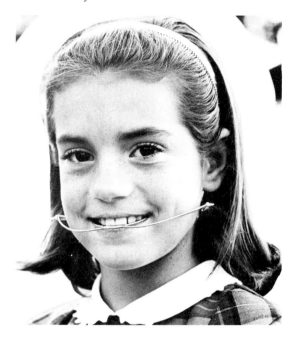

Figure 28.22
Patient wearing a headgear.

elastics will be used between arches to produce an intermaxillary pressure, or force.

A commonly used device is a **headgear.** Various kinds of headgears are used for different problems and different skeletal and dental conditions. The majority of the headgears provide a distal force or a distal and upward force that can be applied to either the maxillary or mandibular arch or to both arches. In a few cases, a headgear is used to provide a mesial, or forward, force to either arch.

When the elastics or headgear devices are to be worn, the patient (as well as the parent) often needs reminding to see that the elastics are worn *constantly,* or the headband is used nightly if the orthodontist so instructs. Often you are in a better position than the orthodontist to encourage the patient.

Study models are widely used in orthodontics as records of progress in treatment. Alginate materials are perhaps most commonly used as an impression material for these models. A detailed and specific method of trimming the models is used, for which the steps and methods are outlined in chapter 33, "Casts and Dies."

The construction of orthodontic appliances involves the use of bands, attachments of many kinds (attached to the bands or arches), arches of various types, and soldering or electric spot-welding equipment. Instruments include contouring and bending pliers, crown shears, band drivers, cementing instruments, mirrors, and explorers. If arch wires are placed lingually to the teeth, the appliance is called a **lingual appliance.** If the arch wires are placed labially to the teeth, the appliance is called a **labial appliance.**

Methods of radiographic cephalometry are used in most orthodontic offices. Lateral head plates in specific positions at specific distances are made as an additional source of information in the treatment of the individual. These large plates involve processing of extraoral film cassettes, often used with intensifying screens to shorten the exposure required.

Your orthodontist may use either or both intraoral and extraoral photography and may use black-and-white or color film. Photography is used as a means of recording case progress and results. These procedures, when used, are so organized that their use is routine, with positioning of both camera and patient controlled for purposes of accurately repeating various views. Lighting also is standardized so that exposures are always the same.

The active movement of teeth and their placement in the dental arch may continue over a period of time. Many orthodontic cases are completed within two years, but some cases may exceed two years.

At the conclusion of active treatment, a **retainer** or **retention appliance** is constructed for each case. A retainer is a device that holds the teeth in correct position until they stabilize. Most of the retainer appliances are removable by the patient. You may have occasion to use your influence to encourage the patient to wear the retainer as instructed. Retainers are not as complex as the original appliances but do require occasional inspection and adjustment. They are frequently a combination of plastic and metal.

Duties of an Orthodontic Assistant

The duties of the orthodontic assistant may be grouped into three main divisions.

Laboratory work:

1. Soldering bands and wires or spot-welding bands;
2. making the retaining appliances;
3. making plaster casts from impressions;
4. trimming plaster casts on a model trimmer precisely as required for records;
5. taking and developing X rays.

Chair Assisting:

1. Seat the patient for impression taking, band forming, or appliance adjustment.
2. Assist in preparing teeth for direct bonding.
3. Prepare cement for placing bands when ready.
4. Remove excess cement from bands and teeth after the orthodontist has cemented the bands.
5. Take photographs, when required, for records.
6. Maintain supply of ligature wires cut to correct length.
7. Keep small envelopes, as required, filled with various sizes of rubber elastics.
8. Make up headgear kits as required.
9. Provide patient instruction about oral hygiene, head gear, and elastic wear.
10. Clean and sterilize instruments and disinfect all surfaces.
11. Provide the proper instruments to the orthodontist for every procedure.

Secretarial Work:

1. Making appointments. The time required for various types of appointments is important. New patient examination, securing history of new patients, consultation with parents, construction of appliances, adjustment of appliances, construction of retainers and removal of appliances, retainer adjustments, and final records—each may require a different block of time.
2. Letter writing. More letters may be written in the orthodontic practice than in general practice. An important letter in any orthodontic practice should be that which is sent to the referring dentist, expressing appreciation for the referral and often including a note on the case involved.
3. Bookkeeping.
4. Ordering supplies.
5. Maintaining an accurate recall file for patients under observation.
6. Maintaining an accurate active treatment file.
7. Maintaining an accurate retention file.
8. Operating a computer.

Pedodontics

As a specialty, **pedodontics**—children's dentistry—is similar in many respects to the general practice of dentistry for adults. The assistant's duties are very similar.

However, the differences that do exist are very important. Duties must be performed with speed and accuracy. The smaller child's attention span is limited. It is necessary to work quickly and efficiently before he or she tires. However, your physical movements near the child must be slow and deliberate, your manner easy-going and relaxed. Quite a combination! Prepare the materials quickly and accurately—but be leisurely and relaxed in attitude. Insert the saliva ejector gently and slowly—but quickly have ready whatever instrument your dentist needs.

Your speech should be calm and reassuring. It is a good idea to refresh your memory about the psychology of the particular age group of the child you have as a patient. If you have memorized the age-group characteristics given in chapter 5 you can pause a moment and review the characteristics before you greet the child patient. After a few weeks of this approach, the psychology will become so routine that you won't have to think of it.

Children are a challenge. They can be the best patients and the most fun if properly approached by the dental health team.

Periodontics

A **periodontist** is a specialist who works with diseases around the tooth. *Peri* is a Greek prefix meaning "around."

The tissues around the tooth that the periodontist usually treats are these:

1. **Gingivae** (or gums)
2. **Periodontal ligaments,** which attach the teeth to the bone socket of the mandible and maxilla
3. **Cementum,** the surface covering the roots of the teeth

The periodontist is interested in the following symptoms:

1. Bleeding of gums during toothbrushing;
2. unpleasant breath that persists;
3. loose, soft gums, red instead of pale pink in color;

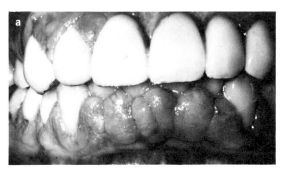
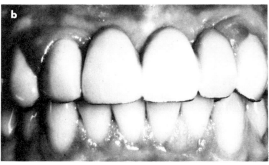

Figure 28.23
Periodontic treatment: (a) Dilantin hyperplasia, preoperative condition; and (b) condition following periodontal treatment.

4. separation of teeth from gums;
5. drifting teeth, or teeth that are changing position;
6. teeth that feel loose, or mobile.

People of all ages have periodontal disease. It is the most common cause of loss of teeth. **Gingivitis** (inflamed gums) is a relatively mild form of periodontal disease. It is sometimes neglected because bleeding and swollen gums (which are its first symptoms) cause very little discomfort. Thus, people are inclined to think that this condition is normal.

If gingivitis is not treated, a more advanced condition of **periodontitis** is the result. (The layman is accustomed to calling this condition *pyorrhea*.) The inflammation spreads around the roots of the teeth, the gums become separated from the teeth, and pockets appear which are collectors of food particles, calculus, bacteria, and pus. When pus develops in a pocket and is not able to drain out, painful abscesses can develop. As the disease progresses, bone around the root of the tooth is lost. Eventually the tooth itself is lost because there is nothing to hold it to the position.

Necrotizing ulcerative gingivitis (Vincent's infection) is a disease in which the gums usually are painful and bleed readily, and the inter-dental papillae have

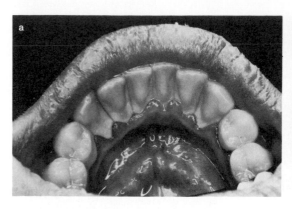

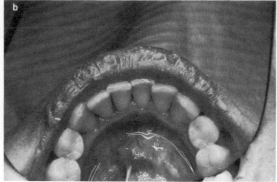

Figure 28.24
Severe calculus and inflammation of gums on lingual aspects of lower anterior teeth: (a) before treatment; and (b) after treatment.

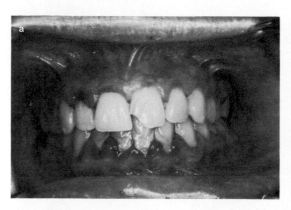

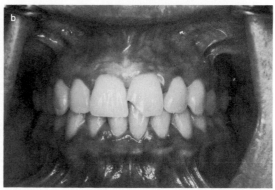

Figure 28.25
Heavy deposits and severe gingival inflammation: (a) before treatment; and (b) after treatment.

been destroyed. These areas between the teeth are concave and covered with a film of white, dead tissue.

Periodontal diseases are caused by the following conditions:

1. Bacterial plaque: a sticky substance coming from saliva that is deposited on the teeth.
2. Calculus (tartar): a calcified or hardened bacterial plaque. This substance irritates the tissues surrounding the teeth.
3. Malocclusions: improper hitting of the occlusal surfaces of the teeth that produces uneven pressures on some teeth.
4. Missing teeth not replaced by a bridge or partial.
5. Bruxism: clenching and grinding of the teeth, especially during sleep—and sometimes during the day.

6. Inadequate nutrition.
7. Worn-out restorations, whether crowns, partials, or bridges.

The periodontist diagnoses the problem for the patient by examination, case history, X rays, and case study. He or she treats the conditions, educates the patient in proper care of the mouth, and has the patient return at regular intervals for examination, making certain that the patient is providing the proper home care. The periodontist uses X rays as necessary to determine the continued health of the part of the mouth that is not directly visible.

In treating the condition the periodontist may select one of many treatment plans. Basically, the causes of the periodontal disease are removed. This means the

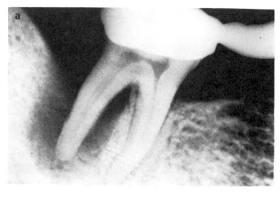

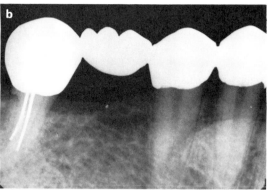

Figure 28.26
(a) X ray of bone loss; and (b) hemisection performed, followed by placement of restoration utilizing the treated tooth as a bridge abutment.

dentist starts with the removal of calculus, then removes diseased gum tissue if any, corrects malocclusions, has missing teeth replaced, and constructs splints or other appliances to control the movement of loose teeth or to correct harmful mouth habits. Most important, the patient is educated to the necessity of proper care of the mouth.

Duties of the Periodontal Assistant

The periodontal assistant aspirates, retracts, serves instruments, and assists at the chair. In addition, this assistant is responsible for the sterilization, preparation, and clean-up of the seven periodontic trays as described in chapter 39.

Prosthodontics

Prosthetics (*Prosthesis,* "a putting to" + *Odont,* "tooth") refers to the artificial replacement of a missing natural part. Thus, an artificial leg is a *prosthesis,* a prosthetic device to replace a missing leg. If a person has lost a tooth or teeth, the dentist may make a **bridge**—a fixed prosthodontic appliance to replace the

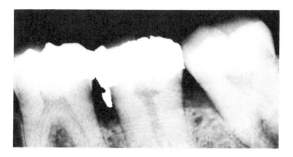

Figure 28.27
X ray of overhang.

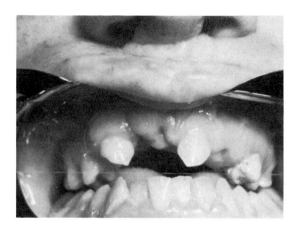

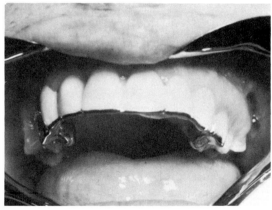

Figure 28.28
(a) The mouth before placement of a fixed bridge; and (b) after placement of a fixed bridge.

missing tooth or teeth. If the patient has lost many, but not all, teeth in one arch, the dentist may make a **partial denture.** If the patient has no teeth left in one arch, the dentist must make a full **denture.** All of the replacements are really prosthetic appliances or, in the dental sense, prosthodontic appliances.

If a person needs full dentures, that person may have emotional problems in adjusting to the idea of losing all the remaining natural teeth. To most people, dentures mean old age. Modern dentistry can create

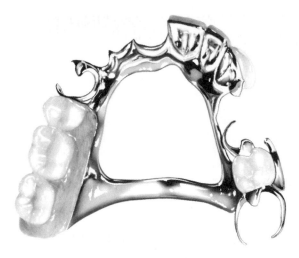

Figure 28.29
A removable partial denture, replacing teeth in a partially edentulous mouth.

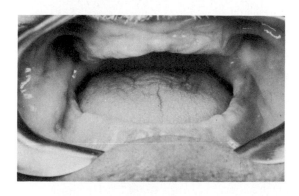

Figure 28.30
The completely edentulous mouth.

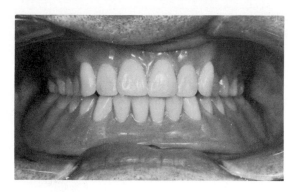

Figure 28.31
Restoration to function and esthetics with removable denture.

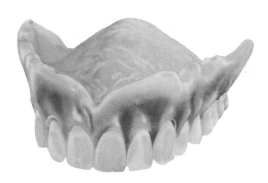

Figure 28.32
A full upper denture.

dentures that are amazingly natural replicas. Therefore, the care and consideration of the dental prosthetic patient includes assisting with the emotional problems. Reassurance and encouragement by staff are essential in working with this patient.

Duties of the Prosthodontic Assistant

In addition to chairside assisting duties of retraction, aspiration, and instrument passing, the prosthodontic assistant will mix impression materials, fill trays, and pour impressions. Preparation for prosthodontics is extensive because instruments, trays, and impression materials must be prepared ahead of time. (See chapters 32 to 34 for a discussion of this special area of work.)

Following a patient's dismissal there are a number of laboratory procedures to be performed. Some must be done immediately, some later on, before the next appointment of that patient. It is important to enter each case on the Laboratory Schedule and follow through to be certain that the prosthetic appliance is ready at the time of the patient's next appointment.

Summary

The duties of the assistant to the specialist will vary from those of the assistant to the general practitioner.

Endodontics is concerned with correct therapy for the conservation of natural dentition for a lifetime. There are seven treatments that are performed in an endodontic practice. The assistant must be well educated in microbiology and sterilization.

The *oral surgeon* removes teeth and treats fractures of the jaw and abnormalities within the oral cavity. The oral surgeon's assistant must maintain and use accurate records, be certain asepsis is maintained where necessary, assist with surgery, perform postoperative duties, and be prepared for emergencies.

The *orthodontist* prevents and corrects malocclusions and reestablishes normal function and pleasing appearance. The assistant has three areas of work: laboratory, chair assisting, and secretarial work.

Pedodontics is dentistry for children, and assistants to the pediatric dentist must not only be prepared to assist at the chair, but must be acquainted with the necessary psychology and techniques of working with children of all ages.

Periodontists treat diseases around the tooth. The assistant must be able to educate patients in home care as well as assist at chairside and maintain asepsis where necessary.

The *prosthodontist* prepares artificial replacements. In addition to chairside assisting and working with impressions, the dental assistant must be aware of techniques of meeting patients' emotional problems caused by artificial replacements.

Study Questions

1. Describe each of the following specialties and explain the areas of work for the assistant:

    endodontics   pediatric dentistry
    oral surgery   periodontics
    orthodontics   prosthodontics

2. What are Angle's classifications?

Vocabulary

apertognathia   open bite

apical curettage   surgical removal of pathological periapical tissue

apicoectomy   removal of portion of root apex

asepsis   free from pathogenic organisms

cementum   surface covering of the roots of the teeth

cleft   partial split

cleft palate   split in palate (roof) of mouth, varying in degree of severity

complete pulpectomy   removal of all pulpal tissue followed by sterilization and filling of root canal

cyst   a closed sac developing abnormally. In dentistry, the cyst is located somewhere in the oral cavity or surrounding tissues

dorsum   upper surface (dorsum of the tongue is upper surface of the tongue)

gingivae   gums

headgear   a device that provides force distally, or distally and upward, to assist in moving the teeth in an orthodontic case

hemisection   amputation of one root and part of the crown of a tooth, usually a lower, allowing the remainder of the tooth to be retained for restorative dentistry

implant   set or fix securely (endodontic implant is a method of stabilizing a tooth by lengthening the existing root with a metallic implant that extends into the surrounding bony tissue)

lesion   a well-defined abnormal change in an organ

luxate   out of place. In dentistry, a tooth may be partially or completely knocked out of its socket and then be reinserted or replanted

pulp capping   superficial treatment of vital dental pulps

pulpotomy   removal of part of vital pulp tissue

pyorrhea   periodontitis

replantation   insertion of a totally displaced, out of its socket tooth, usually following endodontic treatment

retainer   device that holds teeth in correct position until they stabilize

root canal therapy   removal of all pulpal tissue followed by sterilization and filling of the root canal

retrofilling   a method of filling the root canal, particularly the apical portion, from the apex of the root following apical curretage and root resection

Word Elements	
Word Element	*Example*
op, ops, opt prefix meaning: vision, view, eye	*opaque* that which blocks light
pan prefix meaning: all, every	*pantomography* X ray of all the dental arches accomplished on one film
para, par prefix meaning: beside, beyond, accessory to, faulty	*paralysis* loss or impairment of motor function
pathy suffix meaning: disease, of feeling	*sympathy* having common feelings
pedo combining form meaning: child	*pedodontics* branch of dentistry that studies and treats children's teeth
phot combining form meaning: denoting relationship to light	*photography* making images on sensitized material by exposure to light or some other radiation source
phylac combining form meaning: guard, defense	*prophylaxis* prevention of disease
plic combining form meaning: fold, twist	*complication* a change (or twist) not always expected that makes a situation more difficult
plex combining form meaning: strike	*apoplexy* stroke (see Glossary for further definition)
puls combining form meaning: beat	*pulse* rhythmical beating, such as that caused by the heart action and felt in the arteries

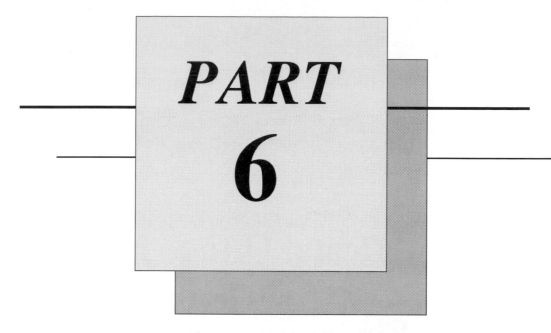

PART 6

The Dental Office: Its Armamentarium and Maintenance

A lawyer can practice law and a teacher can teach almost anywhere there are people gathered together willing to listen. A dentist is unable to perform dentistry (except for minimum services) unless there is a well-equipped and well-maintained office. This office should be attractive as well.

A dentist's education is the most costly of all the professions, and the practice of dentistry generally requires a more expensive installation and higher overhead than does the practice of a physician, an attorney, or any other professional.

The investment in office and equipment in starting a practice is relatively high. Replacement must be considered constantly in view of improved equipment, instruments, and techniques. In order to preserve the equipment and instruments over their useful lives, it is necessary to give considerable thought to their proper treatment and care.

The purpose of this part of your text is to acquaint you with the physical plant with which you and your dentist work—office, equipment, and instruments—and to instruct you in the care of these valuable tools of dentistry.

The Dental Office: Its Atmosphere, Housekeeping, Equipment, and Maintenance

Atmosphere
Components of the Dental Office
Housekeeping and Maintenance
   Daily Routines
   Care of the Laboratory
   Making the Office a Place of Beauty
   Routines for Cleanliness
Dental Equipment—Old and New
Care of Dental Equipment
   The Dental Unit
      Summary of Care for the Older Dental Unit
   The Dental Cabinet
   The Ultrasonic Cleaner
   The Autoclave

Atmosphere

Office atmosphere affects patient relations. People enjoy being in colorful, attractive, clean, well-organized surroundings. Many offices today have background music which helps patients relax and adjust to office routines.

While it is not the responsibility of dental assistants to provide the colorful, attractive surroundings, it is their collective responsibility to see that the office remains attractive and clean. If music is used, keeping the volume at a proper level is also a staff responsibility.

Components of the Dental Office

Dental offices may have several rooms. The dental assistant should know the names and purposes of these rooms. The **reception room** is normally the room a patient enters, a place for relaxation before the appointment. Usually there is a coat rack or closet, comfortable furniture, and reading material. Most dentists provide a small-scale table and chairs for the child patients. This area requires more careful watching because children are inclined to leave the magazine or book where they finished using it.

The **business office** most frequently adjoins the reception room in order that the business secretary may acknowledge entrants to the reception room. Usually there is a counter or window in the reception room that opens into the business area so that the secretary may continue to work between arrivals.

Some dentists have a **private inner office** where they present cases, conduct their professional business, and keep their library of dental journals and textbooks.

The **laboratory** is a room in which all the laboratory preparations to be done in the office are performed.

The **darkroom** is used for X ray developing, washing, and drying.

The **operatory** is the room that is furnished with the necessary equipment to perform all dental operations. There may be several operatories. In an office where there is more than one operatory, each room may be designed for special operations—or they may be exact duplicates.

The dental office today ought to be beautiful, and the colors should be restful and relaxing. We hope that your dentist provides this atmosphere; but regardless of what atmosphere is provided, the dental office must be immaculate, neat, and attractive. The equipment must be in excellent working condition as well as sparkling with good grooming.

This chapter is devoted to helping the assistant maintain the kind of office the fastidious person will enjoy entering. Don't be reluctant about doing some tasks that may seem to be the most menial labor. Sometimes it is necessary to do actual housecleaning. Accidents do happen; occasionally there is need for the assistant to perform janitorial work.

A clean, attractive office, perhaps with musical background of a relaxing nature, provides an atmosphere of congeniality for the dentist, the staff, and the patient.

Housekeeping and Maintenance

The following daily routines are reminder lists of jobs to be done on a regular basis each day. Referral to these lists will help reassure you that the office is at its best at all times.

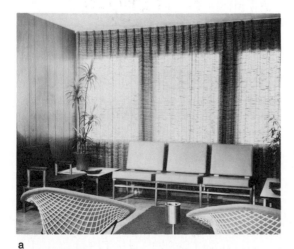

a

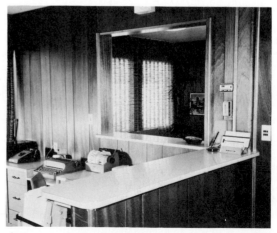

b

Figure 29.1

(a) A dental reception room; and (b) the adjoining business office.

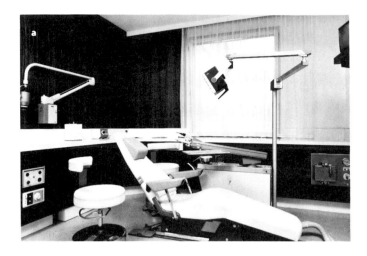
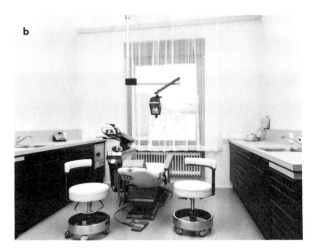

Figure 29.2
(a) A contemporary operatory; and (b) a modern operatory installed in an older office building, including sinks for both dentist and assistant.

Daily Routines

Opening the Office: Open the office one-half hour before the appointment time of the first patient, or at the regular time for office hours to begin, whichever is earlier.

Open enough windows and open all the doors to give the office a thorough airing.

Turn on all necessary switches. Prepare all equipment needed. See that all instruments are sterilized and placed in their proper drawers or on the proper trays. Instruments left in cold disinfectant overnight should be dried and returned to their proper places, ready for use. Rubber bulbs, hoses, or other plastic or rubber parts can be wiped with gauze moistened with a disinfectant or with a disposable disinfectant pad.

Dust *everything* in all rooms carefully; wipe all surfaces of equipment. Extend the arm of the X ray and wipe all crevices with care.

See that everything is neatly and properly arranged, from magazines to equipment.

Illumination in all rooms should be correct for the existing conditions.

When you have finished, walk through all the rooms again as if you had never seen them before. Look around, from the patient's actual position in the reception room and operatory.

Place patients' records for the day in the proper operating rooms.

During the day, keep the office looking as neat as possible. Check it occasionally.

Closing the Office: Clean the instruments and remove debris of the last patient's appointment. Cutting instruments may be left in cold sterilization solution overnight, if necessary. Other instruments may

be prepared for sterilization upon arrival the next workday, unless needed for the first patient; but they should be washed with soap and brush and rinsed whether they are to be sterilized immediately or left until morning.

Whenever possible, setups for the first patient of the next workday should be prepared.

Turn off all equipment.

Elevate chairs completely for easier access to the floor by the cleaning crew.

Check all windows. Be sure that heating or air conditioning is properly set for the night.

Leave no office records out. Appointment book, receipt book, records prepared for the next workday, etc., should be placed together in a closed drawer, cabinet, or filing case.

Cover all office equipment, such as typewriters, adding machines, copiers, and computers.

Any patients for the next workday who have not been contacted by telephone should be called at this time for appointment reminder.

Double-check to see that all sterilizers, units, lights, water valves, and air compressors are turned off.

Take all outgoing mail with you and mail it.

Be certain that the office door is locked.

Care of the Laboratory

The laboratory is the workshop of the dental office for those procedures which require preparation for completion outside the patient's mouth. Since these procedures are directly related to the welfare of the patient, the laboratory should be kept as scrupulously clean as any other part of the dental office. It is frequently as visible to the patient as the operatory. By its cleanliness and general good order, it forms a part of the total impression the patient receives of the dental office.

Making the Office a Place of Beauty

An office can be charming and attractive without losing its efficiency. No matter what the furnishings and decor of the office, the addition of natural or artificial plants and flowers adds a touch of beauty appreciated by most patients.

Whether the dentist or assistant selects the plants, the assistant is responsible for their care. Consult a florist or the public library to learn how to care for any plants with which you are not familiar.

Routines for Cleanliness

Equipment in a dental office will vary in age, type, and condition of maintenance. Breakdown of equipment may be reduced and smoother operation assured by proper maintenance of each piece. A carefully planned schedule for this work takes a minimum of time to execute once the schedule is set up in written form. The list of jobs may seem long, but each item requires only a few seconds or minutes to perform. A come-up file assures your proper care of all items of equipment as they require care.

Most items of equipment listed in this chapter are followed by a series of suggestions for proper maintenance. These suggestions are general. They apply to the equipment produced by most manufacturers. For answers to questions about the care of a particular piece of equipment in your office read the instruction booklet from the manufacturer.

Finishes: Several pieces of equipment in the dental office have similar finishes. The care of each finish is the same regardless of where it is found.

Chrome and stainless steel: Wipe with a clean, damp cheesecloth pad daily. Polish with a dry cloth. If stains or finger marks remain, use a nonscratching cleanser and then polish. Stainless steel will respond well to good soapsuds, a rinse, and a dry polishing.

Enamel: Wipe with a clean, damp cheesecloth pad daily and dry with a soft cloth. Wax lightly every two months. Every six months use a cleaner before waxing the surface. If chipping occurs, touch up the spots with enamel finish, which can be purchased at your dental supply house.

Wood: Furniture generally remains more beautiful when kept waxed. Daily dusting is essential to maintain a clean dental office. Scratches may be hidden with one of the many commercial stains available for that purpose.

Leather surfaces: For normal use apply a cloth dampened with lukewarm water to a mild soap, such as castile, and rub briskly over the surface of the leather. Next, remove soapy film with another damp cloth, since even the film of the mildest soap may cause discoloration if left on the leather. Finally, rub briskly with a dry cloth to bring back the original gloss.

Never use oils, varnishes, or furniture polishes on upholstery leather since most of these compounds contain solvents that attack the finish of the leather.

Occasionally, abnormal conditions of wear, such as the increased acidity in the atmosphere of large cities, necessitate the use of a more effective material for cleaning and preserving the finish of upholstery leather than is possible with the use of soap and water. We recommend an upholstery leather cleaner and dressing.

Plastic surfaces: Wash with a mild soap or detergent, rinse well, and dry. If this procedure is not suitable for a special plastic, the manufacturer's label will so indicate.

Draperies, curtains, rugs, upholstery, slip covers: Watch for signs of soil. The varying conditions of each practice determine the length of time between cleanings. A practice located in the heart of an industrial center may find draperies or curtains soiled in less than a month. A residential, air-conditioned office may find yearly cleaning sufficient.

Commercial cleaning of rugs or draperies is usually preferred. Check to find a reputable cleaner. Be sure that both you and the dry cleaner know the size of the rugs and draperies before they are cleaned. A reminder to the cleaner to be certain that they are returned the same size as they were before cleaning assures you of well-fitting draperies and rugs.

Curtains may be commercially-laundered or home-laundered, as your dentist prefers.

Spots on upholstered furniture should be removed promptly with one of the many detergents available for this purpose. Seasonal dry cleaning may be necessary, depending on the particular type of practice.

Slip covers may be home-laundered or dry-cleaned, as your dentist chooses. They should be cleaned as soon as soiled since they look better and wear longer if they receive proper care.

Pottery and glass: Wash with soapy water, rinse, and polish dry.

Linoleum, rubber tile, asphalt tile, cork, plastic tile: In most offices cleaning services care for floors. However, counter tops are cleaned by the assistants. Frequently these counter tops are made of some form of tile or linoleum.

There are cleaners on the market today that clean these finishes without the use of water. Most of them contain a wax that helps maintain a beautiful finish. The cleaners are labeled for the surfaces on which they may be safely used. A cleaner-wax suitable for one may harm another.

A soapy cloth, followed with a clear-water rinse, is suitable. Be sure to wipe the surface dry when it has been rinsed. The trick is to avoid any excessive quantity of water in cleaning these glued-on surfaces.

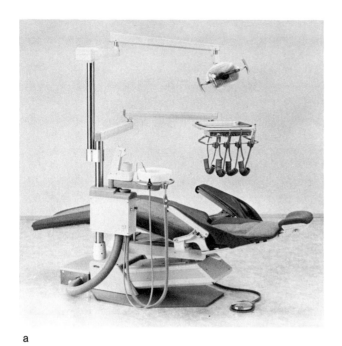

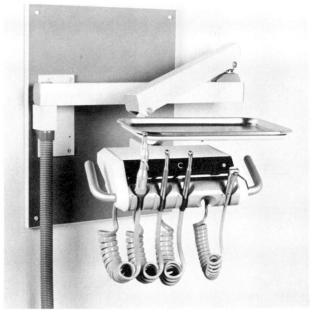

a

b

Figure 29.3
*(a) A contemporary lounge type dental chair and unit; and
(b) the instrument panel with contra-angle, handpiece, and
syringe.*

Dental Equipment—Old and New

The design of dental equipment has undergone more rapid change since the mid-fifties than at any other period in the previous one hundred years. Although many dental offices are still served by the hydraulic-pump-type chair and a floor-mounted dental unit, the contour motor chair coupled with a mobile chair-mounted or cabinet-mounted unit is more characteristic of the modern dental office or clinic.

Dental cabinets may be wall-hung or mobile. Usually the dental assistant's cabinet is mobile. It can then be placed in the position most convenient for the dental assistant. The mounted cabinets will often have an additional sink, one for the dentist and one for the assistant.

All equipment requires expert care, regardless of age. The general instructions given in this chapter for the care of equipment must be supplemented with the specific instructions supplied in manual form with each piece of equipment when it is purchased. Your dentist may have this material available and on file. If not, such information may often be obtained by sending the name of the equipment, the model and serial number, and any other identifying information, to the manufacturer, with a request for the instruction or operating manual.

Care of Dental Equipment

The type of finish used on dental equipment will indicate the care required to keep the piece looking new. Refer to the previous section for directions regarding the proper care of various finishes, such as enamel, chrome, leather, etc.

The Dental Unit

The dental unit will need constant attention to see that it is clean from the patient's perspective. Look at it from the patient's position in the chair. Be sure all the items are clean.

The **evacuator cup** or **cuspidor bowl** should be cleaned as thoroughly as possible between patients, in addition to very thorough cleansing at least daily. A mild soap or cleanser should be used. Remember to examine the cuspidor bowl or evacuator cup from the position of the patient. If you don't there can be unclean areas that are not visible to a person sitting or standing beside the chair but are visible to the person in the dental chair.

In addition to keeping the equipment free from dust, the dental assistant should be aware of the care required to maintain the individual parts of the equipment.

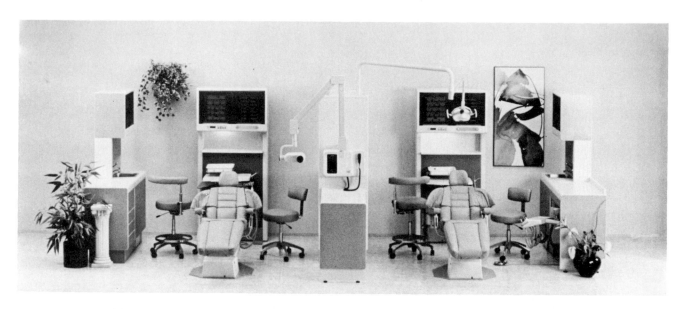

Figure 29.4
Twin operatories, utilizing one X ray.

Whatever the style of the **dental unit,** it usually has the following components:

1. High-speed contra-angle handpiece;
2. low-speed high-torque handpiece with contra-angle;
3. three-way syringe (air, air-water, and water from the same jet);
4. saliva ejector hose;
5. high-volume evacuation;
6. cuspidor or evacuation cup.

Although they are still available, units with a motor-powered belt-driven handpiece have all but disappeared from the market.

An oral evacuator is used to remove water, saliva, scraps of material, or any other foreign matter, from the patient's mouth. It provides a clear field (good visibility) for the dentist's work.

Separation tanks are arranged to trap solid debris, permitting the liquids to be collected in a separate tank or to be automatically directed into a waste line when the motor of the evacuator unit is turned off. *The solid materials must be removed by the assistant at regular intervals to insure proper functioning of the evacuator.*

When the cuspidor is eliminated, usually a second suction line or hose will provide a cup that can be used by the patient to empty his or her mouth when necessary to supplement the evacuator. These occasions will be rare if the low-pressure evacuator is operated in a skillful manner by the dental assistant. The evacuator tip must be used both to remove water and debris from the patient's mouth and at the same time to keep soft

tissues retracted (out of the way). In some areas of the mouth this will seem an impossible problem in dexterity, but it can be developed with practice. The most rapid way to acquire this skill is to observe the manner in which a skilled person manipulates the tip of the evacuator while working with the dentist, then try to repeat the positions yourself.

Dental units that have an **instrument table** attached to an arm may have a gas burner or electric heater coil that is partially enclosed in a metal cup to catch any materials which might drip when heated. Wax drippings may accumulate in this cup when the burner is used; the assistant should remove the drippings and polish the cup with a piece of cotton saturated with chloroform.

All units in the dental office have **water drains.** Each water drain in the dental office will require a **filter screen** to trap the particles of solid waste that accumulate during dental operations. These filter screens which prevent the clogging of the drains must be cleaned regularly. In the conventional, older dental unit, the screen is in the cuspidor bowl (fig. 29.5). In the newer equipment, the screen is in the evacuator cup and/or the lines attached to the evacuation tips (figs. 29.6 and 29.7). Remove and clean the screen whenever a patient has emptied solid materials from his or her mouth, such as pieces of impression materials. In such cases the cleaning operation is best done between patients. Very small scraps of amalgam, however, do not necessitate cleaning the trap until the end of the day.

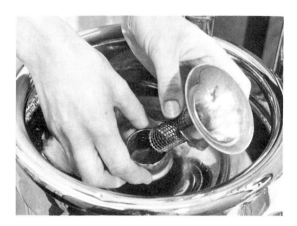

Figure 29.5
Cleaning the cuspidor screen.

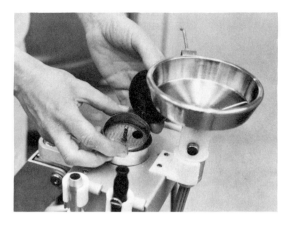

Figure 29.7
Removing the filter screen.

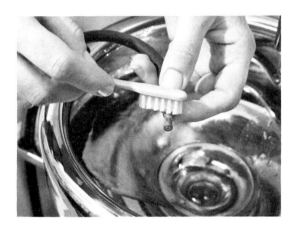

Figure 29.6
Cleaning the saliva ejector screen.

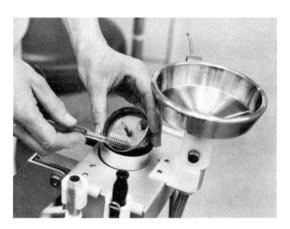

Figure 29.8
Cleaning the filter screen.

The saliva ejector hose in the older, conventional unit is attached to the cuspidor bowl (fig. 29.8). In the newer units, the hose rests in a clamp attached to the unit. The hose has a short rubber collar at the free end into which a saliva ejector is placed (a piece of plastic shaped somewhat like a question mark). Its purpose is to remove saliva from the patient's mouth, when it is required, in order to keep the work area as dry as possible. The saliva ejector is discarded after each use. At the end of the day, flush very warm water through the hose of the saliva ejector; detergent may be added to the water.

All dental units must have water-supply lines. These lines provide the water necessary for dental operations, and all water-supply lines contain filter screens. These **water-supply screens** are usually positioned so that you can remove and clean them regularly without much difficulty. This should be done every three

months, unless this time interval allows a considerable amount of material to collect in the screens. If this is true, increase the frequency of cleaning until only a small amount of debris needs to be removed each time. Much accumulation tends to cut down the flow of water to the necessary devices on the unit and also reduces the amount of suction available for the saliva ejector. To clean the water-supply screen:

1. Turn off the main water valve;
2. place a container under the plug containing the water-supply screen;
3. remove the plug, catching any water which may drain from the pipes;
4. clean the strainer and replace;
5. turn on the main water valve;
6. open the saliva ejector and cuspidor flush valves for a moment to expel any air that may be in the pipes.

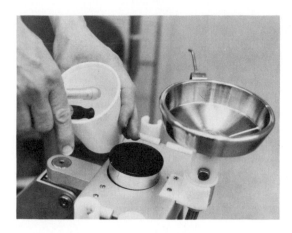

Figure 29.9
Cleaning the water-supply tubing in a newer type unit.

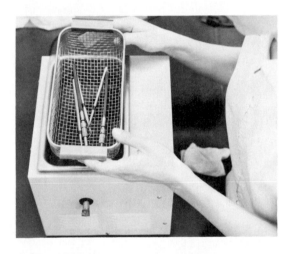

Figure 29.10
A basket of instruments being placed into the ultrasonic cleaner for cleaning.

Remove and clean the **cuspidor trap** of amalgam scrap every day. Place the trap contents on a piece of paper to dry, then into the scrap-amalgam jar.

Every morning wash the **glassware** with soap and water. If it is necessary, use a nonscratching cleanser.

Summary of Care for the Older Dental Unit
Daily:

Clean finish as needed.

Wipe engine arm.

Clean gas-burner or electric-coil cup of wax drippings.

Clean cuspidor bowl thoroughly and repeat as needed during the day.

Wash glassware.

Remove and clean saliva-ejector screen. Flush with warm water through hose.

Remove and clean the cuspidor trap.

Less Frequent Jobs:

Every two weeks oil the dental engine.

Every three months clean the water-supply screen.

Every six months care for the foot controller as directed.

The Dental Cabinet

Dental cabinets should be cleaned at the beginning of each day and recleaned throughout the day. Occasionally, medications, cements, or other materials may be spilled inadvertently. Adhering sticky cements may be cleaned with cotton dampened with xylol. Along with the cuspidor, unit, and chair, the cabinets should be checked for cleanliness before seating the next patient.

The Ultrasonic Cleaner

An excellent device for cleaning instruments prior to sterilizing is an ultrasonic cleaner (fig. 29.10).

The Autoclave

Only distilled water is used in the autoclave. It may need to be replenished during the day. Be sure that you check the water level before each use. Be certain that you fill it or refill it only with distilled water.

Once each month drain all the water from the reservoir. Scrub the inside of the reservoir and the chamber with soap and lukewarm water. Rinse thoroughly and rub dry. Refill with distilled water.

Every six months the autoclave is to be thoroughly cleansed. Prepare a commercial autoclave cleanser and use as directed.

The outside of the autoclave is to be cleaned according to the directions given for chrome and stainless-steel finishes.

All moving parts are to be oiled or greased regularly. Use light oil or silicone grease on the door hinge and center hub of the locking attachment on the door.

Discharge valve screens should be removed and cleaned. Directions come with your particular autoclave.

Check the rubber gasket on the inside of the door, if present. If the gasket is worn so that steam escapes, replace it.

Summary

Office atmosphere is a very important factor in patient relations. Keeping the office clean and attractive is essential to the successful practice of dentistry.

The dental office may be divided into a reception room, business office, private office, laboratory, darkroom, and operatory (or several operatories).

Planning and executing routines for the numerous jobs that must be done to create a clean, attractive office is an important part of the dental assistant's work.

Dental equipment design has changed drastically in the last twenty years. Since the equipment used is expensive and is replaced only infrequently, the office in which you work may have a variety of types of equipment.

Familiarity with the operation and care of equipment in your office is important. Routines to help you maintain it are given in this chapter.

Study Questions

1. Why is it essential to maintain a clean and attractive office?
2. What components are there in a dental office?
3. How can a dental assistant maintain a clean and attractive dental office?
4. Describe the routines for opening the office. For closing the office.
5. Describe the modern dental office equipment.

Word Elements	
Word Element	*Example*
pre prefix meaning: before	*prescribe* to give directions for using a remedy or treatment
pel combining form meaning: drive, force	*repel* to drive or force away
pond combining form meaning: weigh	*ponder* to weigh in the mind
pont combining form meaning: bridge	*pontic* the replacement for a missing tooth in a bridge or partial
pro prefix meaning: forward, forth, for, before, in front of	*process* a projecting part of bone
pros prefix meaning: toward	*prosthesis* an artificial device that replaces a missing part of the body (toward making the body whole)
pyo combining form meaning: pus	*pyogenic* producing pus
pyr, pyro combining form meaning: fire, heat	*pyrotoxin* a poison produced during a fever
pyre combining form meaning: fever	*pyrexia* fever (elevation of body temperature)
rube, rubi combining form meaning: red	*rubella* German measles—a disease characterized by red spots and having oral manifestations

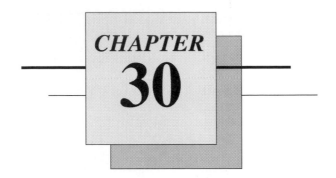

CHAPTER 30

Dental Instruments: Their Use, Care, and Identification

General Instructions About Instruments
The Dental Unit and Its Accessories
The Handpieces
Accessories for the Handpieces
   Dental Burs
   Diamond Instruments
   Dental Prophylaxis Right Angles, Brushes,
     and Cups
   Mandrels
   Stones
Basic Setups
Ten Small, but Important, Items
Rubber Dam
Anesthetic Syringes and Needles
    Preparation of Syringes for Use
    Care of Syringes After Use
Transfer Forceps
Cement Slabs and Spatulas
Mixing Pads

Instrument Sharpening Devices
   Arkansas Stone and Motor-driven Sharpeners
   Care of Sharpening Stone
Hand Instruments
   Instrument Numbering
   Amalgam Instruments
   Cutting Instruments
   Matrix and Matrix Holders
   Gold-foil Instruments
   Plastic Filling Instruments
   Contouring Pliers
Instruments for Five Dental Specialties
   Endodontic Armamentarium
   Oral Surgery Armamentarium
     Color Coding of Surgical Instruments
     Care of Forceps
     Care of Sterile Surgical Instruments
   Orthodontic Armamentarium
   Periodontic Armamentarium
   Prosthodontic Armamentarium

General Instructions About Instruments

This chapter contains descriptions of the use and care of dental instruments and photographs for their identification. Some instruments are larger instruments, such as handpieces. Others are hand instruments: the innumerable objects the dentist uses in the patient's mouth. Some are hard to recognize at first because many look similar.

Instruments are grouped according to purpose and should be studied in connection with their use in the office. Pictures aid in visualizing the small variations in a number of the instruments that basically seem alike. For example, an excavator and a gingival margin trimmer look very much alike, but they are used for different purposes. One has a curved spoon edge, the other a beveled, knifelike edge. However, when you first see these instruments, the variation is not easily recognized. If you confuse them, it could be frustrating to your dentist to be handed the wrong instrument.

Instruments may have a number of assorted sizes and/or shapes for a specific task. For example, there are several differing shapes of explorers, and there are several different sizes of dental mirrors. The illustrations in this chapter attempt to identify for you the general types of each instrument illustrated. Once you see a dental mirror, you can recognize one in your work whether the mirror is a number one or a number five. Therefore, frequently, not all the range of one type of instrument is illustrated. However, by studying these illustrations, you will learn to recognize the many tools of dentistry. Should you later find you cannot remember a specific instrument, look for it in this chapter. The picture will help to identify it.

Clean, sterilized instruments are placed either on tray setups or in the cabinet drawers according to a plan that satisfies your dentist. Ordinarily, instruments used together are grouped together.

If tray setups are used in your office, a group of stainless steel or fiberglass trays are kept in a special section of the work area. Each tray has a specific set of instruments on it for a specific dental operation. When a patient is scheduled for a crown preparation, you have only to pull one of the trays that have been set up for crown preparations and place it in the proper work area. This procedure means faster changeover between patients and allows the dental assistant to replenish the trays in moments that are not pressured.

Instruments are expensive. They are carefully formed, delicate, and not to be subjected to misuse. Flaming, which can ruin the temper of the metal, should be avoided. Without temper the instrument dulls very easily. (**Temper** is sometimes called "the ability to hold an edge.")

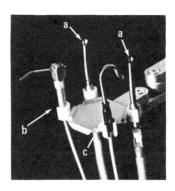

Figure 30.1
A contemporary dental unit arm with (a) evacuator tips; (b) water-air syringe; and (c) saliva ejector located on the assistant's side of the dental chair.

Another misuse of the instrument is to drop it. Dropping can deform the working end. Since the instrument is valuable only so long as it is exactly shaped to perform an explicit task, the slightest malformation ruins it. Please take care of your instruments.

A good assistant is careful to keep all instruments in their proper places, replaces them promptly after sterilization, and is positive that they are clean and, where necessary, sterile.

The Dental Unit and Its Accessories

The **dental unit** may be floor-mounted or mobile. It may have long arms with trays that can be moved to the best position for the operators. There may be two such freely moving trays: one for the dentist and one for the assistant; or one tray may swing into position just below the patient's chest and both the dentist and the dental assistant utilize it. The light may be part of the unit or ceiling-mounted, but the light is essential to the profession of dentistry.

An older-type unit is floor-mounted and stationary. Whether the unit is stationary or utilizes a swinging tray, the unit will contain (or have attachments for) the evacuators (there may be one or two), the three-way syringe, the cuspidor (or cup that replaces the cuspidor), the saliva ejector, and the handpieces.

The **dental light** should be cleaned frequently; the handles should be routinely disinfected between patients.

The **evacuator** has removable tips that should be autoclaved after each use. It is used to keep the site in the patient's mouth free from debris and water. It affords the dentist better visibility of the area being treated. The dental assistant operates the evacuator.

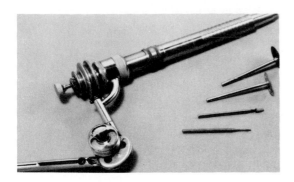

Figure 30.2
Ball bearing handpiece.

The **three-way syringe** delivers water, air, or both, as the operation requires.

The saliva ejector hose is usually mounted on the unit. It is a suction hose into which is placed a small tube that is hook-shaped. The tube is placed in the patient's mouth to remove the saliva that collects during dental operations. This small hook-shaped tube is called the **saliva ejector.** The open end of the ejector is hung over the teeth and lips. This end of the ejector rests on the floor of the mouth where it draws up the nearby saliva.

Saliva ejectors are disposable plastic tubes. A new one is used for each patient and then thrown away after use. They are packaged in sterile wrapping when purchased.

The Handpieces

A **handpiece,** one of the basic instruments of dentistry, is used to prepare teeth for restorations and to clean the surfaces of teeth.

A handpiece is held by the dentist in his or her hand and is used with a variety of burs, stones, wheels, cups, and diamond instruments which the dentist selects and attaches to the end of the handpiece. The dentist then turns on a speed control, usually with his or her foot, causing the bur or tip to revolve at a speed which the dentist can vary. Figures 30.2–30.4 illustrate handpieces.

The **ultraspeed handpieces** are usually air turbine types operating generally at 100,000 to 600,000 rpm. They use compressed air supplied to the handpiece through a very flexible rubber tubing, which is also the means of supplying water spray to the cutting instrument and the area being prepared. This handpiece is necessary in bulk tooth reduction in cavity and crown preparation where slow-speed operation not only is more

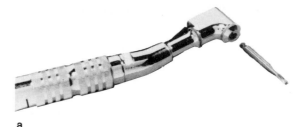

a

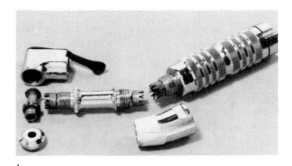

b

Figure 30.3
Latch-type contra-angle: (a) assembled; and (b) disassembled.

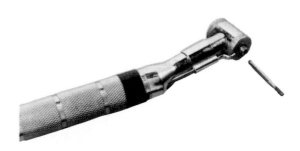

Figure 30.4
Ultraspeed handpiece.

time-consuming and traumatic to the tooth, but does not offer the ease of operation and control of the cutting tip for the dentist.

The handpiece is also described by its shape. There are contra-angles, right angles, and straight handpieces. Their uses vary, but the principle of their operation is the same.

There are several types of handpieces. *The dental assistant should learn the uses and care of those found in the office in which she or he works.* Each handpiece comes with the manufacturer's directions for maintenance. Follow the instructions scrupulously.

Accessories for the Handpieces

Dental Burs

The "drill" with which the dentist prepares a tooth for a restoration is correctly called a **bur.** Dental burs are supplied in two types of material: one is the regular steel bur; the other is a carbide bur. Regular steel burs are used at operating speeds of up to 10,000 rpm. Carbide burs are used at speeds up to 600,000 rpm.

Carbide burs are more expensive than regular steel burs, but they last much longer. They must not be immersed in cold sterilization solution unless the manufacturer specifically indicates that this is permissible.

Manufacturers place a distinguishing feature on their carbide burs: the shank may be colored brown or gold, it may have grooves conspicuously placed around it, it may have other types of markings; or the shape of the bur at the neck may differ markedly. Learn to identify all the brands of carbide burs used in your office so that you will not confuse them with regular steel burs. They are usually stored for use in a bur block different from the block in which regular steel burs are stored.

All burs may be cleaned by brushing well with a **scratch brush.** They must be cleaned thoroughly. Regular steel burs may be sterilized in the dry-heat oven, in oil sanitizers, or in an autoclave. Carbide burs should be sterilized according to the manufacturer's recommendations only.

Burs for contra-angles are supplied with either friction-grip or latch-type shanks. The straight handpiece is designed to hold only the long-shanked burs. The standard latch-type contra-angle will hold standard angle and short-shank burs. A miniature-head latch-type contra-angle is required for miniature burs. Some manufacturers also make a long-shanked bur for contra-angle use. Gear-type contra-angles for slow speed are also available with friction grip. High-speed handpieces, such as air turbines, use burs that have a more slender shank, referred to as a **friction grip** or **Fg type.** These burs are all carbide.

Domestic burs (burs manufactured in this country) are numbered according to a specific numbering system most dentists use. Imported burs may be numbered differently.

Friction-grip and latch-type burs are kept in separate bur blocks, properly labeled. The diagram of burs in figure 30.5 will show you the shapes of burs.

Diamond Instruments

Diamond instruments cut harder structures more quickly than burs and are used particularly to "open" a tooth, i.e., to get through the enamel, or to do major shaping as for a full-crown preparation. They are used

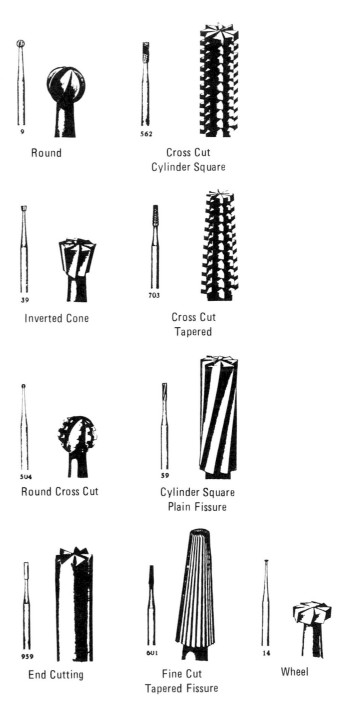

Figure 30.5
Enlargement of bur shapes with an example of actual size.

in a handpiece—usually in those handpieces capable of very high speeds.

Diamond instruments used under a constant stream of water or a water-air spray are very easy to keep clean. If they are used without a stream of water or water-air spray, the job is more difficult and heat is generated that will damage the pulp. The surface of the disc or wheel tends to become clogged with the fine debris of the grinding operation. The longer this debris

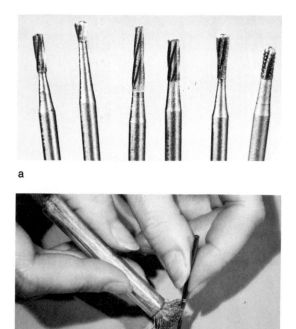

a

b

Figure 30.6
(a) Assortment of burs used in amalgam cavity preparation; and (b) cleaning bur with scratch brush.

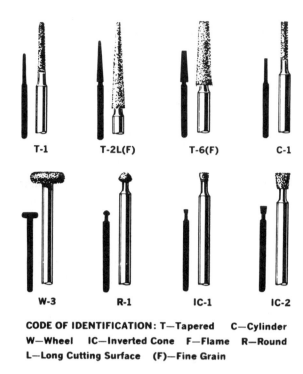

CODE OF IDENTIFICATION: T—Tapered   C—Cylinder
W—Wheel   IC—Inverted Cone   F—Flame   R—Round
L—Long Cutting Surface   (F)—Fine Grain

Figure 30.7
Diamond instruments shown are actual size silhouettes with enlarged view for detail.

remains on the surface of the diamond instrument the more difficult it is to remove and the greater the degree of heat that is generated.

Diamond instruments should be cleaned in the ultrasonic cleaner immediately after use. If an ultrasonic cleaner is not available, immerse instruments for five minutes in a solution of soapy water.

Using a stiff-bristled toothbrush, brush the surface of the instrument until completely free of debris, rinse, and then dry by blowing with the air syringe.

If the debris will not come free, mount the instrument in the slow handpiece, run the engine as slowly as possible, and gently hold a rubber ink eraser against the cutting surface of the instrument, moving the eraser back and forth across the surface until clean. Be careful of your fingers! Rinse with clear water and dry as before.

If, through some circumstance, diamond instruments should become coated with dried blood and mucus that will not brush off, they may be cleaned by soaking in an ordinary paintbrush cleaner.

Diamond instruments that are filled with amalgam may be cleaned most safely by soaking overnight in mercury, then running slowly against an ink eraser.

Keep all diamond instruments in holders for that purpose, clean and ready for use.

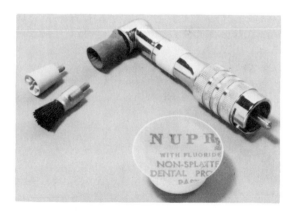

Figure 30.8
Prophylaxis right angle and cups.

Dental Prophylaxis Right Angles, Brushes, and Cups

A patient recall appointment includes a prophylaxis—which, to the patient, means cleaning his or her teeth. A special right angle may be used on the handpiece with cups and brushes that clean and polish the surface of the teeth.

It is possible for prophylaxis brushes and cups to be mounted in the regular handpiece, but the abrasive

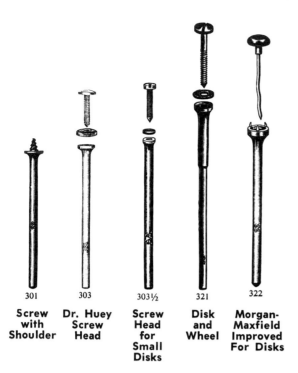

Figure 30.9
Mandrels.

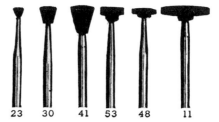

Figure 30.10
Mounted stones.

Stones

The handpiece can be used with mounted or un-mounted stones to do many grinding operations—on surfaces in the mouth, on artificial teeth, on casts, and on any material that needs to be finished.

Several types of stones are used. If the stones are green, they are carborundum; if they are red, they are aluminum oxide; and if they are gray, they are heatless stones, i.e., they produce little heat when being used.

Stones that are permanently attached to a mandrel are referred to as mounted stones; those which must be mounted on a mandrel before they can be used in the handpiece are unmounted stones.

Basic Setups

No matter what dental operation is to be performed, certain instruments are utilized. We refer to them as a **basic setup.** They are placed on the tray for every patient who is seated in the dental chair. A setup includes mirrors, explorers, and cotton pliers.

Dental mirrors: Dental mirrors are supplied with short stems fixed to a circular mirror. There are two types of stems: plain or simple for use with a plain handle, and cone-socket for use with a cone-socket handle. Dental offices usually use one type or the other. The mirror itself is available in two types, plane and magnifying. The plane type gives the same images as a hand mirror, whereas the magnifying type gives an enlarged image. Mirror sizes vary. They are listed either by inches in diameter or by a size number (1–5).

Explorers: Explorers are used most commonly to examine the teeth. Most of them are double-ended, that is, they have a different point on each end. A number on the handle identifies the design of the explorer. When the points become bent or dull, the instrument must be replaced.

Cotton pliers: Cotton pliers are long tweezers with bent, pointed ends. They are used to take materials to and from the mouth.

material used to clean the teeth can work its way into the handpiece and wear it out sooner than necessary. A prophylaxis right angle is designed to prevent this wear from occurring. You may find either used in your dentist's office.

A hygienist may use brushes, rubber cups, and portepolishers for the recall visit.

Mandrels

A mandrel is used to attach small grinding stones or sandpaper discs. It is a rod of metal—a shank that is inserted into the handpiece. A mandrel with no cutting instrument attached to it is equipped with a pin or tiny screw in the end. The dentist attaches a paper disc or an unmounted stone with this pin or screw to the mandrel and then inserts the mandrel into the handpiece. Some stones are mounted stones and are attached permanently to a mandrel. These are simply inserted into the handpiece. There will be some mandrels available if your office uses polishing discs and unmounted stones. Mandrels are available for straight (conventional) handpieces and for (conventional) contra-angles. The latter are shorter than the former.

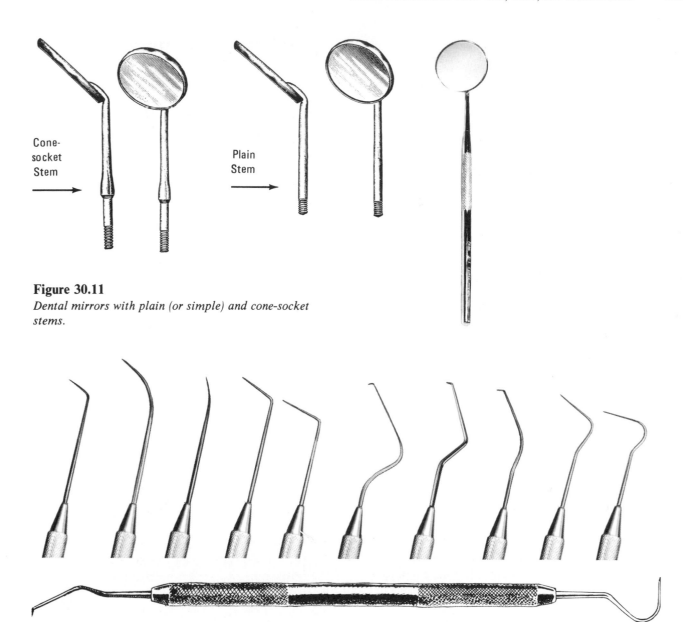

Figure 30.11
Dental mirrors with plain (or simple) and cone-socket stems.

Figure 30.12
A sampling of explorers.

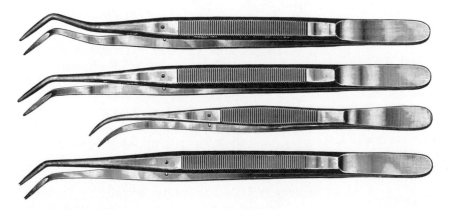

Figure 30.13
Cotton pliers and dressing pliers.

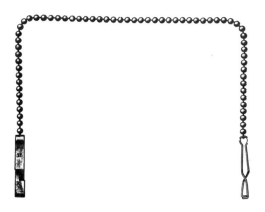

Figure 30.14
Napkin holder.

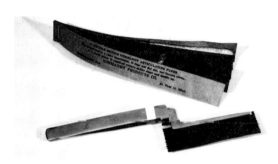

Figure 30.15
Carbon paper (or articulating paper) with holder.

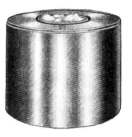

Figure 30.16
Cotton holder.

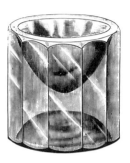

Figure 30.17
Dappen dish.

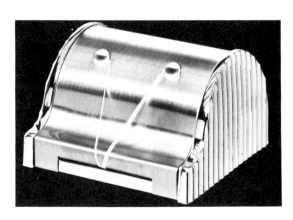

Figure 30.18
A dispenser for dental floss and dental tape.

Ten Small, but Important, Items

Bib or napkin holder: A napkin or bib holder is used to hold a towel or paper napkin across the chest of a patient in order that any debris or splashing from the mouth will not soil the patient's clothes. At each end of the holder is an alligator clip or clasp. Attach the holder to one side of the napkin, lay the napkin across the patient's chest, under his or her chin, slip the chain around his or her neck, and fasten the holder to the other side of the napkin. Be careful that the cold chain does not rest on bare skin. It is an uncomfortable sensation.

Carbon paper: Whenever a restoration is completed, it is necessary to check the articulation to be certain that the teeth are in proper occlusion. Carbon paper is used for this purpose. It has carbon on both sides, and when the patient taps her or his teeth together or bites on this paper, at the direction of the dentist, marks are left that enable the dentist to see whether the restoration needs further carving for correct function.

Cotton holder: This metal receptacle is kept filled with clean cotton for the dentist to use according to need during dental operations.

Dappen dish: This dish has a cup on each end. One is smaller than the other. Small amounts of medicament or prophylactic paste are placed in this dish for the dentist's use.

Dental floss and dental tape dispenser: Dental floss and dental tape are used in oral hygiene as well as in general dental work. The dispenser provides convenience in the use of both materials.

Medicament bottles: Medicament bottles are usually kept in a drawer easily accessible to the dentist.

Bottles should be clearly labeled. Type on white paper the name of the medicament. Trim close to the typing. Put all labels on bottles in a uniform position.

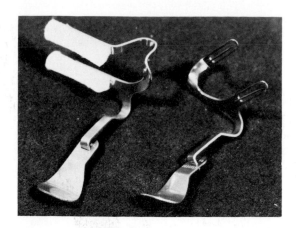

Figure 30.19
Cotton-roll holders.

They may be taped on with a strip of cellophane tape that covers the label completely. Be sure that the label is straight. Replace all labels every six months, or sooner if defaced.

If a label printer is available, effective labels can be made more easily. The tape used is already gummed for application to any surface.

Bottles should be kept clean at all times. It is much easier to keep them clean if no more than one-fourth inch of medicament is placed in any bottle. In the event of spillage, only a small quantity is out of control.

There are exceptions to this rule for quantity of medicaments.

1. Keep a greater quantity in each bottle of solutions that evaporate very quickly, such as alcohol, chloroform, or similar clear solutions.
2. Keep a lesser quantity in each bottle of caustic solutions, such as phenol. These potentially dangerous solutions are used more safely if a cotton pad is kept saturated in the bottom of the bottle so that there is no free liquid to spill and perhaps burn someone.

Check medicament bottles daily to see that there is a usable supply in each.

Self-retaining cotton-roll holders: A device that holds a cotton roll on each side of the lower arch in order to keep the tooth dry is called a self-retaining cotton-roll holder. Each holder uses two cotton rolls. The holder clamps into position by means of a flat brace that slips under the patient's chin and can be locked against the outside of his or her jaw.

The upper arch is kept dry by inserting the cotton roll between the cheek and arch. A cotton roll is not required on the lingual side of the upper arch.

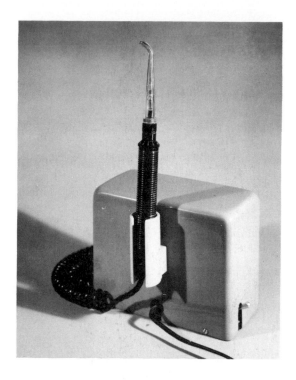

Figure 30.20
A pulp tester.

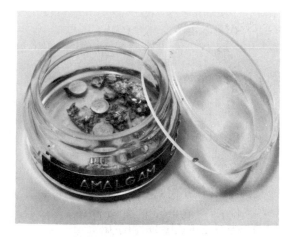

Figure 30.21
Waste receptacle.

Towels: It is the dental assistant's responsibility to see that a clean towel is available at each lavatory where the dentist and the dental assistant wash many times every day. The towels are supposed to be clean. Replace them frequently enough to be certain that they look clean to the patients.

Pulp tester: If there is a question regarding the health of a specific tooth, the dentist may check it with a pulp tester to see whether the tooth is still alive.

Waste receptacle: A waste receptacle should be available for the dentist to deposit any debris or used cotton pellets during dental operations.

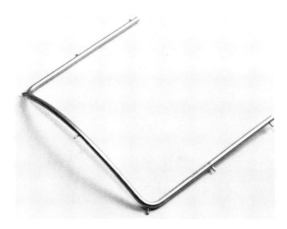

Figure 30.22
Young's rubber-dam frame.

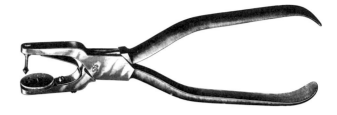

Figure 30.23
Perfected rubber-dam punch.

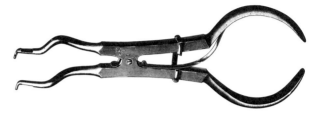

Figure 30.24
Brewer universal rubber-dam clamp forceps.

Rubber Dam

Most dental operations are performed with better visibility and better results when the field of operation is isolated and completely dry. Cotton rolls and cotton-roll holders of various kinds are commonly used for this purpose in addition to low-pressure evacuators or saliva ejectors.

The ideal method of achieving a dry field however, is by applying a rubber dam to the teeth under operation. Rubber dam is supplied either as precut five-inch or six-inch squares or in a roll five or six inches wide, in light or dark color. The dam also comes in various thicknesses. It is usually coated lightly with talc to prevent sticking.

A piece of rubber dam approximately seven inches in length is cut off the roll. The **rubber-dam punch** is used to make a series of small holes in this piece. Holes are usually made for a few teeth to the mesial of the one under operation and at least one to the distal, if one is present. The position of the holes corresponds to a spot in the center of the occlusal or incisal surface of the teeth involved, and in the same relative position to each other hole. That is, if holes were to be punched for a complete set of sixteen teeth in one arch, they would be placed in exactly the same curve as the arch itself. A rubber-dam template may be used as a guide to positioning the holes until sufficient experience is gained.

The rubber dam is lubricated lightly with Vaseline around each punched hole, as an aid in slipping the rubber dam over each tooth. The rubber dam is then placed in the mouth, with the punched holes over the corresponding teeth, and the dam is slipped down over each tooth for which holes have been punched, slipping the edge of the rubber dam through the contact first.

At the cervical area of each tooth, the rubber dam is tucked downward under the free gum margin into the gingival crevice for a good seal against moisture. Saliva, as well as any interference from the tongue or cheeks, is well controlled. A **rubber-dam clamp** is usually placed on the most distal tooth to hold the rubber down in position. A **rubber-dam clamp forceps** is used in placing the clamp. Dental floss is sometimes used in addition to a rubber-dam retainer, or alone, as a ligature around the cervical portion of some or all of the teeth exposed through the rubber dam.

A **rubber-dam frame** or holder is then positioned to secure the sheet of rubber dam. The elastic band of the holder goes around the back of the patient's head and is adjusted to hold snugly. When a saliva ejector has been inserted (sometimes under the rubber dam and sometimes through another hole punched in the dam for that purpose), the field is clear and ready for the operative procedures.

Weights are sometimes clipped to the lower edge of the rubber dam as an aid in holding this edge down, out of the dentist's way.

Gauze napkins, called rubber-dam napkins, are available for use under rubber-dam applications. This gauze is shaped like the piece of rubber dam except for a large opening cut out of the gauze for the mouth, since the gauze is designed to lie between the rubber dam and the skin of the face. The use of a rubber-dam napkin makes a rubber dam much more comfortable for the patient. Moisture that may seep between the skin of the face and the rubber dam is otherwise uncomfortable.

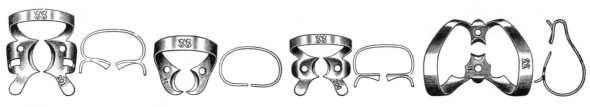

201. Upper Molar.   **22.** For upper and lower bicuspids. Flat jaws. For same clamp with dam-engaging projections.   **206.** For upper and lower bicuspids   **211.** Universal for labial cavities on the twenty anterior teeth

Courtesy S. S. White Co.

Figure 30.25
Assortment of rubber-dam clamps: molar, bicuspid, and anterior.

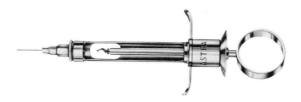

Figure 30.26
An aspirating syringe.

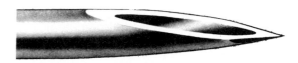

Figure 30.27
An enlargement of the Huber dental needle, showing its construction as a hollow tube, with the scalpel-sharp point at the center line of the long axis of the needle—a factor that aids in patient comfort.

The application of rubber dam is more easily performed with the help of the dental assistant to hold the rubber in position before the retainer is placed, as well as in using a piece of dental floss to help force the rubber dam down between teeth when the contacts are tight.

Observation of the problems involved will show the dental assistant many ways to assist with this procedure.

Anesthetic Syringes and Needles

Syringes: The instrument with which the dentist injects a local anesthetic is called a *syringe.* The most commonly used type in dental offices consists of a barrel with open sides. A plunger mechanism is inserted into one end of the barrel and has a barb on the end to engage the rubber plug in the local anesthetic *cartridge.* The other end of the plunger mechanism has a crossbar or round disc for the dentist's thumb. The end of the barrel containing the plunger mechanism opens in some manner to permit the insertion of the cartridge. This may be a spring device or a screw device. Examine the type used in your office. Learn how it operates.

The other end of the barrel contains the mounting mechanism for the needle. A portion at the end of the barrel is threaded, with an opening in the center through which part of the injection needle extends inside the barrel. This end of the needle perforates the fixed plug

or cap of the anesthetic cartridge and communicates with the solution inside. As the plunger is depressed, the solution is discharged.

Needles for anesthetic syringes: Needles are manufactured in various gauges that are indications of the outside diameter of the needle. The gauges used in dental offices are 25, 26, 27, 28, 29, and 30. Twenty-five-gauge would be the heaviest needle with the greatest diameter; and thirty-gauge would be the finest needle with the smallest diameter.

To insure a sterile and sharp needle every time, presterilized disposable needles are used. Each needle is individually sterile, protected within a two-piece plastic case. It is generally necessary to remove that section that covers the short end, attach the needle to the syringe by holding the remaining plastic sheath, then remove the remaining portion of the plastic sheath when ready for the injection. The ampule is inserted into the syringe barrel prior to attaching the needle.

Local anesthetic solutions are most commonly supplied to the dental office in cans of fifty glass tubes, called **ampules** or **cartridges.** The glass tube, or ampule, is closed at one end by a rubber plug that rests completely inside the tube. This is the movable plug, which faces the plunger when inserted in the syringe. The other end of the ampule is also closed, either with a rubber stopper, which has a shoulder extending over the glass wall, or a metal cap with a small rubber center.

This is the fixed plug, which faces the needle when inserted in the syringe. The fixed plug should be wiped with a solution of 70 percent ethyl alcohol before insertion in the syringe.

Preparation of Syringe for Use

When a syringe is to be used, attach the sterile disposable needle, leaving the plastic cover on.

Open the syringe, insert the cartridge of local anesthetic with fixed plug down, close the syringe, remove the plastic needle cover, and test for delivery. If the solution does not squirt out through the needle, change needles.

If the syringe is to be placed in the operatory some time before use, replace the plastic protective cover on the needle. Place the syringe on the cabinet top, preferably covering it with a disposable tissue so that the patient will not see it.

Care of Syringes After Use

The used carpule is removed from the syringe. Replace the original sheath over the working end of the needle and remove the needle from the syringe. With a pliers, bend and crush the portion of the needle not covered in order to prevent its reuse. Do not stick yourself. The needle is no longer sterile.

Autoclave the syringe.

Transfer Forceps

A transfer forceps is an instrument commonly used in the dental office. It is different from surgical forceps and is used to transfer sterile instruments from the autoclave to the sterile cabinet or storage. The transfer forceps is stored in a sterile container designed for that purpose (fig. 24.6).

Cement Slabs and Spatulas

Cement slabs and spatulas are stored in one of the cabinet drawers. Whenever a cement is required under a restoration, a slab and spatula must be used. These require special clean-up care. If the slab is glass, it must be cleaned for the next use.

Cement is best removed from glass slabs and spatulas immediately after the dentist has used the required amount. Take the slab and the spatula to the sink. Lay the slab in the sink and run warm water on it. Hold the spatula in the stream of water, rubbing it with thumb and forefinger to remove all traces from both sides and edges. Then pick up the glass slab and rub it also with your fingers, under running water, until

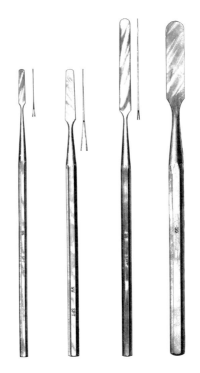

Figure 30.28
Cement spatulas.

all traces of cement are removed. Wash both slab and spatula with soap, then rinse completely with water and dry. Return to storage.

If not cleaned immediately, place both slab and spatula under a light stream of cold water and let stand. The cement will set and, when hard, will flake off quite easily. If slabs and spatulas are not free from scratches, it may be necessary to keep a solution of bicarbonate of soda in which to soak both before rubbing with fingers to clean. Thoroughly rinse off soda solution.

The bicarbonate of soda solution may also be applied to the dry cement with a cotton pellet, if preferred.

Never use one spatula to cut the cement off another spatula. Never use metal to remove cement from the slab. Slabs and spatulas will remain free from scratches and much easier to keep clean if these two rules are followed.

Benzene or fingernail polish remover will remove the rubber-base impression materials from soiled spatulas. Use a gauze to apply and wipe.

Mixing Pads

Another form of slab is a pad of parchment or heavy paper sheets. These parchment mixing pads are made of individual sheets sealed together at the edges. One small area is left unsealed. It is at this point that a clean cement spatula may be inserted and the used sheet of

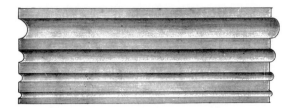

Figure 30.29
Bates Arkansas sharpening stone No. 5, used for sharpening all types of instruments (chisels, gouges, lancets, knives, excavators, and elevators); stone has four grooves—1 mm., 2 mm., 3 mm., and 4 mm.—on one side. The reverse side is flat to be used for the care of all kinds of knives and chisels.

parchment or paper removed by drawing the spatula around the gummed edge in the same manner as you use a letter opener.

Still another form of slab is a pad of clear plastic sheets. These are also sealed on the edges; each sheet is disposable. This particular type is most useful for temporary cements that, as a rule, are very difficult to clean from glass or will soak through the parchment types of pads.

Instrument Sharpening Devices

Instrument sharpening is an important activity in the dental office. Sharp instruments are essential in certain operations.

Arkansas Stone and Motor-driven Sharpeners

Arkansas stone is a sharpening stone used to sharpen instruments. Arkansas stones are available in several shapes in order that many types of instruments can be sharpened.

The Arkansas sharpening stone is commonly found in dental offices as a flat stone; others used are grooved and cylindrical stones of various sizes. These are not motorized but depend on handwork by the operator to produce the desired edge.

Some dentists have their instruments sharpened by a specialist. Others prefer to sharpen their own. Most of the dentists who sharpen their instruments prefer to do so personally rather than have an assistant perform this task requiring special skills. If an individual dentist wishes to delegate this work to an assistant, the dentist will teach the assistant the necessary skills.

The angle at which the instrument is held against the stone determines the bevel of the blade; therefore the dentist must teach the assistant how each instrument is to be sharpened.

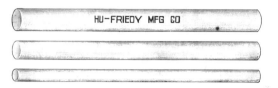

Figure 30.30
Gracey Arkansas files, designed for all types of scalers with a curette type blade: No. 1 is ³⁄₁₆″ × 4″, No. 2 is ¼″ × 4″, and 3 is ⅜″ × 4″.

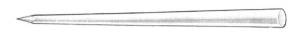

Figure 30.31
Gracey Arkansas cone No. 299; an individual stone for scalers and periodontal curettes.

Care of Sharpening Stone

The Arkansas sharpening stone is of extremely high quality and fine grade and requires good care. Before it is used, oil is applied to produce a finer edge and keep from clogging the stone with debris.

After it has been used, wipe the stone clean with a lintless cloth, apply a few drops of oil, and put the stone away.

Motor-driven instrument sharpeners should be cleaned only according to the manufacturer's instructions. Most of these sharpeners use a synthetic abrasive stone rather than an Arkansas stone.

Hand Instruments

Hand instruments are difficult to recognize quickly until you become familiar with them.

The hand instruments are held in the dentist's hand, so they have a handle. They also have a shank and a working head. The handle varies in size and weight depending on the use of the instrument. The shank is straight or bent at an angle—not always the same angle. The angle is designed so that a specific area in the mouth can be reached with that particular instrument.

You will learn the instrumentation sequence more easily if you recognize that the type of operation determines the basic instrument setup, but that within the basic instrument setup the location of the operation (that is, upper or lower teeth, mesial or distal surfaces, left or right) also introduces some variations in the specific instrument your dentist requires. Therefore, it is

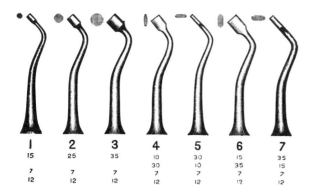

Figure 30.32
Amalgam pluggers.

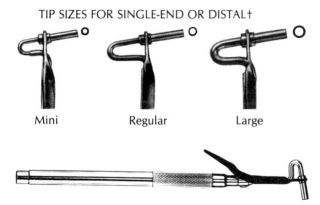

TIP SIZES FOR SINGLE-END OR DISTAL†

Mini   Regular   Large

Figure 30.33
Amalgam carriers.

necessary that you not only know what type of operation is being performed, but that you also know where it is being performed in order to effectively *serve* instruments to your dentist as required. They must be placed in the dentist's hand in the position in which they will be used.

Instrument Numbering

Instruments must be identified, especially for reordering; thus a numbering system has been devised. The numbers indicate important information about the instrument.

The first number toward the operative end, reading from left to right, indicates the width of the blade in tenths of a millimeter; the second number indicates the length of the blade from the center of the angle to the end in millimeters; the third number indicates the angle of the blade with the shaft in hundredths of a circle or centigrades.

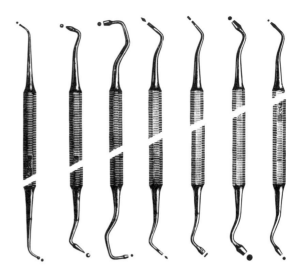

Figure 30.34
Amalgam condensers.

However, some cutting instruments have four formula numbers, and this occurs when the cutting edge of the instrument is at an angle, in which case the second number of the formula indicates the angle of the cutting edge; the third number indicates the length of the blade; and the fourth number indicates the angle of the blade with the shaft.

If *R* or *L* appears in the number of an instrument, this indicates that the instrument is for use on the right or left side of the cavity. The instruments are identical except that their shapes are reversed so that one is usable on the left side and one on the right side *of the preparation*.

Many dental instruments have overlapping uses; that is, a certain cutting instrument may be used for several different dental operations. There are some instruments, however, that are used for specific purposes, such as an amalgam restoration, and are used for no other operation.

Amalgam Instruments

Amalgam carriers are used to carry amalgam to the preparation, where the dental assistant releases the amalgam and the dentist condenses it into the preparation with amalgam pluggers or condensers.

When the preparation is completely filled with amalgam, the dentist carves or shapes the still-soft amalgam with a carver. (Carvers are also used to carve tooth anatomy in wax when making crowns.)

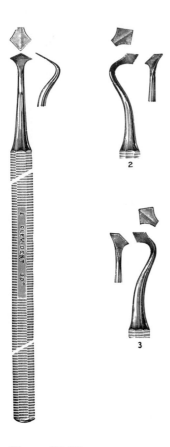

Figure 30.35
Frahm's carvers.

Cutting Instruments

One group of instruments that may be used in any dental restoration is cutting instruments of various types. We speak of them as cutting instruments because they are used to cut either soft tissue or hard tissue in the mouth. Strictly speaking, burs and discs are also cutting instruments, but they are rotary cutting instruments and can be considered with the handpiece with which they are used. This section defines "hand" cutting instruments—those held in the dentist's hand.

Several of the cutting instruments are **chisels** in various forms: hatchets, hoes, enamel hatchets, and gingival margin trimmers. Notice the tiny variations in the working end of each of these instruments and learn to know those which your dentist uses.

Spoon excavators are cutting instruments used to scoop out decay. They have a small curve to their head like a spoon. The edge is sharp and can cut the decay, which is then held in the curve of the spoon.

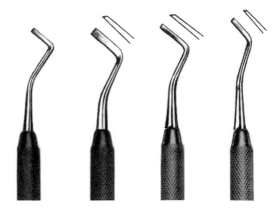

Figure 30.36
Cutting instruments: hatchets.

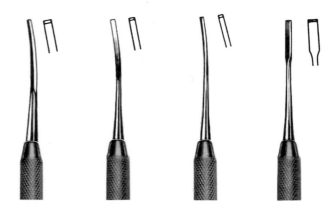

Figure 30.37
Cutting instruments: chisels.

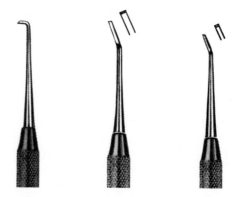

Figure 30.38
Cutting instruments: hoes.

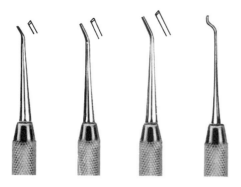

Figure 30.39
Cutting instruments: angle formers.

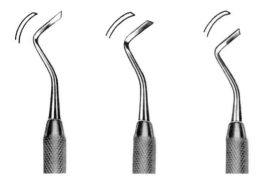

Figure 30.40
Cutting instruments: margin trimmers.

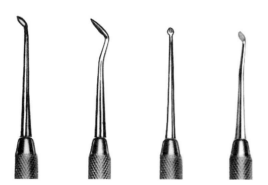

Figure 30.41
Cutting instruments: Cleoid-Discoid.

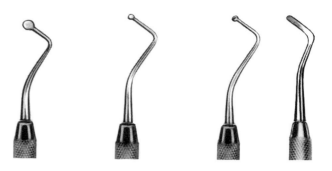

Figure 30.42
Cutting instruments: spoon excavators.

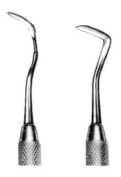

Figure 30.43
Cutting instruments: knives.

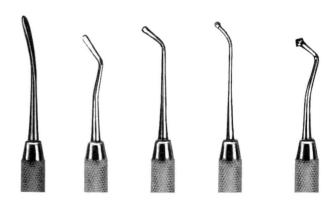

Figure 30.44
Amalgam burnishers.

Trimming knives are very thin-bladed knives used to trim soft tissues. Ideally, they should be resharpened after each use.

Scalers are used for prophylaxis and in periodontics. In the general practitioner's office, the greatest use will be for prophylaxis. These instruments are used to remove deposits of calculus (tartar) from around the teeth. There are many shapes of scalers.

Matrix and Matrix Holders

When an amalgam restoration includes a proximal surface, a matrix band is necessary to hold the amalgam in place until it has been carved and is ready to set. If the location and the complexity of the preparation require it, the dentist may make the matrix band from matrix material. The dentist will usually use a continuous matrix holder, such as the Tofflemire. Most matrix operations, however, can be accomplished with the matrix holder and matrix bands, which are purchased ready to use.

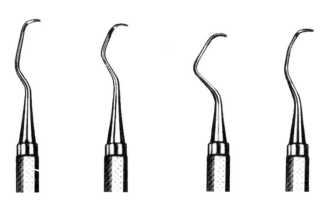

Figure 30.45
A selection of scalers.

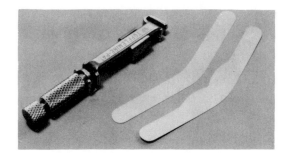

Figure 30.46
Tofflemire matrix retainer.

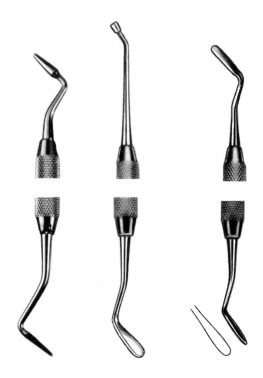

Figure 30.47
Plastic filling/composite instruments.

Gold-foil Instruments

Gold-foil restorations require special instruments. There are gold pluggers, files, holding instruments, annealing instruments, and pellet placers—all for use with gold-foil preparations. There are burnishers that are used for polishing any metal—but especially gold.

Plastic Filling Instruments

Another group of instruments are called plastic filling instruments. Their name utilizes the true meaning of plastic. Plastic means *moldable;* hence, these instruments are used to *shape* plastic material. Amalgam is plastic before it sets; cements are also plastic before setting occurs. The dentist is not asking for a polyethylene bag or a Tupperware cup when he or she asks for a plastic instrument; the dentist means an instrument used for shaping a restoration material that can still be moved.

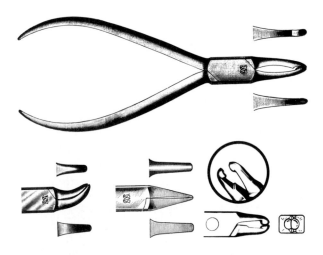

Figure 30.48
Contouring pliers.

Contouring Pliers

Temporary covers, children's steel crowns, and orthodontic appliances usually need to be shaped. Contouring pliers are used for this purpose. Notice there are several different shapes for the heads of these pliers.

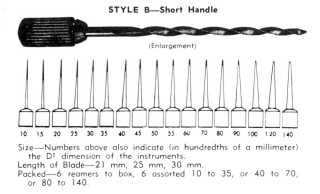

STYLE B—Short Handle

(Enlargement)

10 15 20 25 30 35 40 45 50 55 60 70 80 90 100 120 140

Size—Numbers above also indicate (in hundredths of a millimeter)
the D¹ dimension of the instruments.
Length of Blade—21 mm, 25 mm, 30 mm.
Packed—6 reamers to box, 6 assorted 10 to 35, or 40 to 70,
or 80 to 140.

Figure 30.49
Reamers used for endodontics.

BROACH Barbed, Short Handle

(Enlargement)

XX Fine
X Fine
Fine
Med
Coarse

Figure 30.50
Broaches used for endodontics.

Instruments for Five Dental Specialties

Endodontic Armamentarium

A number of instruments are designed exclusively for Endodontic treatment. Root canals taper from the chamber of the crown of the tooth to the small apical foramen. Roots vary in size and length. Some are relatively straight, but most have varying degrees of curvature. Some are relatively round in cross section while others are broad and oval-shaped. In general the canals within the roots have a shape quite similar to the root itself in cross section. All of these internal spaces must be meticulously cleansed and the canal shaped to an even taper to the apex. When this shaping has been accomplished, it is possible to make obduration conveniently and accurately with gutta percha and sealant cement.

Barbed broaches are instruments with needle-like projections on their surfaces designed to engage soft tissue and debris within the canal for removal and gross cleaning. Reamers and files are instruments with blades designed to cut dentin. By rotating reamers on their axes the walls of dentin can be shaved smooth and the canal shaped to an even taper. The file is used in a push-pull motion to assist in creating a smooth, clean taper.

Spreaders and pluggers are similar instruments. The spreaders are pointed and designed to condense gutta percha laterally in the canal. The pluggers are blunt ended and are used to remove excess gutta percha.

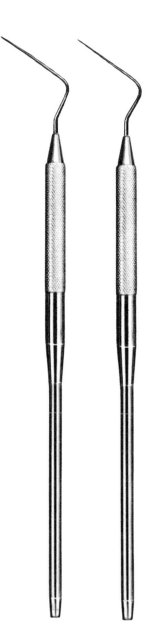

Figure 30.51
Root canal spreaders used for endodontics.

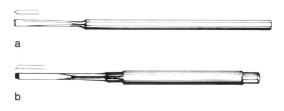

a

b

Figure 30.52
Chisels used for oral surgery: (a) bi-bevel chisel, octagonal handle, 4mm tip; and (b) single bevel chisel, round handle, 4 mm tip.

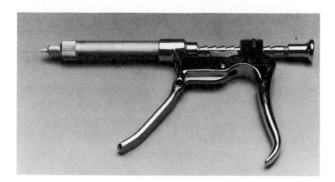

Figure 30.53
Ligmaject syringe.

Oral Surgery Armamentarium

(William P. Frantzich, D.D.S., M.S.D.)

Surgical instruments are used by an oral surgeon or by a dentist with a general practice who performs any oral surgery. The surgical instrument most commonly known to the layman is a *forceps*.

Surgical forceps are used to remove teeth. There are many shapes, each designed to be used in a particular location in the mouth.

Many extraction forceps are available to the surgeon. It is desirable, however, to have a minimum variety of forceps in the armamentarium. If too many types of forceps are available, it is confusing and expensive. A more efficient armamentarium includes a few high quality instruments that can be used on several different teeth. Two or three types of extraction forceps for the upper teeth and the same number for the lower teeth are much easier for the assistant and the surgeon to use.

Other instruments are used in oral surgery, some of which are also called forceps. Examples are tissue forceps (figs. 30.61 and 30.62) and hemostatic forceps (fig. 30.78). Figures 30.52 through 30.78 are examples of some of the instruments that will be found in a surgical armamentarium. Others may be included by some oral surgeons, but these, we believe, are basic.

Color Coding of Surgical Instruments

Color coding is a desirable way to mark instruments. Colored tape can be placed on instruments as an aid in rapid selection. The tape can be autoclaved. An example of the color coding would be blue tape on all instruments used in the upper mouth or maxilla; red tape on all instruments used in the lower mouth or mandible; yellow on all instruments used on the right side of the mouth; and green for the left side of the mouth. This is an aid when an assistant is handing forceps or elevators to the surgeon because the right/left, maxillary/mandibular instruments can be identified rapidly.

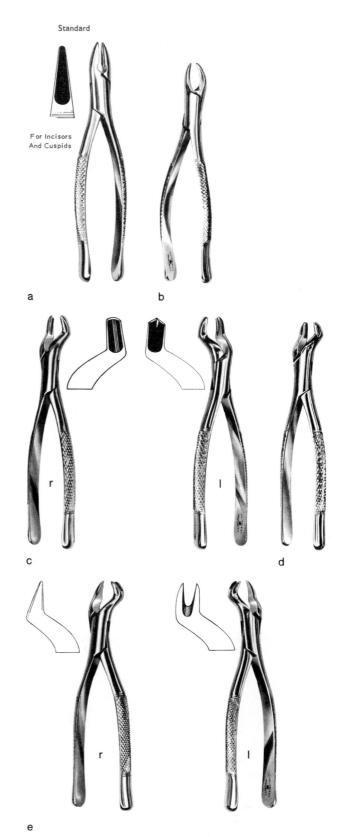

Figure 30.54
Maxillary forceps: (a) anterior forceps; (b) anterior forceps No. 150 (18cm/7'') can be used from second bicuspid to second bicuspid; (c) right and left molar forceps; (d) third molar forceps No. 210; and (e) right and left first molar forceps.

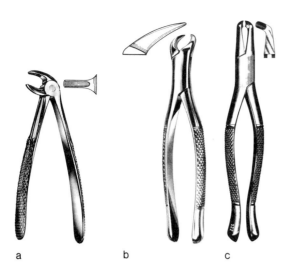

a   b   c

Figure 30.55
Mandibular forceps: (a) incisors, canines, and premolar forceps; (b) molar forceps; and (c) third molar forceps, No. 222.

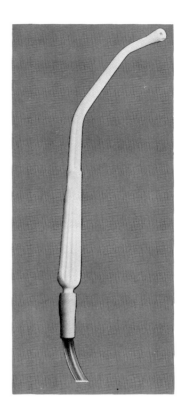

Figure 30.57
Disposable tonsil suction.

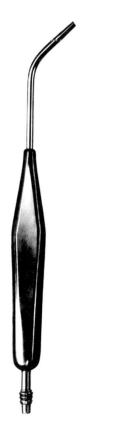

Figure 30.56
Coupland aspirator.

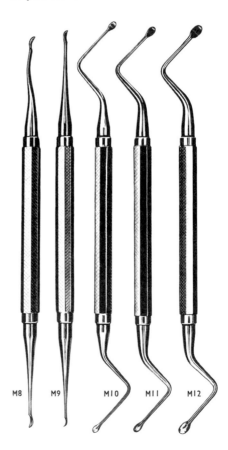

M8   M9   M10   M11   M12

Figure 30.58
Miller bone curettes (surgical).

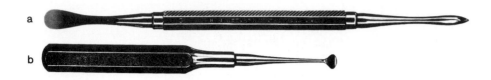

Figure 30.59
(a) Periosteal elevator, Molt 9; and (b) Periosteal elevator, M4.

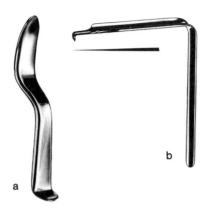

Figure 30.60
(a) University of Minnesota retractor; and (b) Austin retractor.

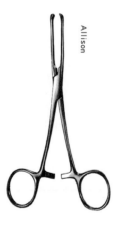

Figure 30.61
Allison tissue forceps.

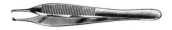

Figure 30.62
Adson tissue forceps with teeth.

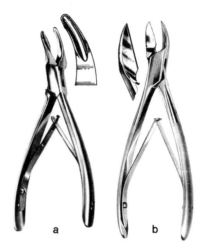

Figure 30.63
(a) End cutting rongeur; and (b) side cutting rongeur.

Care of Forceps

Forceps that are autoclaved for sterilization can be treated with an oil emulsion before processing.

Forceps may gradually become stiff in the joint, making them difficult or impossible to use. Three suggestions for correction of this condition follow. Start with the first. If that method does not succeed, proceed to the second, and finally, as a last resort, to the third.

1. Apply a few drops of dental engine oil to the joint and work it briskly for a minute.
2. Hold the forceps under very cold water and continue to open and close the forceps.
3. Soak the forceps overnight in penetrating oil. This can be obtained at most hardware stores. The forceps should be immersed in the penetrating oil, with the beaks of the forceps opened as wide as possible. Upon removal from the oil, wipe the forceps with a disposable tissue, briskly open and close several times, then wipe with a gauze moistened with 70 percent alcohol. Now sterilize as usual.

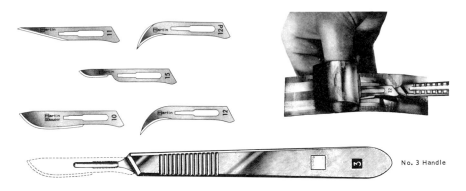

Figure 30.64
Scalpels. Blade No. 15 is most frequently used in oral surgery. Note the blades in the packet are sterile.

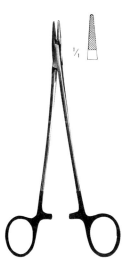

Figure 30.65
Mayo-Hegar fine needle holder (18cm/7").

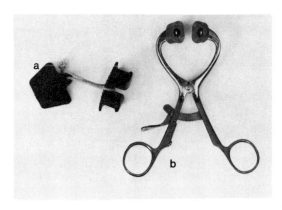

Figure 30.67
Mouth gags: (a) McKesson; and (b) Molt Universal.

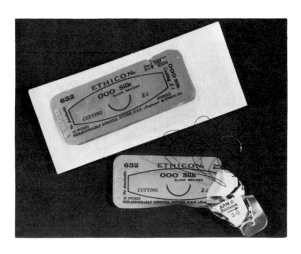

Figure 30.66
Disposable swedged-on suture and suture needles. FS-2 and PS-2.

Care of Sterile Surgical Instruments

All surgical instruments are usually stored in some area where they are protected from contamination. They are transferred from the autoclave to the storage area by means of transfer forceps. The following are the most frequently used methods of storage:

1. Autoclaved, covered-tray setups: one tray for each surgical operation.
2. Autoclaved surgical packs: each pack a complete set of instruments for one single operation. The packs are stored in the surgical cabinet.
3. A centrally located surgical table with an array of surgical instruments.
4. A selection of surgical instruments, including forceps, stored in the surgical cabinet in drawers lined with autoclaved towels.

Figure 30.68
Miller bone file.

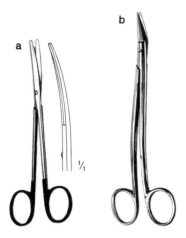

Figure 30.69
*(a) Metzenbaum curved-blunt scissors; and (b) Dean
surgical scissors.*

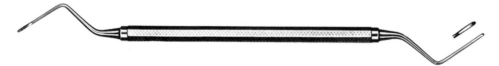

Figure 30.70
Root tip elevator.

Figure 30.71
*Gauze packer used to place medicated gauze strips into
tooth sockets for Rx of dry sockets.*

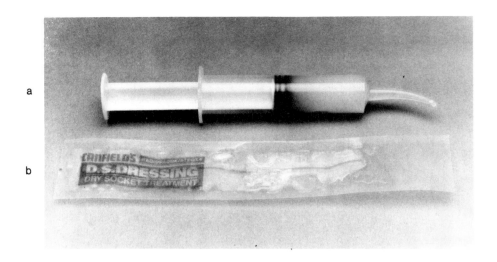

Figure 30.72
(a) Dry socket syringe; and (b) medicated sterile gauze
with radiopaque thread for dry socket treatment.

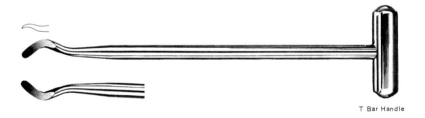

T Bar Handle

Figure 30.73
Potts elevators.

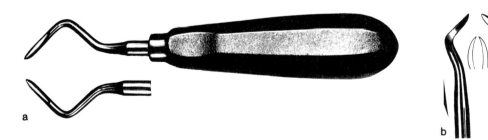

Figure 30.74
Elevators: (a) Schmeckebier Apexo; and (b) additional
elevators for use with 501 handle.

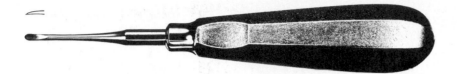

Figure 30.75
Straight elevator.

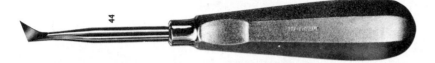

Figure 30.76
Cryer root elevator.

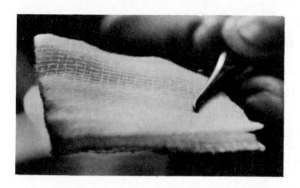

Figure 30.77
Exodontia sponge.

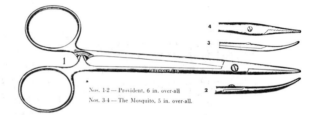

Nos. 1-2 — Provident, 6 in. over-all
Nos. 3-4 — The Mosquito, 5 in. over-all.

Figure 30.78
Hemostatic forceps.

Orthodontic Armamentarium

The orthodontist uses special X ray, casts, and appliances. The special X ray is discussed in chapter 28, "Dental Specialties," and also in Part VIII "Radiography." The materials for appliances are presented in chapter 28, "Dental Specialties." The casts are described and exact instructions for their completion appear in chapter 33, "Casts and Dies."

Instruments commonly used include a variety of pliers: Howe, arch bending, three-jaw wire-bender, birdbeak, band-removing, direct bond removing, distal end cutter, hard wire cutter, band-slitter, pin and ligature cutter, ligature-tying, and separator Alastic. Other instruments are band drivers or amalgam pluggers, scalers, and mouth mirrors.

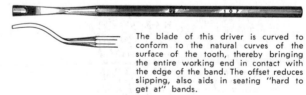

The blade of this driver is curved to conform to the natural curves of the surface of the tooth, thereby bringing the entire working end in contact with the edge of the band. The offset reduces slipping, also aids in seating "hard to get at" bands.

Figure 30.79
Band driver for orthodontic use.

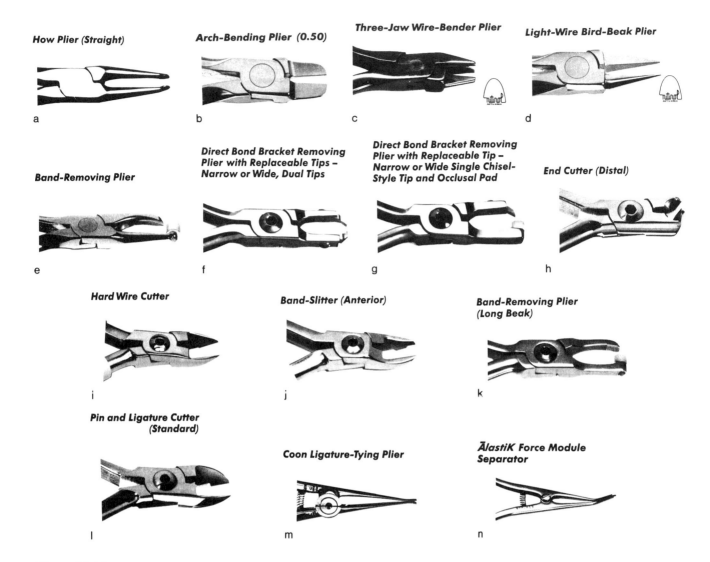

How Plier (Straight)

a

Arch-Bending Plier (0.50)

b

Three-Jaw Wire-Bender Plier

c

Light-Wire Bird-Beak Plier

d

Band-Removing Plier

e

Direct Bond Bracket Removing Plier with Replaceable Tips – Narrow or Wide, Dual Tips

f

Direct Bond Bracket Removing Plier with Replaceable Tip – Narrow or Wide Single Chisel-Style Tip and Occlusal Pad

g

End Cutter (Distal)

h

Hard Wire Cutter

i

Band-Slitter (Anterior)

j

Band-Removing Plier (Long Beak)

k

Pin and Ligature Cutter (Standard)

l

Coon Ligature-Tying Plier

m

ĀlastiK Force Module Separator

n

Figure 30.80
A sample of pliers used by orthodontists:
(a) Howe plier;
(b) arch-bending plier;
(c) three-jaw wire-bender;
(d) bird-beak plier;
(e) band-removing plier;
(f) direct bond bracket removing plier, dual tips;

(g) direct bond bracket removing plier, single chisel tip;
(h) end cutter plier;
(i) hard wire cutter;
(j) band-slitter plier;
(k) band-removing plier;
(l) pin and ligature cutter;
(m) ligature-tying plier; and
(n) alastik separator.

Periodontic Armamentarium

The periodontist, the dentist who treats the area surrounding the teeth, uses probes, scalers, curettes, elevators, sharpening stones, gauze sponges, knives, needle holders, suture scissors, and suturing materials, in addition to the basic setups for operative dentistry. A number of instruments used in general dentistry are also used.

Prosthodontic Armamentarium

A prosthetic device can be fixed or removable. Fixed prostheses include crowns and inlays that replace part of a tooth, and bridges that replace a missing tooth by attaching a pontic to the two teeth on either side of the space left by the missing tooth. These teeth are called *abutments*. A bridge can also replace more than one missing tooth.

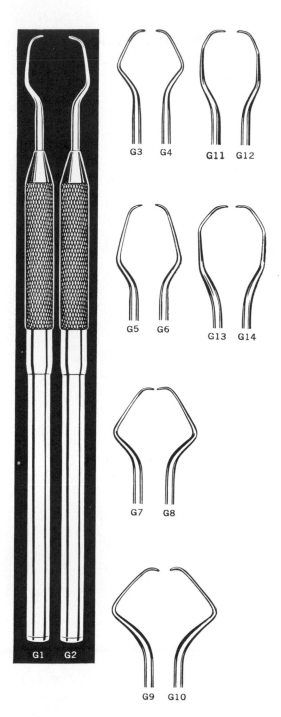

Figure 30.81
Gracey curettes, generally used by periodontists.

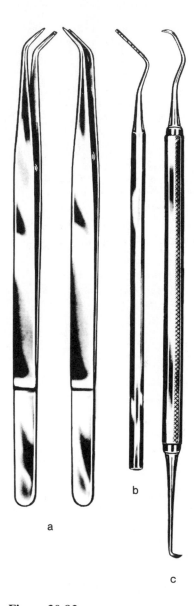

Figure 30.82
Some instruments used by periodontists: (a) pocket markers; (b) pocket probe; and (c) universal scaler.

Instruments for fixed prostheses include **crown and bridge scissors,** which are used to cut copper band and other metals. **Crown forms** are used to make an acrylic cover for a tooth that is prepared and requires protection until the crown has been finished, ready for cementation.

Impressions are taken for both fixed and removable prostheses. In addition to impressions, removable prosthetic devices may require the use of articulators and facebows.

Following surgery there is usually a need for a prosthetic replacement—whether it is a bridge, partial, or full denture. In order to make a prosthesis, the dentist must use **impression trays** to reproduce the dental arch or quadrant. With this impression the dental assistant can make a cast that will permit the dentist to create the reproduction outside the mouth. The trays

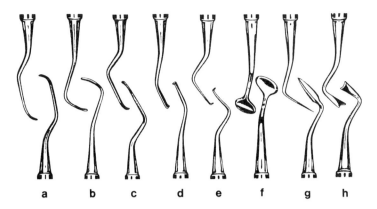

Figure 30.83
Additional instruments used by periodontists:
(a) curettage; (b) curette; (c) curette; (d) hoe; (e) hoe;
(f) heavy-shanked knife; (g) spear-pointed knife; and
(h) triangular tissue retractor.

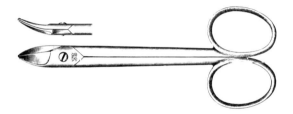

Figure 30.84
Curved collar and crown scissors.

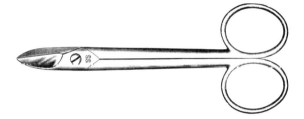

Figure 30.85
Straight crown scissors.

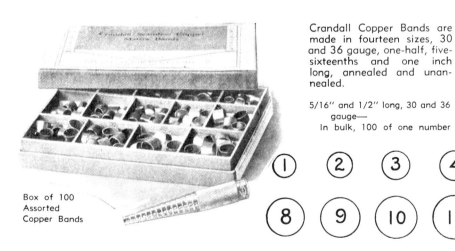

Box of 100
Assorted
Copper Bands

Crandall Copper Bands are
made in fourteen sizes, 30
and 36 gauge, one-half, five-
sixteenths and one inch
long, annealed and unan-
nealed.

5/16" and 1/2" long, 30 and 36
    gauge—
    In bulk, 100 of one number

5/16" and 1/2" long, 30 and 36
    gauge—
    Box of 12 of one number
    Box of 25 of one number
    Box of 100 assorted

1" long, 36 gauge—
    Box of 12 of one number
    Box of 25 of one number
    Box of 100 assorted

Figure 30.86
Crandall copper bands with circles to indicate size of
bands.

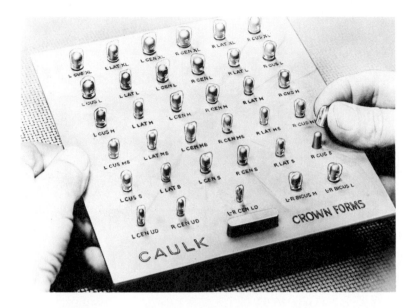

Figure 30.87
Crown forms selection board.

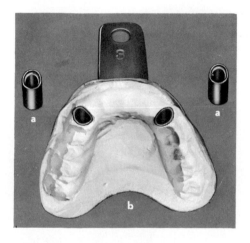

Figure 30.88
(a) Two "thimble" impressions (or copper bands) of synthetic jacket crown preparations; and (b) an impression removed in superimposed plaster tray.

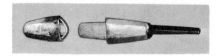

Figure 30.89
Amalgam die made from a thimble impression with a "coping" made to fit the amalgam die.

used must have special care to keep them looking nice for the patient. They are usually aluminun or plastic. If they are not treated properly, they soon become scratched and marred. A patient may feel uncomfortable if a tray inserted in his or her mouth looks as if it is marred and rough, and the patient may wonder where the tray has been. Treat trays gently—according to the following directions.

Impression trays, when returned by the laboratory after use, are usually not thoroughly cleansed. They should first be cleaned of all foreign material. Scrape plaster off when necessary, being careful not to raise rough spots on the surface of the tray.

If compound is sticking on the tray, pass the tray through a gas flame until the compound is softened, then wipe off with disposable tissue or cloth.

Give the tray a very light daubing with Vaseline, flame the tray lightly to melt the Vaseline, wipe with a disposable tissue to remove excess Vaseline. Now sterilize the tray.

To brighten trays periodically, boil in a pan of water containing one tablespoon of detergent to each pint of water.

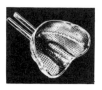
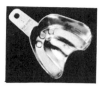

a   b

Figure 30.90
Impression trays: (a) Frigidtrays for use with hydrocolloids, water-cooled; and (b) tray for partials, for use with soluble plasters or other materials.

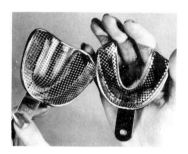

Figure 30.91
Perforated impression trays, upper and lower, for dentulous mouths for use with alginate materials.

Plastic trays, and some special trays made of a very soft, low-fusing metal, cannot be held in a flame. Check with your dentist to see whether the armamentarium includes trays that cannot be flamed.

Articulators are the mechanisms used in the construction of dentures that resemble in various degrees the movement of upper and lower jaws. Many different kinds with varying degrees of complexity are used. One rule applies to all articulators: keep them clean. Dustproof storage is important. One good method is to place each articulator in a clear plastic (polyethylene) bag. The more complex the articulator, the more important it is that it be kept clean and free from dust.

After completion of a denture case, be sure to remove completely all traces of plaster, wax, and other debris. Parts that slide against one another or parts that are hinged should be oiled lightly with a good grade of light oil. When rings or bars are used to mount casts in the articulator, keep them clean by giving them a very light coating of Vaseline prior to use. Check with your dentist on the care you are to give these instruments.

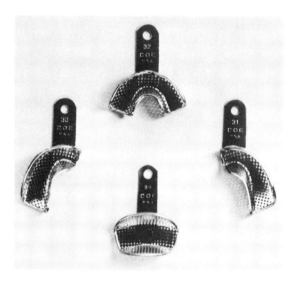

Figure 30.92
Perforated impression trays, partial.

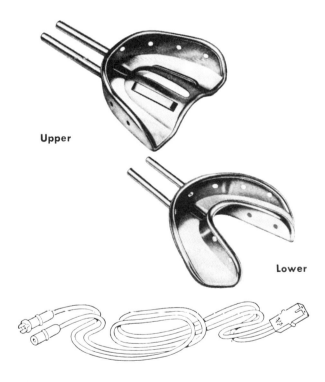

Upper

Lower

Figure 30.93
Water-cooled trays and rubber tubing.

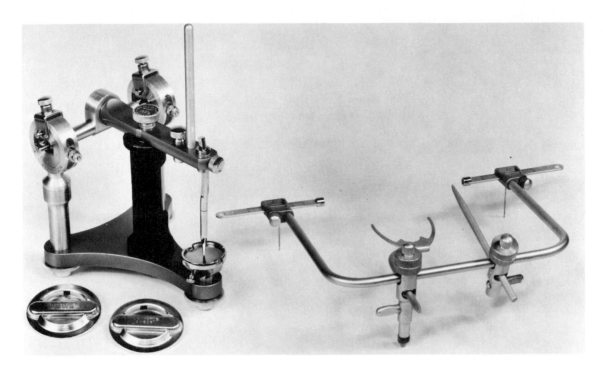

Figure 30.94
Kerr Dentatus articulator and Kerr facebow.

Do not handle any articulator roughly. They should be handled much as you would your most expensive china at home.

The purpose of using a **facebow** is to discover the proper relationship of the patient's upper jaw to the patient's center of rotation of the temporomandibular joints and to transfer this relationship to the articulator. The articulator, a mechanical means of duplicating the movements of the mandible in relation to the maxilla, will then more closely duplicate the actual relationship of the jaws as they exist in the patient. The success of the entire process, of course, rests upon how accurately the original location of centers of rotation is made and how accurately the transfer is made.

A facebow consists of a *U*-shaped rod or bar. At the ends of the *U* are adjustable rods or pointers that slide at right angles from the bar and may be locked at various degrees of extension.

Along that part of the facebow which lies between the two straight end sections are one, two, or three clamps constructed to hold other rods when tightened. One clamp is used to hold a rod that has on its end a forklike smaller *U* about the size of an average dental arch, called a bite fork. A second clamp, if present, may be used to hold a pointer to control the vertical positioning of the facebow by always being placed in contact with a specific landmark on the face, such as the

infraorbital notch or rim. A third clamp, when present, is used as an aid in holding the facebow in proper relationship to the articulator when the actual transfer of the record is to be accomplished.

The dentist first establishes the center of rotation of the temporomandibular joints of a patient by one of two methods.

1. A type of hinge axis locator is used. It has a rod that is placed in the external auditory meatus (the external opening of the ear). The rod has a short arm to which a clamp is attached to hold a pencil in such a position that, as the rod is rotated in a short arc, the pencil inscribes an arc thirteen millimeters in front of the external auditory meatus. With a ruler, another line is then drawn from the upper border of the external auditory meatus to the outer canthus of the eye, intersecting the arc previously drawn. This point of intersection is considered an approximate indication of the center of rotation of the temporomandibular joint. This is marked on both sides of the face.

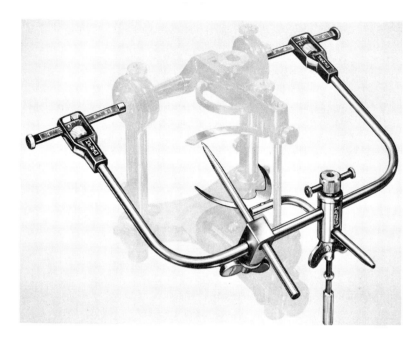

Figure 30.95
The facebow with bite fork and pointer, on a Hanau articulator.

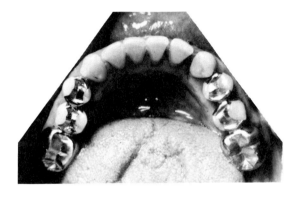

Figure 30.96
Clinical pictures of cast-gold restorations.

2. The dentist may use another device, called a **kinematic facebow,** to more exactly locate the centers of rotation of the temporomandibular joints. This device consists of a mechanism called a clutch that is attached to the lower arch of the dental patient. From this mechanism a pointer arrangement is extended to the area in front of the external auditory meatus. The pointer has some means by which its position in the vicinity of the ear may be adjusted. The dentist will teach the patient how to open and close his or her

jaws with a steady, rhythmic, short arc. As the motion proceeds, the dentist adjusts the pointer until it points to only one spot throughout the movement. This spot will be the exact center of rotation of the temporomandibular joint.

The bite fork is now either embedded in the upper trial denture (if full dentures are being constructed) or covered with a layer of hard pink wax into which the patient makes indentations of his or her natural teeth (if the natural dentition is to be balanced). This is thoroughly chilled in cold water and is reinserted in the patient's mouth. The transfer bow is now slipped onto the bar of the bite fork—loosely, to allow for positioning the sliding rods or pointers at the ends of the *U* over the marks indicating the center of rotation of each temporomandibular joint. The distance each sliding rod or pointer is extended from the *U* bar must be as nearly as possible equal on both sides of the facebow. The *U* bar is then locked tightly to the rod of the bite fork. The second clamp, if present, is tightened when the pointer has been placed on the selected landmark. The entire assembly is removed from the face of the patient. It is now ready for attachment to the articulator and the mounting of the casts.

There may be various other details involved, depending upon the procedure used in a particular dental office, as well as the type of equipment used. These variations may include **jaw registrations,** which may be made in several ways, and perhaps at different stages in the procedures for occlusal equilibration (balancing a natural dentition) or for full-denture construction. A jaw registration is a record of the way the teeth of the upper and lower jaws fit together, necessary in occlusal equilibration and denture construction. It is important to verify the occlusion as work progresses, and the jaw registration permits the dentist to make this verification. Make notes of the particular requirements of your office until you have thoroughly learned the procedures and are able to have the proper materials and equipment ready for use at the proper time.

Summary

If, as you read through this summary, you find that there are comments that do not seem clear, perhaps it will be helpful to review that section of the chapter before you try to answer the questions in the Workbook or go on to the next chapter.

Dental instruments vary in size and shape. Minute differences are important. Learn to recognize the fine points and their uses so that you are a help to your dentist—so that you can anticipate needs and have the correct instrument ready.

Instruments are expensive and delicate. Handle with care. Keep them sterilized or clean, depending on their use. Keep them as you would like to have them kept for use in your own mouth.

A basic setup is a mirror, an explorer, and cotton pliers.

Handpieces are conventional, high-speed, and ultraspeed. Learn to care for them according to the instructions given for each type.

Dental burs are classified for the type of handpiece in which they are used and also by their shape. Learn to recognize them by both classifications.

Diamond instruments cut harder structures more quickly than burs do and are used to open a tooth or do major shaping as for a full-crown preparation.

Prophylaxis handpieces, cups, and brushes are used for cleaning teeth.

Mandrels are metal shanks that fit into a handpiece and on which a disc or unmounted stone can be mounted.

Stones, either mounted or unmounted, do grinding and finishing operations.

The stones used for sharpening instruments are different from the mounted stones put on the handpiece to grind and finish dental prostheses. Learn to care for the sharpening stones used in your office.

Hand instruments have a handle, a shank, and a working head. They are fine, minute heads, and the differences are very important and sometimes hard to recognize. Instruments are numbered in a fashion that identifies them for reordering and also gives important information about the instrument—width, length, and angle of the blade.

Amalgam carriers, pluggers, condensers, and carvers are used only for amalgam restorations.

Cutting instruments are those which are used to cut either soft or hard tissue in the mouth. Some are designed for the right or left side of a preparation. There are chisels, hatchets, enamel hatchets, hoes, gingival margin trimmers, and trimming knives. Spoon excavators are used to scoop out decay; scalers are used for prophylaxis and in periodontics.

Matrix tools are used to make a band fit around a prepared tooth when a temporary wall is needed until the amalgam is packed and carved in the shape of the original tooth.

Special instruments are needed for gold-foil work; pluggers, files, annealing instruments, pellet placers, burnishers, and holding instruments.

Plastic filling instruments are used to shape and trim plastic material before it is set.

Contouring pliers are used to shape temporary covers and crowns.

A pulp tester is used to determine the vitality of a tooth.

Rubber dam is used when the field of operation needs to be kept dry.

Anesthetic syringes need special care, for they must be sterile when used for a patient.

Surgical instruments include several types of forceps as well as other instruments used exclusively for surgery, including elevators.

When surgery has been performed, a prosthesis is usually required, and impression trays are necessary to take an impression in order that the prosthetic device may be prepared.

Finally, articulators and facebows are useful in creating prosthetic devices that may be constructed for the patient who has had surgery and requires rehabilitation. It does not matter whether it is one tooth, several teeth, or full dentures.

Learn the care and use of all these instruments.

Study Questions

1. Discuss handpieces and their care.
2. Explain the use of three handpiece accessories.
3. What is a basic setup?
4. Discuss the care of cement slabs and spatulas.
5. Explain instrument numbering.
6. What are amalgam instruments?
7. What are plastic filling instruments?
8. Describe the endodontic armamentarium.
9. Describe the periodontic armamentarium.
10. Name three instruments used for oral surgery.
11. For what is an articulator used? a facebow? a pulp tester?
12. Describe two instruments used for a fixed prosthesis.

Word Elements	
Word Element	**Example**
rupt combining form meaning: break	**rupture** a tearing apart
sacchar combining form meaning: sugar	**saccharide** a simple sugar, carbohydrate
sequ, secu, sue combining form meaning: follow	**sequence** order of performance
sect combining form meaning: cut	**resection** removal of a considerable portion of an organ, such as a tooth
sep prefix meaning: rot	**sepsis** disease condition in which toxins are disseminated from a focus of infection
sens combining form meaning: feel	**sensitive** able to feel, capable of sending or receiving a sensation (or feeling)
son combining form meaning: sound	**sonometer** an instrument for measuring hearing
super, supr combining form meaning: above, beyond, extreme	**superior** above or upper
spect, spic, spis combining form meaning: look	**inspect** to look at critically
sys prefix meaning: with, together	**system** a set or series of parts that unite to function as a whole

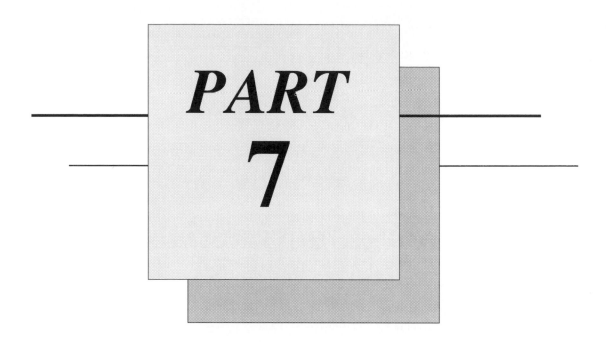

PART
7

Dental Materials and Laboratory Procedures

Now that you have become acquainted with the armamentarium of the dental office, you can profit from understanding the materials that are used in dentistry—and the chairside and laboratory procedures that you will be performing.

The restorative materials of dentistry (used in the mouth), the materials that are used outside the patient's mouth, and the procedures you will use in preparing these materials are discussed in this section. In addition to being familiar with these materials and procedures, you must be capable of working with the materials and skilled in performing the procedures described whether you work with them at the chair or in the dental laboratory.

Procedures associated with certain dental materials are discussed in the proper sequence following basic information concerning that material. However, these procedures, laboratory or chairside, require actual practice under supervision to attain the desired proficiency in their use. It is recommended that your instructor or dentist supervise your work until you have acquired the necessary skills.

CHAPTER 31

Restorative Materials

Biomaterials
Ten Tenets for Restorative Materials
Dental Cements
    Zinc Oxide-Eugenol Cements
        The Ten Tenets Applied to Zinc Oxide-Eugenol
            Cements
        Composition and Purpose of Ingredients
        Care of Equipment
        Mixing the Cement
    Zinc Phosphate Cement
        The Ten Tenets Applied to Zinc Phosphate
            Cement
        Composition and Purpose of Ingredients
        A Word of Caution
        Directions for Mixing the Cement
    Glass Ionomer
    Zinc Silicophosphate Cement
    Zinc Polyacrylate (Zinc Polycarboxylate) Cement
Esthetic Restorative Materials
Dental Amalgam
    Manipulation
    Excess Amalgam
Gold and Gold Alloys
    Welded Gold Restorations
        Annealing Gold
        Protecting Gold
        Purpose of Annealing
        Piece-by-Piece Annealing
        Bulk Annealing
        Noncohesive Gold Foil
Casting Alloys

Biomaterials

One of the most fascinating studies with which the dental profession concerns itself involves the study of the many materials used in the performance of dentistry. No one area in dentistry interrelates with so many disciplines as do **biomaterials.** (*Bio* is from the Greek *bios* meaning "life." *Bio-* means "the relationship to or connection with life.") As the name suggests, these materials are directly associated with living tissues. They are usually used in the mouth and may be temporarily or permanently placed in contact with the teeth and/or surrounding oral tissues.

The environment of the oral cavity is considered restrictive for the following reasons:

1. The oral cavity is constantly moist.
2. The oral cavity is subjected to extreme changes of temperature (hot coffee and ice water).
3. The oral cavity is subjected to pH changes (acid-alkaline foods and beverages).
4. The restorative materials may be placed under the stress and abrasion of masticatory (chewing) forces.

The materials placed in the oral cavity must be unusually adaptable to survive in such an environment.

Consider that an important facet of dental care is the repair and restoration of oral structures damaged or destroyed by injury or disease. Therefore, dental researchers are constantly challenged in their efforts to find the ideal restorative material. Unfortunately, the ideal restorative material has not been developed, and new products seem to appear more rapidly than researchers can properly evaluate. The practicing dentist finds it difficult to evaluate materials before incorporating them into his or her armamentarium because the dentist lacks both time and the laboratory facilities for formal testing procedures.

The American Dental Association recognizes this problem and, in cooperation with the National Bureau of Standards, has established standards or requirements for materials that are to be certified for dentistry. Manufacturers must meet these standards if their products are to be listed by the American Dental Association as certified dental materials. The practicing dentist should restrict selection of materials to the certified list.

As is true of most dental procedures discussed in this book, the discussion of dental materials will be limited to that which is fundamentally necessary for you to know and understand as a beginning dental assistant. If your curiosity is aroused by any individual material or by any particular phase of dentistry, further information is available in many forms to enlarge your knowledge and increase your value as a dental assistant. A text providing a more thorough background in dental materials will be found in the bibliography at the end of this chapter.

The non-dentally-oriented person is usually amazed at the restrictions the oral environment places on materials used to treat or correct oral deficiencies. Anything attached to, or in constant contact with, the oral tissues is subjected to a variety of physical and chemical changes, which require properties of extremely fine dimension. These materials must also be biologically compatible with the oral tissue.

Ten Tenets for Restorative Materials

Ten tenets have been established for a filling material. Any currently available restorative material must be measured against these tenets:

1. **Aesthetics.** To most patients aesthetics is more important than biological or functional considerations, especially in anterior restorations. Aesthetics, therefore, must be a prime requisite of a filling material. To be aesthetically acceptable a material must not only match the variable colors within the crown of a single tooth from incisal to gingival, but it must also match the tooth's translucencies, opacities, and fluorescence. Furthermore, aesthetic appearance should not be lost as the restoration ages.
2. **Toxicity.** The most important biological consideration is toxicity. The material cannot be toxic to the adjacent gingival tissues or the pulp as it sets, polymerizes in the cavity, or after it is set. (Polymerization is the chemical reaction in which smaller molecules combine into larger molecules.) Many manufacturers recommend a cavity liner, or furnish their own, to paint the inside of the cavity and thereby provide the necessary protection.
3. **Solubility.** A material that is soluble in saliva can only be considered temporary in nature. Such a material obviously cannot hold interproximal contact or maintain marginal integrity or contour.
4. **Adaptation.** "Adaptation" and "adhesion" are terms sometimes wrongly, but loosely, used interchangeably. Adhesion is molecular binding; adaptation means modification to fit the conditions of the environment. An adaptable material in

Table 31.1
The Ten Tenets for Restorative Materials Applied to Each Material

Tenet	Zinc Oxide-Eugenol	Zinc Phosphate	Glass Ionomer	Zinc Silicophosphate
Aesthetics	Does not detract; may enhance	Yes	Yes	Yes
Toxicity	No	Needs liner or base for protection	Only in deep area of cavity	Needs liner or base for protection
Solubility	Slightly soluble	Slightly soluble	Soluble	Slightly soluble
Adaptation	For short period: Good	Good	Adhesive	Good
Coefficient of Thermal Expansion	Not of practical importance	As a cementing media: Good	Good	Good
Strength	ZOE alone: Poor Reinforced: Fair	Adequate as a cementing media	Inadequate for masticating surfaces	Inadequate for masticating surfaces
Anti-cariogenicity	No	No	Yes	Slightly
Repairability	Not a consideration	Not a consideration	Guarded	Not a consideration
Manipulability	Good	Good	Good but exacting	Good
Radiopaque	Yes	Yes	No	No

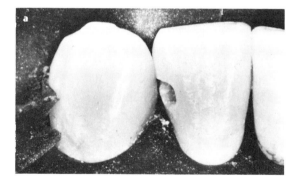

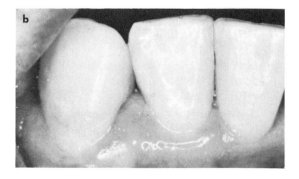

Figure 31.1
(a) Pre- and (b) postoperative anterior restoration.

dentistry, then, is one that will adapt itself to the shape of the preparation in which it has been placed.

There is no material in dentistry today that will indefinitely adhere to vital tooth structure to insure marginal seal, although it would be desirable to have such a material.

Adhesion (the ability to chemically bond to tooth structure) and the maintenance of dimensional stability and contact with the tooth are important for the life of the restoration. The material must not only closely adapt to the enamel and dentinal walls of the cavity, but it must maintain this close contact or seal in a wet environment when subjected to wide temperature variables. A filling that does not accurately fit the cavity will fail quickly because caries can recur at the leaking margins.

5. **The coefficient of thermal expansion** (an expression of the rate of expansion and contraction of a material as related to temperature change.) All things behave differently when subjected to temperature variations. In dentistry the coefficient of thermal expansion is extremely important

Zinc Polyacrylate	Composite Restorative Resins	Amalgam	Cast Gold	Welded Gold
Yes	Yes	No	No	No
No	Needs liner or base for protection	No	Per se: No Cementing media: maybe	No
Slightly soluble	Negligible	Insoluble	Insoluble	Insoluble
Excellent	Good	Good	Fair	Good
As a cementing media: Good	Fair	Fair	Fair	Fair
Adequate as a cementing media	Inadequate for masticating surfaces	Good	Good	Good
No	No	No	No	No
Not a consideration	Yes	Yes	No	Yes
Fair	Good	Good	Fair	Fair
Yes	Some are	Yes	Yes	Yes

when selecting materials for restorations. The material used should closely match the expansion and contraction properties of tooth structure. The patient may drink hot coffee or ice water. As these liquids pass over the tooth, the crown of the tooth and the filling material will expand and contract according to their own characteristics. If the filling material confined in the enamel of the crown or surrounding the tooth has a coefficient of thermal expansion much greater than the enamel, it will expand and contract much more than the enamel when exposed to these temperature extremes. The filling would then be smaller than the cavity prepared for it when the temperature decreases and larger when the temperature increases.

When the filling is smaller than the cavity (because ice water has passed over it), oral fluids, bacteria, and food debris can flow between the filling and the tooth. Discoloration by the debris can occur at this time, and caries-producing bacteria can enter all parts of the cavity. When the patient's mouth is heated by drinking coffee, the filling then expands and the fluids are forced out. However, some

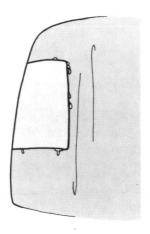

Figure 31.2
Percolation.

residual bacteria and food debris *remain in the spaces between the tooth and filling.* The bubbling of fluids forced out at the margins of fillings subjected to temperature cyclings is called **percolation.**

Now it is understandable that the coefficient of thermal expansion of the filling material should be similar to that of the tooth enamel because an extreme variation would eliminate from consideration an otherwise acceptable filling material.

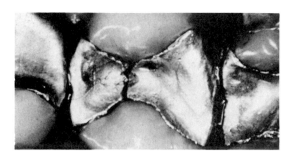

Figure 31.3
Fractured amalgam.

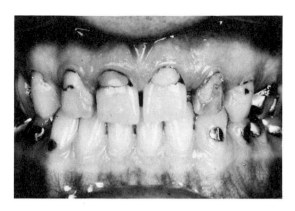

Figure 31.4
Recurrent caries on margins.

6. **Strength.** The strength of a material, whether demonstrated by shear, tensile, or crushing tests, has not been adequately related to masticatory demands. However, a filling material used in areas subjected to stress must be able to withstand incisive or occlusal impact without flow and distortion. It should be as strong as enamel and match its ability to withstand the constant abrasive forces of wear.

7. **Anticariogenic activity.** (*Anti* means "opposite or against." *Cario* refers to caries or decay. *Genic* means "production thereof." Thus, a layman's definition of *anticariogenic* is "opposing the production of caries.") Anticariogenic activity of the material would be a desirable characteristic because it would help to eliminate a recurrence and further invasion of caries at the margins of the restoration.

   Although a material may release an anticariogenic substance such as fluoride when initially placed in contact with the tooth, to remain active it must continually release its anticariogenic substance. Once the material has set or solidified, there can be no release of an anticariogenic component without a breakdown or dissolution of the material. To do so means that the substance must go into solution in saliva. Any material that will continue to go into solution is soluble—and solubility leads to deterioration of the restoration. Thus, a material that has continual anticariogenic activity is also a material that does not make a permanent, strong, satisfactory restoration.

8. **Repairability.** Ideally, a material should be repairable. If a defect occurs in a restoration, it should be possible to repair the defect without removing the entire restoration. It would be advantageous for a filling material to chemically bond to the previously polymerized restoration.

9. **Ease of manipulation.** A dentist wants a restorative material that can be manipulated easily. An acceptable material.

   a. Can be easily prepared and placed in the cavity.

   b. Can be adapted to a cavity.

   c. Can be properly contoured.

   d. Will set in a clinically acceptable time.

   e. Can be polished satisfactorily.

   If a material fails to meet these five qualifications, it will not be as readily accepted by the dentists as one that does meet the qualifications and is of comparable quality.

10. **Radiopacity.** (Not transparent to X ray.) **Radiopaque** materials look white on the X-ray film because X rays do not go through the materials. **Radiolucent** materials look dark because the X rays pass through them. If a restoration is radiopaque, the limitations of the restoration are denoted by radiopacity. Although this quality is not vitally important, it is helpful because radiolucent recurrent caries can then be differentiated from the filling which is opaque on the X ray.

Table 31.1 is a summarization of the application of these tenets to filling materials discussed in this chapter.

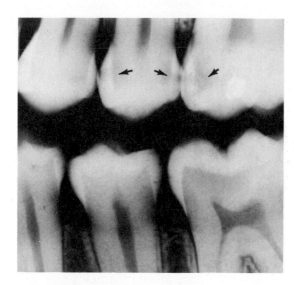

Figure 31.5
Radiopacities and radiotranslucencies.

Dental Cements

Cements are used for a variety of purposes in dentistry: (1) to retain restorations such as inlays and crowns, (2) to seal root canal fillings, (3) as surgical dressings, (4) as impression pastes, (5) as temporary and sedative filling materials, or (6) as protective bases under metallic filling materials.

Cements may be classified as follows:

    zinc oxide-eugenol;
    zinc phosphate;
    silicate;
    zinc silicaphosphate;
    zinc polyacrylate (zinc polycarboxylate);
    glass ionomer.

In addition to these categories, Phillips lists calcium hydroxide cements for pulp capping.[1] Although there are resin restorative materials, they are different from the cementing resin.

Zinc Oxide-Eugenol Cements

If a cavity is very close to the vital dental pulp, but does not actually expose it, a sedative or analgesic substance is placed on the dentin wall immediately over the near-exposure before placing the cement base. For decades the material of choice for this subbase has been zinc oxide-eugenol usually containing calcium hydroxite.

Many cements have been introduced under trade names for pulp capping, pulp protection, and root canal sealers, periodontal packs, and prosthetic impression materials. All of these cements are essentially zinc oxide and eugenol, but they contain other ingredients that enhance their physical properties. They may also serve as a luting (cementing) medium for cast-gold restorations as well as firm protective bases. Although such cements are known as polymer-ZOE or **EBA** (ethoxybenzoic acid cements), they are still considered zinc oxide-eugenol.

The Ten Tenets Applied to Zinc Oxide-Eugenol Cements

Although these cements are not exposed to view as a permanent material is, zinc oxide-eugenols do not detract from the aesthetics of a restoration and, when underlying thin sections of enamel and dentin, may actually enhance the aesthetics by masking undesirable effects of metallic restorations. Tissue adjacent to any material attached to the body and foreign to it must have an other-than-normal reaction. However, zinc oxide-eugenol cements are nonirritating to the point of being sedative. They do not have an exothermic reaction like the zinc phosphate cements and therefore will not irritate the pulp as a result of the setting process in the tooth. The oil base of these cements makes them less soluble in the mouth than zinc phosphate. They are still much too soluble and weak to be considered for restorations. Their adaptation is generally good for the short period they are exposed when used as temporary restorations. Their coefficient of thermal expansion and reparability are not of practical importance since solubility and strength negate their use for purposes other than bases, temporary fillings, cementation, surgical packs, and root canal sealers. They are not considered anticariogenic. One of the major assets of these cements is their ease of manipulation. Most of these cements contain a trace of barium sulfate, making them more radiopaque and distinguishable on an X ray.

Composition and Purpose of Ingredients

The labels of the commercial temporary cements usually denote the same basic common ingredients. The powders contain zinc oxide; the liquids contain an essential oil, usually eugenol.

Preparations vary in the types and amounts of additives incorporated in the powder or liquids to enhance the physical or antibacterial properties:

1. *To increase the adhesiveness, plasticity, and smoothness:* rosin, zinc stearate, and olive oil or Canada balsam
2. *To improve strength:* zinc acetate
3. *To increase the antibacterial effectiveness:* phenol, thymol, thymol iodide, and iodoform

Zinc oxide and eugenol or any of the commercially prepared zinc oxide-eugenol-rosin cements may be used as an analgesic subbase in unusually deep cavities. Other uses include bases under metal restorations, sedative treatments, capping exposed pulps, and temporarily cementing some form of protection over teeth prepared for crown or bridge placement.

Care of Equipment

A zinc oxide-eugenol-rosin cement should be mixed on a paper mixing pad. If a glass slab is used, it should be wiped clean immediately after mixing and washed with a rosin solvent such as xylol or chloroform. Washing with water will not remove the sticky rosin cement. Instruments used with zinc oxide-eugenol preparations must be wiped as soon as possible with a disposable tissue, then with a gauze moistened with chloroform. Wash with soap and water, rinse, and dry.

Mixing the Cement

The cement is supplied in two bottles, one containing powder and the other containing liquid. The consistency of the mix depends on the use for which it is intended. The liquid absorbs a considerable amount of powder; therefore, no more than two drops should be necessary for a subbase. The cement can be mixed rapidly. It is to be as thick as possible for ease of handling.

Place two drops of solution near one end of the mixing tablet.

Place an amount of powder about five times the volume of liquid toward the other end.

First mix about half the powder with the liquid, spatulating rapidly and well into a smooth mix. Then add smaller portions, mixing thoroughly, until the mix is heavy.

Remove excess oil by blotting the mass on absorbent paper or cloth, leaving a soft, puttylike cement that is easily positioned and shaped in the cavity (fig. 31.6).

Ample time can be used for mixing and handling since the material will not harden rapidly. It can therefore be prepared somewhat in advance of use, if desired.

The amount of cement needed should be closely approximated before being carried to the cavity. Too often the placing of the cement base becomes messy because too much cement is placed in the cavity, requiring tedious and delicate removal of the excess. Water acts as a catalyst for zinc oxide-eugenol cements; therefore, a pellet of wet cotton may be used to manipulate the cement in a cavity as well as to remove the excess cement.

Although individual preferences vary, cements mixed for retention of restorations in the cavity should be mixed to a toothpaste consistency in order to permit

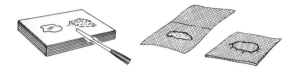

Figure 31.6
Mixing zinc oxide-eugenol cement.

the proper seating of the restoration. Too thick a mix will prevent the restoration from reaching its prescribed position in the cavity and may neccessitate redoing the entire operation.

Zinc Phosphate Cement

Zinc phosphate cement, a material at one time used for restorations, is now used only for thermally protective bases under metallic fillings and as a cement to retain cast restorations such as inlays, crowns, and bridges. This cement contains unreacted phosphoric acid, which is irritating. However, the unreacted free acid is used up within a short time and, consequently, is not a lasting irritant. Cavities receiving zinc phosphate cement bases, or restorations retained with zinc phosphate cement, should be painted with a protective liner to prevent chemical irritation to the dental pulp.

The Ten Tenets Applied to Zinc Phosphate Cement

Zinc phosphate cement is not used as a permanent restorative material per se. It is provided in many shades to offer an *aesthetic* background for cementation of fused porcelain restorations. Its *toxicity* is initially harsh, and a protective liner of cavity varnish or thin paste of zinc oxide-eugenol or calcium hydroxide is necessary for pulp protection. Although it *adapts* well to tooth structure, it has no *adhesion* when set. It is quite *soluble,* has a *coefficient of thermal expansion* within practical limits of tooth structure, is not considered *anticariogenic,* and has *strength* values commensurate with its uses. Although it is quite easy to *manipulate, reparability* is not a consideration with its clinical application. It is *radiopaque* to a degree and can be identified on X ray.

Composition and Purpose of Ingredients

Zinc phosphate cements are supplied as a powder and liquid. The powder is composed primarily of zinc oxide, with some magnesium oxide and traces of other metallic salts composing about 10 percent of the total. The liquid is composed of phosphoric acid and water, buffered with salts of aluminum and zinc. These cements are all balanced by the manufacturer to provide the proper physical properties. *Bottles should be stoppered at all times when not in use to prevent the addition of water to the liquid on humid days or the*

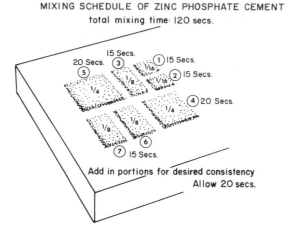

MIXING SCHEDULE OF ZINC PHOSPHATE CEMENT
total mixing time: 120 secs.

Add in portions for desired consistency
Allow 20 secs.

Figure 31.7
Zinc phosphate cement ready to mix.

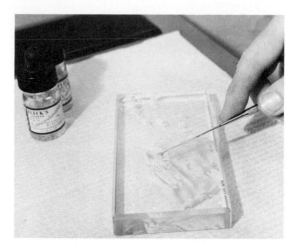

Figure 31.8
Mixed zinc phosphate cement.

evaporation of water on dry days. The balance of acid and water in the liquid must be maintained as manufactured; otherwise the setting time and other properties of the cement will be severely affected. Cloudy-looking liquid indicates that the acid-water ratio is no longer in balance; therefore, dispose of the liquid.

When mixed, the cement sets as a hard, crystalline structure composed of a core of unreacted particles of powder in a matrix of zinc phosphate compounds. The consistency and setting time of the mix can be altered by varying the manner in which the cement is spatulated and varying the amount of powder incorporated into the mix. The necessary consistency and setting time will be determined by the purpose for which the mix is being prepared.

A Word of Caution
The reaction of the powder with the liquid generates heat and is called an **exothermic reaction.** If the cement is mixed too fast or on a warm slab and is placed in the tooth, the heat produced by this reaction could be enough to burn the dental pulp and cause the tooth to abscess. Consequently, the cement slab is always cooled in running water before it is used. It should not be cooled below the dew point, however, which is the point at which moisture from the air condenses on the glass. Should this happen, the cement will have excess water in it and will set much too fast for use. If the cement liquid is placed on the slab long before it is to be mixed, water may evaporate from it, and the subsequent mix will set too slowly for practical use. Therefore, the cement should be spatulated on a cool slab, with small increments of powder added to the liquid at five- to ten-second intervals and the mixture thoroughly spatulated between additions. Total mixing time should be between one and one-half and two minutes. The amount of cement to be mixed as well as its consistency is directed by the use intended.

Directions for Mixing the Cement
Cool and dry the glass mixing slab.

When your dentist indicates it is time to begin, place the required number of liquid drops on the slab. *Stopper the bottle.*

In another place on the slab place the necessary amount of powder. *Stopper the bottle.*

Form the powder into a thin, flat, rectangular shape with the spatula.

Divide the rectangle into halves, then into quarters, then into eighths.

Divide four of the eighths again to make sixteenths.

Place your watch, with a sweep-second hand, near the slab where you can see it easily.

Draw the first sixteenth into the liquid and spatulate with the flat of the blade for thirty seconds.

Add the remaining sixteenths in turn and spatulate each for ten seconds.

Now add the eighth portions, spatulating each for ten seconds, except the last portion, which is spatulated for fifteen seconds.

There should be no unmixed particles of powder or liquid remaining around the edges when each portion is considered to be thoroughly incorporated into the mix.

Setting time may be delayed by first thoroughly spatulating a very small quantity of powder, about the size of a pinhead, into the liquid and permitting this to stand for two or three minutes before proceeding with further additions of powder. Rapid spatulation will hasten the setting time. If a heavy mix is desired, merely add more powder.

An excess amount of liquid is always provided in the bottle. The excess liquid should be discarded when the powder has been used, and a new bottle of each should be opened when the next mix is required.

Powder that has been removed from the original bottle and placed on the slab but not used in the mix should *not* be returned to the original powder bottle.

Glass Ionomer Cement

Glass Ionomer cement is supplied as a powder and liquid or as a prepackaged capsule for mechanical mixing in the amalgamator. The liquid is mainly polyacrylic acid and water with some modifiers to reduce viscosity and enhance setting characteristics. The powder is basically an acid soluble glass prepared with fluoride fluxes.

Glass Ionomer cements are used for cementation as bases and as cervical filling materials. Because the cement is potentially adhesive to tooth structure it lends itself for bonding without cavity preparation. The mixing working time is very limited: 45 seconds mixing; total working time about 2 minutes. The adhesive properties are lost as soon as the mix loses its gloss. (A dull surface indicates that there is insufficient free liquid remaining for interaction with the calcium in the tooth. This interaction is the mechanism of adhesion.) In this respect the glass ionomer is similar to zinc carboxylate cement. The anticariogenic property of glass ionomer is through the powder. The cement has low solubility in acid, lower than zinc phosphate and zinc polyacrylate cement. However, it is very sensitive both to moisture and a drying environment. It needs immediate protection with the varnish which is supplied with the material. Another method of protecting the cement from disintegrating is to place a layer of composite resin on the surface. This is the so-called sandwich technique.

Zinc Silicophosphate Cement

This cement is a combination of zinc phosphate and silicate cement powders. The liquid is still orthophosphoric acid and water buffered to control the physical properties during mixing and setting. This cement is sometimes used to retain restorations and as a temporary filling material.

Zinc Polyacrylate (Zinc Polycarboxylate) Cement

The powder of this cement is principally zinc oxide and magnesium oxide. The liquid is polyacrylic acid and water. When mixed together, the set cement takes the form of zinc oxide particles in a matrix of zinc polyacrylate gel. The liquid and powder should be mixed within thirty seconds on a cool and nonabsorptive surface incorporating all of the powder into the liquid at once.

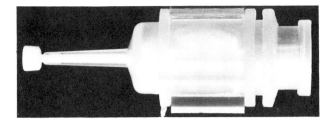

Figure 31.9
Glass Ionomer preportioned capsule.

Esthetic Restorative Materials

Tooth colored materials that can be placed directly into the tooth as a restoration have been in use since the 1800s when silicates were introduced. Powder was an acid soluble glass made with fluoride as a flux, and the liquid was phosphoric acid and water with some buffering agents. Solubility of the set material caused disintegration of the restoration, but the benefit was the release of fluoride in the process. Fluoride acts as an anti-cariogenic agent.

The search for materials with better properties continued; and in the 1940s, the plastics came into use as restorative materials. Some of the shortcomings of these materials are: shrinkage during setting and the contraction and expansion with temperature changes in the oral cavity. These difficulties have been largely overcome with modification of the composition. A stronger plastic matrix was developed and fillers added. These materials are provided as a) a powder and liquid, b) a two paste system, or c) a one paste system. The latter can be initiated to set through exposure to a light source. Depending on the mechanism by which the set of the material is initiated, they are classified as a) chemically curing, and b) a light curing. The light cured composites are the newest and most popular. The light is most often regular visible light, but may be ultra violet light that is focused on the surface of the material after placement in the cavity.

Materials are also classified on the basis of composition. The newest group in use are the BIS-GMA composite resins. By definition a composite is a combination of two distinctly different materials to produce a new product that is different from the original components. As a rule the strength is improved and the dimensional change is minimized resulting in less setting shrinkage and less expansion and contraction with temperature changes. The set material is a resin matrix reinforced with inorganic particles, e.g., glass rods, diamond chips, etc. If barium or strontium glasses are used, the material is radiopaque. The filler particles are surface treated with a coupling agent which provides an improved bond between the matrix and the filler.

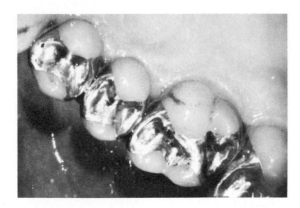

Figure 31.10
Amalgam restoration in patient's teeth.

The size of the filler particles serve as another means of classification: a) conventional composites (also called macrofilled composites) have particles up to 50 microns in size; b) microfilled composites have fillers below the visible light range about 0.04 microns; and c) hybrid composites have a mix of large and small particles.

The resulting properties are related to the size and amount of the filler in the composite. The strength is improved with larger sized particles while the smoothness of the surface is improved with smaller sized particles. When the larger filler particles are exposed, they roll out of the restoration resulting in a rough surface which permits discoloration through food deposits. Microfilled composites polish more easily. However their strength is reduced because less filler can be incorporated into the material since the surface to be wetted by the matrix is larger.

Light cured composites are dispensed from a syringe. This packaging prevents accidental light exposure and is a convenient way of expressing the desired amount of material. One or two turns of the syringe is normally sufficient quantity for a restoration.

The advantage of the single paste system is the elimination of the need to mix it as is necessary with the two paste system. The chance of incorporating air in the mix is avoided, and working time is totally under the operator's control. Once the correct anatomy is established through the shaping of the viscous paste, the tip of the light is directed within 2 millimeters of the surface. When the automatic timer switches off (after 20 seconds), the material is hardened. If the thickness of the material in the cavity is greater than 2 millimeters, it is recommended to cure in layers of about 2 millimeters. When the first layer has been cured, add material and cure again. It can even be cured through enamel.

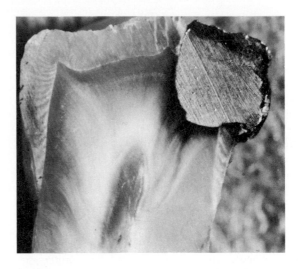

Figure 31.11
Staining from amalgam.

The adaptation of the composite materials to the enamel margins is greatly improved if the enamel is etched, washed, and gently dried before placing the composite. The etchant is an irritating acid whether it is liquid or gel; therefore, the dentin must be protected from it.

There are also dentin adhesion products available but they are still in the early stages of acceptance by the profession.

Dental Amalgam

"Silver filling" is a common term used for amalgam restorations. The material was introduced in France as a "silver paste" in the early 1800s. However, it does not consist of silver alone. In order to produce a "paste," the metal alloy powder has to be mixed with mercury, a metal which is liquid at room temperature. Actually, an "amalgam" is any metal combined with mercury. The composition of the dental alloy powder was the first material used in dentistry to receive a specification by the American Dental Association.

Specification #1 was established in 1919 and requires that the composition of the *alloy* for dental use must be within the following limits.

Silver	65% minimum
Tin	29% maximum
Copper	6% maximum
Zinc	2% maximum
Mercury	3% maximum

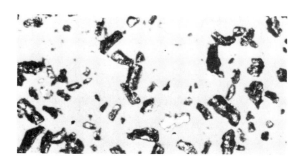

Figure 31.12
Alloy filings.

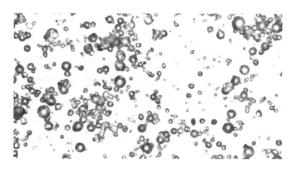

Figure 31.13
Spherical particles.

In 1970 the specification was modified to accept an *alloy powder* which contained a higher copper content. Higher copper content produces a stronger restoration. The new specification is as follows:

Silver	40–60%
Tin	25–29%
Copper	13–30%
Zinc	0– 2%
Mercury	0– 3% permitted

This new alloy is called *high copper alloy* to distinguish it from the original alloy that is referred to as *low copper alloy.* Manufacturers who provide dental amalgam can design their alloy as they choose, provided it remains within the limits of the specifications.

There are two types of high copper alloy in use. One is called *admixed, blended,* or *dispersion* strengthened amalgam. The other is called *unicomposition.* The difference is in the process by which the high copper content is achieved. The admixed type is a mixture of low copper alloy powder with a high copper-utectic powder. The unicompositon refers to the fact that every particle of the alloy powder has the same copper content. The manufacturer determines the composition, shape and size of the alloy powder particles.

After formulating the percent amounts for the alloy, the metals are melted together and either cast into bars called ingots or blown into a chamber of inert gas and atomized into tiny droplets that freeze into minute spheres. Ingots are placed on a lathe, and cut into small filings that are sifted to obtain controlled size. These are referred to as lathe-cut particles. The atomized particles produce an alloy called spherical alloy. The size of these particles is also standardized by sifting through a sized mesh screen. All high copper alloys are spherical because the high copper content makes the alloy too hard for lathe cutting.

During the casting of the ingot and cutting of the filings, changes occur in the alloy. The alloy does not react consistently. It changes as it ages unless it is **annealed.** Annealing is a process that quickens the aging of the alloy, producing material of predictable physical properties. A carefully controlled annealing process stablilizes the alloy so that it does not change when stored. Annealing also makes it possible to have sufficient time to condense the amalgam in the cavity preparation and carve it.

Each of the metals in the alloy has a specific function to perform in the final restoration.

Silver (Ag) is the main constituent of the alloy, and contributes the properties of high expansion, strength, rapid setting, low flow and silver color.

Tin (Sn) is added to counterbalance the silver in the alloy. Tin reduces expansion, slows the setting reaction, and permits more rapid amalgamation and smoother carving.

Copper (Cu) enhances the properties of silver. It improves strength and hardness and decreases flow.

Zinc (Zn) maintains a clean alloy during manufacture. Zinc is known as a scavenger of oxides and is used in many industrial alloys to eliminate oxides that contaminate the metals during the manufacturing process. Newer processes, however, permit the manufacture of dental amalgam alloy with minimal amounts of zinc, since it can be detrimental to the final restoration. Some alloys are, therefore, called zinc-free, but that actually means they contain no more than 0.01% zinc in the alloy.

Zinc is known to react with moisture which can result in delayed expansion of the restoration. Also, the pressure of this expansion on the pulp can cause severe pain.

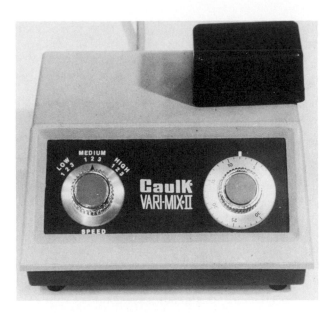

Figure 31.14
Mechanical amalgamator.

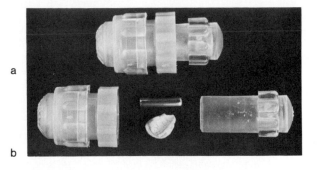

Figure 31.15
(a) Disposable capsule with preportioned alloy and mercury; (b) amalgam, mixed in disposable capsule.

Less mercury results in a stronger restoration. The dentist and the assistant should control the composition of the final amalgam restoration through the process of manipulation.

Manipulation

The first step in the manipulation process is the *proportioning* of alloy and mercury. The preproportioned capsules are the preferred way to minimize human variables. The alloy and mercury are provided in a capsule, either proportioned and kept apart with a membrane until the mixing time, or in a reusable capsule into which the operator places the alloy and mercury (fig. 31.15). The next step is the *trituration* of the powder and liquid. Trituration is the process of vigorous mixing by hand using a mortar (a glass cup with a smooth, rounded bottom) and a pestle (a glass mixing rod, rounded to fit the curve of the cup). The same principle is used with the amalgamator. This is a mechanical device with an automatic timer. It not only saves time (mixes in seconds compared to minutes), but offers control of mixing through standardization of mixing time and speed.

The capsule is placed into the holding arm of the amalgamator, and the speed and time is set according to the manufacturer's recommendation. However, it is prudent to run an occasional trial mix since even the change in the flow of electricity can alter the expected speed of the amalgamator.

An amalgam can expand or contract, depending on its manipulation. The ADA specification No. 1 requires that an amalgam neither contract nor expand more than 20 microns per centimeter.

Amalgam therefore, must not be touched by the hand or come in contact with saliva during manipulation by the dentist or the assistant. It should be placed in the cavity preparation under proper isolation of the operating field to avoid contamination.
Mercury (Hg) in a small amount—up to 3%—is permitted to facilitate amalgamation.

The alloys may be obtained as powders of the lathe cut filings, spheres, or a combination of the two as preweighted pellets, or as disposable capsules with preproportioned alloy powder and mercury kept apart by a membrane until mixing time. If pellets or alloy powder are used, they are mixed with carefully measured mercury of a purity that meets the USP (United States Pharmacopoeia) standards as well as ADA specification #6. This specification requires that there are only minimal amounts of impurities and that the surface is clean.

When pure mercury and an alloy made according to the above specifications are mixed together, chemical and physical reactions occur between the alloy and the mercury. This process is called **amalgamation.** The product formed by this compound is generally referred to as **dental amalgam.** When it is inserted into a prepared cavity in a tooth, it is called an **amalgam restoration.**

The final properties of the restoration are directly related to the amount of mercury in the set amalgam.

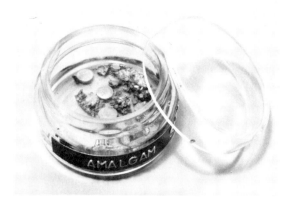

Figure 31.16
Amalgam scrap jar for excess mercury & amalgam scrap.

When mercury comes in contact with the alloy powder, the silver and the tin dissolve in the mercury and two new compounds are formed. They are called the matrix which binds the now smaller particles of the original alloy powder together. These new compounds start to set within minutes with a process called *crystallization.* These crystals grow and touch and push one another apart as they harden. The set amalgam restoration has gone through an initial contraction and then an expansion phase. It is desirable to have a minimum of mercury remaining in the amalgam to avoid too great an expansion.

The excess mercury can be squeezed out with a "squeeze cloth," but the preferred way is to start with the "minimal mercury technique."

It is important that any excess mercury be deposited in a receptacle specifically for mercury. It must not be permitted to fall on the floor where a buildup of mercury contamination in the room would soon constitute a health hazard for everyone.

When the plastic mix of amalgam is placed in the cavity with the amalgam carrier, the condensation process by the operator brings the mercury richer mix to the top. The mix stays plastic for about 3–4 minutes. If more amalgam is needed after that time, a new mix should be prepared. The cavity is always overfilled to allow the mercury rich mix to be "scraped" away. Thus, the stronger mix stays in the restoration.

The amalgam in the restoration, then, is composed of particles of alloy surrounded and bound together by a new alloy formed by the interaction of mercury with the surface particles. The surfaces of filings and spheres need to be coated with mercury in order to react with it, forming the matrix that bonds the filling into one solid mass.

The matrix formed is not as strong as the particles of alloy; therefore, the final restoration should have a minimum amount of matrix to hold the particles together. The more mercury added to the mix, the more

mercury in the final restoration and also more of the newly formed compound of mercury and tin in the set amalgam. This tin-mercury phase, as it is called, is very prone to corrosion and it is weak. The final restoration depends on the amount of the newly formed compounds, the amount of remaining original particles and the density achieved during condensation.

The modern amalgams have no tin-mercury in the final restoration and are therefore stronger and less prone to corrode. The mechanism by which this phase is eliminated is related to the so-called affinity (attraction) of the copper for the tin. In this way tin reacts with copper with preference to mercury and no tin-mercury compound is formed. This is the reason why the modern high copper alloys are sometimes called "tin-free alloys." It is still advisable to use a minimal amount of mercury since the remaining free mercury weakens the final amalgam restoration.

Excess Amalgam

Usually there is some amalgam in excess of the amount necessary for the restoration. It has reclamation value. It should be kept in an amalgam scrap jar (figure 31.16). Scraps recovered from the cuspidor trap are also saved.

Gold and Gold Alloys

Gold may be used in restorative dentistry in several forms. In the pure form it is provided as gold foil, crystalline or mat gold, or as a powder. Small amounts of powder are wrapped in pieces of gold foil for convenient handling. Pure gold is packed in the cavity preparation in a manner similar to amalgam. This restoration in gold may be completely contoured and polished at the same visit because no setting time is required.

Gold alloys are called **casting golds.** They are used to fabricate restorations outside the mouth that are later cemented to the tooth. Gold alloys are produced by combining gold with silver, copper, and small amounts of platinum, palladium, and zinc. By varying the amounts of the metals used in the manufacture of these alloys, casting golds of different hardness and strength for different dental uses are produced.

Welded Gold Restorations

Gold-foil restorations are made from cohesive or noncohesive gold. The pure gold, condensed into cavity preparations, molecularly bonds, forming a solid, **cohesive** restoration. If noncohesive gold is used, it is literally wedged into the cavity.

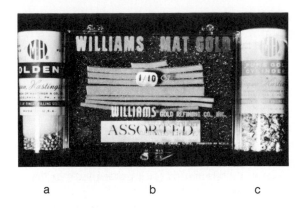

a   b   c

Figure 31.17
(a) Powdered gold; (b) mat gold; and (c) foil.

Decades ago gold foil was commonly used as a restorative material. Now amalgam or cast gold is used in the posterior of the mouth where ability to withstand masticatory stresses is essential. Silicate cement, composites, or fused porcelains are used in the anterior region because aesthetics is the primary concern of the patient. Thus, gold foil has been almost completely replaced; however, some dentists still create beautiful gold-foil restorations. It is therefore important that we understand the process of placing them.

Gold foil is basically in the same physical form as associated with the words aluminum foil, except that gold is capable of being made into the thinnest sheet of metal imaginable, about one-tenth the thickness of an average human hair. This foil is made by hand, "beating" the gold between layers of sheepskin until it has reached the desired thickness.

Gold foil is sold to the dental office as factory-prepared **cylinders** of various sizes, or in **books** of flat gold leaves. Both are sold by weight. In the case of a book, each contains one-tenth of an ounce of gold, and each sheet of foil (which is separated from its neighbor by tissue paper) contains about four grains. Dentists who use gold in this form usually teach the assistant to "roll" gold pellets of the proper sizes from this gold leaf. The most commonly used sizes are 1/64, 1/32, and perhaps 1/16—each fraction indicating what part of a whole leaf each pellet contains. Thus, to make 1/64 pellets, each leaf is first cut in half, each half into quarters, each quarter into eighths, each eighth into sixteenths, each sixteenth into thirty-seconds, and each thirty-second into sixty-fourths—and each sixty-fourth is carefully and loosely rolled into a pellet in such a manner that all edges are turned to the inside of the pellet. If done by an assistant with practice, a "drawer" section full of 1/64 pellets will have pellets that are all nearly identical in size (which is controlled by how tightly the pellet is rolled). These are used as *cohesive gold.*

The leaves of gold foil as purchased in books may also be used to prepare cylinders of **noncohesive** gold. These are generally prepared as one-half and one-fourth cylinders. Experienced operators will use noncohesive gold to build up the larger part of the bulk of a gold-foil restoration, especially in work in the posterior part of the mouth or in large gingival restorations, then complete the restoration with cohesive gold.

Gold foil may also be purchased as ready-prepared gold-foil cylinders of various sizes, supplied in small bottles.

The outstanding feature about pure gold foil is that it can be condensed by hammering (malleting), building up one pellet upon another—actually cold-welding—directly in the tooth that has been prepared to receive the restoration. It is precise, exacting work.

Cohesive gold foil is probably used most commonly by gold-foil operators. In order to cold-weld, this prepared pellet or cylinder must be annealed (heated to a cherry red) before placing it in the preparation, ready for condensing with an instrument called a gold-foil condenser (plugger).

Mat gold is furnished in sheets from which pieces fitting the size of the cavity may be cut, inserted, and condensed. Usually restorations filled with mat gold are completed with gold foil for a denser surface.

Another form of pure gold is furnished in small pellets that are actually pure gold powder of almost microscopic fineness, compacted into small, round pellets and then wrapped in gold foil. The pellet is placed into the cavity preparation following annealing. Due to its density, about one-tenth as many pellets are required to restore a given area as gold-foil cylinders. This powdered form of gold is free from surface impurities, and its cohesiveness permits each pellet to bond molecularly to that already placed as it is condensed in the cavity. To protect the pellets from possible contamination by gases in the air, *the stopper of the vial should be tightly replaced after each use.* As with gold-foil cylinders, these pellets should be annealed by holding them in the clean blue flame of the alcohol lamp until the pellet turns dull red, but no longer. After cooling for three or four seconds, the pellet can be carried to the cavity preparation as directed by the dentist. A nichrome spear foil carrier is used for this purpose. It is made from a piece of 16-gauge nichrome wire that has been sharpened, smoothed, shaped to resemble an explorer, and mounted in a broach holder.

Annealing Gold

Annealing is a very important step in cohesive gold work. Since it is performed by the dental assistant, it is important that she or he know exactly what is desired and what the operation is meant to accomplish. As an

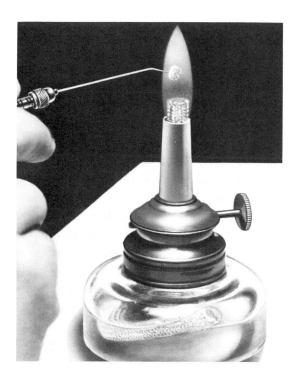

Figure 31.18
Annealing gold foil in alcohol lamp.

operation, it is simplicity itself, but its consequences are basic and far-reaching. If it has been done improperly, even a restoration that is apparently successful will eventually be a failure.

Annealing is a cleansing operation. When gold is absolutely pure and clean, it is inherently cohesive—that is, capable of uniting molecularly throughout the mass of foil. Its laminae (layers of individual foil sheet) will stick together on mere contact. Due to this characteristic, it is possible to weld it in the cold state, instead of using a welding torch such as is used to weld metals in repair shops.

The purity of gold is easily destroyed, however, and when impure, it either cannot cohere at all or does so imperfectly and cannot be welded successfully. Even exposure to the air can make it impure.

Gold may be contaminated by exposure to air because the atmosphere usually contains gases that attach themselves to the surface of the gold foil by molecular attraction. The gases deposit a film of salts on the surface of the gold, and it cannot cohere. Therefore, gold must have its surface thoroughly cleaned just before use. Consequently, it is subjected to annealing which drives off all volatile impurities (those which will evaporate, especially under heat)—leaving it clean.

Protecting Gold

Gold must be protected from the gases that will permanently injure it. Since these gases are present in the dental office, extreme care must be used in storing and

using gold. One way to protect gold from these gases is to coat it with a film of alkaline salts. This protective film, usually of ammonia, is placed there by the manufacturer to prevent deleterious gases from condensing on the foil. The ammonia is then driven off by annealing.

Purpose of Annealing

Annealing drives off all surface atmospheric moisture and whatever film has been formed by the protective alkaline gas in combination with gases that may have settled afterward.

Proper annealing means heating gold foil long enough, at a given temperature, to volatilize all moisture and gases, cleansing all its surface; avoiding injury to the foil in the process; and guarding it against all contamination, from the start of its annealing to its condensation in the cavity.

Underannealing is to be avoided. It leaves impurities on the foil, which prevent its thorough condensation and thus cause the restoration eventually to pit and flake. **Overannealing** is to be avoided no less. It scorches the foil, shriveling the fine edges and rendering it generally harsh and unworkable—with the same harmful consequences as those of underannealing. Scorched foil will not burnish properly. **Contamination** of gold foil during or after annealing may be as harmful as contamination before annealing.

In general, gold foil can be annealed by either of two methods: (1) piece by piece in an open flame or (2) in bulk, on a tray or some other suitable receptacle. Each has its advantages and disadvantages, and either is capable of giving satisfactory results.

Piece-by-Piece Annealing

The method of annealing piece by piece consists in picking up individually each piece of gold foil, of whatever form, heating it directly in an open flame, and placing it in the cavity.

The instrument best adapted for carrying the foil is one with a fine, smooth point. Whatever the instrument, its point should be nonoxidizing, and it should pick up the foil so as neither to crush it nor to cover any portion of it. And obviously it should be cleaned just before use. Simply scrub it with a stiff nailbrush dipped in alcohol, and then dry it thoroughly with a towel.

The foil is passed through the flame at the tip of the inner cone—neither close to the wick nor through the upper portion of the outer cone. Either of the latter may contaminate it with carbon. It is passed through the flame—not held—at a rate that will bring every particle to a dull red. If kept in the flame until it shows a bright glow, it is liable to be overannealed before it can be withdrawn. Heating it to a dull red usually takes

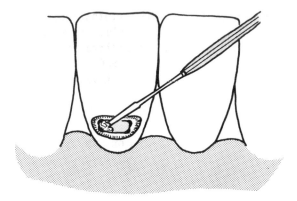

Figure 31.19
Condensing gold foil in cavity.

no longer than a second or two. The exact length of time depends on the size of the piece and the intensity of the flame. Gauging it is entirely a matter of experience. If a piece comes out of the flame looking the least bit shriveled, it is doubtless scorched and is best discarded.

Every annealed piece, in all open-flame annealing, is carried from the flame direct to the cavity. This has the important advantage of precluding all possible contamination of the foil after annealing, whether by atmospheric moisture or gases or by substances that can contaminate it on contact. A common procedure is as follows:

While malleting an annealed piece with one hand, the assistant picks up another piece with the other. When the condensing of the former is finished, she or he then anneals the latter and carries it to the cavity. Repeat the process until the restoration is completed. On reaching the cavity, the foil should have cooled sufficiently not to cause any painful reaction.

Bulk Annealing

A more controlled means of annealing can be achieved by the use of an electrical device designed expressly for the purpose of annealing in bulk. Electric annealers vary, but they all have in common, principally, an outer metal shell housing a heating element, a tray over the latter to hold the gold foil, and a lid that fits over the tray. They all operate directly from an ordinary electric outlet.

Place as many pieces of gold foil on the tray as it will hold loosely—without any two pieces touching each other. To prevent their sliding and sticking together, the tray of a recent electric annealer provides individual compartments for each piece of foil. The current is turned on *after* the foil is in place and *with the lid off*.

It is advisable to keep the annealed foil warm until it is used. For this purpose some electric annealers have a rheostat which permits the current to be regulated

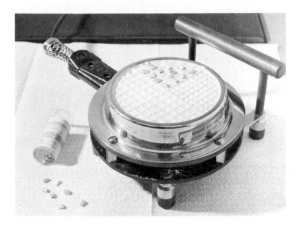

Figure 31.20
Gold foil and electric annealer.

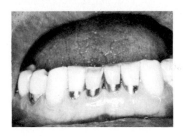

Figure 31.21
Gold foil restoration.

downward. But even one that has no rheostat, provided that its maximum temperature does not exceed 700 degrees Fahrenheit, may be left on—full—without any hazard of overannealing. In the latter case, however, it is necessary that the current be turned off altogether in ample time for the tray to cool before annealing the next batch. Laying out foil on a tray that is hot is extremely difficult.

Annealed foil that remains after the restoration is completed is left on the annealer for the next restoration. Such foil cannot be returned to its usual container because it would stick together and could not be separated. Reannealing does it no harm. There is, of course, the hazard of its being contaminated by gases that are irretrievably deleterious. Since the only protection from them is given by the lid that fits over the tray, even though not altogether foolproof, it is important to replace the lid tightly as soon as the annealer is not in use. If the tray does not have individual compartments for each piece of foil, there is the further hazard that even a slight jarring of the annealer may cause some pieces to slide and stick together.

Noncohesive Gold Foil

Noncohesive gold foil in the form of ropes or cylinders is used by many experienced gold-foil operators. This type of foil is not annealed before use.

Casting Alloys

Cast-gold restorations are not formed inside the mouth as the pure gold fillings are; they are made to conform to a specific shape outside the mouth and are then placed either in or on the tooth that is to be restored. If this casting is cemented into a tooth, it is known as an **inlay,** and the term to describe it is **intracoronal.** If the casting is cemented on part of the tooth or covers the entire crown of the tooth, it is known as a **crown** or **onlay,** and the term to describe it is **extracoronal.**

In order to produce these shapes or forms so that they will accurately fit the tooth that has been prepared, a rather complicated and precise procedure is required. The purpose of this procedure is always the same—the production of an accurate casting that will properly fit the prepared tooth.

The casting gold alloys are generally composed of varying parts of four metals: gold, silver, copper, and platinum. Small additions of other metals, such as zinc, are possibly used by certain manufacturers in adjusting the properties of the particular casting gold designed for a certain purpose.

The most surprising fact is that gold, silver, and copper can be combined to form an alloy that is much stronger than any one of the three by itself. While this does not seem possible, it is correct. Many metals, when alloyed or combined with other metals, make an alloy that has completely different properties than are exhibited by the metals alone.

Improper handling of gold alloys can result in changes in the properties of the alloy. This is best shown in the method of cooling Type C golds after casting. (These gold alloys usually contain a certain amount of platinum, a white metal, which results in an alloy that is less yellow than those of the softer golds, Types A and B.) If the Type C gold is quenched (that is, submerged in water) immediately after casting, the result is a softening of the alloy. If, instead, the casting is allowed to cool on the bench top or in the casting machine for eight to ten minutes after casting and before quenching in water, the result is a hard alloy as Type C golds are designed to be.

The Type A golds are the softer gold alloys. These are designed for use where the restoration will not have much stress placed on it, such as gingival (Class V) inlays. The Type B golds are designed for greater stress, such as Class II inlays, three-quarter crowns or full crowns alone, or those which support one end of a short bridge. The Type C golds are designed for thin three-quarter crowns or full crowns, or those restorations supporting long bridges—restorations that will receive a great deal of stress in relation to their bulk.

The *ten tenets as applied to gold* are shown on the summary found in table 31.1.

Summary

Biomaterials are materials directly associated with living tissues; in dentistry they are usually used in the mouth.

The environment of the oral cavity is *restrictive* because the oral cavity is constantly moist and is subjected to rather extreme changes of temperature and acid. Restorative materials may be placed under the stress and abrasion of masticatory forces.

Standards for certified dental materials are maintained by the American Dental Association and the National Bureau of Standards.

Ten tenets for a satisfactory filling material have been established. See the summary chart for each dental material.

The *restorative materials* of dentistry include dental cements, silver amalgam, gold, and gold alloys. It is important that you understand the procedures used in mixing and using each of these materials.

Dental cements are used for a variety of purposes: to retain restorations, such as inlays and crowns; to seal root canal fillings; as surgical dressings; as impression pastes; as temporary and sedative filling materials; cavity liners; and as protective bases under metallic filling materials. They may be classified as follows: zinc oxide eugenol, zinc phosphate, glass ionomer, zinc silicaphosphate, zinc polyacrylate.

Zinc oxide-eugenol cement is used for temporary covers for crown and bridge work, for sedative treatment, for bases under metal restorations, and for capping exposed pulps.

Zinc phosphate cements are used for bases under fillings and for cementing inlays, crowns, bridges, and jacket crowns.

The *esthetic restorative materials* are classified as chemically curing or lightcuring. The newest group is BIS-GMA composite resins.

Dental amalgam is an alloy. Extreme care must be used in mixing the proper proportions of mercury and alloy when preparing an amalgam restoration.

Gold may be used in several forms. In the pure form, gold is used to make gold-foil restorations.

Annealing is a cleansing operation, and the foil will adhere to other gold when it is pure; thus, contamination of gold foil must be avoided. Proper annealing means heating gold foil long enough to volatilize all moisture and gases, cleansing all its surface, avoiding injury to the foil in the process, and avoiding contamination from the beginning of the process until it is condensed in the preparation in the tooth. Foil may be annealed by one of two methods: piece by piece or in bulk.

Noncohesive gold foil is used by some experienced operators. It is not annealed before use.

Another form of *cohesive gold* for dental use is composed of pellets of pure gold wrapped in gold foil. It is so dense that about one-tenth as many pellets are required to restore an area as gold-foil cylinders.

Casting alloys of gold are used to make a specific shape of restoration outside the mouth. This restoration is then cemented into place in the mouth. It may be an inlay, a crown, or a bridge.

Gold alloys are classified as Type A, Type B, and Type C. *Type A* is the softest of the three and is used for restorations where there is little stress; *Type B* golds are designed for greater stress; and *Type C* golds are used for restorations that will receive a great deal of stress in relation to their bulk.

Study Questions

1. What materials are included as restorative materials in dentistry?
2. Describe the procedures for mixing each of the following:
   - zinc oxide-eugenol
   - zinc phosphate
3. What is an exothermic reaction? Which cement is more likely to need care to prevent this reaction? What would you do to prevent such a reaction?
4. Compare unfilled, filled, and composite plastics.
5. What is dental amalgam?
6. What happens during amalgamation?
7. Discuss making the strongest amalgam restoration.
8. Why is excess mercury deposited in a receptacle specifically for mercury?
9. Discuss the purpose of polishing amalgams and when it is done.
10. What is done with excess amalgam?
11. How can gold be used in restorations?
12. Discuss welded gold restorations.
13. Discuss protection of gold.
14. Discuss the uses of cast-gold alloys.
15. What is the difference between *intracoronal* and *extracoronal*? What other terms are used?

Vocabulary

adaptation   modification to fit the conditions of the environment

adhesion   ability to chemically bond to tooth structure

amalgam   any metal combined with mercury

amalgam restorations   dental amalgam inserted into prepared cavities in teeth

amalgamation   a chemical and physical reaction which occurs between alloy and mercury when they are mixed

annealing   a process that quickens the aging of an alloy, producing material of predictable physical properties

anticariogenic   opposing the production of caries

coefficient of thermal expansion   an expression of the rate of expansion and contraction of a material as related to temperature change

crown   a casting that is cemented on a prepared tooth, covering the entire crown of the tooth

dental amalgam   the alloy of metals specified by the ADA for use in dental restorations (combined with mercury)

dew point   the point at which moisture from the air condenses on the glass: it varies, depending upon the amount of moisture in the air and the temperature of the glass slab

EBA   ethoxybenzoic acid cements

exothermic reaction   chemical reaction that generates heat

extracoronal   a crown or onlay, placed on the tooth

inlay   a casting cemented into a tooth

intracoronal   a restoration that is cemented into a tooth

luting   cementing

mortar   a glass cup with a smooth, rounded bottom

onlay   a term used interchangeably with crown—a restoration cemented onto a preparation, covering the tooth

percolation   the bubbling of fluids forced out at the margins of fillings subjected to temperature cyclings

pestle   a glass mixing rod rounded to fit the curve of the mortar

polymerization   a chemical reaction in which smaller molecules combine into larger molecules

radiolucent   transparent to X ray

radiopaque   not transparent to X ray

trituration   mixing

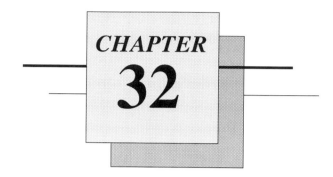

Impression Materials

Special Techniques
Impressions for Cast-gold Restorations
Rubber-base Impression Materials
Hydrocolloid Impression Materials

Special Techniques

Restorations that are constructed outside the mouth require special techniques. Upon completion of the preparation for an inlay, a three-quarter crown, a full crown, or any multiples or combinations of them, it is necessary to construct a wax replica of that portion of the tooth which has been removed. This wax replica is later used to construct the gold inlay or crown and is technically called a **wax pattern.** It does not resemble a dress pattern; that is, it is not a flat piece of wax. It is a sculptured form. It is a pattern in that the inlay or crown will be an exact duplicate of the wax form.

Some dentists do make a **direct** wax pattern, that is, a wax pattern made directly in the mouth of the patient. Direct technique is usually limited to the less complicated patterns, such as patterns for occlusal inlays. It is possible to make direct patterns for all individual restorations constructed in gold should the dentist so desire. If a direct wax pattern is made, no impression is needed.

The majority of dentists, however, use an **indirect method;** that is, a wax pattern is made on a cast, or duplicate, of the patient's tooth or group of teeth. With this method of constructing the wax pattern, the dentist must first make an impression of the prepared tooth in the patient's mouth. A die or reproduction of the prepared tooth can be made by one of several methods.

The die, or exact copy of the prepared tooth in the patient's mouth, is used to construct a wax replacement of the missing part of the tooth. The wax is molded onto the die until all the angles and surfaces are filled accurately. Then wax is added until there is enough wax so the outside of the tooth can be carved to fit properly with the existing teeth in the patient's mouth. (The inlay must properly mesh with the existing surfaces of other teeth in the area.) The wax model must be accurately formed (1) where it joins the remaining tooth structure and (2) where it touches other teeth.

When the dentist is positive the wax model is accurate, it is mounted on a tiny rod or post, called a **sprue pin,** and embedded in dental casting investment, which is plaster mixed with silica. (See chapter 34 for a detailed explanation.) When the investment has hardened, the base and sprue pin are removed, leaving a communicating hole through the investment to the wax model (usually called a wax pattern). This invested pattern is then placed in an oven where the heat burns out all the wax, leaving a **void** (hole) in the investment which is the identical shape of the wax model.

Hot, melted gold (called molten gold) is then forced through the hole left by the sprue pin into the hollow that is shaped like the wax pattern. When the gold cools and hardens, it produces a casting shaped exactly like the wax pattern. The investment plaster is removed, and the casting is cleaned, polished, and cemented to the tooth.

This brief, nontechnical explanation of the process of making a cast-gold restoration outside the mouth should help you understand the overall procedure. Now let us consider the process in more detail, beginning with the making of impressions.

If we regard a prepared tooth or group of teeth as an **original** or **positive shape,** the impression that is taken of an individual tooth or a group of teeth (or of any dental situation for that matter) is a **negative shape.** If you leave an imprint of your hand in a section of modeling clay, that imprint is a negative shape of your hand. If into this imprint or impression you pour or place a soft mix of plaster, permit it to harden, then remove the plaster, this plaster will again have the same curve as the surface of the hand that you pushed into the clay originally. This plaster model (or cast) is a positive copy of the surface of your hand.

The same is true of an impression taken for dental purposes. In order to complete the purpose for which the impression was taken, a positive form must be made from the impression. This positive is known as a **cast** when it involves an entire arch, but more specifically it is known as a **model** or **working model** if a dental restoration is to be constructed upon it. If the impression is of a single tooth for the construction of an inlay or crown, or if the impression is of a quadrant or full arch that contains teeth involved in multiple restorations, the individual tooth model is known as a **die.** In the case of quadrant or full-arch impressions, we shall see later that it is possible to have the dies removable from the model. This means that the individual die may be lifted from the model and replaced to a definite position and relationship by means of some form of notching or keying. This ability makes it much easier to "wax-up" the pattern required for all gold castings.

The direct and the indirect methods of making a wax pattern have already been mentioned. A third method, the **indirect-direct method,** is also used by some dentists. In this method, the pattern is made on the model or die and is then rechecked directly in the patient's mouth prior to proceeding with the laboratory work.

Impressions for Cast-gold Restorations

Many dentists carve wax patterns in the mouth on the prepared tooth. This direct method eliminates two intermediate steps, involving two extra materials, which could contribute to inaccuracies in the final fit of the restoration. Although the direct method can be simply performed with greater accuracy, most dentists and

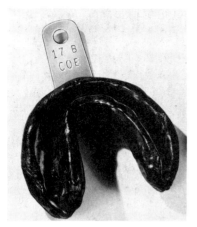

a

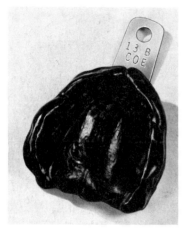

b

Figure 32.1
Preliminary impression in modeling compound (a) lower impression; and (b) upper impression.

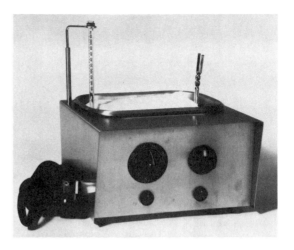

Figure 32.2
Thermostatic compound heater.

technicians prefer to work from models because this method permits greater ease in contouring, carving, and manipulating the materials involved.

Impression compound is a thermoplastic material, the properties of which are governed by the American Dental Association's Specification No. 3. It is furnished in cakes and sticks. The most common use of this material is taking primary impressions for complete dentures, but it is also occasionally used for impressioning single teeth for full-crown restorations.

First, the material must be softened. For individual tooth impressions, it is possible to soften it carefully in an open flame, but a controlled temperature compound heater is usually used for larger impressions. In order to confine the material, the dentist will select a copper band of the proper size, shape it to fit the gingival margins of the prepared tooth, fill the copper band with impression compound, position it on the tooth, and force the softened material under pressure to the tiny recesses at the gingival margin. The

impression must then be cooled. A stream of air from the air syringe or cold water from the water syringe is used. The dentist then removes the copper band containing the impression material and checks it for accuracy. Impression compound is an excellent material for accurate single-tooth impressions; however, it is rigid and cannot be drawn over undercuts in the preparation or contours of the tooth. For that reason it has limited applications for inlay impressions.

Impression plaster is another material that has been used for impressions in prosthodontics. Like impression compound, it is rigid and therefore has little application where cast-gold restorations are involved. It is used sometimes in making **jaw registrations,** which are records of the relationship of the upper arch to the lower arch. A small amount of plaster is placed on the buccal side of the upper and lower posterior teeth when they have been positioned as the dentist wishes. When this portion of plaster has hardened on each side of the mouth, it is carefully removed, trimmed to include only the required area, and used to position casts previously made so they will be in the same relationship on an articulator as the teeth were in the patient's mouth. (See chapter 30 for a discussion of the use of an articulator.)

Rubber-base Impression Materials

The rubber-base impression materials differ from modeling compound and impression plaster in that they are elastic in nature. They are rubbery. The two types of rubber-base impression materials differ in chemical makeup and in the manufacturer's choice of color for the finished product, but otherwise they are similar in texture when set. The silicone-base material is perhaps used somewhat more widely than the polysulfide type.

These materials are supplied in tubes. One tube contains the base material; the other tube contains the catalyst, or material that causes the mix to set. Usually these are of different colors, which make it possible to see more easily when you have a smoothly uniform mix.

Two general consistencies are usually available from any manufacturer—one heavier-bodied for tray use, one lighter-bodied for syringe use.

Either heavy-bodied or light-bodied material is used alone in impressions for complete dentures, and at times for copper-band impressions of individual teeth. The syringe material is used together with the base material when taking impressions for multiple restorations or partial denture impressions.

No special treatment of the rubber surface is required before pouring models in the rubber-base impression materials. This material is dimensionally more stable than the next group of materials to be discussed.

Hydrocolloid Impression Materials

The original hydrocolloid made its appearance prior to World War II. In its final set form it resembles chocolate-colored gelatin with somewhat more density and toughness. This set condition can be changed to fluid again by heating the material. It is therefore a **reversible hydrocolloid;** that is, it can be changed from solid to liquid and back again by heating and cooling it.

(There is also an **irreversible hydrocolloid** material which remains solid once it has set.)

The primary function of the reversible hydrocolloid is taking impressions for restorative dentistry and taking impressions of inlay and crown preparations. It is also used in prosthetics. Although it is a very accurate material, the special heaters, tempering baths, and water-cooled trays make its manipulation more intricate; and consequently it is less popular than the rubber-base impression materials.

The original reversible hydrocolloid is changed from solid to fluid by heating the material in a hydrocolloid conditioner. Boil the material for eight to ten minutes. It will then have acquired a consistency somewhat like thin molasses. At this stage and at this temperature, it is much too hot to place in a patient's mouth. For this reason, the conditioners have tempering baths that permit the material to cool to about 105° Fahrenheit over a period of minutes prior to loading the impression tray and inserting it into the patient's mouth. When seated properly, the circulating water is turned on and the tray is chilled. The resulting impression is extremely accurate when properly taken; however,

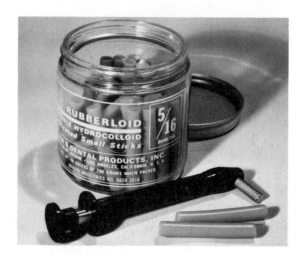

Figure 32.3
Hydrocolloid syringe and material.

unless it is properly managed, hydrocolloid is extremely susceptible to dimensional changes through loss of water by evaporation. Therefore, models should be poured as soon after the impression is taken as is possible. Storage, when absolutely necessary, should only be in an atmosphere of 100 percent humidity—wrapped in a thoroughly wet towel or stored in a humidifier designed for the purpose. Even such storage should not be permitted for extended periods of time.

Read the directions for the proper use of the hydrocolloid available in the office in which you work. There are some variations in temperatures, in treatment with a fixer after the impression is taken and before the model is poured, in the length of time a model may be permitted to remain in the impression, and in the treatment recommended for the combined impression and freshly poured model.

As with the rubber-base materials when used for full-mouth or quadrant impressions of multiple preparations, the reversible hydrocolloids reproduce detail most accurately when a preliminary thinner mix is either painted on the area concerned or is injected with a type of syringe made for the purpose. If syringes are used, they are loaded, sealed from contact with external water, and prepared in the conditioner just as are the full tubes of normal material for tray use.

As with the rubber-base materials, the purpose of the thinner material is to eliminate air in undercuts present in the area to be covered by the tray, as well as to provide the ultimate of fine detail in the impression.

The reversible hydrocolloids are made of agar-agar, a product obtained from seaweed. At the time of its development, most of the desirable seaweed was to be found off the coast of Japan. With the opening of

World War II, this seaweed was no longer available from the previous source, and a search was begun for a substitute impression material.

This search resulted in the development of an *irreversible* hydrocolloid impression material, more commonly known as the **alginates**. This material is prepared in powder form, is mixed with water at a specific temperature (usually 70°) in a mixing bowl for one minute, and does not require a water-cooled tray. The resulting impression paste is seldom used in restorative dentistry but is the most frequently used for primary impressions for complete dentures and for primary and final impressions for removable partial dentures. Since it also forms a gel, as do the reversible hydrocolloids, it is susceptible to the same dimensional changes and handling characteristics. Models should be poured immediately, or proper storage should be instituted for brief periods only. The irreversible hydrocolloids are easy to work with and therefore are very commonly used in dental offices.

However, most offices will use either the rubber-base impression materials or the *reversible* hydrocolloids for impressions of multiple restoration procedures.

The elastic impression materials, in general, do not lend themselves to making amalgam dies. The very dense die stones that have been developed provide a technique for making models with removable dies that has been found entirely satisfactory; but as with all dental procedures, preciseness and care must be used if a good result is to be obtained. A material must always be used in the manner for which it is designed.

Summary

Restorations that are prepared outside the mouth are made by taking an impression in the mouth and then working with a model outside the mouth.

Materials that are useful for impressions are:

1. *Impression compound,* used by dentists for primary impressions for complete dentures and for individual full-crown preparations.

2. *Impression plaster,* which has been used in prosthodontics.
3. *Rubber-base impression materials,* which are elastic in nature; they are supplied as pastes and are dimensionally more stable than hydrocolloid materials.
4. Hydrocolloid impression materials, which are both reversible and irreversible. The *irreversible hydrocolloids* are easy to work with and are commonly used in dental offices for full-mouth impressions but generally are not used for dies for gold castings. The *reversible hydrocolloids* are used, as are the rubber-base impression materials, for impressions involving multiple restoration procedures.

Study Questions

1. Distinguish between direct and indirect wax patterns.
2. Explain an impression and its use.
3. What is a die?
4. Describe briefly the process of making a gold restoration outside the mouth.
5. Describe the use of
   a. impression compound.
   b. impression plaster.
   c. rubber-base impression materials.
   d. both kinds of hydrocolloid impression materials.
6. Discuss the uses of rubber-base impression materials, reversible hydrocolloid materials, and irreversible hydrocolloid materials.

Vocabulary

jaw registration   records of relationship of upper arch to lower arch
die   exact copy of a prepared individual tooth
molten gold   hot melted gold
sprue pin   tiny rod or post to hold wax pattern
wax pattern   replica of a part of a tooth that has been removed
direct w.p.   made directly in the mouth
indirect w.p.   made on a model of the tooth outside the mouth

CHAPTER 33

Casts and Dies

Casts: Basic Instructions
   Artificial Stone and Plaster
     Mixing Artificial Stone
     Mixing Plaster
   Boxing Casts
   Pouring Casts
   Separating Casts
   Trimming Casts
Orthodontic Casts
Restorations
Dies (Positives of the Impressions)
   The Stone Die
   Electroplating
   Lubricating the Die
   Copings
Indirect Inlay Technique
   Step One: Mixing an Impression Tray for Single
     or Multiple Inlays
   Step Two: Making the Impression in the Custom-
     Made Tray
   Step Three: Pouring the Model
   Step Four: Cutting the Removable Dies and
     Completing the Castings
Fixed Prostheses Impression Techniques
Copper-Band Impressions
Removable Prostheses
   Denture Casts
   Trial Bases
   Occlusal Rims
Emergency Denture Repair

Casts: Basic Instructions

Restorations that are constructed outside the mouth are the subject of chapters 32, 33, and 34. The second skill to be learned is making a model or wax pattern from the impression we learned to take in chapter 32.

Dies on which to fabricate (make) wax patterns for cast-gold restorations may be made of artificial stone or amalgam. Amalgam is used only occasionally for individual copper-band compound impressions. The artificial stone or die stone is a material similar to plaster but is much more dense, providing a hard, smooth surface that will withstand the manipulation necessary when carving wax patterns. Although plaster can be used in preparing study casts, it is too porous and weak to be used for dies.

Artificial Stone and Plaster

Artificial stone and plaster[1] are supplied in almost any amount, by weight, from five-pound cans to hundred-pound barrels. Do not purchase larger quantities than can be used in a period of two or three months and, naturally, no more than the dental office is equipped to store.

Plaster is most commonly supplied in white. Die stones are supplied in several contrasting colors, varying with the particular brand or use intended. The color coding of these materials quickly indicates which material has been used to pour a given cast.

Both die stones and plaster are made from a similar variety of natural gypsum. The gypsum is mined, crushed, and fed into kilns where it is heated to drive off some of the water of crystallization to form what is called a **hemihydrate,** which is then prepared in a powder form and packaged.

The rough, irregular, and porous particles of plaster require a relatively large amount of water for mixing when compared to the more regular shape of die-stone particles. The artificial stones require about half as much water for mixing as does plaster. Although the final product is stronger when less water is used, you must have sufficient water to separate the particles and wet them thoroughly in order to manipulate the mix and pour a cast from it. The water added replaces that driven off when the gypsum was heated. In addition, the particles are porous, and water must penetrate and fill these pores. Therefore, an excess of water must be present. The effect is somewhat the same as if many small sponges were stirred under water. The final product of the reaction is gypsum. In other words, when water is added to the hemihydrate, the original calcination reaction is reversed—and gypsum, the original product, is again attained. It is by no means as dense as the product mined from the ground, however, because excess water is necessary for the mixing. It is

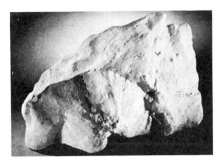

Figure 33.1
Natural gypsum rock as it is mined.

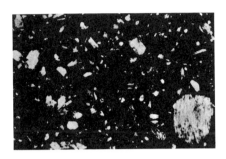

Figure 33.2
Photomicrograph of plaster particles.

obvious that the final gypsum product must be porous in order to contain this excess water. *It should now be evident that the less water used in mixing a gypsum material, the stronger the final product will be.* The less amount of excess water, the denser the gypsum and, consequently, the greater its strength.

Since plaster is chemically the same as dental stone, why is stone so much stronger and harder when it has set?

The particles of hemihydrate used in the dental stone show a fairly smooth and regular surface, and they are quite free from porosity. Therefore, when the dental stone is mixed with water, much less water is required to separate the particles since they are neither porous nor rough.

In contrast to plaster—which requires approximately sixty cubic centimeters of water per 100 grams of plaster for mixing—stone can be easily mixed with twenty-eight cubic centimeters of water per 100 grams of the powder. In fact, as little as twenty-five cubic centimeters of water per 100 grams of stone can be used, although the mixture is very thick and requires vibration to make it flow. Very strong, hard casts can be obtained with this heavy mix.

Special die stones have particles that are slightly larger in size. The larger-size particles are more easily displaced by the water and therefore require less water to make a mix of the same consistency.

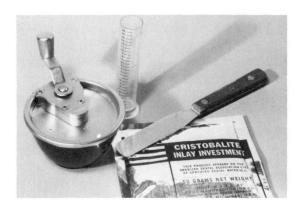

Figure 33.3
Premeasured powder, mixing bowl, and measuring cup for water.

You should note that a relatively slight difference in the water content of the mix with a dental stone results in a considerable difference in the strength of the final product. In certain instances, an *increase* in water content of as little as one cubic centimeter per 100 grams of stone may result in a *decrease in strength* of as much as 1,000 pounds per square inch. While this difference in strength is not as great in mixing plaster, it does make a noticeable difference to mix plaster with as little water as possible.

When plaster is used, you can judge reasonably well the proportion of water to powder after some familiarity with the "feel" of mixing correctly proportioned mixes. Such guesswork should not be used in the case of stone.

Unless the amounts of water and powder are being properly measured, the chances are that the resulting cast will be deficient in strength, hardness, and accuracy—with possibly critical and costly consequences.

Fortunately, most die stones are prepackaged. Therefore the powder is already weighed, and only the correct volume of water must be measured and added.

A few words of caution should be given concerning the use of a stone in connection with the hydrocolloid technique. The hydrocolloid is apt to soften the surface of the stone when the latter is allowed to set in contact with it. This effect can be definitely minimized if certain precautions are observed.

1. If a "fixer" is required by the manufacturer, it should always be used according to the directions supplied.
2. Be sure that there is no water clinging to the impression when the cast or die is poured. The surface of the hydrocolloid can be dried by blotting it with an absorbent, *but under no circumstances should it be dried by an air blast.*

3. Separate the impression from the stone cast or die approximately one hour after it has been poured. If it is separated too soon, its surface will not be hard; and if it is allowed to set too long in contact with the hydrocolloid, it will be softened. If it is absolutely necessary to leave the stone in contact with the impression for a prolonged period, the impression and cast should be kept in 100 percent humidity. However, the best method is to separate at the end of an hour as previously stated.

All stones may lose their properties if they are not stored properly. By all means, store them in a dry place. Since they are **hygroscopic,** they absorb moisture to a degree. Once they take up moisture, a deterioration sets in. The first evidence of deterioration is an increase in setting time. Later, a longer setting time is observed, and finally a stage is reached when the stone will not set at all.

Such changes may be slow and not easily observed. An increase in the setting expansion and a decrease in strength may occur before any change in setting time is evident. Therefore, the can of stone should be kept tightly shut at all times, and it should always be stored in a clean, dry place. Before every use shake up the contents while still in the container.

Mixing Artificial Stone

To prepare artificial stone for pouring a cast, the following materials are required:

1. Plaster bowl
2. Plaster spatula
3. Water measure (50 cc. graduate is convenient)
4. A common teaspoon
5. Scale for weighing
6. Waxed paper cups for weighing
7. Six-inch-square glass slabs for each cast
8. Artificial stone
9. A vibrator (if available)
10. The impression which is to be poured

For the average single-arch impression, 42 cc. of water will be ample. This amount of water is poured into the mixing bowl.

With a spoon, place sufficient artificial stone from the storage bin or can into the paper cup on the scale to weigh 150 grams. Sift this powder into the water in the mixing bowl by using the spoon. When all the powder has been sifted into the mixing bowl, place the bowl with its contents on the vibrator and vibrate for five to ten seconds. Then spatulate the contents of the mixing bowl until a uniform, creamy mixture is obtained. Again vibrate the bowl with its contents for ten

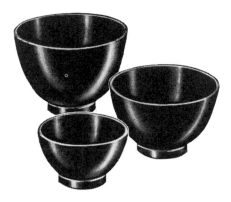

Figure 33.4
Hygienic flexiboles.

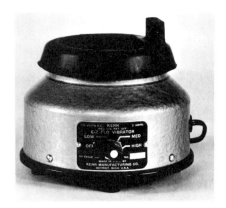

Figure 33.5
Kerr E-Z Flo vibrator.

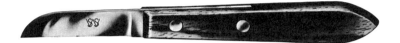

Figure 33.6
Office knife, 5A.

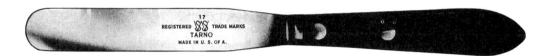

Figure 33.7
Plaster spatula No. 7.

to fifteen seconds. If no mechanical vibrator is available, rapidly jar the bowl on the laboratory bench for one minute.

Special forms of artificial stone are often used to make special types of cast and dies for indirect crown, bridge, or inlay construction. Specific instructions for mixing these special types accompany the material when purchased. These directions should be followed explicitly to secure the required results.

Mixing Plaster

Plaster is available in two types. **Natural-setting** is used for the pouring of models in the laboratory. Setting time is between fifteen and twenty minutes. **Quick-setting** is used for some purposes in taking impressions directly in the mouth. Setting time is from three to five minutes. Either flavored or plain plaster is available.

The timing involved in preparing plaster of the quick-setting variety for an impression in the mouth is extremely important, as is the method by which it is spatulated and handled prior to the impression. These details are best learned by practice if this type is used in your office.

The transition (change) of the soft mixture of plaster with water to a hard, set material is a controllable process. That is, the time required for the transition may be altered by various means. Cold water used for the mix will delay setting; warm water will hasten it. Adding a pinch of table salt will hasten setting, as will the addition of powder made by grinding previously-set plaster. Spatulation helps hasten the setting, other conditions being the same.

Mixing bowls used for preparing plaster and artificial stone are frequently made of flexible plastic for easy cleaning.

A plaster or laboratory spatula is used to spatulate both materials. Spatulas that have become sharp-edged from long use should be discarded. They tend to cut the bowl, making the removal of old plaster or stone difficult.

To prepare plaster for pouring a cast, the following materials are required:

1. Plaster bowl
2. Plaster spatula
3. Water measure (100 cc. graduate is convenient)

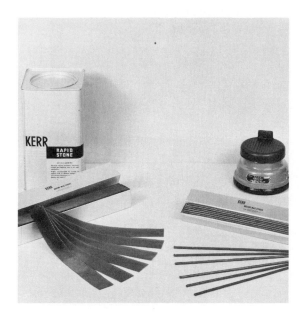

Figure 33.8
Material for boxing and pouring impressions.

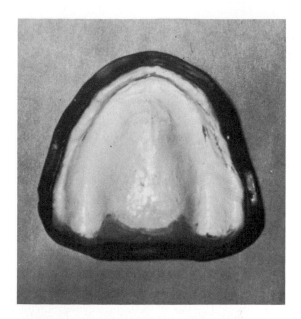

Figure 33.9
Maxillary impression with beading applied ready for boxing.

4. Plaster
5. A common teaspoon
6. Six-inch-square glass slabs, one for each impression to be poured
7. A vibrator (if available)
8. The impression that is to be poured

For an average single-arch impression, 60 cc. of water will be ample. This amount of water is poured into the plaster bowl. To begin with, use the coldest water available in order to provide the greatest amount of time possible in which to work. The reason for measuring the water is simple economy. There is no object in wasting dental materials at any time. With a little care, a more accurate amount of material may be used with less waste.

Generously heap a teaspoon with plaster from the storage bin or can. Shake the plaster smoothly and rapidly off the spoon into the 60 cc. of water. Repeat until the water has absorbed all it will apparently take. This quantity of water will need approximately one-half cup of plaster to make a mix of moderately heavy consistency.

The spatula is then used to stir the mix smoothly, with as little air as possible incorporated into the mix. Spatulate until the mix of plaster is thoroughly smooth. Add more plaster, if required, to make the mix just heavy enough so that it will not drop off the spatula when it is lifted above the bowl and turned over.

This point should be reached without wasting time. If you spatulate a thin mix long enough, it will begin to thicken—it will be starting its initial set. This stage is too late to pour the cast well.

When the mix is at the desired consistency, place the plaster bowl on the vibrator and vibrate well to remove as many entrapped air bubbles as possible. If no mechanical vibrator is available, rapidly jar the bowl on the laboratory bench for one minute. The material is then ready for use. (See "Pouring Casts.")

Boxing Casts

Boxing an impression is simply the enclosing of the impression and its supporting tray with sides made of waxed sheets or strips. The wax strips enclose the plaster or artificial stone which forms the base of the impression. Boxing wax strips are available for this purpose. This particular wax is soft, pliable, and sticky enough for two ends to stick together with finger pressure.

Boxing also makes a more accurate and dense cast by vibrating the water to the top of the boxing wax, leaving the denser stone where the teeth are. Hydrocolloid impressions are usually not boxed because the time involved causes the impression to dehydrate and also because it is very easy to distort portions of the hydrocolloid with the boxing material.

Final impressions for complete dentures are nearly always boxed before pouring. Casts for removable partial dentures that are made from alginate or reversible hydrocolloid are usually poured by using the double mix method. The stone or plaster is vibrated into the impression until it is filled to the peripheries and then it is allowed to set without inverting the impressions. After the initial set is reached (about ten minutes for stone), the filled impression is inverted onto a mound of stone on a glass slab.

The trimming required to reduce the overall size of a poured cast is reduced by the use of this procedure, and since the material used is confined within the box, less plaster or artificial stone is required to make an adequate base for the cast.

Any impression can usually be boxed successfully if the dentist has trimmed it enough to expose the outer surface of the tray in which it was taken. Care must be taken with materials such as hydrocolloid and alginate to prevent distortion of the impressions. Impressions taken in modeling compound will not distort during the application of boxing wax.

An upper impression requires boxing material around its outer periphery only. This is easily accomplished. To hold the boxing material in place, it is **luted** (sealed to the tray with a warm instrument) with care to avoid damage to the impression material through the use of too much heat.

A lower impression is in the shape of a *U* and requires more effort to box well. The open section between the two arms of the *U* must be fitted with a piece of boxing material, which must then be well luted to the tray. Then another piece of boxing material is wrapped around the periphery of the tray, luted to the tray, and luted to the section that closes the opening between the arms of the *U*.

Pouring Casts

Impressions taken in impression plaster must be coated with a film of some material that will aid in separating the cast from the plaster impression material. The impression may be coated with tincture of green soap or with a commercial separator, made for this purpose, applied shortly before the impression is poured.

When an impression is boxed and the material of choice has been prepared, the cast is ready to be poured. The vibrator is turned on. A small quantity of the plaster or stone is picked up on the end of the plaster spatula. If the impression is an upper, the first addition of plaster or stone is made on the palate area while the impression tray is held snugly in contact with the vibrator plate. For a lower impression, the material is added at one or the other end of the *U*-shaped arch—the **heel area.** The plaster or stone will flow off the spatula even when mixed to a very heavy consistency.

Applied in small quantities to the palatal portion of the impression, the material will flow from the higher portion of the impression into the lower portions. When the impression has been partially filled with the plaster or stone, the remaining mix may be applied at the edge of the boxing material and allowed to flow down into the boxed impression until a satisfactory amount to provide a base for the impression has flowed in. The object in flowing the cast material into the impression is to prevent trapping of air in the lower portions of the

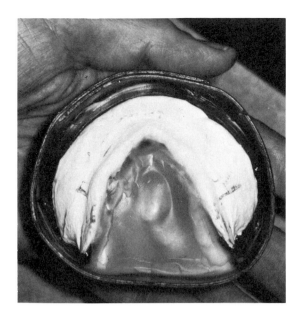

Figure 33.10
Mandibular impression boxed and ready to pour.

impression, especially when teeth are present on the cast, as well as to free any air bubbles that remain in the mix of plaster or stone.

If no mechanical vibrator is available, the cast material may be flowed into an impression by the use of a serrated instrument handle drawn across the handle of the tray, much like a violin bow is used on a violin. The serrations will create sufficient fine vibration to aid the flow of material.

Impressions taken in alginate or hydrocolloid materials must be treated according to the manufacturer's instructions upon completion of the pouring process. These materials otherwise absorb water from the plaster or stone, resulting in a soft, chalky surface on the finished cast.

The poured impressions should be given ample time to set thoroughly before separation is attempted. The average time required for the material used in your office will be indicated on the container in which it is supplied. The recommendations of the manufacturer should always be followed to insure the best results with the product. Excessive time is not recommended.

If boxing is not possible with an impression, the low portions of the impression are filled with the cast material, using the vibrator as indicated previously. When the impression has been filled to as high a level as possible, the remaining plaster or stone is placed in the center of a six-inch-square glass slab in the form of a mound. Care must be taken not to trap air. The filled impression is inverted over this mound of plaster or stone and gently seated until the periphery (edge) of the impression has been adequately covered with the cast material. All excess material is removed from the slab with the plaster spatula.

Separating Casts

Separation of casts from alginate or hydrocolloid impressions is easily accomplished. The boxing material, if used, is stripped from the base of the cast. Hold the tray firmly in one hand, and with the other hand grip the base of the cast and gently but firmly start the cast at one edge to permit air to enter between the cast and the impression material. It teeth are present on the cast, care must be taken to prevent breakage by not removing the cast at too great an angle. Once started, the cast should be lifted directly out of the impression.

If the impression is taken in modeling or impression compound, it is best inserted (after thorough setting is accomplished) in the compound heater set at a temperature of five degrees less than is required to prepare the impression compound for use. Care should be taken not to leave the poured impression in the water at this temperature for any longer time than is required. After five minutes' immersion at the proper temperature, gently try separating the cast from the impression. If the compound is still too firm to allow separation, replace it in the compound heater and repeat the trial each minute thereafter. Five to ten minutes is usually sufficient time. If watched properly, the compound will leave the cast very cleanly. If left in the bath too long, the compound may stick to the cast to some extent. While the cast is still warm from the heat of the bath, this remaining impression compound may be removed by "picking" it off with a piece of stick compound that has been softened in the flame of the laboratory burner.

If a compound heater is not available, a pan of water may be used for the same purpose to separate casts from impressions taken in modeling compound. Greater care must be exercised to prevent overheating the compound.

Immediately after separation, the casts should be trimmed and the patient's name written on the cast with an indelible pencil to provide a definite identification.

Trimming Casts

Properly boxed impressions will provide casts that require little if any trimming. A **cast trimmer** consists of a rotating disc, with a very gritty surface, attached to a motor and provided with some means of wetting the disc as it rotates. These are available in a large laboratory size and in a small dental-office size. The harder the material used to form the cast, the more desirable it is that any excess be avoided that will require trimming. Final finishing can be done with sandpaper after the cast is thoroughly dry.

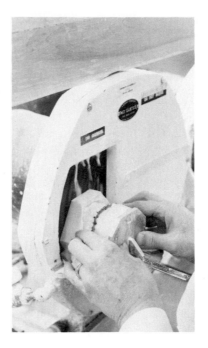

Figure 33.11
Dental assistant using a cast trimmer.

Orthodontic Casts[2]

An orthodontic cast is used for record purposes, often to show before and after conditions of an orthodontic case. The actual base of cast is called the **art portion** and the rest of the cast (showing the teeth and jaws) is called the **anatomical portion.** The art portion should be approximately ⅓ the total height from occlusal plane to the bottom of the cast; the anatomical portion is then ⅔ of the total height. The following directions and illustrations show how to make beautiful casts for orthodontic cases.

1. Trim the base of the lower cast (fig. 33.12). To do so,
    a. the cast should be wet, and
    b. the base should be trimmed parallel to the occlusal plane.
    c. Art portion should be ⅓ total height, anatomical portion: ⅔.
2. Trim the heel of the lower cast. This is a very important step. Study Figures 33.13, a–d and follow these directions:
    a. Use a divider to measure equidistant from midline at anterior teeth to an arc passing ¼ inch behind the last molar (whichever molar is farthest back).

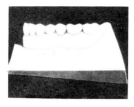

Figure 33.12
Trim base of lower cast.

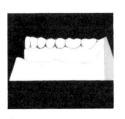 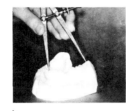 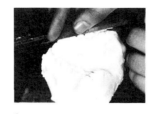 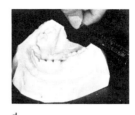

a   b   c   d

Figure 33.13
(a)–(d) Trim heel of lower cast.

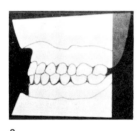 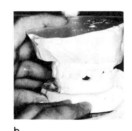

a   b

Figure 33.14
(a)–(b) Trim heel of upper cast.

b. Sight through the central grooves of the premolars and molars and make a mark intersecting the arc just scribed by the divider.

3. Trim the heel of the upper cast, following these directions:

a. Place upper and lower casts together, with teeth in occlusion (fig. 33.14, a).

b. Mark upper cast to correspond to the heel of the lower cast.

c. Trim the heel of the upper cast separately until you are close to the marks you just made.

d. Place the casts in occlusion for the final cut to minimize the danger of damaging the occlusal surfaces through handling (fig. 33.14 b).

4. Trim the top of the upper cast parallel to the base of the lower cast (fig. 33.15, a–c).

a. Because the casts are wet, the teeth are easily damaged so trim the upper cast separately.

b. Place the casts in occlusion on a flat surface. You are going to mark the casts for this cut. Scribe a line 2½ inches from the flat surface on which you have placed the casts. Be sure to mark all the way around the upper cast.

c. Make a final cut with the teeth in occlusion.

5. Trim the sides of the lower cast to a 55° angle with the heel (fig. 33.16, a–c).

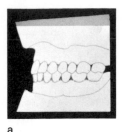
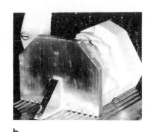
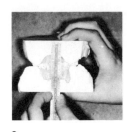

a　　　　　　　　b　　　　　　　　c

Figure 33.15
(a)–(c) Trim top of upper cast.

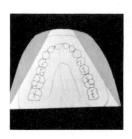
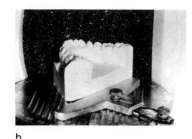
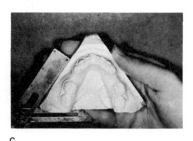

a　　　　　　　　b　　　　　　　　c

Figure 33.16
(a)–(c) Trim sides of lower cast 55°.

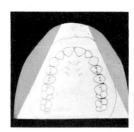
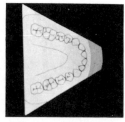
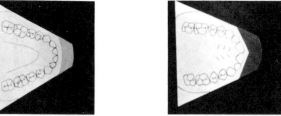
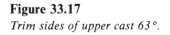

Figure 33.17
Trim sides of upper cast 63°.

Figure 33.18
Trim lower front round.

Figure 33.19
Trim upper front pointed.

    a. Check the angle with a hand instrument set for this purpose.

    b. Make the cut to within ⅜ inch of the premolar teeth, or to the base of the mucobuccal fold.

6. Trim the sides of the upper cast to a 63° angle with the heel (fig. 33.17).

    a. Check the angles with a hand instrument set for this purpose.

    b. Make the cut to within ⅜ inch of the premolar teeth, or to the base of the mucobuccal fold.

7. Trim the front of the lower cast to a curve (fig. 33.18).

    a. This rounded section should extend distally to the center of the lower canine on each side.

8. Trim the front of the upper cast to a point (fig. 33.19).

    a. The point should coincide with the median line of the upper teeth.

    b. Each cut extends distally to the center of the upper canine.

    c. The angle formed by these two cuts will vary because the angle depends on the shape of the upper arch of this particular patient.

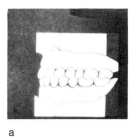
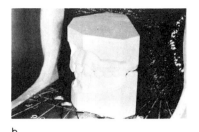

a   b

Figure 33.20
(a)–(b) Trim heel points to ½" 125°.

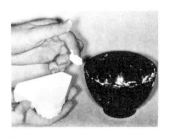
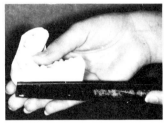
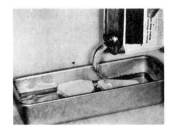
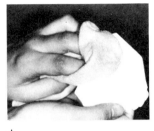

a   b   c   d

Figure 33.21
(a)–(d) Finishing the casts.

9. Trim the heel points to a plane ½ inch in width at an angle of 125° with the heel of the casts (fig. 33.20, a, b).
    a. Place the casts in occlusion for each corner cut.
10. Finish the casts (fig. 33.21, a–d).
    a. Fill all holes by working soft plaster into the cast with your finger. (a)
    b. Smooth the art portion of the cast by using a file. (b)
    c. Let the casts dry thoroughly.
    d. Soak for 30 minutes in a soap solution or other cast-finishing solution. (c)
    e. Shine the casts by rubbing with a chamois or soft flannel. (d)

Restorations

We come now to the replacement of missing teeth. The processes are complicated and require great accuracy. While the dentist will be performing many of the steps, some of the preparation will be your responsibility.

The several replacements include inlays, crowns, bridges, removable partials, and full dentures.

An **inlay** (intracoronal) replaces part of a tooth. It is cemented in place and restores the individual tooth to full function. If more tooth structure has been lost, the tooth receives a **crown.** A crown (extracoronal) replaces the entire outside of the tooth, leaving the center intact.

If a tooth must be removed, it is replaced with a **bridge.** A bridge can be made for one tooth or for several.

A bridge replacing one missing tooth is called a **three-tooth bridge.** It consists of two **abutments,** or supports, and a **pontic,** or replacement for the missing tooth. The abutments, of course, are placed on the natural teeth that are nearest the space left by the missing tooth in the mouth. The total length of a bridge is designated as the number of abutments plus the number of pontics.

Upper posterior bridges generally have a different type of pontic than a lower posterior bridge. Since a smile lifts the corners of the mouth upward, usually a porcelain or acrylic portion is made, called a **facing,** on the pontics of an upper posterior bridge. In the lower arch, food is passed between the tongue, cheeks, and lips during mastication. To provide for better mouth hygiene, lower posterior pontics are often made without facings and with some opening between the pontic and the ridge below it—somewhat as though the pontic is a hammock suspended between the abutment teeth. This type is referred to as a **hygienic pontic.**

When preparation of the teeth for support of a bridge has been completed, it is necessary to construct by some means an accurate model of the abutments, the ridge area between the abutments, the relationship of these two items to each other, and the relationship of the opposing arch to the area involved in the bridge.

Many different techniques are used to secure these impressions. A dentist may take individual impressions of the abutments, construct the abutment crowns, and have an appointment with the patient at which these abutments are placed in the mouth and a relationship impression taken in plaster. The bridge is then finished from this impression.

A removable **partial** replaces several teeth, usually not together. It is removed to clean it. Figure 28.29 illustrates a partial denture.

A **full denture** is made for someone who has no teeth. To assist in the restoration techniques, you will need to know about **Dies** or Positives of the impressions. Dies are replicas of the teeth that are being replaced either partially or completely. Dies may be used in the construction of inlays, crowns, bridges, or partial dentures.

After you are familiar with the making and use of dies, we will consider the techniques involved in the construction of the replacements: whether they be inlays, bridges, or dentures.

Dies (Positives of the Impressions)

The Stone Die

An individual tooth impression of rubber base inside a copper band is first wrapped with a sheet of softened wax or a piece of masking tape so that the "root" portion will be approximately ½″ long.

The special die stone is then prepared according to the manufacturer's directions and either vacuumed to remove the entrapped fine air bubbles or vibrated onto a piece of paper toweling and squeezed to remove excess water, as well as to reduce the likelihood of bubbles.

Removable dies of individual teeth can be incorporated into quadrant or full arch impressions. Die pin spotters are commercially available that will permit the pouring of multiple removable dies with only one mix of stone. Each manufacturer has specific instructions for the best use of the product.

Electroplating

Some dentists still perform another operation in the preparation of dies before they are used for constructing the wax pattern. This additional operation consists of giving the impression a coating of copper by electroplating processes. It is considered an effective way of securing a better working surface on the die. When the amalgam, stone, or other material is packed into the impression after the impression has been electroplated with copper, it is allowed to set hard in the usual manner. Upon separation, the copper shell that has been deposited in the impression forms the outer surface of the die. The thickness of the copper is controlled by the length of time the impression is plated

and the amount of current used during this period of time. The process is always begun at a slow rate, which can be increased once the initial film of copper has been deposited, until the thickness has reached the point preferred by the dentist. Copper-plated dies are used very well with a light coating of microfilm as a separating medium.

Lubricating the Die

The amalgam die is coated with microfilm or similar separating media. A die of artificial stone may be soaked or vacuumed in a mixture of 50 percent glycerin and 50 percent water, dried, and then given a light coating of microfilm. These surface coatings facilitate removal of the wax pattern after it has been shaped on the die and is to be sprued. Without such a coating, the wax pattern is almost impossible to remove without fracturing. The lubricant used should be water-soluble; never use machine oil. It should be a thin lubricant. Do not use too much. Any oily lubricant, or too much of any kind of lubricant, can result in a rough casting.

Copings

After the dentist has made individual dies of crown preparations in the construction of a bridge, he or she may decide to make copings for the abutment teeth. A **coping** is made as a thimble that fits over each crown preparation. It is placed in the mouth over the crown preparation to check the gingival fit. When the dentist is satisfied that the gingival fit of each coping is accurate, he or she places the copings over each crown and takes a plaster impression, embedding them in the plaster. The impression is allowed to set and is then removed from the mouth as any other plaster impression would be. Now the individual dies of the crown preparations that were previously made are set in the copings in the impression, and a working cast is poured. When the cast is separated, the dies will be in their proper relationship because the copings will have held them accurately in place.

Indirect Inlay Technique

Step One: Mixing an Impression Tray for Single or Multiple Inlays

Whenever an individual inlay is to be made for a patient, a series of preparations must be completed. A stone model of a section of the mouth is made prior to any dental procedures. This stone model is then used to make a custom tray. This special impression tray is prepared for either single or multiple inlays. We have illustrated the steps in this process so that you may more easily understand what is expected of you.

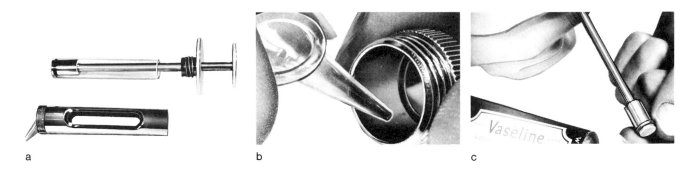

a   b   c

Figure 33.22
(a)–(c) A syringe used for elastic impression materials. (a) The syringe before assembly; (b) insert the plastic tip into the tip retainer; and (c) lubricate the rubber ring washer with white petrolatum jelly.

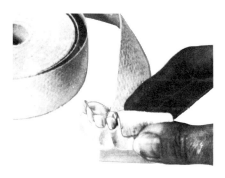

Figure 33.23
The liner material, moistened and folded over the teeth.

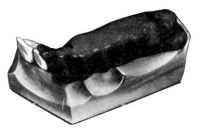

Figure 33.24
The second piece of liner placed on the teeth.

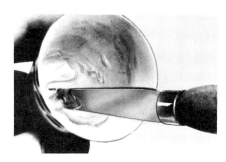

Figure 33.25
Combine powder and liquid in a 30-second mix.

1. The first task for you will be to assemble the syringe that is used to place the light-bodied impression material. (See fig. 33.22, a-c.) To assemble the syringe for use, first insert the plastic tip into the tip retainer (b). Screw retainer into metal barrel, then lightly lubricate the rubber ring washer with white petroleum jelly (c). Then insert the plunger into the plastic sleeve and push forward until the plunger is flush with the end of the plastic sleeve. Now set the syringe aside until the elastic impression material has been mixed.
2. From the roll of liner material, cut two pieces, one shorter than the other. Moisten the shorter piece and fold as shown in figure 33.23 and place over the teeth.
3. Moisten the second piece of liner material and adapt it lengthwise (fig. 33.24). Remove the liner from two small areas to provide stops to prevent the tray from setting too far down when the actual impression is taken.
4. In a mixing bowl, combine powder and liquid and mix for thirty seconds (fig. 33.25). Allow it to stand until it is nonsticky (fig. 33.26). Now you can preform this tray to the approximate size (fig. 33.27).
5. Adapt material over the liner and form a handle (fig. 33.28). Note the operator is forming a handle at the left end of the illustration. In seven to ten minutes remove the tray and strip out the liner material (fig. 33.29).

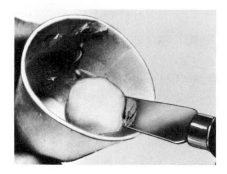

Figure 33.26
Tray material ready to use.

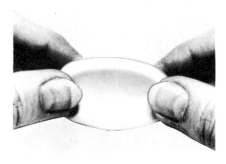

Figure 33.27
Preform the tray.

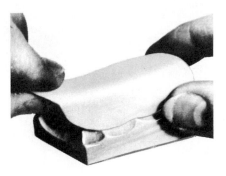

Figure 33.28
Forming a handle for the tray.

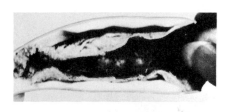

Figure 33.29
Remove tray and strip out liner material.

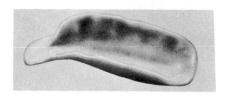

Figure 33.30
The completed tray.

6. The custom-built tray is now completed (fig. 33.30) and only needs to have adhesive applied lightly to all inner and peripheral surfaces. The adhesive must be allowed to dry before using the tray.

Step Two: Making the Impression in the Custom-Made Tray

1. Layout the base and catalyst for the light-bodied impression material and mix in 45 to 60 seconds. Load the syringe that you prepared in Step one so that you complete the mixing and loading in not more than 1 1/2 minutes (fig. 33.31).
2. Put the entire mix of light-bodied impression material in a dappen dish (fig. 33.32).
3. Insert the sleeve of the syringe with plunger into the dappen dish and with locking disc forced against plastic sleeve, draw the plunger back slowly to fill the sleeve (fig. 33.33).
4. Now wipe the end of the sleeve clean of excess material (fig. 33.34).
5. Place the filled plastic sleeve in the metal barrel of the syringe and screw locking disc

down as far as possible. Tighten securely (fig. 33.35).
6. Next, mix the heavy-bodied material base and catalyst for approximately one minute (fig. 33.36).
7. Your dentist may ask you to spread heavy-bodied material over all adhesive-covered surfaces of the tray, using the remainder of the mix to fill the tray. Avoid trapping air in the material (fig. 33.37).
8. While you are preparing the tray, the dentist will dry the prepared teeth, inject light-bodied material into all preparations in the mouth (fig. 33.38).
9. The last small amount of light-bodied material is ejected by the dentist between teeth in an area not involved in the impression, to provide a means of checking the set of the material (fig. 33.39).

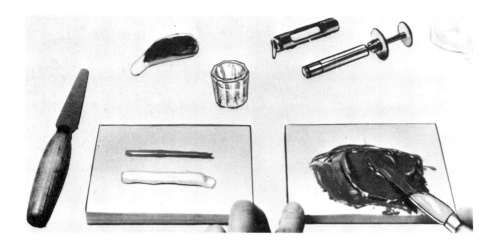

Figure 33.31
Equipment assembled for making light-bodied impression material.

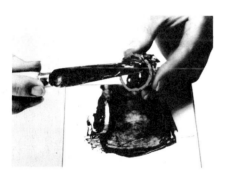

Figure 33.32
Transfer the mix to a dappen dish.

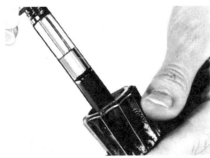

Figure 33.33
Fill the syringe with the mix.

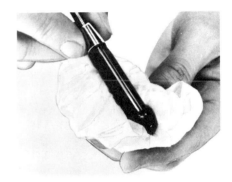

Figure 33.34
Clean the syringe.

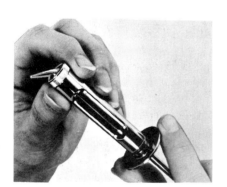

Figure 33.35
Assemble the filled syringe.

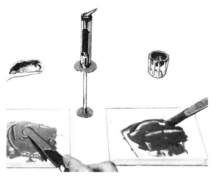

Figure 33.36
Mixing the heavy-bodied material.

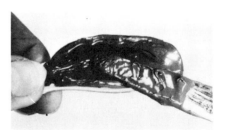

Figure 33.37
Spreading the heavy-bodied impression material over all adhesive-covered surfaces.

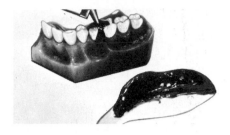

Figure 33.38
Injecting the light-bodied material into all preparations.

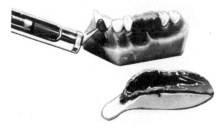

Figure 33.39
The small amount of light-bodied material injected between the teeth away from the impression area.

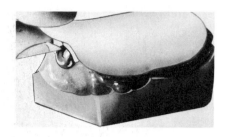

Figure 33.40
The dentist seats the tray immediately.

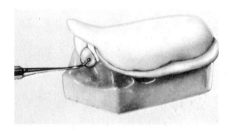

Figure 33.41
The dentist checks the set of the material.

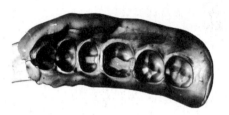

Figure 33.42
The finished impression.

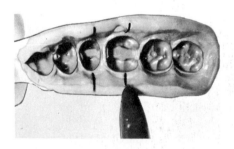

Figure 33.43
Guidelines for locating prepared teeth and positioning dowel pins.

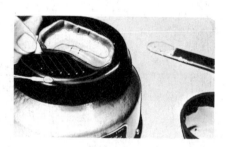

Figure 33.44
Pour impression using medium vibration.

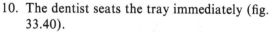

10. The dentist seats the tray immediately (fig. 33.40).
11. Ten minutes after beginning the mix of light-bodied material the dentist checks the small amount for set, removes the tray from the mouth and gives it to you (fig. 33.41).
12. Take the impression and rinse it well. Then blow it dry before pouring the model (fig. 33.42).

Step Three: Pouring the Model

Casts and dies can be poured in die stone, or the impressions can be electroplated. The series of illustrations included illustrate only the stone model technique.

1. With a ball point pen or pencil, draw guidelines on the impression to locate the prepared teeth and position dowel pins (fig. 33.43).
2. Mix enough die stone to fill the impression tray 3 to 5 millimeters above the gingival of the teeth. Vacuum mixing is best, but the mix can be completed by hand spatulation.
3. Pour the impression, using medium vibration. Make small additions of mixed stone until the impression is filled 3 to 5 millimeters above the teeth (fig. 33.44).

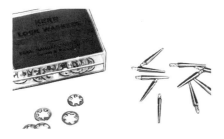

Figure 33.45
Dowel pins and lock washers illustrated.

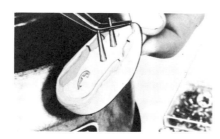

Figure 33.46
Setting the dowel pins and lock washers into the soft stone.

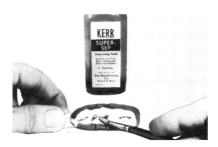

Figure 33.47
Apply separating fluid over all areas of dies that are to be removable.

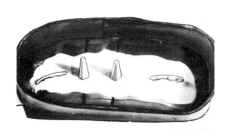

Figure 33.48
Box impression preparation ready for final pouring.

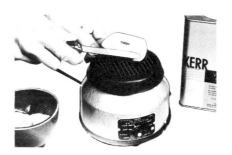

Figure 33.49
Pouring the second mix of die stone to complete the model.

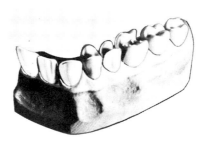

Figure 33.50
After the stone is set, separate the model from the impression.

4. Use dowel pins to produce removable individual dies. Lock washers provide the anchorage between the two pours of stone (fig. 33.45).
5. Rest your hand on the vibrator with the switch on low. Line up dowel pins with markings on the impression and set them into the soft stone. Set the lock washers halfway down in sections that are not to be separated. The upper half will then project into the space that will be filled with the second pouring of stone (fig. 33.46).
6. Allow the first pour of stone to set, then apply one or more coats of separating fluid only over areas of dies that are to be removable (fig. 33.47).
7. Box the impression in preparation for the final pouring of stone (fig. 33.48).
8. To make it easy to locate the dowel pins later, place a piece of utility wax across the ends of them. Make a second mix of stone and complete pouring the model (fig. 33.49).

Step Four: Cutting the Removable Dies and Completing the Castings

1. When the second mix of stone is set, separate the model from the impression (fig. 33.50).
2. Cut through the first pour of stone with a 2/0 gauge saw blade (fig. 33.51).
3. Notice the angle of the cut in figure 33.52. The cuts must be either vertical or converging at the base of the first pour of stone to permit withdrawal of dies.
4. Remove wax from ends of dowel pins. Tap dowel pins lightly to help remove the die from the model (fig. 33.53).
5. Remove the dies. They are now ready to be trimmed (fig. 33.54).
6. Remove excess stone from gingival margins of dies with a sharp blade (fig. 33.55).
7. Lubricate the dies with microfilm (fig. 33.56).

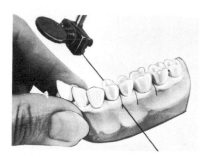

Figure 33.51
Cutting through the first pour of stone.

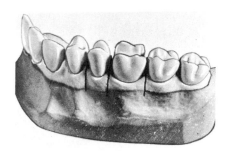

Figure 33.52
Cuts that will permit the withdrawal of the dies.

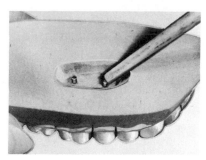

Figure 33.53
Removing the die from the model.

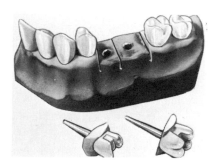

Figure 33.54
Dies removed and ready for trimming.

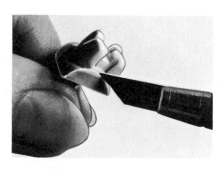

Figure 33.55
Clean the excess stone from gingival margins.

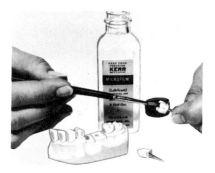

Figure 33.56
Lubricate dies with microfilm.

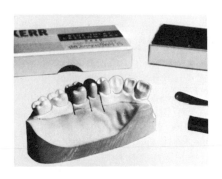

Figure 33.57
Wax patterns on dies.

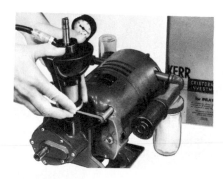

Figure 33.58
The vacuum investing unit.

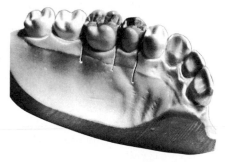

Figure 33.59
Unpolished castings on stone dies.

8. The wax registrations made by the dentist at the time of treatment are now placed on the dies and the wax patterns completed (fig. 33.57).
9. The now completed wax patterns are removed from the dies, sprued and invested as described in chapter 34 (fig. 33.58).
10. The unpolished castings are seated on stone dies (fig. 33.59).
11. This is how the polished castings look (fig. 33.60).

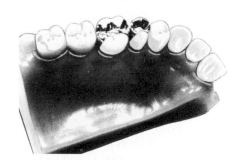

Figure 33.60
The polished castings.

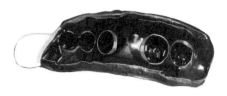

Figure 33.61
The rinsed and dried completed impression.

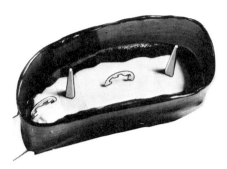

Figure 33.62
The model poured with the first mix of stone.

Fixed Prostheses Impression Techniques

Impressions for fixed bridges are taken in the same manner as those for single or multiple inlay impressions.

In constructing the bridge, however, it is sometimes desirable to keep the abutment teeth and the included ridge area of the cast in one solid piece. (This is especially true in the most common bridge, that which replaces one missing tooth, a **three-tooth bridge.**) To accomplish this goal it is necessary to make the teeth adjacent to the abutment teeth (beyond the bridge area) removable so that the wax patterns can be carved. Starting with the completed impression follow these directions to prepare the model for this method of bridge construction.

1. Rinse and dry the completed impression. Use a pencil or ball point pen and draw guide lines to the teeth adjacent to the abutment teeth in order to properly position the dowel pins (fig. 33.61).
2. Prepare the first mix of stone. Pour model just as you did in steps 3–7 in the section titled *Pouring the Model* (figs. 33.44–33.48). When the stone is set, paint separating fluid over areas of the teeth that are to be removable. Complete the pouring for the cast (fig. 33.62).

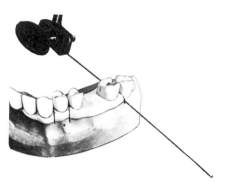

Figure 33.63
Sectioning the model so adjacent teeth can be removed.

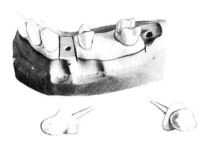

Figure 33.64
The model with the adjacent teeth removed.

3. When the stone is set again, remove model from impression and section it so that the teeth adjacent to the abutments can be removed (fig. 33.63).
4. Remove adjacent teeth. Leave the entire bridge space attached to the main body of the model. Lubricate the dies, wax, invest, burn out, and cast the bridge (fig. 33.64).
5. Finished fixed bridge is shown on stone model in figure 33.65.

Copper-Band Impressions

Another technique with which you may be requested to assist is the preparation of an impression made in a copper band.

1. The dentist will have prepared the copper band to fit properly in the patient's mouth. Reinforce the copper band by plugging one end with impression compound (fig. 33.66).

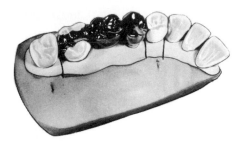

Figure 33.65
Finished fixed bridge on stone model.

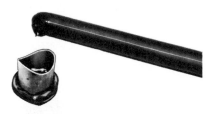

Figure 33.66
A copper band for impression technique.

2. Paint the inside of the band with adhesive (fig. 33.67).
3. Mix the impression material within 30 to 60 seconds. While your dentist is drying the tooth, load the band carefully. Avoid trapping air. When the dentist has completed the impression, it is blown dry and inspected. Pour the die according to your usual laboratory procedures (fig. 33.68).

Removable Prostheses

Denture Casts

Denture casts are of two types: complete denture or partial denture. Complete denture impressions will be impressions of **edentulous ridges**—the ridges without teeth present. Partial denture impressions may include any number of teeth—they are **dentulous** impressions. Study casts may be poured in plaster, and working casts are generally poured in artificial stone of the type preferred by the dentist.

Complete denture impressions can be boxed in the same manner as other impressions. Care must be taken, however, to include all the area desired for the construction of the denture. Since no teeth are present, the limits of the cast are dictated by other anatomical landmarks.

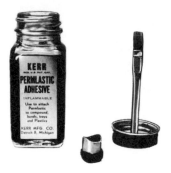

Figure 33.67
Paint the inside of the copper band.

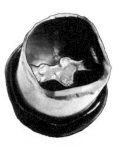

Figure 33.68
The copper band impression.

Either the dentist or the dental assistant (where state law permits) takes impressions with alginate for study casts.

Study casts made from these impressions are used to form a special tray for taking the final impression. This individualized tray may be made from acrylic resin tray material adapted directly to the cast or by using a wax spacer. Other tray materials are vinyl or double thickness shellac base plate material. When the tray is prepared, the dentist makes the final impression of the edentulous ridge areas, using any of several impression materials: rubber base, silicones, zinc oxide and eugenol impression pastes, poly-ether, impression plaster, mouth softening wax, etc. The final cast is poured in these impressions in the same manner as with any other impression material. Of these impression materials, plaster is the only one that requires a separating medium. To facilitate separation when zinc-oxide pastes are used, the cast and impression are immersed in water at about 160° for ten minutes, after which separation is easily accomplished because the zinc oxide paste and the base material will be softened to some degree to facilitate peeling it from the cast and tray. *Remember to mark the casts with the patient's name immediately after separation and trimming.*

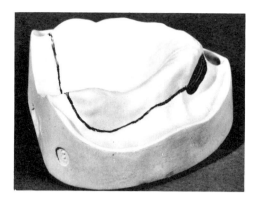

Figure 33.69
Making an individual impression tray.

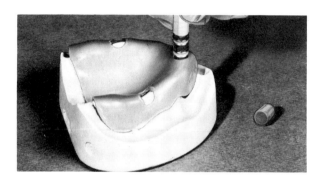

Figure 33.70
Wax spacer adapted over the cast.

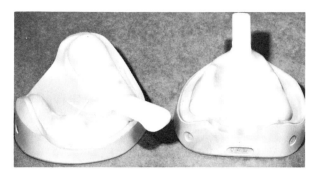

Figure 33.71
Completed lower and upper individualized trays adapted to casts, showing handles attached.

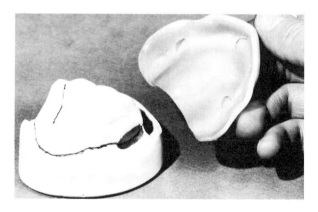

Figure 33.72
Completed upper tray separated from the cast.

Casts for partial dentures must be separated very carefully from the impression material, especially if isolated teeth are present in the arch. These can be very easily fractured during separation unless the cast is withdrawn from the impression in a line parallel to the long axis of the teeth. Trial bases may be constructed for partial denture procedures, particularly if more than half the teeth are missing from the arch involved. If less than half the teeth are missing, the dentist very frequently will arrange some form of bite registration at the time the impressions are taken.

Trial Bases

Trial bases are then constructed for complete denture cases. They can be fabricated from vinyl, acrylic resin, gutta-percha base plate material, or shellac base plate material. It is imperative that the material of choice be very accurately adapted to the cast. To avoid distortion of the trial base or damage to the cast, undercuts are blocked out (usually in wax) prior to adapting the trial base material.

Occlusal Rims

A wax **occlusal rim** is next applied to the trial base. One type of wax occlusal rim material is supplied in 4 1/2″ bars of wax about 1/2″ square in cross section. These are softened in warm water. (The softening temperature is usually about 125° unless otherwise stated on the box in which the wax rims are supplied.) They are then molded into a curve to correspond with the curve of the dental ridge on the cast. (Another type comes already molded into the curve.) Melted wax is used to fill in the spaces and angles between the baseplate gutta-percha and the wax bite rim until a smooth contour is established. When well filled in, the wax surface may be "flamed" slightly and wiped with a dry towel to produce a shiny, smooth surface.

After dentures are processed by the commercial laboratory, they are frequently remounted in the articulator to recheck articulation of the teeth. If the original mounting has not been preserved by the laboratory, then a new base to hold the finished denture must be made. Since most dentures will have some areas that are **undercuts,** they could not be removed from a plaster

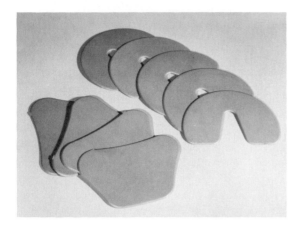

Figure 33.73
Trial base plates.

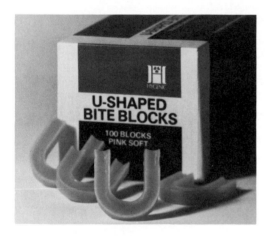

Figure 33.74
Occlusal wax rims.

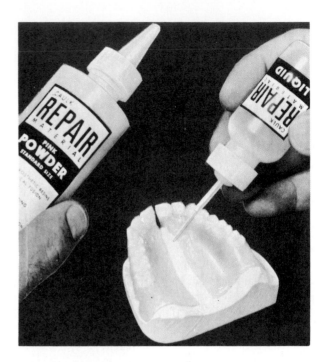

Figure 33.75
Adding powder and liquid to a denture fracture.

base that is poured directly into the denture. To facilitate removal from these temporary bases, the tissue side of the denture is lightly coated with Vaseline; then all the undercut areas are filled in with wet pumice or wet cotton patted into place with the finger. When the plaster base is made over this preparation, the denture can be easily removed when desired and can be easily cleaned (fig. 33.74).

Emergency Denture Repair

One of the common denture emergencies is the breaking of the denture along the midline. The repair of this breakage can be accomplished as follows:

1. Lock the two halves into their proper relationship by placing short applicator sticks or wooden matchsticks across the arch, luting each end to the teeth with sticky wax. (The same process may be used if the denture is broken into more pieces, which occasionally occurs.)
2. Eliminate undercuts with wetted cotton or pumice.
3. Gently fill the tissue side of the denture with plaster. The line of fracture must be completely supported by plaster, however.
4. After the plaster has set, remove the pieces of the denture from the cast and wash them clean.
5. Widen the area of the fracture, using a vulcanite bur in a dental lathe or handpiece.
6. Cover the plaster that is in the area of the fracture with tinfoil, carefully burnishing it into place with a piece of cotton. An alternate method is to give the plaster a coating of **liquid foil** made for this purpose.
7. Reposition the pieces of the denture on the cast.
8. Now, by alternately adding repair powder and liquid, replace the area cut away through the fracture (fig. 33.75).
9. Thoroughly cure according to directions with the material you use. (The cure may be hastened by immersing the cast and denture in water.)
10. Trim and polish the repair area to create a smooth joint with the original denture parts.

Summary

Two of the materials used to produce a positive cast or model from an impression are *plaster* and *artificial stone*. Each type of stone and plaster has specific uses in the dental office. They must be properly stored and carefully used. Be accurate in measuring water and powder when mixing them.

Directions for mixing plaster and stone vary and are given specifically in this chapter. Be sure you care for the bowls and spatulas when you are through with the mixing process.

An impression may be *boxed*.

All casts should be properly poured and separated. Orthodontic casts should then be trimmed.

Casts are mounted on an articulator to provide a working relationship for construction of inlays, crowns, bridges, and partial or complete dentures.

Single tooth impressions are used to construct an *individual stone die*, a positive cast of the impression of the tooth. The die stones are also used with elastic impression materials.

Some dentists also *electroplate* the impression. It gives a better working surface on the die.

Several materials can be used to lubricate the *die* so that it will permit the *wax pattern* to slip off without fracturing when the pattern has been completed.

Custom trays for impressions for both single and multiple inlays and bridges are also made. Four techniques for different procedures are illustrated. Pouring casts with removable dies is also illustrated.

Complete and *partial denture casts* must be handled carefully. Impression trays and trial bases may be constructed for complete denture cases.

Emergency repairs of dentures with laboratory supplies available in the dental office are often made.

Study Questions

1. Explain the uses in the dental office of artificial stone and plaster.
2. Describe the difference in mixing artificial stone and plaster.
3. Explain the process of boxing.
4. Describe the steps in preparing casts.
5. Describe the preparation of orthodontic casts.
6. Define *die*.
7. What materials are used to make a die?
8. What is the purpose of copings?
9. Describe four techniques for constructing custom trays.
10. Describe an emergency denture repair.

CHAPTER 34

Basic Principles of Casting to Dimension

Successful Casting Technique
Wax Patterns
   Spruing the Pattern
   Thickness of Sprue
   Attaching the Sprue
   Mounting the Pattern on Crucible Former (Sprue
      Base)
Two Methods of Investing
   Introduction
   Investing the Pattern (Without Vacuum)
      Lining the Casting Ring
      Cleaning the Pattern
      Mixing the Investment
      Painting the Pattern
      Filling the Ring
   Vacuum Investing
Removing the Crucible Former and Sprue
Burning Out the Mold
   Too Rapid Burnout
   Overheating the Mold
   Incomplete Wax Elimination
   A Practical Burnout Technique
Melting the Gold
   Gas-Air Blowpipe Technique
Casting
Fluxing
Cleaning Residue Buttons
Correct Casting Temperature
Heat Treatment
Pickling
Finishing and Polishing

The process of constructing restorations outside the mouth includes three important stages. In the last two chapters we have learned to take an impression of an area in the mouth after it has been prepared for the restoration; then we learned to make a wax model or pattern, invest it, and burn it out. The hardened investment material now contains a hole shaped like the inlay or crown that is to be made of gold alloy.

The next process, to cast the gold alloy into the hole in the investment material, is the subject of this chapter.

Successful Casting Technique

A successful inlay casting technique[1] must produce accurately fitting inlays. To do this it must utilize the dimensional changes of the wax, investment, and gold in such a manner that the shrinkages and expansions balance out, with the net result that the casting is neither smaller nor larger than the wax pattern that was originally made to fit the preparation. There are a number of ways the shrinkages and expansions can be made to counterbalance each other. Theoretically, it should be possible to measure exactly the amount of shrinkage or expansion of each material and the effects on these dimensional changes of variations in manipulative procedure. With the aid of these data, it is possible to select a combination of materials and technique that would invariably produce the required accuracy. From a practical standpoint, the problem is not as simple as this, and a certain amount of trial and error is necessary. Nevertheless, a basic understanding of the properties of the materials used and of the effects of variations in manipulative procedure does make it possible to establish a satisfactory technique with a minimum of experimentation and to standardize the various steps so that consistent results will be obtained.

The principal shrinkage to consider is the casting shrinkage of gold that, in common with most materials, expands when heated and contracts when cooled. Since the gold must be liquid to cast, the mold is filled with expanded metal that shrinks as it cools to room temperature. Unless compensated by an expanded mold, the casting will be too small. The casting shrinkage of gold alloys was studied at the National Bureau of Standards, and the results were published in Research Paper No. 32. It was found that in every case the net casting shrinkage was less than the free thermal contraction of the metal from its solidifying temperature to room temperature. This was thought to be due, at least in part, to the fact that at very high temperatures the metal was quite weak and might actually be weaker than the investment, so that if there was any interlocking between the casting and the investment mold, the cooling metal would be held and stretched by the

investment and thus prevented from shrinking its normal amount. This suggests that thin castings and those which, because of their irregular shape, would be well locked in the investment mold might show somewhat less shrinkage than bulky castings or those with fewer irregularities. This may explain why bulky castings appear to require more compensation than thin ones, and one-surface inlays more than two- or three-surface inlays. It may also explain why the tests made at the Bureau of Standards on gold rods 12/100 of an inch in diameter and 3¼ inches long, cast under dental laboratory conditions, showed a net linear casting shrinkage of 1¼ percent, while more recent tests made on much shorter and bulkier rods, cast in abnormally weak investment molds, showed shrinkages ranging up to about 1⅗ percent. There is also evidence that casting golds with varying compositions have slightly different casting shrinkages, but these differences appear to be so small as to be of little practical significance.

Other factors that might make the casting too small include possible shrinkages of the impression and die materials in the indirect method, and thermal contraction of the wax pattern. Impression materials, for instance, have relatively high rates of contraction on cooling, which can result in serious inaccuracies if uncontrolled. However, if the compound, hydrocolloid, or rubber-base impression material is used with a very careful technique, the impression can be made to fit the preparation at a temperature low enough to minimize the effect of its normal shrinkage on cooling. Similarly, the impression should be guarded against temperature changes during the interval between removal and completion of the die.

If the die is to be made of amalgam, avoid an alloy that shrinks on setting and use one that has a very slight setting expansion. Most of the gypsum-base die materials have a small setting expansion, which is desirable. If the impression is copper-plated before the die is poured, the setting expansion of the die material has no effect on the size of the die. Wide variations in the temperature of the plating solution will, of course, cause corresponding variations in the size of the impression being plated.

Pattern waxes also have high rates of thermal expansion and contraction so that if the pattern is made to fit the preparation at one temperature and invested at a lower temperature, shrinkage will be produced. Such shrinkage can be avoided by investing the pattern at the same temperature at which it was made or compensated for by providing additional expansion of the mold. The thermal expansion of the wax and the setting expansion, hygroscopic expansion, and thermal expansion of the investment are the principal compensating means available for offsetting unavoidable shrinkages.

Inlay wax has a high rate of thermal expansion so that if the pattern is made to fit the preparation at approximate room temperature, and then invested at a higher temperature, a relatively large expansion will be introduced. This was one of the earliest methods used in compensating for the casting shrinkage of gold. Unfortunately, it presents a number of practical difficulties, chief of which is the fact that when a wax pattern that has been formed to the preparation and chilled under pressure is reheated, it not only expands but also tends to warp due to the release of internal strains. Although progress has been made toward overcoming this fault, the danger of warpage still appears to be a real hazard; and consequently, thermal expansion of the wax pattern as a major means of compensation has been largely abandoned.

The setting expansion of investments varies from brand to brand and also with the water/powder ratio. Generally speaking, the thicker the mix, the more the expansion. The amount of the setting expansion for various water/powder ratios is usually published by the manufacturer and may run as high as ½ percent. While this type of expansion does affect the size of the mold, it is doubtful if the full theoretical amount is effective in compensating casting shrinkage. In the case of full and three-quarter crowns, MOD inlays, and similar patterns, there is a tendency for the wax pattern to restrain the setting expansion of the investment. In order for this expansion to take place unrestrictedly, the wax pattern should move uniformly with the investment. This could occur theoretically if the heat evolved by the setting investment were just enough to expand the wax thermally as much as the investment itself expands due to its setting reaction, but it seems doubtful if this exact balance is achieved. Therefore, the wax pattern will be stretched by the force of the expanding investment or the investment will be compressed by the resistance of the confining wax pattern. What actually takes place is probably a combination of three things: (1) some thermal expansion of the wax due to the heat of the setting reaction, (2) some stretching of the wax by the force of the setting reaction, and (3) some compression of the investment by the resistance of the wax pattern. Consequently, the full amount of the setting expansion will rarely be effective in expanding the mold, and the degree to which it is effective may vary depending upon the type of pattern and the physical characteristics of the wax and investment used. There is also a tendency for the metal inlay ring to restrain the setting expansion radically and force it to take place toward the open ends of the ring, causing distortion. However, the use of a liner to serve as a cushion and permit free expansion in all directions can eliminate this effect.

Hygroscopic expansion of the investment occurs when the investment sets in contact with water, and for some investment compositions it is much greater than ordinary setting expansion. The exact mechanism of this expansion is obscure, but it is known that the amount varies with the formula of the investment, the water/powder ratio, the temperature of the water in which the investment is immersed, the amount of time after mixing at which it is immersed, and the length of time it is kept immersed. The usual procedure is to invest the pattern and immediately immerse the ring in water at approximately 100° F. and allow it to stay there until the investment has set. A commercial investment especially designed for this technique is stated by its manufacturer to have an "effective hygroscopic expansion" of about 1⅖ percent after thirty minutes' immersion at approximately 100° F., after which there is no further change. However, there is some uncertainty as to how much of this expansion is actually effective in enlarging the mold, because the same factors that tend to restrict ordinary setting expansion are also operative here, though to a much more limited extent. The temperature of the water bath will expand the wax pattern, but the amount of this expansion is ordinarily much less than the hygroscopic expansion so that the difference will be reflected in stretching of the wax and compression of the investment. Although the softened wax offers less resistance to stretching, it seems probable that it would still have sufficient strength to compress the investment to some extent, especially in the early stages of the setting reaction. To be considered, also, is the possible danger of warpage of the pattern due to the higher temperature of the wax and the release of internal strains as previously described. While the exact amount of the enlargement of the mold by hygroscopic expansion is indefinite, it is certain that if an additonal ⅘ to ⁹⁄₁₀ percent thermal expansion were added by heating to approximately 1300° F., the mold would be overexpanded, and the casting would be too large. For this reason the mold is cast at a lower temperature, usually about 800° to 900° F., at which temperature the thermal expansion of the investment is only about ³⁄₁₀ percent. At this relatively low temperature, a much longer time would be required to carbonize and eliminate the wax by burning it out in the usual manner. This problem is met in one of three ways: by heating the ring rapidly while the investment is still wet so that the water in the investment will boil and flush out the wax; by flushing out the wax by placing the ring in a pan of boiling water; or by removing the wax with a suction device made for the purpose. Properly controlled, the hygroscopic technique yields excellent results in the form of well-fitting castings with smooth surfaces.

Thermal expansion of investment is perhaps the most easily and accurately controlled of the various expansion means available for compensating the casting shrinkage of gold. Again, the amount will vary over a wide range, depending upon the type of investment, the water/powder ratio, and the temperature at which the casting is made. It may be as much as 1⁷⁄₂₀ percent. Data on the thermal expansion for various water/powder ratios over the commonly used range of temperature are available from most investment manufacturers. Since the metal ring and the investment do not expand at the same rate when heated, it is advisable to line the ring with material to serve as a cushion that will allow the investment to expand freely. If this is done, the maximum thermal expansion should be fully effective in enlarging the mold.

Most of the investments intended for this technique are heated to approximately 1300°F. to develop thermal expansion that, combined with the usable setting expansion, will completely compensate for the average 1¼ percent casting shrinkage of gold. There is one type of investment that develops sufficient thermal expansion at 800° to 900°F. so that the mold may be cast at that temperature or at 1300°F., depending on the wax elimination technique followed.

From the foregoing discussion it is clear that in spite of the great advances in the common fund of knowledge on this subject and the enormously improved materials and techniques that have been provided, there are still factors common to all inlay techniques that are not completely provided for and understood. Inlay casting is not yet an exact science. Nevertheless, enough is known of the properties of the materials used and the effects of variations in manipulative procedures to enable the operator to make enlightened choice of materials and techniques and, with some experimentation, to make such adjustments in his or her procedure as may be necessary to meet individual requirements.

For efficient and practical operation, a standardized technique should be adapted to the need and equipment of the office and made routine. With the various steps in the technique standardized as far as possible, it will be reasonable to expect consistently satisfactory results. Furthermore, it will be relatively easy to detect and correct any errors that might creep into the technique.

Inlay castings that come out too small or too tight indicate that more compensating expansion is needed. If the operator is presently using a low-heat technique, a study of the curve in figure 34.1 will show what would happen if the burnout temperature were increased. Assuming the investment has a thermal expansion curve as shown in figure 34.1 and the burnout temperature was about 800°F., we see that the thermal expansion of the mold is less at that temperature than at any other between 600° and 1650°F. Increasing the burnout

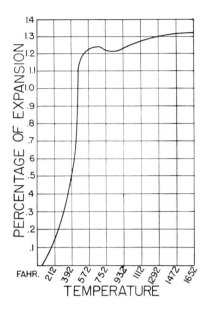

Figure 34.1
Thermal expansion curve of Cristobalite inlay investment.

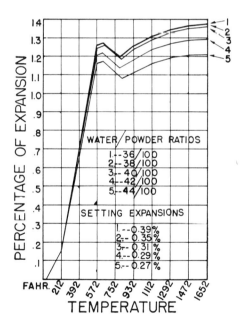

Figure 34.2
Thermal expansion of Cristobalite inlay investment, using different water-powder ratios.

temperature to 1000°F. or over would increase the amount of expansion. Referring to figure 34.3 (the thermal expansion curve of another widely used investment), we see that thermal expansion is also increased as the mold temperature is increased.

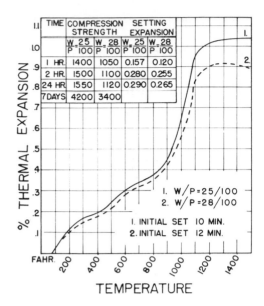

TIME	COMPRESSION STRENGTH		SETTING EXPANSION	
	W_25/P_100	W_28/P_100	W_25/P_100	W_28/P_100
1 HR.	1400	1050	0.157	0.120
2 HR.	1500	1100	0.280	0.255
24 HR.	1550	1120	0.290	0.265
7 DAYS	4200	3400		

1. W/P = 25/100
2. W/P = 28/100

1. INITIAL SET 10 MIN.
2. INITIAL SET 12 MIN.

Figure 34.3

Physical properties of Ransom and Randolph gray investment.

Both figures 34.2 and 34.3 illustrate another method of gaining mold expansion: by decreasing the water/powder ratio. The thicker the mix, the greater the thermal expansion at any temperature. It is true, furthermore, that the thicker mixes produce greater setting expansion.

Figure 34.4 shows the hygroscopic expansion curve of an investment developed especially for this technique. As can be seen, the greater the length of time—up to thirty minutes—that the investment is allowed to set in water, the greater the expansion. The expansion may also be increased by using a thicker mix, by increasing the temperature of the water bath, or by immersing the investment sooner after mixing.

Figure 34.5 shows the thermal expansion of this same investment, and it is evident that the expansion can be increased by raising the burnout temperature up to 1400°F. Between about 950° and 1200°F. this investment expands very rapidly so that a small variation in temperature causes a relatively large variation in the size of the mold. To avoid this wide and hard-to-control variation, it is preferable to cast either below

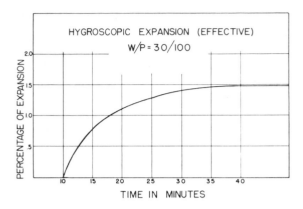

Figure 34.4

Effective hygroscopic expansion of Ransom and Randolph hygroscopic investment.

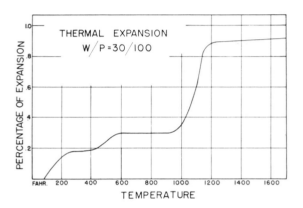

Figure 34.5

Thermal expansion of Ransom and Randolph hygroscopic investment.

950° or above 1200°F. It should be noted, however, that heating the mold to temperatures above 1350°F. is inadvisable since the plaster binder in the investment tends to break down at these excessive temperatures, liberating corrosive sulphur compounds that attack the cast metal.

If inlay castings are overexpanded and loose, less mold expansion is required, and the adjustments in the technique would be just the opposite of those described for increasing expansion.

Table 34.1

Condensed Step Chart for Thermal Expansion Technique for Cristobalite Inlay Investment (based on procedures recommended by the investment manufacturer)

Description of Step	Cristobalite Inlay Investment	
	Control Technique Kerr *Control Powder* added to Cristobalite in definite proportions will produce controlled reduction in expansion where desired.	Low Burnout Technique Cristobalite Only
Preparation of inlay ring	Place a single thickness of liner, lapped, and ⅛″ short at both ends. Moisten thoroughly.	Line with single thickness of liner, lapped, and ⅛″ short at both ends. Moisten thoroughly.
Water temperature	Room	Room
Mixing ratio	Proportions under Control Technique are automatically delivered by Kerr Scale.	15–17 cc. water to 40 gms. investment. When mixing, add investment to water.
Mixing technique	Hand spatulate; vibrate bowl 30 sec. then mechanical mixer 30 sec. (or use vacuum equipment as directed).	Hand spatulate; vibrate bowl 30 sec. then mechanical mixer 30 sec. (or use vacuum equipment as directed).
Investing pattern	Paint carefully with camel's hair brush. This painting may be blown off and pattern repainted. Do *not* dust with dry investment.	Paint carefully with camel's hair brush. This painting may be blown off and pattern repainted. Do *not* dust with dry investment.
Filling ring	Fill inlay ring with same mix and insert painted pattern with slight wavy motion.	Fill inlay ring with same mix and insert painted pattern with slight wavy motion.
Setting time	Allow to set 30 min. or longer.	Allow to set 30 min. or longer.
Wax elimination and burnout	Place flask into furnace preheated to 850–900°F., sprue hole down. Raise temperature to 1200–1350°F. in 30–45 min. Cast into red hot mold. *or* Flask can be placed into cold furnace and heated to 1200–1350°F. Longer time is required.	Place flask into furnace preheated to 850–900°F. Cast in approximately one hour and after discolored investment has regained a white color.

Table 34.2
Condensed Step Chart for Thermal Expansion Technique for R & R Gray Investment (based on procedures recommended by the investment manufacturer)

Description of Step	R & R Gray Investment	
	Single-mix technique is suggested for all two-surface inlays and ¾ crowns for anteriors.	**Double-mix technique** is suggested for MODs, ¾ crowns for posteriors, full crowns and single occlusal inlays.
Preparation of inlay ring	Place a wet liner loosely in ring, lapped for half circumference.	No liner required.
Water temperature	Room	Room
Mixing ratio	14 cc. water to 50 gms. investment.	For first mix, 7 cc. water to 25 gms. investment.
Mixing technique	Spatulate mechanically (or use vacuum equipment as directed).	Spatulate mechanically (or use vacuum equipment as directed).
Investing pattern	Paint carefully with fine brush; vibrate gently to eliminate entrapped air.	Paint pattern, then dust with dry investment and vibrate gently until powder is absorbed. Repeat 3–4 times. Allow to set 5–10 min.
Filling ring	Pour investment into ring and carefully vibrate painted pattern into filled ring.	Fill ring with second mix, made 16 cc. water to 50 gms. investment. Immerse painted pattern momentarily in water and insert in ring.
Setting time	Allow to stand for 10–15 min.	Allow to stand for 10–15 min.
Wax elimination and burnout	Heat invested ring until entire sprue hole shows dull red color (1200–1300°F.) Cast *immediately*.	Heat invested ring until entire sprue hole shows dull red color (1200–1300°F.) Cast *immediately*.

Table 34.3
Condensed Step Chart for Two Hygroscopic Techniques (based on procedures recommended by the respective investment manufacturers)

Description of Step	R&R Hygroscopic Investment	Beauty-Cast Inlay Investment
Preparation of inlay ring	Place one layer of liner ⅛″ short at crucible end.	Place a single thickness of liner ⅛″ short at both ends of ring to provide investment seal; then wet.
Mixing ratio	15 cc. water to 50 gms. investment.	15 cc. water to 50 gms. investment. No change in W/P ratio is necessary when using vacuum equipment.
Mixing	Spatulate mechanically (or use vacuum equipment according to directions).	Add powder to water, hand spatulate to wet, then spatulate mechanically 50 turns. (If vacuum equipment is used, follow manufacturer's instructions.)
Investing pattern	Paint with fine brush; vibrate gently.	Paint with brush; vibrate with serrated instrument on crucible former.
Filling ring	Place ring around painted pattern and fill, gently vibrating.	Place ring around painted pattern and fill slowly, using spatula; vibrate to place.
To obtain hygroscopic expansion	Immerse immediately in water bath at approx. 100°F., water covering the ring.	Immerse immediately in water held within 2° of 100°F.
Setting time	Allow to remain in water for 30 min. or longer.	Let set for at least 30 min. under water.
Wax elimination and burnout	Place wet ring at 800° to 950°F. Heat 45 min. or longer, depending on size of pattern. Cast immediately. *or* Place ring in water and heat to boil. Discontinue heating and with rubber bulb (e.g. chip blower) or with manufactured wax evacuator, remove the wax. Place wet ring in furnace at 800° to 900°F.; heat 30 min. Cast immediately.	Place ring in furnace and bring to 900°F. in 40 min. *or* Burnout directly in a hot furnace at 900°F. for at least 40 min. Cast any time thereafter. If a good grade of inlay wax is used, it is not necessary to eliminate the wax with boiling water or any other method before burning out.

Wax Patterns

The waxing-up of the pattern is accomplished by the use of the gas burner, wax spatula and carvers, and inlay wax. Inlay waxes are specially compounded to burn out of the mold cleanly, leaving no residue harmful to the casting of the gold into the form left by removal of the wax (fig. 34.6).

With a hot spatula, inlay wax is melted, run into the preparation, and pressed against the walls of the die with the fingers to insure adaptation. It is essential that all grooves and angles in the preparation be reproduced in the wax, and a convenient way to insure this is to flow a thin film of **soft wax** into the cavity first and then build up the remainder in the harder inlay wax. Pressure must be applied continuously to prevent the wax from shrinking from the margins as it cools, and this pressure applied to the hard wax effectively forces the softer wax into all corners of the die.

The pattern is built up to approximate shape, removed from the die, and its inner surface is checked for accuracy. If satisfactory, it is replaced, the die is seated in the model, and the contacts and occlusion are established. The contact areas on the model, if present, should be lubricated and the wax pattern softened with a hot spatula to permit the excess to be squeezed out as the die is seated. If it is undersize, the contacts should be built up by adding wax. The occlusion is established

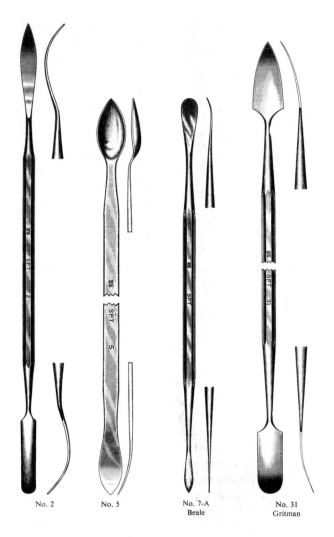

Figure 34.6
Wax spatulas.

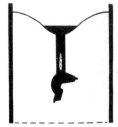

Figure 34.7
Correct positioning and spruing for centrifugal casting.

by closing the articulator or by the marks established on the wax registration and adjusting the wax to the bite. The die is then lifted from the model, and the carving is completed. Remove all surplus wax and carefully create the proper contours and occlusal carvings, using as one guide the general shape already developed in the pattern through the articulation of the waxed die.

Check all margins carefully and replace any missing portions, using a hot spatula, but do not flow wax beyond the margins as it may get into an undercut area and cause distortion of the pattern when removed from the die.

Smooth the pattern by polishing the wax with a piece of soft cloth, rubbing the surface gently toward the margins. It is advisable to make a final check under a magnifying glass with a good light.

Since the wax pattern is the basis of every gold casting, much of the hard work in finishing and polishing can be eliminated before the casting is made by paying particular attention to the waxing procedure. Obviously, it is much easier, faster, and less costly to shape, smooth, and finish a wax pattern than a gold casting, and any additional effort spent in perfecting the pattern will be rewarded later by a considerable saving in time and gold.

Spruing the Pattern

The method adopted for spruing the wax pattern is much more important to the success of the inlay than is generally realized (fig. 34.7). Although the fundamental principles are simple and easy to follow, many inlays are ruined by failure to carry out this primary step correctly.

Thickness of Sprue

A very common error, which results in **shrink-spot porosity** or **pitted castings,** is the use of *too thin* a sprue. When molten metal is cast into a mold, the outer surface of the casting cools fastest and freezes first, forming a shell of solid metal around a molten center. As the metal continues to cool, this shell increases in thickness, and finally the thinner sections freeze solid while there is still molten metal at the center of the thicker sections. If the sprue is thinner than the casting proper, it will solidify completely while the bulkier casting is still partially molten. The molten metal in the casting continues to cool and shrink, and since no more metal can be supplied from the button because the sprue has already solidified, this shrinkage produces voids or pits known as shrink-spot porosity. This type of porosity is not a peculiar defect of the inlay golds or of dental alloys generally. It has to be provided for in all foundry practice and is a simple demonstration of the fact that metals in their solid state occupy less space than when they were fluid. Consequently, if a solid metal is required to occupy the same space that it filled in its fluid form, it can do so only if it adds to its volume by "acquiring" porosity.

To avoid this type of defect, the sprue should be thicker than the pattern so that the inlay will freeze first and the sprue will remain molten to feed additional metal to the inlay until it has frozen solid. In centrifugal casting, the use of a thick sprue is practicable; but in pressure casting, if the sprue opening into the crucible is thicker than fourteen gauge, molten metal is likely to slip down and block off the sprue before casting pressure is applied. However, a reservoir added to the sprue will get around this difficulty and will concentrate the shrink-spot porosity harmlessly outside the inlay. The reservoir should be thicker than the thickest part of the pattern and placed as close as possible to the pattern, never more than $\frac{1}{16}$ inch away. The very short length of sprue between the reservoir and the pattern should be thickened with wax. Such a reservoir is conveniently made from the end of a stick of inlay wax cut off about ⅛ inch long, or by wrapping a ⅛ inch strip of sheet casting wax around the sprue.

Attaching the Sprue

Shrink-spot porosity will also occur when a bulky section of a casting is separated from the sprue by a thinner section. Naturally, the thinner section freezes first and so prevents the sprue from feeding additional metal to the bulky section as it solidifies. For this reason the sprue should always be attached to the thickest part of the pattern. When there are two bulky sections separated from each other by a thin section, as in an MOD with heavy mesial and distal legs connected by a thin occlusal isthmus, it is helpful to attach a sprue to each bulky section.

The wax pattern must be securely attached to the sprue so that it will not break away and be lost during investing, but forcing or melting the sprue deeply into the pattern may cause serious distortion. To avoid such distortion and yet assure firm attachment, place a small amount of sticky wax on the pattern and insert the sprue into the sticky wax.

Mounting the Pattern on Crucible Former (Sprue Base)

In mounting the sprued pattern on the crucible former, it should be adjusted so that there is not more than ¼ inch separating the bottom of the casting ring from the nearest part of the wax pattern (fig. 34.8). The reason

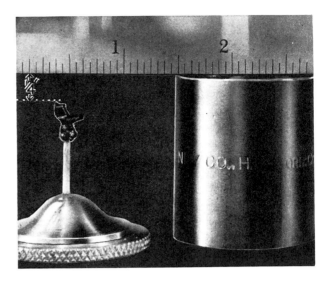

Figure 34.8

Correct spruing and positioning of pattern for pressure casting, using Ney crucible former and heat-resisting Ney inlay ring.

for this is that the air in the pattern chamber is of necessity forced out through the investment as the molten metal enters; and if the bulk of investment is too great, the escape of the air may be so slow that the gold will freeze before the mold is completely filled. This is one of the principal causes of incomplete castings with rounded or short margins.

The crucible former should be clean and free of old investment or other debris. This debris could produce a rough crucible, or the loose particles might be flushed into the pattern chamber with the gold and cause a defective casting. It is also advisable to lubricate the crucible former lightly with a thin oil or with Vaseline to prevent the investment from sticking. If the crucible former is rubber, this lubrication is not necessary.

The shape of the crucible former is also an important factor. A very shallow flat-bottomed crucible does not concentrate the gold over the sprue hole, and much of it may remain in the crucible instead of being forced down the sprue, resulting in an incomplete casting. When a centrifugal casting machine is used, this type of crucible may cause spilling of the gold. A deep, steep-walled crucible is satisfactory for centrifugal casting, but if used for pressure casting where the gold is melted directly in the investment crucible, the gold at the bottom is not readily reached with the blowpipe flame, and melting is difficult. The crucible former illustrated in figure 34.8 is flared at the top for easy access of the flame and has slightly steeper walls at the bottom to concentrate the gold over the sprue hole. Consequently, it gives excellent results with both centrifugal and pressure casting machines.

Two Methods of Investing

Introduction

Investing of wax patterns may be accomplished in either of two ways: (1) by hand or mechanical spatulation of the investment material, beginning the application of the investment to the pattern by painting with a small brush, then vibrating the balance of the investment material into the casting ring, or (2) by mixing the investment material under vacuum and investing the wax pattern also under vacuum.

The actual casting of gold into the prepared mold is also commonly done in either of two general ways: (1) by use of a simple centrifugal casting machine, or (2) by casting with vacuum casting equipment.

Either method of investing wax patterns—investing without vacuum or investing under vacuum—may be followed by the use of a simple centrifugal casting machine to make the casting.

Vacuum investing, however, can be and often is used together with vacuum casting equipment.

Investing the Pattern (Without Vacuum)

The particular investment material that your dentist desires you to use, the technique to be followed in investing the pattern, the equipment available in your office for this purpose, and the technique for burning out the pattern—all are factors that will dictate the method you will use in the dental office in which you are employed. There are several investments, several techniques of investing a pattern, several methods of burning out a pattern, and several methods of casting gold. Some of these techniques will be discussed.

First, a technique depending chiefly on the thermal expansion of the investment to compensate for the casting shrinkage of the gold will be outlined here. This technique requires the use of a high-expanding investment, a number of which are available. Each should be handled according to the instructions supplied by its manufacturer.

Lining the Casting Ring
In this technique it is advisable to use a liner in the inlay ring. The investment and the metal ring do not expand at the same rate when heated, and the lining serves as a cushion that allows the investment to expand freely and tends to prevent distortion or cracking of the mold due to this unequal expansion. The ring with liner should be dipped in water to moisten the liner (fig. 34.9).

Cleaning the Pattern
Just before investing, the pattern should be thoroughly cleaned with a half-and-half mixture of green soap and

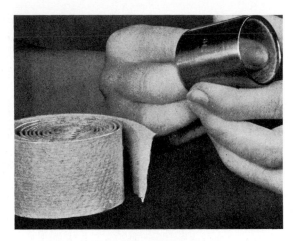

Figure 34.9
Liner being placed in inlay ring to cushion the unequal expansion of investment and ring.

hydrogen peroxide, then rinsed in room-temperature water, and thoroughly dried. This procedure is essential in obtaining castings that are free from surface bubbles and nodules. If the pattern is not clean, the investment will not adhere readily to the wax surface, and a rough casting is quite likely to result. If you wish to use one of the wetting agents available for reducing surface tension, it should be applied to the pattern at this time, carefully following the manufacturer's directions.

Mixing the Investment
In mixing the investment it is advisable to use a good mechanical spatulator because this method produces a smoother mix, freer from entrapped air bubbles, than hand spatulation. Air bubbles in the investment are likely to collect on the wax pattern and, when cast, produce a rough surface and prevent the inlay from seating. It is also important to use the exact proportions of investment powder and water recommended by the manufacturer. Too thin a mix may have insufficient expansion and is likely to crack during the burnout, causing fins and rough surfaces. Too thick a mix is difficult to apply to the pattern and may result in damaged margins and entrapped air.

Painting the Pattern
Paint the pattern carefully with the investment mix, being sure to carry it into all grooves and angles. A good method is to apply the investment with a small brush held lightly against a vibrator. As the brush is vibrated, the bristles work their way into all corners and cover all areas of the pattern thoroughly with investment, eliminating any air that might be entrapped in the investment. After the first coat has been applied in this manner, the bulk of the investment may be gently blown

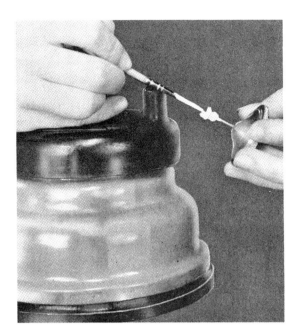

Figure 34.10
Painting the pattern. The brush is held lightly against a vibrator.

off the pattern and the process repeated as an additional precaution to assure thorough painting and a smooth casting (fig. 34.10).

Filling the Ring

After the painting is completed, it is sometimes suggested that the invested inlay be dusted lightly with dry investment powder to absorb excess water, as well as to harden the mass so that it will hold its shape while investing is completed. The ring is now seated over the invested pattern and onto the crucible former and is filled to overflowing with the balance of the mixture. Pour the investment so that it runs down the side of the ring, filling it from the bottom up to avoid trapping air or washing the painted investment off the pattern.

Vacuum Investing

Vacuum investing of wax patterns results in some differences in technique even before the actual investing is done.

For purposes of standardizing, it is recommended that a 50-gram ring (an inlay casting ring which will contain a 50-gram mix of investment material) be used for all casting. In addition to the fact that it will not cool down as fast as a smaller ring when removed from the burnout oven for casting, it is also unnecessary to be constantly changing the balance weight on the casting machine to balance different size rings.

When vacuum investing, it is advisable to use a thinner mix of investment and water than is usually recommended.

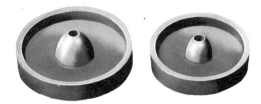

Figure 34.11
Sprue bases.

Many dentists prefer to eliminate the use of liners in the casting ring for most castings, since it has been found that expansion is greater under vacuum investing because practically all air is drawn out of the investment. Air forms tiny voids, creating cushions into which expansion is partly dissipated. With practically all air eliminated, the mass of investment is more dense. Expansion is then greater because the grains of investment are compressed closer together and the expansion is not dissipated into tiny air voids. If additional expansion is desired on any particular case, one may readily obtain it by immersing the casting ring in a pan of 90° to 100° water immediately after removing the ring from the vacuum unit (the hygroscopic technique). The higher the temperature of the water, the greater will be the expansion obtained.

The crucible former or sprue base used in vacuum investing is formed of rubber in order to seal one end of the casting ring. Spruing position and thickness of sprue are the same as in the method discussed in earlier pages, if casting is to be accomplished in a simple centrifugal-type casting machine (fig. 34.12).

Removing the Crucible Former and Sprue

Allow the investment to set until it is hard, usually for at least one-half hour. Then trim the surplus investment from the bottom of the ring so that it will seat properly in the casting machine. Remove the crucible former by gently rapping the base. Trim off any rough edges or overhanging ledges of investment around the periphery of the crucible and carefully flush out the crucible with running water to remove all loose particles of investment that otherwise might be carried into the pattern chamber and cause a defective casting. The sprue is heated over a flame to loosen it from the invested wax pattern and is then removed with tweezers or pliers. Be careful to use a straight pull and not to drag or break the surrounding investment (fig. 34.13).

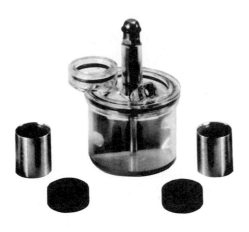

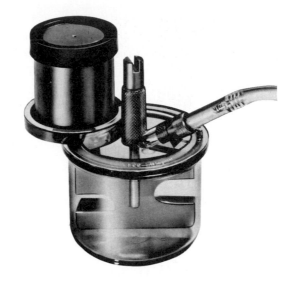

Figure 34.12
The Whip-Mix Vac-U-Spat investing machine.

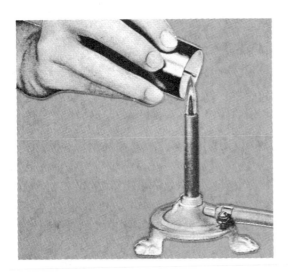

Figure 34.13
Heating the sprue to loosen it from the invested wax pattern before removal.

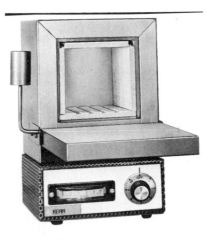

Figure 34.14
The Kerr electric furnace.

Burning Out the Mold

There are numerous methods of burning out the mold, but since the technique described employs a high-expanding investment, a so-called high-heat burnout is used. The method requires the use of a heating device capable of heating the mold uniformly to a temperature of 1300° to 1350°F., or a dull red, and provided with means for controlling both the rate of heating and the final temperature. An experienced and careful technician can obtain good results with simple equipment, but it should be remembered that the burnout is one of the most important steps in the entire technique. Failure to carry out this operation correctly, through carelessness or lack of adequate equipment, is a frequent cause of defective castings. The following paragraphs describe the most common errors and a method of avoiding them (fig. 34.14).

Too Rapid Burnout

One common defect, usually traceable to incorrect burnout technique, is a casting with "fins" or "feathers" caused by cracks in the investment around the pattern that become filled with the cast gold. This condition frequently results from starting the burnout before the investment has had time to set thoroughly, while it is still too weak to stand heating without cracking, or from

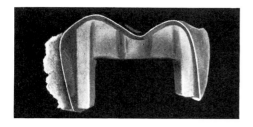

Figure 34.15
Casting with fin from cracked investment.

too rapid heating during the initial stage of the burnout. It may also be caused by mixing the investment too thin (fig. 34.15).

Overheating the Mold

Black or badly discolored castings that do not clean up readily when pickled are also the result of incorrect burnout technique. Many technicians believe that any discoloration of the surface of the casting as it comes out of the investment indicates some fault either in technique or in the materials used, but this is not necessarily true. Most casting golds oxidize at high temperatures, and it is therefore natural for some surface oxidation and discoloration to take place as they cool in the investment. This normal oxidation is easily removed by pickling and does no harm. However, the black casting that does not clean up in acid pickling solution is not normal and indicates an error in the burnout—usually that the investment mold was too hot when the casting was made.

The binder in most investments is plaster or some similar form of gypsum, which chemically is calcium sulphate. At high temperatures the calcium sulphate slowly decomposes and gives off sulphur or sulphur compounds, which readily combine with most base metals to form metallic sulphides. If the investment mold is cast at a temperature high enough for this reaction to occur, the sulphur combines with certain metals in the casting gold, especially copper and silver, forming a surface film of sulphides. This type of discoloration usually can be removed by boiling in nitric acid solution, which is a better solvent for the sulphides, or by repeatedly heating the casting to a dull red and exposing it to air and then pickling it in sulphuric acid. The heating and exposure to air break up the sulphides and form oxides, which are dissolved away in the ordinary pickling solution.

It is usually possible, though troublesome and inconvenient, to salvage an inlay that has been badly discolored by casting into an overheated investment mold. However, there is another serious consequence of this error in burnout technique. The sulphur given off by overheated investment attacks the metal inlay ring, the heating element of electric furnaces, and other metal parts, causing rapid deterioration. This is a frequent cause of abnormally short lives of inlay rings and the metal parts of heating devices.

Incomplete Wax Elimination

Black castings that will not pickle-clean easily may also be caused by incomplete elimination of the wax pattern as a result of heating the mold to too low a temperature for too short a time. Under these conditions a thin layer of carbonized wax remains in the pattern chamber and sticks to the surface of the casting, causing it to be quite black. Since carbon is insoluble in acid, pickling will not clean the casting. This type of discoloration can be removed by holding the casting in the flame of a Bunsen burner, which burns off the carbon or oxidizes the metal underneath it; and then pickling to dissolve the oxides.

Frequently, incomplete wax elimination will have an entirely different result. The wax residue combines with the oxygen of the air in the pattern chamber to form carbon monoxide gas, which is a reducing agent. This gas prevents oxidation of the surface of the cast gold, with the result that the inlay comes out of the investment bright and shiny. However, when this occurs, the formation of the gas is likely to be so rapid that enough back pressure is created to slow up the entry of the gold so that it freezes before the mold is completely filled. This causes incomplete castings with margins rounded or short. Consequently, inlay castings that are abnormally shiny should be looked on with suspicion and carefully checked for margin deficiencies.

A Practical Burnout Technique

The foregoing description of several common burnout errors readily suggests the simple precautions necessary to avoid them.

1. Do not start the burnout until the investment has thoroughly set.
2. Heat the mold slowly at first, at least until the investment is dry.
3. Heat the mold to a high enough temperature and for a long enough time to completely eliminate the wax. Be careful at the same time not to allow it to get too hot.

To observe the first precaution, allow the investment to set for at least one-half hour, or longer if a very slow-setting investment is used. If allowed to stand overnight, it is advisable to soak the ring in water just before starting the burnout to prevent roughness on the surface of the casting.

When starting the burnout, place the ring in the cold oven of the electric furnace. If a gas furnace is used, see that the flame is turned low or that the ring is placed high above the flame. The heat should be regulated from time to time if necessary. The important point is that the rate of heating should be reasonably uniform and such that the investment mold reaches 1300° to 1350°F., or a dull red, in not less than one hour. The heating device must then be regulated to maintain that temperature for at least an additional one-half hour. Under no circumstances allow the mold to exceed this temperature and do not use a heating device not equipped with a rheostat, gas regulator, or other suitable means for obtaining this necessary temperature control.

To help eliminate the wax completely, the mold should be burned out with the sprue hole down so that the wax can run out instead of soaking into the investment. The casting should be made as quickly as possible after the ring has been removed from the furnace to avoid a drop in temperature and consequent shrinkage of the mold.

Melting the Gold

The most widely used melting equipment is the blowpipe supplied with artificial or natural gas and compressed air. Where neither artificial nor natural gas is available, numerous substitutes may be used including hydrogen, bottled gases such as propane, and acetylene. In some localities the available natural gas used with compressed air does not produce enough heat to melt the higher-fusing inlay golds efficiently so that it is advisable to use oxygen in place of compressed air. Each of these fuels has its individual characteristics and requires its own method of handling, but all of them will give good results if used with care and understanding.

Gas-Air Blowpipe Technique

Because it is widely used to melt gold and because it is important to handle the gas-air blowpipe flame correctly, it is illustrated and described in detail. When properly adjusted, this flame has a dark blue inner cone near the tip of the blowpipe, a center cone of lighter blue, and an outer sheath of dark purplish blue. The dark blue inner cone consists chiefly of a stream of compressed air mixed with unburned gas. It is relatively cold and strongly oxidizing and, therefore, should not be directed against the metal being melted. The light blue center cone is the area of almost complete combustion and is, therefore, the hottest part of the flame. This part of the flame should contact the gold and cover it as completely as possible for rapid melting and protection from oxidation. The purplish outer

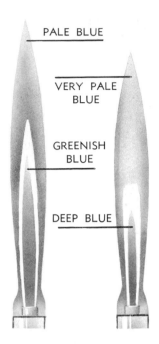

Figure 34.16
The gas-air blowpipe flame.

sheath is made up of the products of combustion, burning gas, and oxygen absorbed from the surrounding air. It is cooler than the center cone and oxidizing in its effect and should not be used in melting (fig. 34.16).

If at all possible, use a reducing flame. Never have a noisy, hissing flame. To get a reducing flame, turn on the gas first, then add air, or oxygen, until the yellow has just disappeared. Notice that the reducing flame is pale blue on the tip while the oxidizing flame is very pale blue.

The effects on the molten metal of the three principal parts of the flame can be graphically demonstrated. Simply hold the blowpipe close to the button of gold so that the dark blue inner cone touches the metal and note the rapid formation of a scum of oxides. Then withdraw the blowpipe slowly until the light blue center contacts the metal, noting that the oxide film disappears and the metal becomes noticeably hotter and more fluid. As the blowpipe is withdrawn until only the purplish blue outer flame touches the gold, the oxide film reappears, and the metal seems to become more sluggish. It is helpful for the beginner to actually carry out this experiment with the blowpipe to become familiar with the characteristic appearance of molten gold when the flame is being used correctly and incorrectly. The experienced technician often moves the blowpipe back and forth slightly to be sure that he or she is using the correct part of the flame.

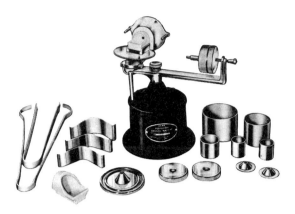

Figure 34.17
Kerr Centrifico casting machine.

Casting

When a centrifugal casting machine is used, the gold and the fire-clay crucible can advantageously be preheated with the blowpipe or in the burnout furnace before the ring is placed in the casting machine to save time in melting and avoid unnecessary cooling and possible shrinkage of the mold before casting (fig. 34.17).

Fluxing

Regardless of how carefully the blowpipe is handled, some oxidation of the metal will nearly always occur during melting. For this reason it is important to protect the gold with a good casting flux. Ordinary borax, frequently used for this purpose, is unsatisfactory. Although it forms a covering and protects the metal to some extent, it also dissolves and slags off any oxides that may be formed. The oxidizable metals present in casting golds (principally copper and a small amount of zinc) are important ingredients added by the manufacturer in the exact amounts required to give each alloy the desired properties. If any part of these metals is lost by being oxidized and then dissolved in the borax, the balanced formula of the alloy will be upset and its properties impaired. For best results it is essential to use a reducing flux which forms a protective covering. Flux also contains an effective reducing agent to convert the oxides back to clean copper and zinc, returning them to the molten button. The original composition and properties of the alloy are thus retained. This flux should be applied as soon as the gold starts to turn red and is hot enough for the flux to stick to it. More flux should be added just before casting.

Cleaning Residue Buttons

Before reusing sprues and residue buttons cut from previous castings, they should be thoroughly cleaned of investment and surface oxidation. The most satisfactory method is to melt down the button on a clean charcoal block with liberal applications of **casting flux** and then plunge the hot button into sulphuric acid pickling solution. Asbestos and fire clay blocks are unsuitable for this purpose because it is practically impossible to keep them free from small beads of metal that become entangled in adhering flux and contaminate metal subsequently melted. A charcoal block, however, is easily scraped clean just before using, and in addition, the charcoal has a valuable reducing action that, in combination with the reducing action of casting flux, breaks up the metallic oxides and converts them back to clean metal. The flux slags off adhering investment; and if a great deal of investment is present, it is advisable to remove the slag with a clean slate pencil during the melting operation. When the hot button is finally plunged into pickle, the sudden cooling crazes and cracks off the glasslike flux, and the acid dissolves any surface oxidation.

Correct Casting Temperature

It is, of course, essential that the gold be completely melted before an attempt is made to cast, otherwise it will not flow freely into the mold. It is also important to avoid heating the metal to unnecessarily high temperatures, since such temperatures promote excessive oxidation and absorption of gases and tend to produce rough castings that are weaker and more brittle than normal. A practical method of judging the right casting temperature is to shake the crucible slightly and cast when the metal rolls freely.

Heat Treatment

Soft and medium-hard golds are not affected by heat treatment, but the hard and extra-hard types can be hardened appreciably by slow cooling or left in a softened condition by rapid cooling. If the inlay is not to be soldered subsequently (which would destroy the effects of a previous heat treatment), these hardening or softening treatments can be carried out conveniently and effectively by regulating the time the casting is allowed to cool in the investment after casting. For softening, the mold should be plunged in water one to two minutes after casting; for hardening, it should be allowed to cool for three to six minutes before quenching. Plunging instantaneously, while the casting is very hot, may cause serious warpage, but air-cooling to room temperature will do no harm. However, investment is removed more easily if the ring is plunged while still warm.

Pickling

After removing the casting from the ring, brush away adhering investment and boil the casting in pickling solution to remove surface oxidation. Sulphuric acid is preferred for this use because it is a very effective solvent of oxides, and its fumes are not as objectionable as those of hydrochloric or nitric acid. The solution should consist of approximately equal parts of acid and water; and in making up the solution, *the acid should always be poured into the water.* If water is poured into sulphuric acid, it will boil violently and may splatter and cause serious burns.

The acid should be hot for rapid and effective pickling. It is common but definitely poor practice to heat the casting and plunge it into cold acid to speed up the pickling. Because the resulting sudden and uneven cooling may cause serious warpage of the inlay, this procedure should be avoided.

Pickling solutions should be stored in glass-stoppered bottles and kept clean at all times. One of the possible causes of discoloration of a gold casting in the mouth is a contaminated pickling solution. After a period of use, any pickling solution will have base-metal salts dissolved in it. If iron or any other metallic tweezers are used in handling the inlay, and if the tweezers are in contact with the inlay while it is immersed in the acid, then base metal can very easily be thrown out of solution by an electrolytic action, and the surface of the casting may be contaminated.

For example, after some use, the solution will contain dissolved copper salts, among others, and a thin copper plating can be given the inlay if it is handled in acid with metal tweezers. This copper "flash" is extremely difficult to entirely remove from the casting, even with thorough polishing. Therefore, when the inlay is placed in the mouth, the copper discolors, and this discoloration is frequently mistaken for tarnish of the gold.

To avoid this complication use two pickling dishes and discard the tweezers. Place the inlay in one dish, cover it with acid, and boil. When the pickling is completed, pour the *acid only* into the second dish, leaving the inlay in the first dish. Flush this dish out with plenty of running water and then remove the inlay.

Because metal ladles also contaminate the acid, it is preferable to use a nonmetallic dish. When the solution becomes dirty and discolored from the dissolved flux and oxides or investment, discard it and make up a fresh solution. After the casting is removed, it should be dipped in a solution of ordinary soda and water to neutralize the acid.

Finishing and Polishing

Before attempting to seat the casting on the die or tooth, the inner walls should be carefully checked. Any nodules or surface roughness that might interfere with seating should be removed with a small, sharp bur. The sprue is then cut off with a separating disc, and the inlay is checked for marginal fit, occlusion, and contact. The method of carrying out these steps depends on whether the direct, indirect, or a combination of these techniques is being followed. The casting is then ready for final finishing and polishing.

The importance of a smooth, highly polished outer surface cannot be overemphasized. It is common knowledge that natural teeth acquire deposits of solid matter from the saliva, but the fact that the same deposits also form on inlays, fillings, and other hard-surfaced objects in the mouth is frequently overlooked. These deposits become stained and discolored and are frequently mistaken for "tarnish." Rough, poorly polished surfaces hold the saliva and greatly accelerate the formation of deposits; while smooth, highly polished surfaces allow the saliva to wash across freely and tend to remain clean and bright. While such deposits can usually be removed from accessible areas of gold inlays by thorough cleaning with toothbrush and dentifrice, it is obviously a much better practice to minimize the cause of their formation of giving the inlay a high polish.

A practical method of obtaining a high polish is to start with a heatless stone, followed successfully by a sandpaper or separating disc, rubber wheel, tripoli on felt cones and wheels, and, finally, rouge on a soft chamois buff. In each step, the coarser marks left by the previous abrasive should be completely removed before going on to the next finer abrasive. The polishing should be done toward the margins in order to spin them into closer contact with the cavity walls and to avoid nicking and injuring delicate margins. After the final polishing, the inlay should be boiled with a soapy cleaner and water to remove all traces of rouge and dirt.

If the technique is followed carefully, the inlay will have a smooth, high-luster surface with minimum tendency to acquire a deposit and become discolored. It should be remembered, however, that a good polishing job must be a thorough one.

Summary

A proper casting technique uses several ways of counterbalancing the normal shrinkage and expansion problems.

The principal shrinkage occurs in the change from liquid gold alloy to solid gold alloy. Impression and die materials may also shrink. Some die materials expand; pattern waxes and certain investment procedures can also cause expansion of the finished casting.

The variable factors can be controlled by a systematic approach to the entire procedure from beginning to end. Use a standardized technique.

The first step is to build a wax pattern. Since the wax pattern is the basis of every gold casting, much hard work in finishing and polishing can be eliminated before the casting is made by perfecting the wax pattern.

The method adopted for spruing the wax pattern is much more important to the success of the inlay than is generally realized. The thickness of the sprue is important. It is necessary to attach the sprue correctly. Directions for mounting the pattern on the crucible former should be followed meticulously.

Although there are two methods of investing (with and without vacuum), only investing without vacuum is discussed since vacuum investing is rarely performed by dental assistants. After the investing is completed, it is necessary to remove the crucible former and sprue. The mold is then burned out. There are problems with burnout technique that make it necessary to follow three precautions to avoid such problems.

In melting the gold it is necessary to learn to use the flame correctly.

Care must be exercised to follow directions accurately throughout all stages of casting and also through pickling, finishing, and polishing. A good polishing job must be a thorough one.

Study Questions

1. Discuss proper casting techniques.
2. Discuss shrinkage and expansion of materials.
3. How can the variable factors be controlled in casting?
4. Discuss the building of a wax pattern.
5. Why is the thickness of the sprue important?
6. Describe two methods of investing.
7. Discuss three precautions to take during burnout.
8. Describe casting.
9. What steps follow casting?

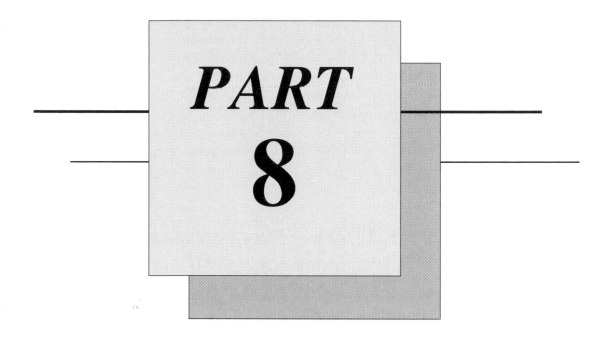

PART 8

Radiography

—Radiography—Roentgenography—X ray—
—Names you will encounter in your studies, your
conversations, and your practical work in the dental
office—they all refer to one and the same thing.

Dr. Roentgen discovered something unusual that he called X ray because its character was and remains so puzzling. X ray has become of utmost importance. Since its original discovery, other scientists have renamed X ray to honor Dr. Wilhelm C. Roentgen, its discoverer. They call it roentgen ray.

In scientific communications we correctly refer to *roentgen ray*. In lay communication, that is, with patients in the office, it is correct to say *X ray*. Somewhere between X ray and roentgen ray, the term *radiograph* has also been developed, probably because it is radiant energy.

Regardless of which term you find in your readings—roentgenography, radiography, or X ray—each refers to the same subject.

It is the purpose of this section to acquaint the dental assistant with radiographs—their use, hazards, care, and techniques for processing.

Acknowledgement is made of the gracious consultations given in the preparation of this section by J. Donald Hauptfuehrer of the University of Illinois College of Dentistry, Department of Radiology.

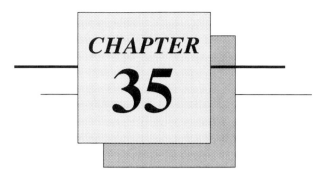

CHAPTER 35

Radiography: Elementary Knowledge

Part One: Theory
More Than the Eye Can See
What Are X Rays (Roentgen Rays)?
The Creation and Use of X Rays
Geometry of Shadow
Recording the Image
   Exposure
   Sensitivity
Part Two: Safety
Potential Dangers of X Ray
Hazards
   Primary Beam
   Scattered Radiation
Protection
Part Three: Dental X-ray Machine and Dental Film
The Dental X-ray Machine
   The Tube
   The Head
   The Timer
   Operating the Machine
The Panoramic X Ray
Dental Film—Intraoral and Extraoral
   Film Description and Management
   Intraoral Film
   Extraoral Film
   Panographic Film
   Getting Acquainted with the Actual Film
   Protecting the Film

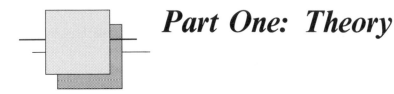

Part One: Theory

More Than the Eye Can See

When a dentist examines a patient's teeth to detect any carious lesions, he or she can see all the lesions on the exposed surfaces of the teeth. However, it is impossible to see the surfaces of the teeth that touch each other. If there are any carious lesions on these surfaces, the lesions will become unnecessarily large before they can be seen. Sometimes the caries reaches the pulp chamber of the tooth before it is discovered visually.

It becomes evident that something more than the eye is needed to examine the mouth. Radiographs (X rays) have been developed and are used commonly for patient examination. Bitewing radiographs are frequently obtained to examine the surfaces of teeth that the dentist cannot see. If any caries is present, it can be read on the radiograph. A full-mouth radiograph is taken regularly for the well-educated and well-cared-for dental patient. The frequency with which this diagnostic measure is used is determined by the dentist. These radiographs show not only the surfaces of the teeth that touch each other, but the roots of all teeth in the mouth and the area immediately around the roots. If there is a cyst, impacted third molar, an abscess forming around a root tip, or some other abnormality, the radiograph is a diagnostic aid. The dentist can diagnose the problem and prescribe the necessary treatment with greater accuracy. If a tooth must be surgically removed, the radiograph is of vital importance to the oral surgeon prior to removal and, frequently, postoperatively (after removal).

Considering these facts, you can understand that complete diagnosis of conditions within the mouth cannot be made without the use of radiographs. It is one of the necessary tools of dentistry. *It can be a dangerous tool if improperly handled, however.*

Regulations governing the use of radiographs vary in different states. In some states the dental assistant may take the radiographs; in other states she or he may only assist the dentist by operating the timer. In most offices, however, it is the dental assistant who *processes* the radiographs, *mounts* them, and places them with the rest of the examination record of the patient.

A **dental radiograph** is a photographic record produced by the passage of X rays through the tissues

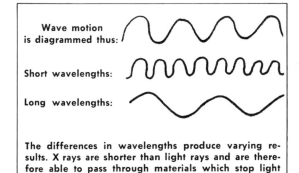

Figure 35.1
Schematic illustration of wavelengths.

of the mouth to a film. The dentist studies this photographic record as an aid to diagnosis.

It is important to make high-quality radiographs. The operators must understand what they are doing, and why, in order to achieve this essential high quality.

What Are X Rays (Roentgen Rays)?

A **roentgen ray** is electromagnetic radiation produced when electrons strike a metal target in a vacuum tube. Like light, X rays are a form of radiant energy; they can be measured because they travel as a wave motion (fig. 35.1).

X rays penetrate materials that absorb or reflect light because they have such a very short wavelength (about 1/10,000 the length of light waves). X rays have the same properties as light rays, but they have them in different degrees; therefore, X rays behave differently from light rays. Three characteristics of X rays are important to dentistry.

1. They penetrate many materials that either absorb or reflect light.
2. They can be seen on photographic film. (They can take a picture.)
3. *They can produce biological changes and even kill*; thus, we must be exceptionally careful in using X-radiation.

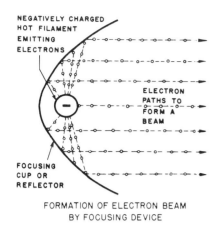

NEGATIVELY CHARGED
HOT FILAMENT
EMITTING
ELECTRONS

ELECTRON
PATHS TO
FORM A
BEAM

FOCUSING
CUP OR
REFLECTOR

FORMATION OF ELECTRON BEAM
BY FOCUSING DEVICE

AN ELECTRON SOURCE

The three requirements for the production of x-rays are all met in the x-ray tube. The cathode serves as the electron source. Electrons are emitted from the filament, a coil of tungsten wire, as it is heated to a high temperature. Because the filament gives off electrons in all directions, some means must be used to focus them on the target, directing their travel in a convergent stream across the x-ray tube. A reflector, or focusing cup, within the cathode structure, into which the filament is placed, focuses the electron beam much as light is focused by a flashlight reflector.

A TUNGSTEN TARGET

There must be a target for the electron beam to strike before x-rays are actually produced. In radiographic tubes the target proper is made of tungsten since it is a metal relatively efficient in x-ray production and one that will stand high temperatures without melting.

To help dissipate the large amounts of heat generated at the target, the tungsten is usually embedded in a large mass of copper. Copper conducts the heat away from the tungsten, dissipating it into oil, in the case of an oil-immersed tube.

FUNDAMENTALS OF AN X-RAY TUBE

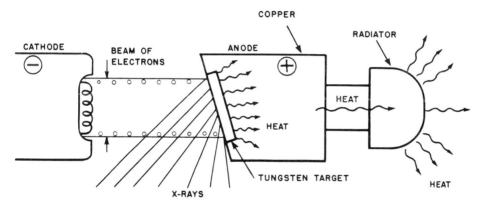

CATHODE   BEAM OF ELECTRONS   ANODE   COPPER   RADIATOR

HEAT

HEAT

X-RAYS   TUNGSTEN TARGET   HEAT

Figure 35.2
Schematic drawing of X-ray tube.

The Creation and Use of X Rays

Electrons are minute particles of negative electrical charges that can be made to move rapidly. If electrons collide with a metal target at a high speed, X rays (or X-radiation) are produced.

An **X-ray tube** is designed to be an efficient means of producing X rays. In an X-ray tube, the rapidly moving stream of electrons is directed against a metal target. When the electrons strike the target, they are stopped. A small portion of their energy is made into X rays; the rest is changed to heat.

In dental radiography, an X-ray tube is a sealed glass bulb from which all air has been pumped. It contains a cathode and an anode. The **cathode** is a filament of tungsten wire inside a focusing cup that directs the electrons to the target on the anode side of the tube (fig. 35.2). The **anode** is a copper bar with a tungsten button in it. The anode is made of copper because copper conducts heat well and helps absorb and remove the tremendous heat generated by the electrons when they strike the target.

Remember that only a small portion of the electron energy becomes X rays; the rest is heat. Something must be done with the heat. It is a waste product to be dissipated. X-ray heads are either oil-cooled or gas-cooled. The oil-cooled tubes are completely immersed in oil, and the heat transfers from the copper bar to the oil. The gas-cooled tube is cooled by a similar process, using gas instead of oil. The heat is a waste product. Only the X-radiation is of use in radiography.

The **tungsten button** is called the target at which the stream of electrons is directed. There is an area on the target called the **focal spot,** which the electrons strike. The smaller the focal spot, the better the detail of the X ray.

The number of electrons produced to form X rays is very important to good dental radiography. The number of electrons is determined by the heat of the cathode filament. (One type of X-ray machine uses a heater in addition to the cathode. The cathode heats the heater; the heater produces the electrons. However, regardless of its construction, either the heat of the cathode or the heat of the heater that is heated by the cathode produces electrons.) As the temperature of the cathode filament is increased, more electrons are produced.

The number of electrons that form the stream is measured in **milliamperes,** which is an electrical term referring to the amount of electrical current being carried by the conductor (the copper wire). Thus, in X ray, the **milliamperage** refers to the amount of current flowing within the X-ray tube head. The hotter the cathode filament becomes, the more electrons are produced. The more electrons available, the greater the intensity of the X ray. Thus, when you adjust the milliampere control on the X-ray machine, you are watching the effect in the milliammeter of the increase or decrease in the number of electrons being hurled against the target. The milliammeter measures the amount of electrical current available. This really means that you determine with the milliammeter the **current flow** to be used in taking the photograph (which regulates *how many* electrons will hit the target).

Kilovoltage is another electrical term to be understood. Kilovoltage controls the *speed* at which the electrons travel, which is very important to the quality of the radiographs produced.

When the electrons travel at greater speed, the X rays produced are of shorter wavelength, which gives them greater penetrating power.

What do we mean by **penetrating power?** It simply means the ability to pass through an object. Thus, with greater penetrating power, the waves can pass through an object of greater thickness and density. The waves that pass through the object record the image on film, therefore, the X-ray waves that have the greatest penetrating power are most desirable in dentistry. The longer X-ray waves are *absorbed* by the tissue rather than being able to pass through it.

Other factors that must be considered are the thickness and density of the object to be X-rayed. Obviously, two pieces of identical matter of different thickness will absorb X-radiation in different amounts. For example, a two-by-three-inch sponge one inch thick will absorb more water than a two-by-three-inch sponge ½ inch thick. Thus, thickness of the bone will determine the amount of X radiation absorbed and the amount allowed to pass through. In addition, the density of the material will affect the absorption rate. Bone is denser than soft tissue. Some bone is denser than other bone. Thus, cortical bone (denser) absorbs more X-radiation and allows less to pass through the spongy bone. Spongy bone allows less radiation to pass through and absorbs more radiation than soft tissue. Soft tissue absorbs more than air spaces. Adult bones have greater calcium content and thus absorb more than the bones of young people, other considerations being equal.

The degrees of difference in absorption of X rays by the various tissues in the mouth give a radiograph

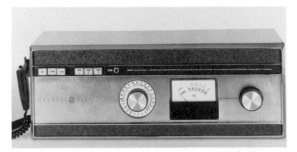

a

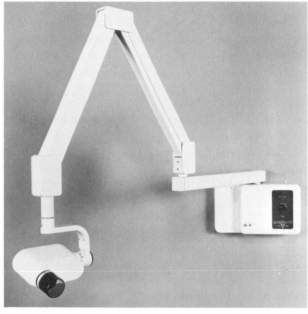

b

Figure 35.3
(a) Controls for an X-ray machine; and (b) gendex wall-mount X ray for intraoral radiography.

its different shades of gray that make it an aid to diagnosis. The film is blacker (more exposed) where there is tissue and lighter where there are bones and teeth. The degree of darkness varies with the degree of denseness and thickness of the tissues through which the X ray must pass before reaching the film.

In technical discussions this degree of difference is spoken of as "an area-to-area variation in the intensity of the X rays which emerge from the subject." It simply means that the denser part of the bone lets fewer X rays through; therefore, a variation in darkness on the X-ray film exists. It is called **subject contrast.** (The heavier the bone, the lighter the shade of the X-ray film.)

There should be subject contrast on a radiograph. However, if the equipment is not properly operated, the contrast can be so poor that the radiograph is unreadable or of such poor quality that diagnostic value is questionable.

To summarize, then, higher milliamperage produces a greater number of electrons, which means a greater total quantity of X rays. Likewise, decreasing the milliamperage decreases the quantity of X rays. The X-ray intensity of the image created on the film directly corresponds with the milliamperage setting. More milliamperage equals more blackness; less milliamperage equals less blackness, but over a range of milliamperage settings, *these various intensities of the parts of the image on the film will have an identical relationship to each other.* For example, let us assume that a given milliamperage setting is used to produce a film image that contains three different degrees of X-ray intensity as projected through the subject: one area is twice as dense as the second area, the second area is twice as dense as the third. If the milliamperage setting is reduced and the X ray of the subject is repeated, the overall intensity of this film image will be lighter, but the three areas will be as before: the first area will be twice as light (more dense) as the second area, and the second area will be twice as light as the third area on the film.

The kilovoltage setting controls the penetrating power of the X rays. Higher kilovoltage moves the electrons more rapidly. Faster-moving electrons mean greater penetrating power. Thus, the higher the kilovoltage, the more penetrating the X rays.

There are two additional effects that are not always desirable, however: (1) the entire range of X rays produced, if affected by the increase in kilovoltage setting, including the total production of "soft" or unused rays, will result in more radiation to the patient but no more effective exposure of the film; and (2) overall subject contrast is reduced when the kilovoltage is increased.

There is no universal agreement among dental radiologists on the ideal combinations of film, milliamperage setting, and kilovoltage setting to secure the best results. Distance (from target to film) is also a variable factor, depending on the particular technique your dentist wishes to use. Distance, milliamperage, and kilovoltage control the image intensity.

Geometry of Shadow

One objective in taking dental radiographs is to obtain as accurate an image of an area as possible. It is sometimes said that an X ray of a tooth is essentially the same as a shadow of the tooth. Sharpness and size of the radiographic image are two factors that contribute to the accuracy of the image. Thus, the smaller the focal spot and the nearer the film to the object being photographed, the more accurate the picture. If one tooth is farther from the film than its neighbor, the shadows of the teeth will be magnified in direct relation to their relationship to the film. If you will place a single light bulb in a holder about six feet from a wall, this principle can be more easily understood. Consider the light bulb as the target in the X-ray tube, and the wall as the X-ray film. Hold your clenched fist (the tooth) between the light source and the wall—first six inches from the wall, then a foot from the wall. When your fist is six inches from the wall, the shadow (the radiographic image of the tooth) is smaller than the shadow of the fist held one foot from the wall. In other words, the tooth closer to the film will show on the film as a smaller shadow than the tooth farther from the film. The difference in size can be figured mathematically if you know the difference in distance from the film (fig. 35.4).

We have mentioned that the distance from the target to the film is a variable factor, depending on the X-ray technique used by your dentist. The eight-inch target-film distance has been used for many years and is still commonly used. Long cone techniques using target-film distances of sixteen inches are used for purposes of obtaining more true radiographic images, but due to problems of dental office design, the additional cone length is not always as convenient to use since there is limited space for maneuverability of the X-ray head.

You should understand the manner in which distance affects the radiographic image, however, not only because eight-inch target-film distance and sixteen-inch target-film distance techniques are used for periapical and bitewing films, but also because different distances are used for other dental X-ray procedures. An occlusal film packet may be used for a radiograph of the maxillary incisor region, a radiograph of the maxillary canine-molar region, or a radiograph of the maxillary arch. Each of these uses a distance of nine inches. The corresponding radiographs of the mandibular areas use a distance of ten inches. Sheet films, with intensifying screens, may be used for large-area radiographs of the mandible or of the temporomandibular articulation at distances of fifteen inches or greater. When necessary, even lateral headplates can be made at distances of seventy-two inches, using a dental X-ray machine.

Distance also affects the intensity of the X rays reaching the film. The relationship of intensity to distance is known as the **inverse-square law.** This law states that the intensity of the radiation varies inversely as the square of the distance from its source. For example, let us say that the correct exposure at eight inches is one second. For the second area to be photographed imagine that it is physically impossible to place the X-ray machine head so that the distance is still eight inches. It has to be sixteen inches away. You can have the same intensity of X rays reaching the film if you will leave the milliamperage and kilovoltage settings exactly the same and increase the exposure time by the square of

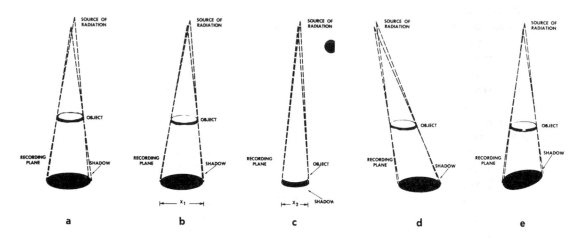

Figure 35.4

Diagrams showing geometrical effects on image sharpness: (a) unsharpness caused by a large focal spot and long object-recording plane distance; (b) improvement in sharpness produced by a small focal spot; (c) superior result of a small focal spot and minimum distance between the object and recording plane. Notice the enlargement (X₁) caused by the distance of the object from recording plane as compared to the more accurate size (X₂) produced when the object is close to the plane; (d) a true enlargement because the object and recording surface are parallel even though the source of radiation is not vertically above the object; and (e) distortion results when the object and the recording plane are not parallel.

the increase in distance. Sixteen inches is twice as far away from the source (target) as the original eight inches; therefore, the exposure is two squared (2 × 2), or four times the exposure at eight inches, making the new correct exposure four seconds. A change in distance from target to film does not alter the subject contrast. The same is true in changing milliamperage. A change in kilovoltage, however, will result in a change in subject contrast, together with a change in the intensity of the X rays.

The factor of distance of the object from the film is important because it affects the quality of the X-ray photograph that your dentist must read for accurate diagnosis of the conditions within the mouth. If the film is placed close to the object to be X-rayed and in a plane parallel to it, the image is more likely to be accurate. If the object to be photographed is not parallel to the film, it will be distorted because part of it is farther from the film.

Accurate image formation is obtained by observing five rules.

1. The smallest practical focal spot is used. Usually this is controlled by the manufacturer of the dental X ray, and you don't need to think about it.
2. The longest focus-film distance which is practical is used.
3. The film is placed as close as possible to the area to be photographed.
4. The central ray of the X ray is directed as nearly at a right angle to the film as

possible. The position of the film in the mouth will affect somewhat the possibility of using a right angle. You simply can't change the anatomy of the head of an individual, and often it will be impossible to aim at a perfect right angle.
5. The film should be parallel to the area being photographed insofar as it is practical.

Recording the Image

Photography is really the basis for radiography. A special film is used, but the essentials for photography—radiant energy, photosensitive film, and a chemical process that makes an invisible image visible and lasting—are present, as well as the object to be photographed.

Gelatin containing a silver compound forms an emulsion that is found on one or both sides of a base. This base and emulsion sandwich is actually the X-ray film.

The emulsion is exceedingly sensitive, and whenever X rays are absorbed by it, a physical change occurs that is so fine that special chemical solutions must be used to make this change visible. The special chemical solution is called a **developer,** and it causes the exposed grains of silver compound to change to tiny masses of black metallic silver. Since the unexposed grains are unaffected, the silver particles suspended in gelatin make the visible image on the film.

Exposure

A radiograph is obtained when the film has been **exposed** to the area to be recorded by having X-radiation pass through the area to the film, thus physically changing the silver in the emulsion coating on the film.

The intensity of the X-radiation and the length of time the rays act on the film determine the darkness of the image on the film. When the area to be X-radiated is dense, the time the X rays are allowed to penetrate the area must be increased, while the time necessary for penetrating an area where the bone is less dense is of shorter duration. For example, the lower incisor area takes the least amount of time for exposure, while the upper molar region takes the greatest amount of time.

Every manufacturer of dental film provides a table of exposure for their film that you can follow when exposing radiographs.

Sensitivity

The rapidity with which film responds to exposure is known as **sensitivity.** When little exposure is needed, the film is very sensitive and is known as high-speed film.

All dental film manufacturers make a regular film and a high-speed film. One of the advantages of high-speed film is that less X-radiation is used to make a photographic record, thus decreasing the X-ray dosage to the personnel and patient. Another advantage is that there is less chance that the patient will blur the image by moving.

Learn to produce the radiographic results that your dentist desires with the equipment he or she has available for your use.

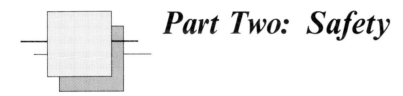

Part Two: Safety

Potential Dangers of X Ray

The potential danger of X ray, both to the personnel operating the equipment and to the patient whose teeth are X-rayed, must be thoroughly understood, and necessary precautions must be taken for the complete protection of all persons in the dental office. The use of X rays in dentistry contributes to the total radiation exposure of humans. This exposure must be kept within safe limits since the effect of radiation is cumulative over a period of time; that is, the dose you will receive tomorrow adds to the dose you received today, and they add to the amount you received yesterday to build a total X-radiation dosage.

Since the use of radiographs is essential to diagnosis in dentistry, it is important to continue using them. Proper precautions will result in adequate protection. But you must know how to eliminate the dangers to yourself and others and be careful to see that you *do eliminate them.*

Many pioneers in the field of radiology died because the dangers of X-radiation to the unprotected operator were not understood. Today, detailed information for the protection of personnel is available in NCRP Report Number 5, available from the National Council on Radiation Protection and Measurements. The report is titled *Dental X-ray Protection.*

What are the risks to the patient and office personnel from an overdose of X-radiation? Repeated doses of X-radiation build up the effect of X rays on the tissues of the body. When the radiation goes beyond the limits that the body tissues can tolerate, the tissues begin to break down. Continuation of the breakdown will eventually result in death when it is a vital organ or fluid that is affected. X-radiation is also known to cause biologic changes by affecting the reproductive organs of certain humans, which in turn affect the unborn children. Some of the tissues of the body are radiosensitive, which means that these cells are very sensitive to X rays. Cells of the blood, hair, skin, nails, and reproductive organs are some of the tissues most sensitive to X-radiation. However, any tissue may be injured by over exposure. You have only to think what would happen to you if the cells of the blood were overexposed to X-radiation and began to break down. Continued breakdown would result in the inability of the blood to function at all.

One of the first symptoms of overexposure is skin erythema. It looks somewhat like sunburn. If the erythema, or reddening of the skin, is not heeded, further stages of the condition include scaling of the skin, a loss of hair, brownish pigmentation, stiffening of fingers, cracking of tissue over joints, longitudinal splitting of the nails, piling up of outer layers of the skin, and sores that fail to heal. These may become chronic and may eventually become cancerous.

Hazards

What are the hazards and how can we eliminate them?

Primary Beam

The first hazard, obviously, is the direct roentgen beam itself. It comes from the X-ray head. This beam is needed to photograph the area that your dentist wishes to study. The head of the machine is aimed at the patient's face. Most of the rays enter the patient's tissue and record the desired image on the film. However, anything in front of that tube receives the rays. The finger that holds the film in position receives as much dosage as the rest of the area. Therefore, **anyone habitually exposed to working in radiology (dentist or assistant) never holds the film in place.** Film holders are available that eliminate the need for anyone to hold the film packet in place. Some of the holders help reduce the dosage of X ray to the patient.

Should your dentist not employ film holders, and a patient is unable to hold the film for any reason, a relative or friend—not the dental assistant—should hold the film.

The roentgen rays from the focal spot on the target of the X-ray machine are primary beams and are most dangerous for repeated exposures.

It is important to understand where the X-ray beams are traveling in order to remain out of their path.

X rays radiate from their source in all directions. Since they are needed in only one direction to take the picture, the X-ray tube is designed so that the X-radiation can escape only through one opening—a sort of window in the tube housing. The X rays that escape through this opening are of different wavelengths and penetrating power.

We speak of the X rays escaping in only one direction. Obviously something must be able to stop the rays from traveling. Generally, lead is used. It is found in the X-ray tube housing to keep the X rays from escaping anywhere but through the one opening designed for the purpose.

The primary beam (the greatest number of X rays) leaves the target of the machine in a cone-shaped path. The size of the beam increases as the distance from the target increases. The plastic cone of the X-ray machine does not limit the beam; it only aids in visualizing the field due to the open-end cone.

Closed-end plastic cones are conceded to be a source of secondary radiation. In some states open-ended metal or lead-shielded cones are required by law.

X-ray machines that are currently being sold have a lead-lined or metal-lined cone that contains the X rays more effectively, permitting the rays to travel only in the desired direction.

Scattered Radiation

Scattered radiation is a danger to be considered carefully in any dental office. Scattered radiation is of two types: leakage and secondary.

Leakage radiation: Some of the X rays have bounced off the target in the X-ray tube in all directions. Modern tubes and heads of X-ray machines are protected, but where leakage from the head of the X-ray machine occurs, it must be considered dangerous to the operator.

Secondary radiation: This radiation is "new radiation which is created by primary radiation acting on or passing through matter."[1] Secondary radiation, then, is the radiation that is emitted in all directions from the patient's head while being radiographed.

A lead apron is required in some states to be placed over the patient during radiography. The apron is used to protect the patient from the secondary radiation that is emitted from that patient's head during filming. The primary beam from the X-ray machine is very well controlled and strikes only the area of the mouth at which it is aimed. It is the secondary radiation, the new radiation created by the primary radiation as it passes through the area of the mouth, which is dangerous to the patient—or *anyone else in its path.*

Protection

Everyone in the dental office can be protected from overdosage by observing a few safety rules. The NCRP report states that the exposure of persons other than the patient can be limited by a combination of three measures.

1. Increase the distance of the individual from the source.
2. Reduce the duration of exposure.
3. Use protective barriers (shielding) between the individual and the source.

The bulletin further states that protective shielding and distance are the factors most easily controlled in the dental office. Protective shielding includes that which is built into the X-ray machine and barriers used in the office, such as thick concrete walls, lead-lined walls, or movable lead shields.

The patient can be protected by techniques of radiography and by careful record of the total exposure of the patient, with determination to eliminate any unnecessary use of X ray. (If the patient has had a cumulative dosage that is dangerously high, the necessity of radiographs versus the health hazard without them is a decision that the dentist must make.)

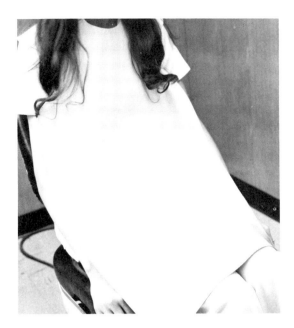

Figure 35.5
A patient protective apron to be worn during filming of radiographs.

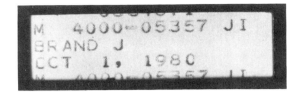

Figure 35.6
Film badge.

Although everyone can be protected from overdosage, uncertainty frequently exists about the dosage the personnel are receiving. Scattered radiation and the individual's lack of awareness of personal habit patterns are factors affecting the dosage received. One way to be certain that an individual employee is not receiving a dangerous amount of X-radiation in the course of a day's work is for the office to subscribe to a film-badge service.

The service provides a film badge for each employee to wear (fig. 35.6). Each week the badges are collected, and the service determines the amount of radiation and the energy level of the radiation. The energy level indicates whether the radiation is gamma or X ray. The service also determines whether the radiation passed through lead, plastic, copper, or aluminum. Thus the service tells you the *amount* and *type* of radiation to which you have been exposed. If there is leakage radiation in your office, it will be easy to recognize that your X-ray machine needs some attention.

Today, in some areas, legislation compels any owner of a radiation source to monitor the amount of radiation reaching personnel. (An X-ray machine is a radiation source.) Where passed, this legislation means that each dentist must provide film-badge service or some equivalent method of verifying the X-radiation dosage received by all personnel.

Some persons believe that a paper clip or penny attached to a film packet worn in a pocket is a method of determining the exposure to X-radiation. (The film is developed at the end of a week. If there has been too much radiation leakage, the penny or paper clip will show on the film.) Actually, this method is ineffective because it doesn't tell the amounts of exposure or the type of radiation.

The rules, then to protect everyone in the office from an overdose of X rays are these:

1. Use of the fastest available film to cut the amount of time the rays are in operation in your office.
2. Lead apron is mandatory for the patient (fig. 35.5). Dentist and assistant should be protected by walls or shields when possible.
3. Use a long cord for the controls or have the controls in another room.
4. Never hold the film for a patient.
5. Never have your hand on the tube housing or pointer cone while the machine is filming the patient.
6. Wear a film badge.

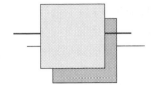

Part Three: Dental X-ray Machine and Dental Film

The Dental X-ray Machine

If you ever have a chance to visit the Smithsonian Institute in Washington, D.C., please do treat yourself to a trip through the dental section. There you will see early dental equipment—including an ancient X-ray machine with its high-tension wire strung out in the open. One look at it and you can really appreciate the efficient machines in use today.

A specific type of X-ray machine is used in the dental office. It is usually labeled 40 to 70 or 100 kvp, which means that its voltage range is 40,000 to 70,000 or 100,000 volts. This high range is necessary for dental radiology. The machines used for medical radiology and therapeutic or industrial radiology are quite different in construction and voltage. Some are low-voltage machines, but some may use 3,000,000 volts.

We are concerned with only the dental X-ray machine. Its basic electrical parts are a high-voltage circuit, a low-voltage circuit, an X-ray tube, a control circuit, and a timer.

Not all dental offices have the latest equipment. You may find that the X-ray machine in your office is not of the very latest type. Some machines operate with a narrow, fixed range of kilovoltage (usually a fixed kilovoltage of 65, a milliamperage of 10, and target-film distance of eight inches). The newer machines have adjustable kilovoltage controls. The selection is usually from 40 to 70 or 100 kv, a milliamperage range of 5 to 15, and timers that permit exposures of extremely short duration. The new equipment also allows the use of either an eight-inch or sixteen-inch target-film distance. There will be two meters to check: the kilovoltmeter and the milliammeter.

The dental X ray has a **high-tension transformer** that steps up the 110-volt alternating current (which your office receives from the electrical outlet) to the desired 40,000 to 100,000 volts necessary for radiography. There are two circuits involved in the transformer: the primary circuit is connected through a control device called the voltage compensator or autotransformer; the secondary circuit is connected to the X-ray tube terminals. The **autotransformer** is a manual control that you turn to the voltmeter reading you want.

Another transformer, the **filament** or **stepdown transformer,** is used to provide current for the filament. It reduces the line voltage to about twelve volts, which heats the tungsten filament in the cathode to produce the electrons.

The Tube

We have already described the dental X-ray tube and its operation in the production of radiographs.

The Head

Recent developments in head construction of X-ray units have changed the appearance and safety of the head. Formerly, the closed-end cone was all plastic, and plastic acts as a source of secondary radiation. The new heads have a cylinder-shaped cone rather than a pointed one. The cylinder contains metal that prevents scattered radiation from escaping. (One leading manufacturer advertises the head cylinder as lead-lined acrylic; another as lead and stainless steel.)

The purpose of the cone is to allow the operator to align the beam accurately with the area to be radiographed. The new cylindrical cones are designed to accomplish this necessary function even though they are not shaped to a point as the older-model cones are. Diaphragms and filters are used to further restrict the X-ray beams and block soft radiation. It is conceded that some operators find it more difficult to see angulation with open-ended cones, but compensation is possible with film holders and specific training.

Adaptations for older machines are available. The pointed cone is discarded, and the replacement cylindrical cone is attached to the X-ray machine (fig. 35.7).

The Timer

The X-ray unit has a timer on it that allows you to set a pointer at the desired number of seconds or fractions of a second for exposure and then push a button. The timer automatically allows the machine to produce X rays in the amount of time for which you have set the indicator. It increases markedly the accuracy of the time factor in radiography. The only errors with such a device are caused by faulty equipment or inaccurate setting of the time indicator by the operator. The directions with the X-ray machine that your dentist owns will explain what to do if you have made an error in setting the timer.

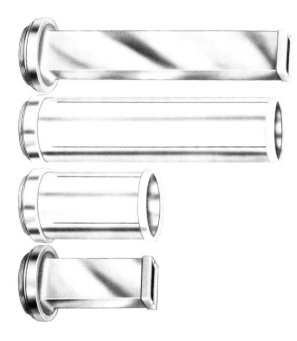

Figure 35.7
Adaptation devices for pointed cone X rays: called PIDs by the manufacturer.

Operating the Machine

As with all work in the dental office, an orderly routine is important in operating the X-ray machine.

1. Turn on the switch. Warm-up may be required for some machines. Some manufacturers recommend turning the machine on in the morning and off at the end of the day.
2. Check the milliammeter setting to see that the current is reaching the machine.
3. Check the kilovoltmeter setting.
4. Set the timer to the desired number of seconds or fraction of a second.

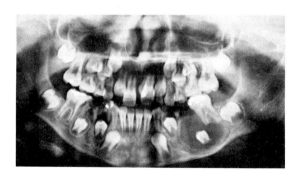

Figure 35.9
Radiogram made with the Orthopantomograph.

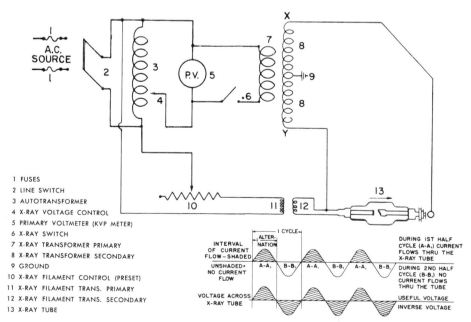

1 FUSES
2 LINE SWITCH
3 AUTOTRANSFORMER
4 X-RAY VOLTAGE CONTROL
5 PRIMARY VOLTMETER (KVP METER)
6 X-RAY SWITCH
7 X-RAY TRANSFORMER PRIMARY
8 X-RAY TRANSFORMER SECONDARY
9 GROUND
10 X-RAY FILAMENT CONTROL (PRESET)
11 X-RAY FILAMENT TRANS. PRIMARY
12 X-RAY FILAMENT TRANS. SECONDARY
13 X-RAY TUBE

A basic x-ray unit consists of the three types of transformers, the x-ray tube and several additional devices. The circuit is shown above. For explanatory purposes the basic circuit is separated into the filament circuit, the high-voltage circuit and the timing circuit.

Figure 35.8
Schematic drawings of the basic dental X-ray unit.

5. When your doctor signals you that he or she is ready, press the release button and hold it depressed. The timer will count off the seconds or fraction of a second.
6. Observe the milliammeter during the exposure. If it is not operating, the image will not appear on your film. Usually the required milliammeter reading is ten.
7. When you have finished the series of radiographs for one patient, turn off the machine if so instructed.

The Panoramic X Ray

The panoramic X ray is used for a generalized overview of the oral cavity. The patient sits or stands with his or her chin on a chin rest (fig. 35.11). The tube and film move around the patient's head, recording an X ray of the oral cavity on one large sheet of film contained in a cassette mounted in the machine (fig. 35.10).

The panoramic radiograph is intended as a survey-type film that enables the dentist to see more anatomy. It is a screening view. The periapical film may still be necessary for operation. If a dentist uses the panorama approach to roentgenographic study, the usual procedure is a panoramic view and posterior bitewings. If anything on the panorama indicates the need, individual periapical films are made of those areas.

One of the advantages of the panorama is that the radiation dose is less than for a full mouth taken on individual periapical films. In addition, the problem of holding films correctly, either with bite blocks or by the use of the patient's finger, is eliminated. Film confusion is lessened because films are identified in the cassette. Films need not be mounted, thus a tedious, time-consuming, and difficult job is eliminated.

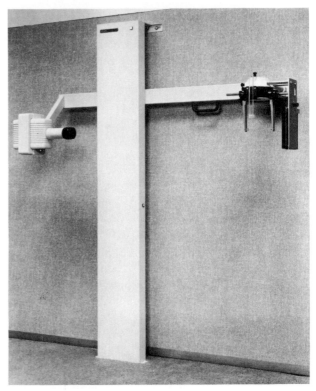

a

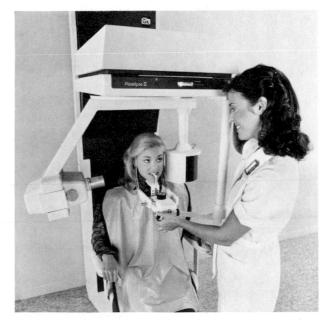

b

Figure 35.11
(a) Panoramic X ray for use with patients either sitting or standing (Panelipse II by Gendex); and (b) Cephalometric X ray (GX-CEPH by Gendex).

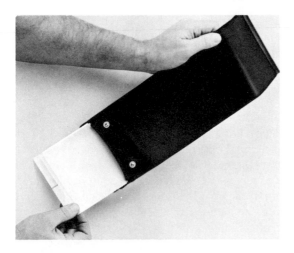

Figure 35.10
A panoramic X-ray cassette for film.

Dental Film—Intraoral and Extraoral

Two general classes of film are used for dental radiography. They are **intraoral** and **extraoral**. In this usage, *intra* means "inside" and *extra* means "outside": inside the mouth, outside the mouth.

Intraoral radiography is the type most commonly used by the general practitioner of dentistry. This technique allows the examination of teeth, surrounding tissue, and some limited examination of the maxillae or mandible.

There are three types of intraoral film: periapical, interproximal (or bitewing), and occlusal. **Periapical films** are used to examine the entire tooth and its surrounding tissues. **Interproximal films** examine the surfaces of the teeth that touch each other and the tissues and bones in those areas. We call them "bitewing X rays" in the dental office. **Occlusal films** are used for areas of the maxillae or mandible to discover pathology, root fragments, unerupted teeth, fractures, and other conditions.

In addition to providing total oral cavity view with the panograph machine, other types of extraoral radiographs are used to give the dentist additional information that may be needed for certain conditions. They are used for further examination of the mandible and maxilla and, in addition, of the temporomandibular joints and articulation, and of the facial bone and profile. These radiographs may be used in the study of injury, bone disease, presence of foreign bodies, development of the jaws, and presence of abnormalities. Orthodontists use facial profile radiographs (cephalometry) to measure bone structure and unerupted teeth, record conditions of the patient, and later to observe changes due to treatment or growth. They may be used in prosthodontics to record the relationship of the soft tissue of the face and the natural relationship of the teeth prior to their removal in order that the prosthetic devices may restore as much natural appearance as possible—and that the patient may be allowed to see that the natural appearance has been restored.

Film Description and Management

Dental film itself is composed of an emulsion, that is, gelatin containing a silver compound coated on a tinted base that is made from a cellulose derivative. The base is about 0.008 inch thick. It is stiff and flat to the degree necessary for proper manipulation. If the base is coated on both sides with emulsion, it provides maximum film speed, which means less radiation for patient and operators. Speed means shorter exposures. Shorter exposures also have an added advantage: the patient is less likely to move and blur the image; therefore, less retakes are needed with faster film.

Standardization is occurring in film production. All manufacturers now put the film speed on the outside of the package. Perhaps film speed will be standardized and classified by number in the near future. The correct number for the speed of the film can be used on all film packets.

The large sheets of emulsion-coated base that are to become dental film are cut to the size used for one of the several types of dental films. They are then either made into a packet for the intraoral work or packaged for extraoral use.

Intraoral Film

Periapical film is manufactured in three sizes: No. 1, or standard film, is about 1¼-by-1⅝-inch; child's film, or No. 0 or 00, is about ⅞-by-1⅜ inch. Some manufacturers make an in-between size for older children (six years to eleven or twelve years of age) that is about ¹⁵/₁₆-by-1⁹/₁₆-inch. Standard periapical film is used for older children and adults. It usually shows three or four teeth and the surrounding bone and tissue, including the apex of the root. Children's film is used for small children.

Bitewing film is made in a variety of sizes to accommodate the variations in the size of dental arches and the multiple uses of the film.

A tab or flap is used with bitewing film to hold it in proper position for these X rays. The tab fits between the lower and upper arches and is held firmly in place by the patient when the patient closes his or her teeth as the film is placed.

Occlusal film is about 2¼-by-3 inches and is used to show larger areas that cannot be seen on a periapical film. The film is held in place in the mouth, much like a cracker, by gentle pressure of the teeth.

Extraoral Film

Extraoral film is usually a five-by-seven-inch or eight-by-ten-inch sheet. The five-by-seven-inch size is used for the lateral jaw technique; the eight-by-ten-inch size is used for skull views. Sometimes a larger size is also used for these views.

The film is supplied in boxes of various sizes. Each film is placed between a folded sheet of black paper. All the films are wrapped in light-proof paper that usually has a tinfoil backing and are then placed in a cardboard container and sealed. This container must not be opened except in a darkroom that is equipped for safely handling such film. In order to use this film, a film holder can be made of cardboard to hold the film in a lightproof container while exposure is made.

If it is desirable to reduce the time exposure and still use the same emulsion, a cassette is used instead of a film holder. It is usually an aluminum case in which two intensifying screens are placed.

An **intensifying screen** is a device that helps obtain the image on the film with less radiation than is possible with X-ray film alone. A screen is a smooth cardboard or plastic sheet coated with tiny fluorescent crystals mixed in a suitable binder. X rays can make certain substances give off visible light. These substances are phosphors. Two of them, calcium tungstate and barium lead sulfate, both of which give off blue light, are used to make intensifying screens. Each fluorescent crystal that absorbs X-ray energy gives off blue light and ultraviolet light radiation. The intensity is directly related to the intensity of the X rays in that part of the image. Therefore the differences in intensity of the X ray are transformed into differences in intensity in the blue and ultraviolet light. The film is highly sensitive to this light. It means that the light helps make the image faster than the X-ray beam alone can make it. Usually there are three types of intensifying screens: (1) fast for high intensification, (2) average for balance between speed and definition, and (3) slow for better image sharpness. Average screens usually are used for extraoral radiography. These screens, placed in the cassette, must contact the surface of the film perfectly, and the cassette must be lightproof.

Suitable marking equipment is needed to identify the X rays and the side visualized. This is important since an X ray may be used as evidence. The question may arise as to how your dentist knows that this particular film is actually an X ray of the patient involved in the court action. A code number or actual printing of a patient's name on the X ray will remove any doubt. No method is available for intraoral film marking as yet.

Panographic Film

The panographic film is placed in a cassette with an intensifying screen. One manufacturer uses a wraparound film cassette that is a lighttight vinyl envelope. Another manufacturer uses a flat metal box as the cassette.

Care of the intensifying screen is important because anything that affects the screen also affects the film image. The screens must be protected from damage and dust. Chemicals dripped into the cassette can leave a stain on the screen which will block the light and prevent the exposure of the underlying part of the film. Be certain the cassette and screens are clean at all times. Screens may be cleaned with a *damp* (not wet) sponge or with alcohol.

Getting Acquainted with the Actual Film

For all practical purposes, periapical film will acquaint you with dental X-ray film. To the layman, an X-ray film is a white paper-covered object that is placed in

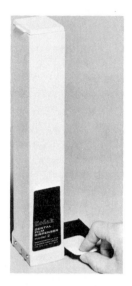

Figure 35.12
Film dispenser.

the patient's mouth when an X ray is to be made. To the dental personnel, this packet consists of the outer wrapper, which is sometimes in two pieces, a piece of black paper, a thin sheet of lead foil, the film itself (the emulsion-coated base), and another piece of black paper.

Take a packet apart. See and feel each part. Close your eyes and learn to distinguish the various pieces by touch so that you will recognize them when you develop X rays in the darkroom. The larger five-by-seven-inch or eight-by-ten-inch film will feel the same as the periapical-size film itself. Thus you can discern its texture from the wrappings in which the larger films are packaged just as you differentiate the periapical, occlusal, or bitewing films from their wrappings.

Protecting the Film

Film must be protected from the X rays that escape in the dental office during the filming of a patient's mouth. Thus, it is kept in a film storage box that is lined with lead to protect the film.

There are two commonly used types of storage boxes. One is approximately ten inches long, six inches wide, and four inches deep, with a removable lid. The other type is a wall mounted metal container that will hold more than one package of periapical film stacked vertically. Individual films are removed from the bottom of the film safe, and provision is made for refilling as needed (fig. 35.12).

In the first type of storage box mentioned, more flexibility is available for storing different sizes of films. The various sizes of film used in the office may be kept separate from each other by the use of cardboard boxes within the film storage container.

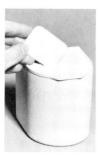

Figure 35.13
Receptacle for exposed film.

It is also important that the film exposed during radiography of a patient be stored in a lead container in order that stray radiation does not spoil the radiography already recorded on the film (fig. 35.13).

Summary

X rays are necessary to complete diagnosis in dentistry. They can be dangerous and therefore must be properly used.

A dental radiograph is a photographic record produced by the passage of X rays through the tissues of the mouth to a film.

Three characteristics of X rays important to dentistry are:

1. They penetrate many materials that either absorb or reflect light.
2. They can be seen on photographic film.
3. They can produce biological changes and even kill; thus, we must be exceptionally careful in using X rays.

We need to understand the construction of an X-ray tube and its correct operation. Vocabulary to understand includes milliamperes, kilovoltage, penetrating power, subject contrast, geometry of shadow, exposure, and sensitivity.

The potential danger of X ray must be thoroughly understood, and necessary protection should be afforded all persons who come in contact with X ray.

Symptoms of overdose of X ray must be recognized.

Hazards to be memorized:

1. Direct roentgen beam
2. Scattered radiation
   a. Leakage radiation
   b. Secondary radiation

Six rules should be observed to protect everyone in the office from an overdose of X ray.

The parts of the X-ray machine with which you should be especially familiar are the tube and the timer.

There are seven steps in operating the X-ray machine that should be memorized.

The panograph X ray automatically records a full-mouth roentgenogram of a patient whose chin is resting on a chin rest. The full mouth X ray appears on one sheet of film. Less exposure is required than for the group of individual periapical films required for a full mouth series of X rays. However, detail may not show as clearly in all areas. The panograph may indicate the use of a periapical film for a particular area.

Two general classes of film are used for dental radiography. They are intraoral (inside the mouth) and extraoral (outside the mouth).

Three types of intraoral film are periapical, interproximal, and occlusal.

Extraoral radiography is used to give the dentist added information that he or she may need for certain conditions.

Dental film is composed of an emulsion coated on a tinted base. High-speed film is more desirable since it means less exposure to X rays and less danger of the patient moving and blurring the image.

Films are made in various sizes. You should be familiar with the sizes used in your office.

Extraoral film is usually a sheet five-by-seven-inches or eight-by-ten-inches. This film is usually used in a cassette instead of a film holder.

An intensifying screen helps obtain the image in a shorter period of time than is possible by the film alone.

Extraoral film should be marked with an identifying number or name.

It is wise to get acquainted with X-ray film by taking a packet apart.

Film must be protected both before and after exposure from the radiation that will be found in the dental office during the exposure of other films. There are lead-lined containers for used and unused film.

Study Questions

1. What value are X rays in dentistry?
2. Give three important characteristics of X rays which must be considered when using them.
3. Define or explain these terms:

cathode	kilovoltage
anode	penetrating power
focal spot	subject contrast
milliamperes	geometry of shadow
exposure	sensitivity
emulsion	

4. Discuss "an area-to-area variation in intensity of X rays which emerges from the subject."
5. Give five rules for accurate image formation.

6. Describe the potential dangers of X ray.
7. What precautions must be taken in the dental office against dangers of X ray?
8. List and describe the hazards in the use of X ray.
9. Describe the symptoms of X-ray overdose.
10. What are the six rules to be observed to protect the office personnel and patients from an overdose of X ray?
11. Discuss the X-ray head as it is manufactured today.
12. What is the purpose of a timer?
13. Describe the operation of a standard X-ray machine.
14. Describe a panoramic X ray and state its purpose.
15. Discuss the different types of film and their purposes.
16. How is film protected? From what must it be protected?

Vocabulary

anode   copper bar with tungsten button in it

bitewing X ray   interproximal X ray

dental radiograph   photographic record produced by passage of X rays through the tissues of the mouth to the film

developer   chemical solution that causes exposed grains of silver compound to change to masses of black metallic silver during development of X-ray film

extraoral   outside the mouth

film badge   a badge that indicates the amount and type of radiation to which wearer has been exposed

intensifying screen   a device that helps obtain an image on X-ray film in a shorter period of time than is possible with X-ray film alone

interproximal films   X-ray film used to examine surfaces of teeth that touch each other and the tissues and bones in those areas

intraoral   inside the mouth

inverse square law   states the relationships of intensity to distance

kilovolt   electrical term that measures the speed at which electrons travel

leakage radiation   radiation that has escaped from the X-ray tube in directions not intended for use

milliampere   electrical term referring to amount of electrical current being carried by the conductor

occlusal films   X-ray films used for areas of the maxillae or mandible to discover pathology, root fragments, unerupted teeth, fractures, and other conditions

panoramic X ray   intended as a survey-type film which enables dentist to see more anatomy, a screening view

penetrating power   the ability of a beam to pass through an object

periapical films   used to examine the entire tooth and its surrounding tissues

primary beam   direct roentgen ray beam

roentgen ray   X ray

scattered radiation   leakage radiation

secondary radiation   new radiation that is created by primary radiation acting or passing through matter

sensitivity   rapidity with which film responds to exposure

CHAPTER 36

Radiographic Techniques

Part One: Intraoral and Extraoral Techniques
Quality Radiographs
Intraoral Procedures
   The Relationship of the Patient to the X-ray Tube
   Periapical Short Anode-film Procedure
   Periapical Long Anode-film (Long Cone)
      Procedure
   Bitewing Technique
   Occlusal Technique
Extraoral Procedures
Seven Steps for Better X-ray Exposures
Part Two: Processing of Film
Automatic Film Processing
Hand Processing of Films
   The Darkroom or Processing Room
Care of X-ray Developing Tank and Solutions
X-ray Processing Solutions
   X-ray Developer
   X-ray Fixer
Procedure for Developing X Rays
   To Develop the X Rays
Ten Steps for Excellent Processing of Radiographs
**Part Three: Processed Film . . . Its Use, Care, and
      Storage**
Mounting Radiographs
Distinguishing Bitewing X Rays
Distinguishing Periapical X-ray Series
Panoramic X Ray
Filing X Rays and Records
Four Steps in Preservation of Radiographs

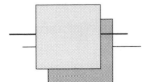

Part One: Intraoral and Extraoral Techniques

Quality Radiographs

The quality of radiographs depends on the skill with which they are produced. A poor radiograph prevents or interferes with the making of an accurate diagnosis. Since the purpose of the radiograph is diagnosis, we should not expose human beings to unnecessary radiation unless the results of the exposure will be radiographs of excellent quality.

This chapter is devoted to a discussion of the techniques that will produce excellent radiographs. Whatever part you play in their production (depending upon the laws of your state and the wishes of your dentist), it is imperative that you develop expert skills in the execution of your duties from proper preparation of the patient for X rays to hanging films to dry. While some states do not permit the dental assistant to take X rays, it is the belief of the authors that this function may become more broadly legalized as a function of the dental assistant.

Certain steps must be followed to secure good radiographs. It is necessary to select the correct film, properly prepare and position the patient, correctly place the film, see that it is properly retained, position the X-ray head, make the correct exposure, remove the film, and place the film in safe storage before the next film is exposed. Intraoral radiographs add one step after removal of the film: wipe off all moisture; then place the film in safe storage before proceeding with the next exposure.

The patient should be routinely asked when the last X-ray studies had been made and whether the patient has been exposed to X-ray or gamma-ray radiation for industrial, experimental, medical diagnostic, or therapeutic reasons.

The patient should remove such items as glasses, dentures, removable partial dentures, or removable bridgework. Any of these objects will produce shadows on the X ray. These shadows may obscure details that should be observed or may cause confusion in diagnosis.

Intraoral Procedures

The Relationship of the Patient to the X-ray Tube

The plane of occlusion of the teeth to be visualized on the radiograph should be parallel to the floor. The sagittal plane (vertical, midline plane) of the body should be perpendicular to the floor. Thus the spine should be straight—at right angles to the floor—and the occlusal plane of the teeth should be parallel to the floor.

Mouths vary, and it is sometimes necessary to make adjustments in the film techniques to accommodate the differences in individuals. Some mouths have narrow dental arches, some have high vaults.

Angulations, as indicated on charts of recommended X-ray tube positions, are now properly read on the angulation scales on the X-ray machine. Having the patient properly positioned makes these scales on the machine effective and useful. For example, if the patient is to have an upper central incisor radiographed, he or she is seated with the upper arch horizontal. The X-ray tube head is adjusted to a vertical angle of forty to forty-five degrees. The X-ray film is placed, any necessary adjustment is made in tube angulation for variation in vault shape, and the exposure is made.

If, however, the patient is seated with the upper arch sloping toward the distal twenty degrees (let us say), the tube-head angle would have to be increased to sixty to sixty-five degrees for an average range. If the exposure were made at the recommended angulation but with the patient incorrectly oriented to the tube head and no visual correction or adjustment made, the resulting X-ray visualization would be elongated to the point of worthlessness.

The general rule for the vertical angle of the central ray is that the central ray must be projected perpendicularly to a plane bisecting the angle formed by the longitudinal axis of the tooth and the plane of the film packet.

Ninety percent of the jaws are fairly symmetrical and can be photographed by the use of the rule. Individuals with a high vault may need to have the angle *decreased* about five degrees because the high vault causes the packet to be more nearly vertical in position.

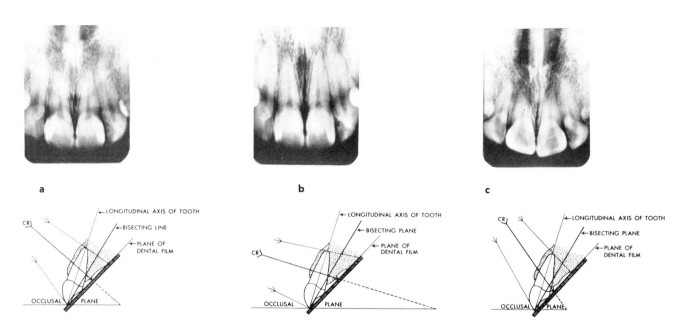

Figure 36.1
Vertical angle of the central ray affects results: (a) diagram shows proper projection of central ray to obtain image of correct proportion on film; (b) when central ray is projected from too low an angle (as in diagram), images are enlongated on film; and (c) when central ray is projected from too high an angle (see diagram), images are foreshortened on film.

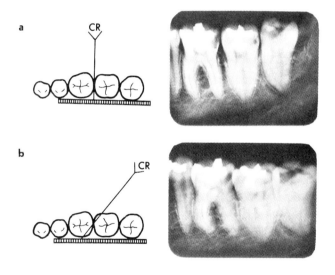

Figure 36.2
Horizontal angle of the central ray affects results: (a) diagram shows correct horizontal angle for projection of central ray to obtain film with distinct images without overlapping; and (b) diagram shows incorrect horizontal angle of central ray projection, which results in images that are badly overlapped and blurred on the film.

If the vault is low, the angle may have to be *increased* five degrees because the low vault causes the packet to be less vertical in position. When an individual's mandibular area is not symmetrical, it may be necessary to increase the vertical angle about five degrees when the teeth are buccally inclined or the mouth is shallow. If the teeth are more vertically positioned or the floor is deep, the angle is decreased about five degrees.

The central ray must also be correctly projected at a horizontal angle. The beam must pass through the spaces between the teeth without overlapping the adjacent tooth structures (fig. 36.2). Thus the central ray must be positioned correctly both vertically and horizontally.

Periapical Short Anode-film Procedure

Average angles: Figure 36.2 gives directional information for placing films properly in the average mouth. The average angles are a guide in placing films, which may then be varied if the mouth is nonsymmetrical.

Bending of films: Whether or not a film should be bent when placed in a patient's mouth has been the subject of considerable discussion. It would seem that the films must be bent in order to permit the film to occupy the positions given in figure 36.2.

Table 36.1
Correct Placement of Films for Best Results In Various Regions of the Mouth

Region	Long Axis of Film	Center of Film	Anterior Edge of Film	Occlusal Edge of Film	Approx. Vert. Angle*
Upper molar	Horizontal	Over 2nd molar	Over middle of 2nd premolar	¼" below occlusal surface	35°
Upper premolar (bicuspid)	Horizontal	Over interproximal space between molars	2nd incisor region	¼" below occlusal surface	45°
Upper canine (cuspid)	Vertical	Over canines		⅛" below nasal edge	45° to 60°
Upper incisors (centrals and laterals)	Vertical	Over interproximal space between 1st incisors		⅛" below incisal edge	50° to 60°
Lower molar	Horizontal	Over 2nd molar	Over middle of 2nd premolar	¼" above occlusal surface	−5°
Lower premolar (bicuspid)	Horizontal	Over interproximal space between premolars	2nd incisor region	¼" above occlusal surface	−35°
Lower canine (cuspid)	Vertical	Over canine		⅛" above nasal edge	−35°
Lower incisors (centrals and laterals)	Vertical	Over interproximal space between 1st incisors		⅛" above incisal edge	−35°

*If the jaws are edentulous, it may be desirable to increase the above approximate angles by 15° in the upper and decrease them −15° in the lower. If a child's mouth is to be visualized, increase in the above approximate angles may be desirable.

The packet must not be bent so that the bend occurs over the center of the region of interest because the image will then be distorted. This distortion will make the film valueless for the purpose of interpretation.

In bending the film packet, great care must be taken so that the packet is not sprung. If this occurs, light may leak in around the packet and expose the emulsion. The packet must not be bent to such an extent that a crease is produced. The emulsion is extremely sensitive to pressure, and a sharp bend will result in increased pressure along a definite line. When the film is processed, a clear line will cross the film over the region of the bend.

Since there is adequate depth or height in the molar region, no bend is necessary. However, in the premolar region the film must be bent at the anterior radicular edge away from the side of the film, which will be placed next to the teeth, so that the film may occupy the correct position in the mouth and not gouge into the anterior portion of the floor or the roof of the mouth. Since the canine occupies the corner of the arch, the film must be adapted to the curvature of the arch, and the anterior radicular edge of the film must also be bent away from the tube side of the packet. In the anterior region, the film must be gently curved on the long axis so that it will fit this region of the mouth.

Placement of the film: The correct positioning of film in the patient's mouth is of utmost importance. The center of the film must be placed so that it is over the center of the region of interest. This might be the premolar region or it might be a single tooth, as for example, the first molar.

When increased vertical angulation is necessary for the production of a shadow of a tooth equal in length to the tooth itself, the buccolingual diameter of the tooth will cast a shadow on the film that will add to the length of the shadow of the tooth. Therefore, in the molar and premolar region the occlusal edge of the film must be ¼-inch below the occlusal plane of the upper teeth and ¼-inch above the occlusal plane of the lower teeth so that the entire occlusal surface of the tooth can be visualized on the X ray. Since the anterior teeth do not have large buccolingual diameters at the level of the occlusal plane, the occlusal edge of the film need be placed only slightly above or below the incisal edge of the anterior teeth.

Table 36.1 outlines the position for the film packet in order to produce a satisfactory X ray of each region of the mouth. It is important, in all regions of the mouth, to place the packet in such a way that the occlusal edge of the packet will be parallel with the occlusal or incisal edge of the teeth.

The anterior edge of the film is mentioned in table 36.1 because it is frequently easier to place the anterior edge of the film over a certain tooth or region than to place the center of the film over the center of the region of interest. The vertical angulations are only approximate and over a long period of time have been found to produce satisfactory X rays in the majority of instances. Occasionally, even though these angles are used, elongation or foreshortening results. If unsatisfactory results are produced, this condition may be corrected by taking a second picture and increasing or decreasing the vertical angle in a positive or negative direction by at least fifteen degrees as described in the section on the geometry of shadows.

The placement of film must be deftly carried out so that the delicate structures of the mouth are not lacerated or the patient's gag reflex stimulated.

Procedure for placing films in the upper molar region varies according to the side to be examined. For the upper right side, the film is carried in the mouth so that it is parallel with the occlusal plane. It is pushed back in the patient's mouth on the occlusal surface of the upper teeth until the posterior edge of the film contacts the tissue over the anterior border of the ascending ramus of the mandible. With your right hand, grasp the patient's left palm and guide his or her thumb so that it presses the film packet firmly against the roof of the mouth and the lingual surface of the teeth. If this procedure is carefully followed no gagging will result.

For the upper left molar region, the same procedure is followed, except that the patient's right thumb is guided into the mouth to hold the film firmly against the lingual surface of the teeth and the roof of the mouth.

If the film is not back in the mouth far enough, grasp it between the thumb and forefinger and slide it back so that it occupies the position outlined in table 36.1.

Placement of the packet in other regions of the upper jaw presents no appreciable difficulty, provided that the films are adapted to fulfill the requirements stated previously.

Great care must be taken to have the patient relax the tongue and muscles of the floor of the mouth in order to place films for the lower jaw. To accomplish relaxation is frequently difficult. One way of teaching the patient is to insert one forefinger under the tongue and the other forefinger on the outside of the face underneath the floor of the mouth. Your forefinger then bounces up and down on the muscles of the floor of the mouth. The patient will know which muscles to relax. The film packet is ready for placement following the attainment of a relaxed state of the floor of the mouth.

To place film for the lower right side, displace the tongue with your right index finger and place the film with your left hand. Remove your right hand and place the patient's left forefinger on the film so that it is held firmly against the molar teeth and gums. When placing film for the lower left side, the same procedure is followed except that the duty of each hand is reversed.

The easiest and most direct technique for the retention of film is to have the patient use his or her thumb to hold the film against the upper teeth and use a forefinger to hold it against the lower teeth so that an exposure may be made.

Bite blocks are used with very satisfactory results. The film is inserted in a small groove in a block, which is then placed between the teeth. The block is held steady by the pressure of the upper and lower jaws on it. This technique has some advantage over the finger-thumb method since the film does not slip as readily in a bite block.

Wipe all moisture from each film packet as it is removed from the mouth.

Periapical Long Anode-film (Long Cone) Procedure

The **long target-film technique** differs from the short target-film technique in three basic ways.

1. The distance between the target and the film is increased from approximately eight inches to at least sixteen inches. A special extension cone is used. The central rays of the X-ray beam are at the center of the cone.
2. The film is placed in the mouth so that the mean plane of the film and the tooth are as nearly parallel as possible. It involves the use of special film-holding devices. Because the film is more nearly parallel to the tooth, the vertical angles are much smaller than those used in the short target-film technique.
3. Contrast and penetration are controlled by increasing or decreasing the kvp setting on the X-ray machine.

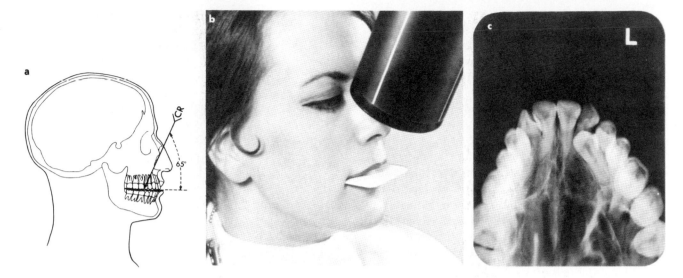

Figure 36.3

Occlusal film technique, maxillary incisor region: (a) projection of central ray (CR);
(b) placement of packet and cone; insert occlusal packet with nonslip side toward upper arch,
long axis coincident with median plane; direct central ray at vertical angle of +65° through
bridge of nose to center of packet; patient slowly closes mouth to immobilze packet with
gentle end-to-end bite; and (c) resulting radiograph.

In order to have an exposure time that is practical, ultraspeed film should be used. With sixteen-inch film-target distance and ultraspeed film, the exposure times become approximately equal to those used for techniques using the short film-target distance and intermediate-speed film.

Since ultraspeed film is more sensitive to variations in exposure factors, it is desirable that the X-ray unit be equipped with a filament stabilizer whenever it is to be used with the extension-cone technique.

Bitewing Technique

Bitewing technique has very definite advantages, and also disadvantages. It is designed for the specific purpose of visualizing the coronal portion of the tooth. It is excellent for locating interproximal and occlusal caries. It may be helpful in studying the alveolar process and alveolar bone at the neck of the tooth. Since only the coronal portion of the tooth is visualized, any change in the apical structure cannot be seen.

The film is placed so that it is parallel with the long axis of the teeth. Special film designed for the bitewing technique may be purchased; or a film for this technique may be made inexpensively by fastening an index tab to the tube side of the packet of a regular periapical-type film. When this method is used, be sure to use water—not saliva—to moisten the index tab. A paper loop is available for this purpose.

For the molars, place the film so that the tab is on the occlusal surface of the lower teeth. Carry the film as far posteriorly as possible. Ask the patient to close carefully so that the teeth touch the tab, using the tongue to hold the film close to the lingual surface of the teeth. A vertical angle of +5 degrees and correct horizontal angle will produce a satisfactory result.

When X-raying the premolar area, the anterior radicular edges of the film must bend away from the tube side of the packet so that these edges do not dig into the roof or floor of the patient's mouth.

Bitewings in the anterior region are not especially valuable because the long axes of the upper and lower teeth are not parallel. Angulation that produces suitable X rays of the upper teeth produces elongation of the lower teeth, and vice versa. A good periapical film of the anteriors usually will produce better results.

Occlusal Technique

Occlusal films are used when the small periapical films do not permit complete visualization of the region that is to be inspected roentgenographically. Occlusal films are 2½-by-3-inches in size.

Insert the film in the mouth in much the same way as you would a cracker. The packet is held in the occlusal plane by gentle pressure of the teeth.

Extraoral Procedures

Extraoral radiographs often supplement the information that your dentist obtains from periapical, occlusal, and bitewing radiographs. In some instances the extraoral radiographs are used without the intraoral examinations. (For example, the orthodontist uses facial profile radiographs to record changes due to treatment or growth.)

Extraoral radiography is used for examination of the mandible, maxilla, temporomandibular joints, and the facial profile. These radiographs are used more frequently by orthodontists, oral surgeons, and sometimes prosthodontists, in addition to institutions such as hospitals and clinics.

These films require special handling because their packaging is different from the film packet used for intraoral radiography.

Extraoral technique requires equipment in addition to that necessary for the intraoral technique. Various sizes of film are used. For the lateral-jaw technique, five-by-seven-inch film is used; for postero-anterior views, eight-by-ten-inch, or larger, film is used.

The panograph is included as an extraoral radiographic technique. One panoramic X ray, the Ortho-pantomagraph, has an attachment that permits the combination of the panoramic and cephalometric X-ray procedures on the same machine.

Seven Steps for Better X-ray Exposures

1. Be certain that the patient's head is correctly positioned.
2. Remove the film from its storage box.
3. Place the film packet correctly.
4. Align the central X ray accurately.
5. Select the correct exposure from your chart.
6. Make the exposure.
7. Store the film in a safe box where it will not receive further radiation.

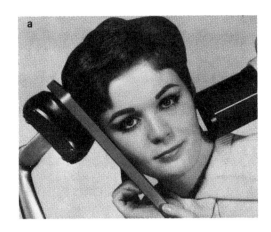
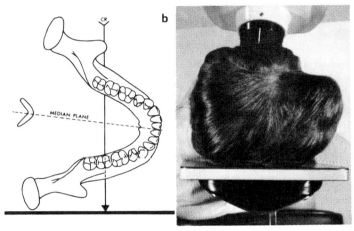
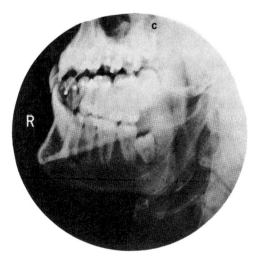

Figure 36.5
Extraoral film technique, ramus of mandible; (a) patient seated sideways with arm of chair lowered; film holder placed on headrest and chair back so that film is at +45° with horizontal plane; film holder held in position by patient using both hands at lower corners; (b) patient's right cheek in contact with front of film holder, median plane of head slightly rotated until zygomatic arch is touching film holder with lower border of mandible parallel to approximately +25° through lower second molar area on side being examined, to center of film; and (c) resulting radiograph.

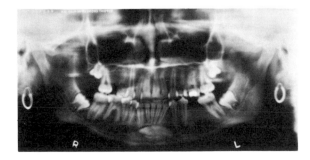

Figure 36.4
A panoramic film.

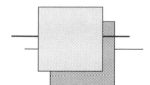

Part Two: Processing of Film

Changing the image on the film so that it can be seen is a process referred to as **developing** or **processing** the film. The process is accomplished by the use of chemicals, and at least the beginning stages must be performed in the dark. Thus **darkroom** evolved as the term for the place where exposed film is developed. Sometimes reference is made to the **processing room.**

Advances in technology have created the development of automatic processing in which the assistant places the film in an opening in a machine. The entire process is then automatically accomplished, with the finished film emerging from the machine minutes later.

Automatic Film Processing

The automatic developer is described as a mechanical link in a system designed to process dental X-ray films; it offers mechanical and chemical control of the process. It maintains solutions at proper temperatures and transports the film mechanically through these solutions at a specific speed, ending with a drying cycle.

We will describe one processor, but the principles of operation are similar regardless of the manufacturer.[1] The developer consists of three sections: film loading section with an electrical control panel; film processing section with plastic tanks, solution recirculation pumps, the roller transport system, temperature control devices, and the replenishment system; and a film dryer section containing air heaters, a blower system, and the receptacle for processed, dry radiographs.

Automatic processing is desirable because quality radiographs can be made in less time. Drying time also is cut with automatic processing. The entire automatic process is less than ten minutes.

Chemicals for the automatic processor are not the same as those for hand processing. They are purchased especially for the automatic processor, and the manufacturer's directions for use must be carefully followed, both for original filling of tanks and for replenishment.

Hand Processing of Films

Inasmuch as many dental offices still use hand processing and darkrooms, it is important that the process be explained thoroughly.

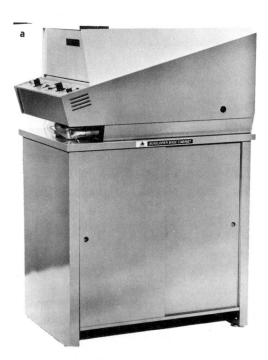

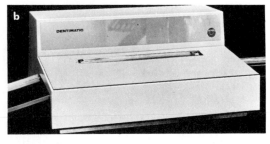

Figure 36.6
Automatic processors: (a) S. S. White processor described in text; and (b) Siemens fully automatic processor.

The Darkroom or Processing Room

A darkroom must be exactly what its name implies—a place that can be made totally dark. This does not mean it cannot be painted in bright colors. It usually is a small, windowless room containing only the necessary special equipment for developing X rays. Order must be maintained so that it is possible to find what you need in very low illumination. It must be kept absolutely clean if high-quality processing is to occur. It must contain a minimum of the special equipment, but some darkrooms will contain very elaborate equipment.

LEGEND

1 KODAK Darkroom Lamp with ML-2 Filter

2 Electric fan

3 Rack for drying films

4 Storage rack for intraoral hangers

5 Bulletin board

6 Exposure and Processing Chart for KODAK Dental X-ray Films

7 Drip pan

8 Shelf

9 Timer

10 KODAK Utility Safelight Lamp, Model C (fitted with opalized glass)

11 Gooseneck faucet

12 Loading area

13 Splashboard

14 Hot- and cold-water valves

15 8 x 10 dental processing tank

16 Utility sink

17 Supply cabinet for chemicals, cassettes, and other accessories

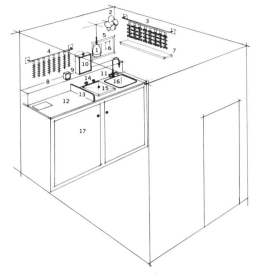

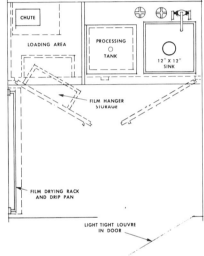

Figure 36.7
The components for an X-ray processing room.

Figure 36.7 is a model processing room. Note the seventeen items that are listed for this particular room. Not all these items are actual necessities, but they certainly help make the task easier. Let us look at the processing components that are necessities and at some that are helpful.

A normal electric light is necessary for use when films arc not being processed, in addition to a darkroom lamp, which is necessary for use during processing (fig. 36.7 [1]). This allows some dim illumination of the room, yet will not affect the X-ray films being processed, because the light rays that are harmful to film are filtered out. Counter-top safelight [10] for viewing wet films may also be used.

Racks for holding X-ray films [3] during processing and drying are necessary. The sizes your office uses will be determined by the types of radiographs your dentist takes.

A timer [9] is a necessity to time the development and washing of films.

A sink [16], equipped with hot and cold running water and a way of providing hot and cold water to processing tanks, is essential; as is a drain for the tanks.

A bulletin board [5] is convenient for posting your list of films and the developing chart [6] for the film that your office uses, but these lists can be taped on the wall if no bulletin board is available.

Some experts believe that it is better not to use an electric fan [2] in the darkroom because a fan stirs up dust in the room, and this dust may mar your films. An electric dryer is more desirable. However, proper cleaning can eliminate most dust.

Care of X-ray Developing Tank and Solutions

X-ray developing tanks are generally made to hold one gallon of developer and one gallon of fixer in separate compartments, with a larger central compartment connected to the water supply line and to the drain. The tank may be made entirely of hard rubber, a hard-rubber shell with stainless-steel one-gallon inserts to hold the solutions, or entirely of stainless steel. The tanks generally are made so that the containers for the developer and fixer are removable from the tank shell for easier cleaning.

When solutions need to be changed, they are drained by removing the plug that faces the central compartment on each side—one for the developer compartment and one for the fixer compartment. This allows the used developer and fixer to escape down the drain in the central compartment.

Always use the same compartment that previously contained the developer for the fresh developer, and the other for fixer. If your tank has steel inserts that are removable, remove, clean, and replace only one at a time to prevent reversing their positions.

The compartments for developer and fixer, when emptied, are scrubbed with a stiff brush and a solution of a strong detergent; the interior of the main tank is also scrubbed; then all are thoroughly rinsed with clear water.

Seat the rubber plugs very firmly. The developer and fixer compartments may now be filled with their fresh solutions.

X-ray Processing Solutions

Proper preparation, use, and storage of X-ray developing and fixing solutions are of extreme importance in the production of quality radiographs.[2]

You know that when a film packet is exposed to X-radiation a change occurs in the silver salts in the emulsion. The change causes the formation of a latent image (one to be developed). This image can be converted into a visible one by the chemical action of a **developer.** The film is then rinsed and placed in a **fixer** solution, which prevents the developing action from continuing so that your picture does not become entirely black and unreadable. The fixer solution changes the undeveloped silver salt particles to another salt that is water-soluble and transparent. If the film is thoroughly washed, the white particles are washed off, and the film is transparent where it should be transparent. If you do not wash the film thoroughly, it becomes milky white again and is not transparent. Thus, it is very important to wash the film thoroughly.

X-ray Developer

An X-ray developer, like a photographic developer, contains four kinds of ingredients.

1. The **developing agents,** which free the silver from the silver halide crystals.
2. The **preservative,** which prevents the developer solution from oxidizing in the presence of air.
3. The **activator,** which softens and swells the gelatin of the emulsion and provides the necessary alkaline medium so that the developer can readily attack the silver halide crystals.
4. The **restrainer,** which inhibits the fogging tendency of the solution. Like the activator, it also controls the rate of development.

When mixing developer solutions, the manufacturer's directions on the label *must be followed carefully* to obtain best results. Cleanliness is essential. Any chemicals spilled or splashed should be wiped up at once. Tanks must be kept in good condition by thoroughly cleaning after discarding old solutions. All traces of scum, dirt, and sediment must be removed.

Observe these general recommendations when mixing solutions.

1. In most instances, city water supplies are satisfactory. Chlorine produces no bad effects, but water should not be used that has a high calcium content or that contains metallic impurities or hydrogen sulfide. Temperature of the water in which the chemicals are to be dissolved should never exceed that recommended in the manufacturer's directions.
2. The container reserved for mixing the developing solution may be a clean crock, tank, or other suitable vessel of inert material. Stainless steel, hard rubber, glass, enameled iron, and glazed earthenware are satisfactory, but wood or reactive metals such as aluminum, galvanized tin, zinc, and copper are not suitable as either mixing containers or developing tanks. Stainless steel tanks should have welded rather than soldered seams, for solder will react with the developer solution to fog the radiographs produced.
3. Pour the water into the container first, then add the chemicals. When powdered chemicals are used, add them slowly, stirring vigorously.

4. When the chemicals are entirely dissolved, add sufficent cold water to bring the solution to the correct volume and temperature. Solutions should be at the optimum temperature of 68°F. before they are used.
5. Use separate stirring spoons or paddles for mixing developer and fixing solutions.
6. Cover tanks when not in use.

Development difficulties of various kinds may result if proper solutions and correct procedures are not used.

Lack of activity of a fresh developer solution may be the result of incorrect mixing or error in dilution.

High activity occasionally occurs, although it is less likely than low activity. It may be caused by incorrect mixing, such as the use of too small a volume of water, or by too high a temperature.

Crystallization is due to insufficient dilution when mixing or storing solutions at too low a temperature. The first difficulty can be avoided by proper mixing; the latter can be corrected by raising the temperature.

The solutions employed in developing X-ray films are most effective when used within a comparatively narrow range of temperatures. Below 60°F. some of the chemicals are definitely sluggish in action, which slows the action of the developer. Above 80°F. they work too rapidly. Within these limits, changes in temperature can be compensated for by varying the development time. A temperature of 68°F. is most practical from the standpoints of uniformity of chemical activity and time required.

After the temperature of the developer has been determined, the films should be left in the solution for the exact interval that is required. Consult the manufacturer's directions. Guesswork should not be tolerated. An accurate timer and thermometer should always be used.

One of the advantages of time-temperature technique is that it provides a definite check on the accuracy of the exposure used. If a radiograph is too dark after fixation, exposure was too great; if the radiograph is too light, the film was underexposed.

Agitation: When films are first placed in the developer, they should be agitated for a second or two beneath the surface of the developer in order to break loose any air bubbles that might be clinging to their surfaces. These bubbles would cause round spots on the radiograph.

Replenishment: Developer replenishment should be practiced to maintain developer activity. Increasing development time as the developer loses its activity is not a good procedure for two reasons: (1) It is inaccurate, because no one can judge how much activity has been lost and compensate by establishing a new time factor that will be accurate. Radiographs will be of top quality only when the developer is fresh. (2) There will always be a loss of quality near the end of the useful life of the developer. Radiographs can be of excellent quality if more developer is added as the level of the solution is lowered through use and evaporation. The replenisher solution should be mixed according to the directions on the container label.

Discarding developer: Developer solutions should be discarded on schedule so that the radiographic quality will remain high. Developer used past its useful life will produce developer fog, which seriously impairs the interpretative quality of the radiograph. Replenishing the developer does not eliminate the necessity to change the solution on schedule. If many radiographs are processed every day, discard the developer every two weeks. If fewer radiographs are processed, a three-week interval may be acceptable, but the developer should seldom be used longer.

Storage of developer solution: Developer is exhausted by use and by exposure to air since both cause oxidation. All air should be excluded from stored developer solutions since exposure to air is detrimental to the solution.

One excellent method of storing developer is in six- or eight-ounce bottles. Each bottle is completely filled so that there is no air included in the bottle. There can then be no oxidation. When it is time to replenish the developer, one entire bottle of solution is added to the tank. The rest of the solution, stored in other six- or eight-ounce bottles, is not opened and thus remains fresh.

This method is far superior to storing all the solution in one large bottle that acquires more air each time the solution is poured from it to replenish the tank.

X-ray Fixer

An X-ray fixer solution also contains four kinds of ingredients.

1. The **clearing agent** chemically changes the unexposed silver halide crystals remaining after development.
2. The **preservative** prevents decomposition of clearing agent and assists in clearing the film.
3. The **hardening agent** shrinks, tans, or hardens the gelatin emulsion to prevent excessive swelling and softening.
4. The **acidifier** provides the necessary acid medium and makes possible the correct action of the other ingredients.

Clearing time is the interval between placing the film in the fixer and the disappearance of its initial opaqueness.

Fixing time is the total interval the film must remain in the solution to chemically change the undeveloped silver salts and to harden the gelatin. This should be at least ten minutes, but films should not be left in fixer solution for prolonged periods or overnight, for the image itself will gradually lose density.

Mixing fixer solutions: When mixing fixer solutions, the manufacturer's directions on the label must be followed carefully in order to obtain best results. Cleanliness is absolutely necessary.

Temperature: It is desirable that the developer, rinse water, and fixer be maintained at a constant temperature.

Agitation: Fixing time is shortened and nonuniformity of the image prevented if films are agitated in the fixer. Thus, a greater volume of the fixer solution is brought into contact with the films in a given period, and rinse water is more rapidly removed.

Discarding fixer: The usefulness of the fixer solution ends when it has lost its acidity or when too long a time is required to change the unexposed silver salts. Use of an exhausted fixer should be avoided to assure production of excellent quality radiographs. A good rule is to discard the fixer solution at the same time that the developer solution is discarded.

Procedure for Developing X Rays

Materials required:

1. X rays to be processed correctly labeled with the patient's name
2. Film holders for the number of X rays you are to develop
3. A pencil
4. Developer
5. Fixer
6. X-ray washing equipment
7. Timer or watch with a sweep-second hand

It is extremely easy to confuse the identity of X rays during processing and mounting. To exchange X rays of two different patients can be most dangerous and embarrassing. Be very careful to keep X rays correctly identified at all times.

Most dentists use a type of X-ray packet containing one piece of film, but some packets are available with two pieces of film. It is possible to take two identical X rays with such a packet. Discover just what film packets are used in your office before you begin to develop X rays.

X-ray film, while still wrapped in the packet, is not harmed by light. When unwrapped, however, it is sensitive to most kinds of light and must not be exposed in this manner anywhere but in a darkroom. This room is so designed that no light can reach the unwrapped film except the special illumination provided by a safelight designed for the purpose. This safelight, while very dim, will give you enough light to work in after your eyes have become adjusted.

To Develop the X Rays

With the ordinary light on in the darkroom, place the packets that you have to process—still wrapped in groups with the name of the patient written on the bundle—on the work top.

Place a pencil beside the films to be developed.

Place as many film holders as you need on the work top. The holder is usually a metal bar about twelve inches in length. The top end of the bar is curved to form a hook. A series of clips are arranged along each side of the metal bar. The individual films are attached to these clips. Another excellent type of holder has an arrangement of slots into which the films are placed.

At the top of the holder you may have noticed a white piece of plastic. The patient's name is written on this in pencil. If more than one patient's X rays are to be mounted on one holder, the names are written in the order in which the films are mounted on the holder.

The length of time for which the film is left in the developing solution is very important. On the bottle or can in which your developer is supplied to your office, you will find a recommended time-of-development scale. In general, the warmer the solution, the more quickly the film is developed. A floating thermometer should always be kept in the developer in order to indicate its exact temperature whenever you need to develop X rays. Find this temperature. Then, checking with the time-of-development scale, determine the length of time needed to develop the films you are about to do.

Developing solutions should not be used at temperatures in excess of 78° F. because the X-ray film may be damaged. If the temperature of the water in the central compartment is such that it cannot cool the solutions to less than 78° during the hot summer months, ice may be placed in it to accomplish this purpose. Do not put the ice directly into the developer or fixer. Unless it is confined in a plastic bag, the ice is placed in the central water compartment.

Fresh developing solutions are more active than solutions which have been used for a period of time. When first using a fresh solution, developing time should be exactly as recommended by the manufacturer at the temperature of your solution. As the solution gets older, when one-half minute more than the recommended time is needed to secure good development of the film, the solution should be discarded and fresh developer put in the tank. It should be changed every three weeks, or more frequently.

Turn on the darkroom safelight. Turn out the ceiling light in the darkroom. Pick up a package of films belonging to one patient. The patient's name and the number of films that are his or hers have previously been written at the top of a hanger. If there are four, for example, these four films are mounted, two on each side, at the top end of the hanger. If the first pair of clips are quite close to the top end of the holder, never use them. They may be out of solution when part has evaporated.

Separate a film from its wrappings, black paper, and foil. With forefinger and thumb open a clip, and with the other hand place an end of the film in the clip. Release the clip, then give it a firm squeeze to be certain that it has gripped the film securely. This is necessary to prevent the film from coming loose and dropping to the bottom of the X-ray tank while processing. If your holders have slots instead of clips, slide the film into the slots. Hold the film by its edges.

Do not place films on the lowest pair of clips unless the lower end of the hanger has been bent at a sharp angle to hold it away from the side of the tank when immersed. Unless this has been done, films placed on this pair of clips often develop improperly because they are held flat against the side of the tank, and the solution cannot circulate around them.

When the holder is loaded with film, hold it in one hand and plunge it up and down in the developer compartment three or four times before finally hooking the hanger over the edge of the tank. Place the cover on the tank.

Set the timer for the proper length of time. Since this is a matter of minutes, you can go on to other duties until you hear the timer bell indicate that the films must be removed from the developer. Leave the room with safelight only. Close the door. When the timer rings, the films must be removed immediately to prevent ruining them by overdevelopment.

Reenter the darkroom, closing the door behind you. The safelight is on. Remove the cover of the tank. Lift the hanger out of the developer and dip it four or five times into the water in the central compartment. Shake off the excess water. Plunge the hanger four or five times into the fixer compartment of the tank, then hook the hanger over the edge. Replace the cover on the tank.

The room light may be turned on now. It does not need to be turned off again, provided the cover of the tank fits well and is not removed until fixing is completed. The manufacturer of the fixer you use gives the recommended minimum period of time for proper fixing of film. Somewhat longer periods of time, such as one-half hour, are not harmful, provided the temperature of the solution is not permitted to become too high.

When fixing is completed, the film must be washed to remove all traces of fixing solution that has soaked into the film. Washing can be done in either the central compartment with the water running continuously or in a separate pan placed in the sink under an open faucet. If a pan is used, one end should be raised slightly, and the water should enter the pan at this end. If the washing is done in water that is circulating vigorously, one-half hour is sufficient; otherwise allow one hour.

Upon completion of washing, hold the hanger firmly and shake off all excess water, then hang where the film may dry undisturbed. Do not touch the film until all trace of water is gone. The hanger clip points will be the last areas to dry.

Ten Steps for Excellent Processing of Radiographs

1. Stir developer.
2. Check the developer temperature.
3. Select the correct developing time.
4. Open the film packets.
5. Attach films to correct hanger.
6. Set timer and develop films.
7. Rinse them.
8. Fix them.
9. Wash them thoroughly.
10. Dry them.

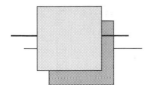

Part Three: Processed Film... Its Use, Care, and Storage

When the radiographs are completely dry, they should be prepared so that the dentist can read the film for each patient.

Mounting Radiographs

The first step is to mount the radiographs so that the films are more easily seen in relationship to each other. Prepare yourself for this task by gathering a few materials at your desk. You will need an X-ray mount for each patient whose X rays are to be mounted. An **X-ray mount** is a cardboard, celluloid, or both cardboard and celluloid card designed with openings or slots to hold the X-ray films in an orderly manner. They are available in many different sizes and combinations to suit the individual dental office.

You will also want the X-ray hangers, with the patient's X rays *still clipped to the hangers,* and a pen or pencil to write the name of the patient and the date of the X rays on the mount.

Again, we repeat: it is extremely easy to confuse the identity of X rays during processing and mounting. To exchange X rays of two different patients can be most dangerous and embarrassing. Be careful to keep X rays correctly identified at all times.

Remove from the hanger only those X rays belonging to one person. Mount them and write the patient's name on the mount, in pen or pencil, before removing the next group of X rays. The celluloid tab on the hanger has each patient's films correctly identified. Following this procedure will help you keep that identification accurately.

Any group of X rays of a given patient are mounted in sequence; that is, each area shown in any one X ray is the neighboring area of the one mounted next to it.

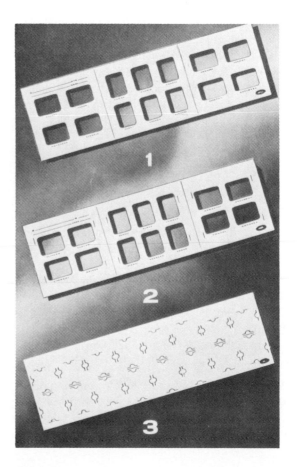

Figure 36.9
Complete film X-ray mounts, all for same purpose, depending on dentist's preference: (1) frosted backing cardboard mount; (2) clear backing mount; and (3) an all celluloid mount.

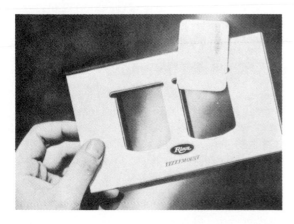

Figure 36.8
Film X-ray mount, Rinn Eezeemounts.

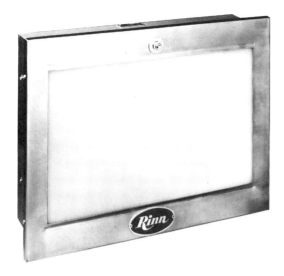

Figure 36.10
Recessible X-ray viewer on which X rays are placed on the glass panel with illumination from behind which permits viewing all details for accurate diagnosis.

Each X-ray film has a small, raised dot in one corner. When the film is mounted, this raised dot usually stands out on the side away from the face of the mount. (Some dentists prefer to reverse this mounting position, however.) Do not confuse clip marks from the hanger used in developing with the raised dot that the manufacturer places on the film.

Distinguishing Bitewing X Rays

Examine a mounted set of bitewing X rays and learn to recognize these landmarks:

1. The slight curve upward from the canine area toward the molar area, formed by the biting (occlusal) surfaces of the teeth.
2. The upward curve of bone at the end of the lower arch.
3. The appearance of the area behind the upper molars as compared with the appearance of the area behind the lower molars.

Now dismount this set of X rays, mix them up, and turn them over thoroughly; then see if you can mount them correctly. Repeat this by remounting a set that you have not seen in the mount.

Distinguishing Periapical X-ray Series

Compare a complete X-ray series with the bitewing X rays to recognize the same landmarks. Then learn these additional features:

1. The root differences between upper and lower teeth.
2. The way in which the root tips usually curve toward the back (distal) of the mouth.
3. The mental foramen in the lower premolar area.
4. The canal in the lower jaw through which the nerve and blood vessels pass.
5. The difference in size of upper anterior teeth as compared with lower anterior teeth.
6. The darkened area (sinus) usually visible above and between the roots of the upper premolar and molar areas.

Dismount this set of X rays, mix them thoroughly, and see if you can mount them correctly. Practice with several old complete X rays and have your work checked for accuracy.

X rays of a complete set of teeth are the easiest to mount correctly. With practice, you will soon be able to progress to mounting X rays that have few teeth visible to help you orient yourself.

Panoramic X Ray

Film sheets of panoramic X rays are often unmounted, although there are mounts for them. The sheet of film can be stored in the patient's record envelope or in a separate X-ray envelope that is placed in a file for X rays. This envelope is the same size as the film and thus requires a special-size file drawer.

Filing X Rays and Records

After your dentist has finished diagnosing the patient's dental needs from the radiographs that you have mounted, the films must be stored since they are a permanent part of the record of each patient.

Most dentists keep an X-ray film mount for each patient, with the current X rays in it. The method of filing these may vary, however.

The cardboard mount has lines on the upper border for the name of the patient and the date of current X rays. If the date is written in pencil, it can be erased and kept current through the years.

There are two commonly used methods of filing X rays in mounts. Some offices file them in a file drawer reserved for X rays only, either alphabetically by name or numerically by the patient's number. The mounts are filed as cards would be filed. For the alphabetical file, the name of the patient is written in ink, last name first, on the line provided in the upper left-hand corner. The patient's number precedes the name if the office uses a numerical file. The penciled date is written on the next line.

The complete X-ray mounts are filed in one drawer, or at least under one set of alphabetical guide cards. The bitewing X-ray mounts are filed in another drawer, or under a separate set of guide cards.

The patient's mounts are removed from the file for an appointment and are returned to the file at the close of the appointment.

Some dentists prefer to keep the X-ray mounts in the patient's record envelope in accordance with the principle of having all records of the patient kept together.

In either case, when the X rays are no longer current (that is, when new X rays are taken), they are removed from the mounts and placed in an envelope. A coin envelope works nicely. The patient's name and date of the X ray are written in ink on the outside of the envelope. These envelopes are usually kept in the patient's record envelope as part of the permanent record. The new films are then placed in the mounts.

Four Steps in Preservation of Radiographs

1. Mount the dry radiographs in proper mountings with accurate identification.
2. Have your dentist read them for diagnosis, using the X-ray viewer.
3. Keep them available during patient's visits.
4. File them properly when work has been completed.

Summary

The quality of radiographs depends on the skill with which they are produced. A poor radiograph prevents accurate diagnosis. It is essential that the correct film be selected, the patient properly prepared, the films correctly placed, the correct time used for the exposure of the film, and proper care taken of the film after exposure.

Short-target techniques are commonly used in the dental office, but long-target techniques are also important and use of eight-inch and sixteen-inch techniques are to be encouraged.

Intraoral techniques include periapical, bitewing, and occlusal radiographs. Panoramic X-ray procedures produce an overview of the oral cavity for which a special machine is used. Some dental offices use the panorama and posterior bitewings for the routine dental examination, adding periapical films of doubtful areas. Other extraoral techniques are used to supplement information gained through the use of the intraoral techniques. In some instances the extraoral radiographs are used without intraoral examinations. The common uses for extraoral radiographs are examination of the mandible, maxilla, temporomandibular joints, and the facial profile. The extraoral radiographs are more commonly used by orthodontists, oral surgeons, prosthodontists, hospitals, and clinics. The extraoral film receives special handling.

Review seven steps for better X-ray exposures.

It is necessary to develop or process the exposed X-ray film. The processing can occur with an automatic developer into which the assistant places the exposed film and then removes it some minutes later, or the film can be hand-processed. Hand processing is subject to more error than automatic processing.

If hand processing is performed, a darkroom must be utilized. A darkroom is a place that can be made totally dark for the development of X rays. The special equipment necessary to develop X rays is kept in this room.

The mixing and the care of solutions used for the development of the radiographs are very important parts of dental assisting.

Learn to care for the solutions properly and to develop X rays carefully. Follow the instructions given you either in this chapter, by your dentist, or on the direction sheets that come with your X-ray developer and fixer.

Properly developed X rays are the first step to good diagnosis. Care should be taken in mounting the radiographs so that they may be read easily and correctly.

For properly mounting X rays you will need the following materials:

Mounts for complete and bitewing X rays.
X-ray hangers with patients' films still on them.
Pen.
Medium pencil.

Be careful to correctly identify all X rays.

Mount them in sequence.

Learn the identifying landmarks for both bitewings and full-mouth X rays.

Panographs are usually left unmounted.

Proper storage of X rays following use is desirable. They may be filed numerically or alphabetically in an X-ray file or kept in the patients' folders, depending on your dentist's preference.

Study Questions

1. On what does the quality of radiographs depend?
2. What three basic differences are there between long target-film technique and short target-film technique?
3. List the types of intraoral film.
4. For what purposes is extraoral film used?
5. What dental specialties most commonly use extraoral film?
6. Explain the purpose of processing film.
7. Describe automatic processing.
8. List the advantages of automatic processing.
9. Describe the steps in hand processing of film.
10. Describe the care of developer for hand processing.
11. Describe the care of fixer for hand processing.
12. What is the procedure for developing X rays by hand processing?
13. List the ten steps for excellent processing of radiographs.
14. Describe an X-ray mount.
15. Describe mounting periapical films.
16. Why must an X ray be positively identified?
17. Discuss the characteristics of bitewing X rays.
18. Discuss the characteristics of periapical full-mouth films.
19. Discuss panoramic X-ray storage.
20. Discuss two methods of filing periapical X rays.
21. What are the four steps in preservation of X rays?

Vocabulary

darkroom   room where X rays are developed in total darkness

developer solution   makes the latent image visible by its chemical action

extraoral   outside the mouth

fixer solution   stops developer action

intraoral   inside the mouth

latent image   one to be developed

radiograph   X ray

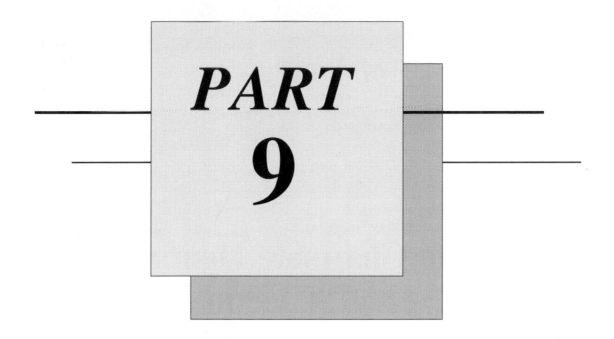

Operatory Procedures

This section is devoted to a general discussion of work and conduct with adults and children in the operatory, followed by a chapter on four-handed dentistry and then a chapter delineating a series of basic requirements for most operatory procedures. Each dentist may vary the requirements for certain procedures, but the materials and instruments that are considered basic requirements are listed. Your dentist may wish to go through this section of your text and write in his or her preferred instrumentation and materials for each operation.

You can then memorize the instruments and materials needed for a particular operation and be certain that they are available whenever the dentist is likely to need them.

CHAPTER 37

The Chairside Dental Health Team

Contribution of the Chairside Assistant
Risk Management
Waste Management
General Rules for Conduct in the Operatory
Preparing the Patient
   Care of the Patient's Dental Appliance
Tray Setups
Color Coding Instruments
Assisting with Preparations
Dismissing the Patient
Assisting with Children
Oral Examination Technique

The appointments have been made, the case studies presented, the telephone answered, most of the detail tasks discussed, and now it is time to enter the operatory and actually assist at the chair.

Contribution of the Chairside Assistant

The chairside assistant begins the association with the patient by readying the chair for patient comfort and placing a bib for protection. When the dentist enters the operatory, the assistant follows the dentist's directions. Often the routines have been so well prepared that no verbal directions are given.

The object of having a chairside assistant is to relieve the dentist of every task that someone else can do. Once the dentist begins preparation in the mouth, the necessity to look away to find an instrument or material creates eye strain and loss of time. If it is possible for the dentist to continue to look at the work-site, he or she avoids these two problems. The assistant proves to be valuable every time she or he can do for the dentist that which would cause the dentist to look away from the work-site. The chair assistant becomes a second pair of hands and eyes for the dentist. This team relationship has resulted in the concept known as **four-handed dentistry.** This concept embodies the most important work relationship in dentistry today. Four-handed dentistry is discussed in detail in chapter 38. The material in chapter 37 explains some general ideas useful in preparing for four-handed dentistry or in a dental office in which four-handed dentistry is not practiced.

In some offices the chair assistant has an assistant—a coordinating assistant or floater whose duties include keeping the chair assistant supplied with all necessary materials. The coordinating assistant takes impressions to the laboratory and cares for them. The chair assistant remains seated and receives from the coordinating assistant the same care that the chair assistant is giving the dentist. This concept developed the term, **six-handed dentistry:** (the dentist, the assistant, and the assistant to the assistant).

This chapter explains routines and duties generally necessary in every dental office. These duties are necessary for effective office management.

Risk Management

Today we are deeply concerned about infectious diseases. The dental operatory is a site for the quick spread of such infectious diseases as hepatitis and AIDS because the field is the patient's mouth. The transfer of disease from the patient to you, the dentist, or the next patient is so likely that it is essential to protect *everyone*.

The spread of infection can be controlled. It means that the dentist and the assistant *must* wear *protective eye wear, masks* and *gloves.* Cleanliness is the first step. It is very important everywhere, but it is mandatory in the operatory. Not just the operatory, either; *you* must be clean. Good grooming is essential. You will have accomplished it routinely by now. Hands must be clean before you start the day's work.

In the morning before you begin chairside assisting and again after lunch before you resume chairside assisting, it is wise to give your hands a thorough washing according to the hospital standards. Follow the directions given in chapter 24, "Microbiology and Sterilization," (1) in the morning after you have given the office its morning cleaning but before you begin chairside assisting and (2) on your return from lunch before you resume chairside assisting.

We learned in the section on microbiology that residue around soap dishes, water in which soap brushes are left standing, and the residue on the dispensers of liquid detergent or soap cultivate the growth of bacteria. Thus, at all times you should see that soap bars are set so that they drain dry. The dispenser for powder or liquids should be frequently scrubbed clean and brushes thoroughly rinsed. In addition, the wash basin itself must be scoured and kept shiningly clean.

Prepare the wash basin and soap so that they are clean and free from accumulations that encourage the growth of bacteria. This preparation can be made in the morning cleanup routine that precedes your preparations for chairside assisting.

Hospital scrub procedures require sterile brushes, which is a good idea. Your fingernail brushes can be autoclaved regularly.

In addition to thoroughly cleaning your hands, you are to wear glasses and a mask. Last, put on a new, clean pair of disposable gloves. These gloves are destroyed when you finish the cleanup of the patient. A new pair is used for the next patient.

It is essential to protect the patient as well as yourself and your dentist. Thus, strict observance of sterilization and cleanliness procedures in managing instrument and operatory cleanup is mandatory.

Waste Management

Used medical products (syringes, needles, blood bags, surgical blades, bandages, vials) washed up on the Atlantic Ocean beaches in New York and New Jersey creating an awareness of the serious threat posed by medical waste. These products had been thrown into the trash, and the waste haulers had dumped their trash loads into the ocean where much of the trash did not disintegrate. Bathers were even cut by used needles and surgical blades.

Thus, Congress began legislation to control the disposal of all medical waste, and at this writing, a plan for proper disposal has been implemented. The trial program includes New York, New Jersey, and the Great Lake States where medical waste must be properly handled.

Some states have developed their own plans and have been allowed to drop out of the federal program. The acceptable plans require the proper sorting, labeling, wrapping, transporting, and disposal of the ten types of medical waste listed below. The management and disposal of these types must be reported on a regular basis to the appropriate agency of the federal or state government.

1. cultures and stocks of infectious agents and associated biologicals
2. pathological waste
3. human blood and blood products
4. used sharps (syringes, needles, surgical blades)
5. contaminated animal carcasses
6. surgery or autopsy waste
7. laboratory waste
8. dialysis waste
9. discarded medical equipment
10. isolation wastes

The first five types must be reported by everyone. Types 6 to 10 may be excluded if it is determined that they do not present an environment or health hazard, either presently or at some future time.

The object of the program is to track the disposal of these wastes. All users of medical products are required to dispose of the waste they generate according to the directions from the EPA (Environmental Protection Agency) and to report the disposition regularly to the tracking agencies of the federal or state governments.

The importance of this information in the dental office is that this requirement must be met. All medical waste must be properly sorted, labeled, wrapped, and given to a disposal firm that has been approved by the EPA for disposing of medical waste.

The entire staff of each dental office will be expected to follow the regulations. Your dentist will receive instructions. The follow-through will be the responsibility of the entire staff. The EPA intends to track the disposal of medical waste and penalize anyone who does not comply. The trial program will be completed in June 1991. At that time, in view of the serious threat posed by medical waste, the EPA intends to develop a regulatory program for all fifty states.

(Material in this section is derived from the Federal Register for March 24, 1989, pages 12326–12337,

"Standards for the Tracking and Management of Medical Wastes" and the Minnesota Department of Health bulletin describing the Minnesota Infectious Waste Control Act of 1989.)

General Rules for Conduct in the Operatory

1. No conversation should deal with any subject other than the patient, the work in hand, or dental education. The patient is not assumed to be interested in what your young brother or sister, friend, or spouse said to you this morning or last night that was so funny.
2. Any message to the dentist while working on a patient should be indicated in a note held out of the patient's line of vision—just behind and to the left of the patient's head. If urgent, and beyond the scope of a note, indicate by note just the word "office" or "lab." The dentist will then go to the private office or laboratory as soon as possible to receive the message. Use this method only for urgent, confidential messages.
3. Be pleasant but never familiar with either the patient or the dentist.
4. Be sympathetic toward the patient.
5. Concentrate on the job you have to do.
6. Speak to and refer to the patient by name. The patient should not be referred to as *he* or *she* when the patient is present.
7. Keep your hands away from your person when working at the chair.
8. When the dentist is with you at the patient's side, your contributions to any conversation should be a minimum. If the dentist leaves the chairside, you should take up the duty of conversation. If you also must leave the patient, ask him or her to excuse you. If any wait is involved for the patient, see that reading material is provided (preferably material related to dentistry).
9. Assistance at the chair is primarily to help the dentist perform his or her duties more rapidly. Whenever you must leave the chairside during operations requiring assistance, accomplish the task as quickly as possible and return.
10. Maintain a pleasant expression in the operatory. However, be sure that you do not laugh for any reason at a time when the patient is not ready or able to share a laugh with you.

Preparing the Patient

Everything is in readiness for the patient. The patient's file is in its place, the radiographs are placed on the viewbox, and the instruments are ready. The operatory sparkles with cleanliness and is attractive; you have viewed it from the patient's point of view. It is time to seat the patient.

The dental assistant should enter the reception room, rather than merely extend her head and shoulders through the doorway or service window. A hand extended to the younger child may be helpful.

"Will you come in please, Mrs. Jones?"

"It's your turn now, Jimmy."

Your words should be carefully phrased to help the patient respond favorably to the trip into the operatory.

Lead the way to the proper operating room.

Ask men to remove jackets or to loosen neckties and shirt collars. Place women's purses or packages in a place visible to the patient but where they will not be in the way. A shelf for this purpose in each operatory is ideal and can usually be placed well toward the front, or on the front wall, about four feet from the floor.

Invite the patient to be seated and adjust the dental chair for her or his comfort.

Learn to adjust the dental chair used in your office. Practice until you are skillful. Comfort of the entire body allows the patient to relax. Dentistry becomes less difficult for the comfortable, relaxed patient.

Most chairs have marks indicating the average position of the headrest, the height of the backrest, and the angle of the backrest to the seat. Ask your dentist to show you how these are used. Know how to make the chair as comfortable as possible.

Place the bib over the patient. The bib chain should not rest on the bare skin at the neck unless unavoidable, and it should not be placed over a coiffure. If a full-length drape or throw is used, it is placed before the bib is put into position.

Give women a disposable tissue for removing lipstick. Often no words are necessary, but request removal of lipstick if the patient does not remove it.

If the patient is a stranger, introduce the dentist: "Mrs. Jones, may I present Doctor Smith?" Or, "Mrs. Jones, have you met Doctor Smith?"

Use the patient's name first. Pronounce the dentist's name clearly and distinctly.

Whenever possible, listen to patient-dentist conversation. Do so without having it be obvious to the patient. You may overhear an item you should note on the patient's record as a contact on the patient's next appointment. Pay attention to all sounds and words in the operatory. Awareness of everything occurring in the operatory is essential to good assisting.

Be fully prepared for all work scheduled for the patient's appointment.

When you and your dentist are ready to start performing dentistry, allow the patient to see you remove a new pair of gloves from the supply box and put them on. The patient is then assured that you are protecting the patient as well as yourself.

Care of the Patient's Dental Appliance

At an appointment for operative work or for prophylaxis recall to check a patient's remaining natural teeth, the patient is asked to remove his or her full denture, partial denture, or removable bridge after he or she has been seated in the dental chair. The dentist will make this request if he or she finds it desirable, although some patients will remove these appliances voluntarily when seated. Sometimes the dentist prefers to see the appliance while it is still in the mouth, and the dentist then removes it after this examination.

The assistant should carefully take the appliance, rinse it under the cold-water tap, and place it in a bowl of water until the appointment is over.

Bring the appliance back to the patient wet and lying on a folded disposable tissue on the palm of your hand. Let the patient pick up the appliance.

Do not forget to return appliances. Patients very easily fail to remember the appliance is missing until they are out of the office. It is embarrassing for most patients to return and ask for their appliances.

Tray Setups

In many offices today all the instruments necessary for a specific dental operation are placed on a tray immediately after they have been sterilized. They are placed in the order of their use, neatly arranged. A storage area holds the group of trays. The number of similar trays for each dental operation will vary with the frequency of use. Each tray is labeled for quick identification.

When the day's work schedule indicates the next patient is to have a crown preparation, a tray for crown preparation is removed from the storage unit and placed in the operatory. In this way, change-over time between patients is kept at a minimum. The dental assistant simply removes the tray of used instruments and replaces it with a tray of sterilized instruments for the specific operation to be performed.

Color Coding Instruments

Some offices use a color coding system with tapes. For example, all instruments to be placed on crown and bridge trays have a narrow gold ring taped on them, amalgam instruments are ringed with blue, and so on.

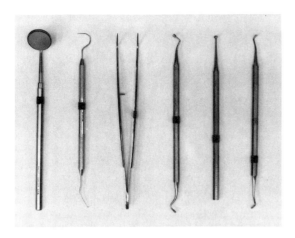

Figure 37.1

Sequence of use of instruments shown by placement of the identification band on the handle.

If storage of trays is in each operatory instead of a general storage area, an identification can be made with tape to indicate the correct operatory for each instrument. If the office has more than one operatory, one ring indicates the first operatory, and two bands indicate the second operatory. The trays are also marked on the edge with one or two stripes of color.

It is also possible to indicate the sequence in which the instruments are used by the placement of the color bands. For example, let us say five instruments are used in a specific operation. The color band is placed at the top end of the first instrument used in the preparation, ¼ inch farther down the handle of the second instrument, ½ inch down the handle of the third instrument, etc. When the instruments are placed in proper order on the tray, the rings form a diagonal line across the instruments (fig. 37.1). The dental assistant knows immediately whether or not the instruments have been placed correctly. The same process can be used for operatory two by considering the two bands a unit.

The cleanup and sterilizing of instruments can be performed at a time when the day's schedule permits. The sterilized instruments and trays are then replaced in their proper storage units. If they have been labeled by color coding, tape writing, or banding, the dental assistant can quickly reassemble the trays and return them to the storage cabinet.

Assisting with Preparations

If your dentist practices four-handed dentistry, this section is not for you. Turn to chapter 38 to learn four-handed dentistry. If your dentist does not utilize the concept of four-handed dentistry, these instructions are important for you to observe.

In dentistry, **preparation** is the term used to designate the shape a dentist makes in a tooth, with burs or other instruments, into or onto which the restorative material of choice is placed. The headings used in some of the following pages on operative procedures refer to the work associated with preparing a tooth to receive a restoration or crown of the particular type named.

The instruments required for a certain operation should be placed on the work surface (bracket table, cabinet top, or tray) before the operation is begun. A minimum number of drawers need be opened or instruments found once work has started. Keep all instruments lying in an orderly manner on the work surface. The working end of the instrument should always be visible. It is amazingly difficult to locate a particular instrument when it is lying tangled in a group of handles pointing in all directions. You keep the instruments in order. Place to one side the instruments that have been used and will no longer be required. Keep the instruments needed for the next step most conveniently placed.

Your dentist will endeavor to work in an orderly manner and to do each type of operation in the same sequence. Following orderly procedures will speed operating time and will make it much easier for you to be of real assistance at the chair. There will be variations at times from a customary sequence, but over a long period of working together, even these variations take on a pattern of uniformity. You will be able to anticipate his or her needs and will always have the correct instrument in its proper working position.

Remember: *Your purpose is to conserve the dentist's time and energy. Try to time your moves in such a way as never to delay progress of treatment.*

Always observe which tooth is being prepared. The location of the tooth is the factor that accounts for most of the variation in procedure.

Study the sequence in which your dentist uses instruments during each type of operation. Try to have each successive one held out to the dentist close to the front of the patient's chin. Also, be ready to receive the instrument the dentist has been using. Hold instruments so that the dentist can recognize which instrument you are holding and can take it from your hand *in the position required for use in the mouth.* When the handpiece is to be used, it is helpful to remove it from its hanger and bring it to the location at the front of the patient's chin. When its use is completed, it should be received from the dentist and restored to its hanger.

If the dentist wishes, the dental assistant should learn to place and remove carbide burs or diamond instruments used in the air turbines. The higher-speed handpieces, such as the air turbine, require less change of instruments than is required by the slower belt-driven handpieces.

The assistant should watch for things that may be uncomfortable to the patient: wet chin, uncomfortable headrest, dry lips, saliva ejector pulling soft tissue, or pressure from evacuator tip pinching lips on teeth.

Instructions for serving and receiving instruments are discussed in chapter 38, "Four-Handed Dentistry."

Dismissing the Patient

When work has been completed, the patient must be dismissed, i.e., taken from the chair to the reception room door—graciously, unhurriedly—yet without preventing your dentist from continuing to the next patient. Most of this procedure becomes your job.

The dismissal begins at the chair when all dental procedures have been completed. When the dentist leaves the patient at this point, the dentist should not be obligated to have any more conversation with that patient. The assistant should plan to be present to take over promptly, and will receive from the dentist any necessary information for future appointments.

If any debris is present on the patient's face, assist in removing it. For example, some of the impression pastes are difficult to remove.

Return all possessions: dental appliances first, then packages or purses stored on the shelf, or suit coat if removed at the chair. Now show the patient to the powder alcove or mirror.

When the patient is satisfied with his or her appearance, proceed to arrange any further business that you may have with the patient. You should know the details of the patient's account and how it is being handled in the event that it is necessary to make new arrangements or change existing arrangments for the account. The patient may require information about the account.

Keep in mind the advisability of assisting elderly individuals whenever possible, and also parents with small children.

Try never to let a patient leave the reception room without saying "Goodbye, Mrs. Jones" at the moment the patient is about to leave. If you must leave the patient before that moment, make the farewell definite and warm. The assistant should be standing in the reception room when these words are said, not inclining her or his upper body through the doorway indicating haste to return to other duties.

Assisting with Children

Some special emphasis should be given to chair assisting for young children. It is somewhat different from working with adults. Special attention to the psychology of the young child is most desirable if your office works with children. (See chapter 5, "Fundamental Principles of Human Relations.")

Dental work for children necessitates efficient chairside assisting, as well as good management of appointments. One of the chief reasons for unpleasantness in performing dentistry for children arises from failure to start the child's relationships with the dental office at a sufficiently early period in the child's development. The recommendations given to parents officially by the American Dental Association have gradually lowered the recommended age level for the first dental appointment to age two. Activity of the American Society of Dentistry for Children has been largely responsible for this improvement.

Most children enter a stage of negativistic behavior at about two to two and one-half years of age. If a direct suggestion is made to them, the answer is a vehement "No!" This is the period in which the child is trying to establish himself or herself as an individual. The child wants to assert himself or herself, make choices, and thus be a "person." Unless the child is very phlegmatic, he or she does not respond cooperatively to new experiences such as a visit to the dentist. As a common result, neither the child nor the dentist enjoys the visit. On the other hand, if the child can be brought to the dental office prior to this stage in his or her behavior pattern, at the age of eighteen or twenty-two months, for a prophylaxis and examination visit involving the use of a revolving instrument on the teeth and an explorer and mirror in the mouth, the child is usually more interested in the procedure than he or she is in objecting to it. Cases of rampant dental caries are thus observed at a more opportune time for treatment. However, the average youngster will require no treatment of a pain-producing nature. His or her experience is one of pleasant investigation and observation. Occasionally, the child will shed tears at the beginning of the appointment, but curiosity soon overcomes fear. Frequently, he or she is not willing to leave the chair at the conclusion of the appointment. Seen at frequent intervals thereafter, the youngster whose relationship with the dental office has been so advantageously begun rarely turns into the problem type of patient. Dental care is pleasant for everyone.

Many youngsters are first brought to the dental office because they are experiencing pain. The dental assistant can be a great influence in promoting cooperation. However, a child will not be led to believe that the assistant is sympathetic unless the assistant expresses a genuine liking for children.

Most dental offices that do have child patients have some arrangement to give the child a gift. The present is usually a small toy or novelty, given up to a certain age level.

The practice of using these toys or novelties as rewards for good behavior is not approved by child psychologists. *The toy or novelty should be a present to the child from the dentist simply because the dentist likes the child.* Properly used, such presents to children are a tremendous help in cultivating a pleasant attitude toward the dental office, but they should be presented impartially, without regard for behavior. The gift gives the child a pleasant memory of the office, regardless of the treatment he or she may have had in other respects. The uncooperative child very frequently will make an intense effort to be more cooperative at succeeding appointments when this procedure in handling gifts is used.

The dental assistant may be in charge of purchasing the novelties. Select those which are not harmful, dangerous for the child, or of danger to anyone around the child. Noisemakers of any kind are not appreciated by parents.

When young children are in the dental chair, it is extremely important to be thoroughly set up before starting. The entire procedure should be completed as rapidly as possible and without interruption. Young children cannot hold their mouths open easily for any great length of time. The strain on them is lessened directly in proportion to the speed with which the operation is completed.

To most young children, the operatory is full of mysterious and unfamiliar equipment. If the child exhibits an apprehensive attitude toward the equipment, gently and slowly show the child the various parts, how they move, how they sound—with no effort made to explain their use. Touch his or her cheek with the evacuator tip, if one is to be used, to show its gentleness and yours. The child will frequently begin to ask questions at this point, and the conversations should then be led to things of interest to the child outside the dental office. The object of this approach is to de-emphasize the dental equipment as much as possible and to present a legitimate distraction.

Most children get along better without the presence of the parent in the operatory, although occasional youngsters will do better if a properly instructed parent is there. Most dentists prefer to have the parent remain in the reception room.

Never leave a young child alone in the dental chair. When the dentist takes over at the chair, it is also your signal to keep silent in order that the child's attention may be given to the dentist alone. Keep a friendly expression always.

Everything done around a young child should be unhurried, calm, and performed with a friendly manner.

All effort is directed toward giving the youngster the feeling that what is being done is usual and commonplace as eating lunch at home. By your actions and words give the youngster the impression that he or she is expected to accept it as usual and commonplace, too.

You do not go into elaborate explanations, solicitous statements, or make apprehensive expressions when you are about to serve lunch to a youngster at home. If you were to do so, the child would immediately begin to wonder what undesirable plans you had. The same is true of the dental office and its procedures. If the parent, the assistant, and the dentist are able to treat a dental appointment as a casual thing that calls for no unusual reactions, children are inclined to accept it as such.

Commonly, however, the child has heard (and remembered) little remarks made by adults concerning their dental visits or dental needs—sometimes dental pains. Perhaps the child has heard older children tell of the terrors of their visit to the dentist. When the day arrives that the child is in the dental office, all these expressions and fears return, magnified a thousandfold due to the element of the unknown.

Children have vivid imaginations. However, if a child is properly approached, imagination can be made an assistance in the dental office.

All the effort of the dental office should be devoted to giving or restoring the casual, friendly, "it's fun" attitude of the normal, well-adjusted child.

Oral Examination Technique

An oral examination is made of each new patient and also of regular patients at the time of their recall examinations and prophylaxis appointment.

When the dentist is ready to proceed with this part of the examination, sit at the patient's left, facing the dentist, so that you may hear the dentist more easily. It is helpful to have the dental assistant aware of which part of the mouth is being examined to prevent charting errors due to incorrectly designating *left* or *right*.

Some dental offices use the patient's examination card to enter the notes of the examination, others may use a paper pad or clipboard with paper on which these notes are written for later entry on the patient's card. If a separate piece of paper is used, the patient's name and the date, including the year, should be noted at the top for identification.

Record the information necessary to complete the charting. Remember to write legibly and accurately. Record every item the dentist mentions and indicate any need for slower dictation.

Summary

Managing the risks associated with infectious diseases, such as hepatitis and AIDS, requires the appropriate procedures for cleanliness and sterilization in the operatory. Protective eye wear, masks, and gloves are mandatory for both the dentist and assistant.

Proper management and reporting of dental-medical wastes must be achieved.

Note the general rules for conduct in the operatory. The assistant is to *assist* the performance of dentistry and keep attention centered on the patient.

Learn to adjust the dental chair correctly and seat the patient properly. Pleasant attitude and concern for the comfort of the patient are essential.

Care for the patient's dental appliance and remember to return the appliance at the close of the appointment.

Tray setups, if used, will speed the setup and cleanup of the operatory.

Assisting with preparations is exacting work, and the dental assistant should learn the requirements for serving her or his dentist: maintain the correct lighting, keep a clear field of operation, and present instruments and materials as needed.

The purpose of dental assisting is to conserve the dentist's time and energy.

Dismissal of the patient begins at the chair, with the dental assistant accepting the responsibility for the patient's appearance. The assistant removes debris that would be difficult for the patient to remove. Dismissal continues through providing an opportunity for the patient's personal grooming, accepting payments for services, making new appointments, and ushering the patient out of the reception room. It may include helping with outer clothing.

Assisting with children is different from working with adults. Careful attention to the proper attitudes and remarks is essential.

Oral examination requires that the assistant make notes while the dentist examines the mouth. Charting is an important part of this examination and should be carefully learned according to the dentist's choice of method.

Study Questions

1. What is *risk management?*
2. Explain the requirements in risk management.
3. Explain *waste management.*
4. Detail the correct scrubbing procedures.
5. What are general rules for operatory conduct?
6. Discuss the preparation of the patient for the dentist, beginning with the patient seated in the reception room.
7. What is important in assisting with preparations?
8. Describe dismissing the patient.
9. What is important to remember in assisting with children?
10. Describe *oral examination.*

CHAPTER 38

Applying Principles of Four-handed Dentistry In Daily Practice

Anthony DiAngeles, D.D.S., M.P.H.

Introduction
Dimensions of Four-handed Dentistry
Principles of Work Simplification
Concepts of Motion Economy
The Functional Operating Position
Seating and Positioning the Patient
Zones of Activity
General Precautions in Patient Care
Oral Evacuation
    The Evacuator Tip
    Control of the Evacuator Tip
    Tissue Retraction
    Placement of the Evacuator Tip
Use of the Air-Water Syringe
Instrument Handling and Transfers
    Pre-prepared Trays
    Techniques of Instrument Transfer
    Basic Instrument Grasps
    Instrument Transfer
    Syringe Transfer

Introduction

This chapter is designed to familiarize the dental assistant with the basic philosophy, methods, and skills necessary for effective four-handed dentistry. Proper application of these principles will result in increased efficiency and productivity for the dental team, comfort and high quality dental services for the patient, and a reduction in the physical and mental stress associated with chairside clinical procedures.

In the preceding chapters of this text, the reader has become familiarized with a broad range of topics describing the fundamental organization of a dental practice, the role of the dental assistant as a member of the oral health team, specific and general aspects of the oral structures in health and disease and the armamentarium and procedures utilized in diagnosing, preventing, and treating various oral diseases and conditions.

A thorough understanding of this information is essential for the dental assistant to fulfill her or his role and to achieve the goals and objectives of the practice or institution in which she or he is employed. It is difficult to select one area as being more important than another, because each area of knowledge tends to complement and reinforce the other. The material to be described in this chapter draws upon many of the preceding topics and focuses on an analysis of those skills necessary for effective chairside dental assisting. For many assistants, mastery of these skills is critical because the skills comprise the most significant portion of their daily activities. Placing this chapter near the end, then, really signifies both a summary and synthesis of all earlier knowledge and a beginning for translating this knowledge into a skillful dynamic that characterizes the modern dental assistant.

Dimensions of Four-handed Dentistry

The role of the dental assistant has changed dramatically. The emergence of the concept of four-handed dentistry signalled not only a marked improvement in the delivery of dental services, but a greater involvement of the dental assistant in the provision of these services. The original intent of four-handed dentistry was to increase the productivity of dentists while minimizing the stress and fatigue associated with practicing dentistry. Its broadened definition has come to encompass an entire manner of practice, in which office design and administration, dental equipment selection and its placement, and personnel selection and training all create a maximally efficient and effective dental work environment.

Principles of Work Simplification

Much of the success of four-handed dentistry is based on the principles of work simplification. The major objective of work simplification is to make work easier. Dentistry is a demanding profession that requires precise skills involving a large armamentarium of instruments and materials, effective management of patients and human resources, and efficient coordination of the activities of the dental team. Application of work simplification principles to all aspects of dental practice can result in a less stressful, more productive work environment for the dentist, dental assistant, and patient.

Four generally agreed-upon components that govern work simplification have evolved from industrial studies. These components are defined as: (1) *eliminate,* (2) *combine,* (3) *rearrange,* and (4) *simplify.*

Eliminate. In analyzing the individual steps in any given procedure, it is often possible to reduce the numbers of instruments, equipment, and motions used to accomplish a particular task. This reduction will result in saving the time of the patient and conservation of both time and effort for the dental staff. There are many instances in which elimination can facilitate activities in the dental office. The following examples illustrate this point:

1. Infrequently used instruments and materials should be removed from tray set-ups and the immediate chairside environment to decrease clean-up time as well as to provide a less cluttered work area for the assistant. The seldom used instruments and materials can be stored outside the immediate work area and incorporated only when indicated.

2. Numerous unnecessary motions can be eliminated during instrument transfer. For example, in many offices placing of amalgam involves the assistant passing the amalgam carrier to the dentist, and after placement of the amalgam, the dentist exchanges the amalgam carrier for a plugger. This sequence is repeated as often as necessary to fill and condense the restoration. If, instead, the assistant carries and places the amalgam in the preparation, the dentist is able to continue using only the amalgam plugger, thereby eliminating a number of instrument transfers. Not only are the number of steps in the procedure reduced, but also the number of motions and the fatigue associated with amalgam

placement. In many dental offices amalgam restorations comprise a major portion of the daily activities. Elimination of these unnecessary transfers over the course of a day, week, or month results in a significant saving of time.

Combine. When the functions performed by two instruments or two pieces of equipment can be incorporated into one instrument or one piece of equipment, both time and cost can be saved. Similarly, when two steps in a procedure can be combined and accomplished in one step, both time and effort are saved.

If one carefully analyzes instruments it is not surprising to realize that frequently one end of a double-ended instrument is used almost exclusively. Consequently, there may be two or more double-ended instruments on a tray set-up that are only partially used. With the wide variety of dental instruments on the market it is feasible to find a dental manufacturer who combines the frequently used ends of two instruments into one double-ended instrument. In doing so, one reduces the number of instruments to be purchased and sterilized, and the number of instrument transfers from two to one.

Another example of work simplification can be demonstrated in the application of the rubber dam. The general sequence involves placing a ligated clamp on the selected tooth, applying the rubber dam over the clamp, and then securing the rubber dam frame. By *combining* these three steps into one outside the mouth, it is possible to carry and place the pre-prepared clamp, dam, and frame in the mouth in one motion.

Rearrange. An important premise of four-handed dentistry is that all aspects of the work environment be adapted to the needs of the dental team. For many years the converse was true. The dental team had to adapt to equipment and office design ill-suited to four-handed dentistry. Frequently, availability of modern equipment and materials is insufficient to assure smooth and efficient working habits. Proper placement and positioning of equipment and instruments is essential in reducing unnecessary motions and steps as well as in supporting the desired operating positions of the dental team.

Simplify. Simplification really represents the final process in analyzing how work is accomplished in the office. After the principles of eliminating, combining, and rearranging have been accomplished, all activities are viewed from the perspective of whether they, in fact, represent the most direct and efficient approach. Simplification suggests that unpredictability and unnecessary complexity have been removed from a task, permitting establishment of an efficient work routine.

Such a routine allows all members of the dental team to perform their functions smoothly, sequentially, and expeditiously.

To summarize then, proper application of the principles of work simplification is a fundamental tenet of effective four-handed dentistry.

Concepts of Motion Economy

Any discussion of dental practice, and in particular four-handed dentistry, will include reference to motion economy. Minimizing extraneous movements helps to conserve time as well as to reduce fatigue.

A classification of motions evolved from early studies on time and motion in dentistry. This classification has become an essential part of our descriptive language. Motions are classified into five categories ranging from the simplest to the most complex.

Class I   motions involving only the fingers
Class II motions involving the fingers and wrist
Class III motions involving the fingers, wrist, and elbow
Class IV motions involving the entire arm from the shoulder
Class V   motions involving the arm and twisting of the body

It is desirable to minimize the number of Class IV and V motions in the chairside work environment. These movements require a greater expenditure of both time and energy. In addition, a constant refocusing of the eyes from the higher intensity illumination of the oral cavity to the lower intensity illumination of the operatory is required whenever the dentist employs Class IV and Class V motions. The cumulative effect of this constant refocusing may result in both stress and fatigue.

Prior organization and arrangement of equipment and supplies will do much to eliminate the need for Class IV and Class V motions during patient treatment. Effective instrument transfer techniques (to be discussed later) will also reduce the number of Class IV and Class V motions.

A thorough understanding and constant application of the principles of work simplification and motion economy will greatly enhance the effectiveness and efficiency of both the dentist and dental assistant.

The Functional Operating Position

Any chairside dental procedure begins with proper positioning of the patient and seating of the dentist and dental assistant so as to achieve a "functional" operating position that will provide (1) access to the operating field, (2) good visibility, and (3) comfort for the dental team and patient.

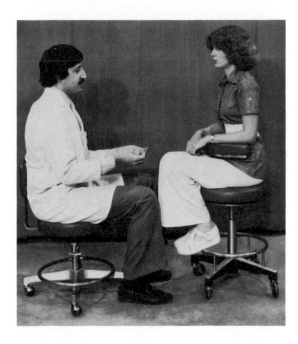

Figure 38.1

Proper functional positions for both the dentist and dental assistant.

It is critical that this functional operating position be established and maintained. It represents the pivotal point around which all other activities in the operatory are focused. The functional operating position of the dental team is supported and maintained by: (1) placing the patient in a supine position, (2) use of a dental mirror, (3) use of high-speed evacuation, (4) effective instrument transfer, and (5) proper positioning of equipment and materials.

Figure 38.1 illustrates the functional operating posture for both dentist and dental assistant. The following list represents some general guidelines that both describe and define this posture of the dentist and dental assistant.

1. The back and neck should be kept relatively erect.
2. The shoulders should be maintained parallel to the floor.
3. The upper body should be fully supported by sitting completely on the seat of the stool.
4. The upper arms and elbows should be kept close to the upper body.
5. The forearms are maintained parallel to the floor.
6. The thighs are maintained parallel to the floor by proper adjustment of stool height.
7. For the dentist, use of a properly adjusted backrest will give additional support to the back.

8. For the assistant, the support arm is adjusted to support the upper body just below the rib-cage, and/or used as a rest for supporting the forearms and elbows.
9. For the dentist, feet should be kept flat on the floor.
10. For the assistant, feet should rest flat on the stool footrest.

Major and/or frequent deviations from this posture may cause strain and fatigue, and over a long period of time may produce impairment of body functions. If you must deviate from the functional operating position, be certain that it is for brief periods only. If you must lean forward, do so from the hips, not from the neck and shoulders. In this way your head is being supported by the spinal column and musculature of the entire upper body, and not just by the neck and upper shoulder muscles.

Seating and Positioning the Patient

To further explore the functional operating position, it is necessary to analyze the positions of dentist and dental assistant relative to the patient. In general, the patient is seated so as to accomodate the dental team. Rather than bending, twisting, or reaching in order to gain access or visibility, the dentist or dental assistant should request the patient to move his or her head. Remember, the patient is in the chair for a short time, whereas the dental team is at the chair all day. The dental team members cannot change their working positions for every size and shape of patient. To do so would most likely result in constant fatigue.

Placing the patient in a supine or modified supine position is essential for maintaining the functional operating posture of the dental team.

To place a patient in the supine position, the following sequence is suggested:

1. Raise the arm of the chair.
2. Position the chair seat at a level comfortable for being seated.
3. Lower the chair back approximately 30° from the upright position.
4. After the patient is seated, raise the chair sufficiently to allow the dentist's legs under the chairback when it is lowered.
5. Tilt the seat back until the patient's calves are parallel to the floor.
6. Slowly lower the chair back until
   a. the maxillary arch is in a plane perpendicular to the floor, and
   b. a line from the patient's nose to knees is parallel with the floor (fig. 38.2).

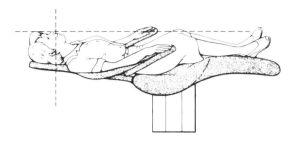

Figure 38.2
Proper placement of patient in the supine position. Note imaginary line from nose to knees is parallel to the floor and imaginary line through maxillary arch is perpendicular to the floor.

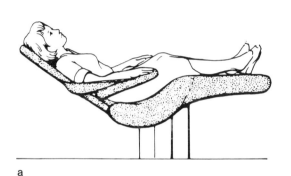
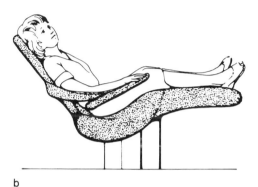

a   b

Figure 38.3
(a) Proper placement of patient for work in most areas of the mandibular arch; and
(b) placement of patient for work in mandibular right posterior area.

7. Ask or assist the patient to move his or her head to the top of the chair and to move the whole body toward the dentist so there is no unoccupied chair between the dentist and the patient. This positioning reduces the need for the dentist to bend or reach in order to gain adequate access or visibility.

8. Lower the entire chair until it is on or slightly above the dentist's lap. The patient's mouth should now be at elbow level for the dentist and the dentist should be able to maintain his or her forearms parallel to the floor.

For the majority of dental procedures, this is the position of choice. All work on the maxillary arch and much on the mandibular arch can be accomplished with the patient in the supine position. However, access to some areas of the mandibular arch require a modification in the supine position. By lowering the chair seat and raising the chair back until the mandibular arch (when mouth is open) is approximately parallel to the floor will permit improved access and visualization to the posterior mandibular areas (fig. 38.3a and b).

Zones of Activity

Up to this point, the seating positions of the dental team and the patient have been discussed separately and *statically* (without activity in dentistry). The following discussion will explore the dynamic relationship of these seating positions to one another during dental treatment. (*Dynamic* here refers to a continuous productive activity.)

A useful guide for describing this relationship is to view the patient's mouth as the focal point of activity in the dental operatory. If one then superimposes the

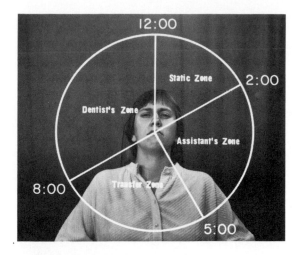

Figure 38.4
Zones of activity as defined by clock positions.

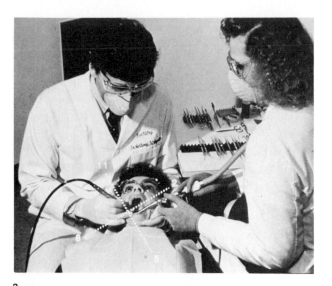

a

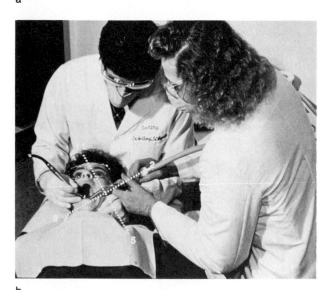

b

Figure 38.5
(a) Proper position of dental team and equipment within the zones of activity; and (b) dentist violating designated zone of activity.

face of a clock over the center of the patient's mouth, the area around the mouth may be divided into four zones of activity (fig. 38.4). The four zones are:

Dentist's zone, the area of primary activity for the dentist
    8 to 12 o'clock for right-handed dentist
    12 to 4 o'clock for left-handed dentist

Static zone, the area in which equipment, instruments and supplies infrequently used during a procedure are kept
    12 to 2 o'clock for right-handed dentist
    10 to 12 o'clock for left-handed dentist

Assistant's zone, the area of primary activity for the chairside assistant. It permits the assistant to sit in direct line with the operating field in a 3 o'clock position, with her or his legs parallel to the dental chair back. It is in this zone that the assistant's mobile cabinet is located, allowing immediate and easy access to frequently used instruments and supplies.
    2 to 5 o'clock for right-handed dentist
    7 to 10 o'clock for left-handed dentist

Transfer zone, the area of greatest shared activity of the dental team. The majority of instrument transfers occur at or just below the patient's mouth, and it is equally accessible to both the dentist and the assistant.
    5 to 8 o'clock for right-handed dentist
    4 to 7 o'clock for left-handed dentist.

If the dental team is to operate efficiently, any interference with the primary function of each zone must be avoided. Compromise of the primary function of the various zones by activity or equipment may result

in a loss of access, visibility, and/or comfort to the dentist or assistant. For example, movement of the dentist to the static zone will require the assistant to position herself or himself away from the operating field, resulting in reduced access and visibility and increasing the number of Class IV and Class V motions (fig. 38.5a and b).

Figures 38.6–38.8 illustrate favorable functional operating positions for the dental team.

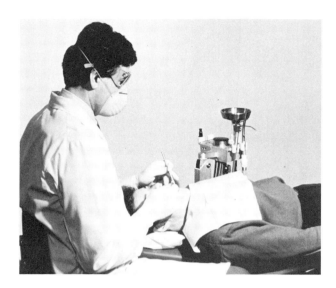

Figure 38.6
Proper position for dentist.

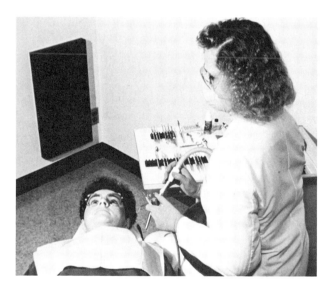

Figure 38.7
Proper position for dental assistant. Note assistant in direct line with patient's mouth.

General Precautions in Patient Care

The dental team must be ever alert to the comfort and safety of the patient. Consideration of the following will do much to insure a pleasant appointment for the patient:

1. When placing the patient in the supine position or returning the patient to the upright position, always lower and raise the chair back slowly so as to not induce dizziness.

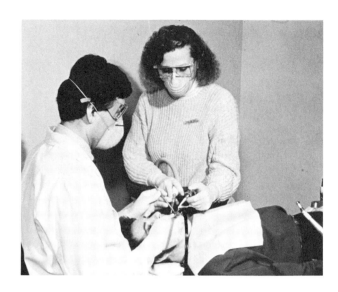

Figure 38.8
Proper position of dental team and patient. Note assistant 4" to 6" above eye level of the dentist for improved access and visibility.

2. Several medical conditions can be aggravated by placing the patient in a supine position. Be certain that the patient's medical history is free from contraindications.

3. After the patient is seated, remove any dental prostheses and wrap them in a moistened paper towel or place them in a container with water.

4. Patients who wear eye glasses should be asked to leave them on, as debris is sometimes splashed onto the face from the cutting effects of the ultraspeed handpiece. Patients who do not wear glasses should be provided with a pair of plastic safety glasses or asked to close their eyes during the cutting procedures. Both dentist and chairside assistant must always wear eye glasses (safety or prescription) when working. Damage to the eye from particulate matter and/or bacterial splash is a constant hazard for dental personnel.

5. Exercise continual caution to prevent patients from swallowing or aspirating any object. Effective isolation, use of the rubber dam, capable evacuation, and careful working technique will do much to reduce this potential hazard.

6. Sometimes it is advisable to place a cushioned inset under the patient's neck or small of the back for additional support and comfort. This is usually done when a

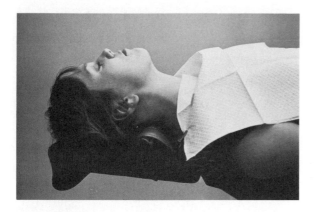

Figure 38.9
Patient's neck supported for greater access to maxillary posterior areas.

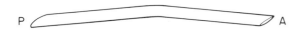

Figure 38.10
Evacuator tip. End P is used for posterior areas, end A for anterior areas.

small patient is moved to the top of the chair and loses the lumbar support provided by the chair contour, or when a patient is asked to arch his or her head back towards the dentist to afford greater visibility and access (fig. 38.9).

Oral Evacuation

Placement of patients in the supine position and use of the ultraspeed handpiece with water coolant requires dental assistants to be highly skilled in the techniques of high volume evacuation. The primary goals of high volume evacuation are to: (1) prevent rapid accumulation of debris and fluids in the patient's mouth, and (2) to insure a clear operating field. Consequently, effective oral evacuation should result in comfort for the patient and increased visibility for the dentist.

The Evacuator Tip

The working end of a high volume oral evacuation system is the evacuation tip. The most commonly used tip is a metal or plastic tube bevelled on both ends with a slight bend in the middle (fig. 38.10). Perhaps one of the most common errors of the inexperienced dental assistant is selecting the wrong end of the tip. The end designated *P* is used primarily for evacuation in the posterior areas of the mouth, whereas end *A* is utilized for evacuation in the anterior areas. Figures 38.11a–c

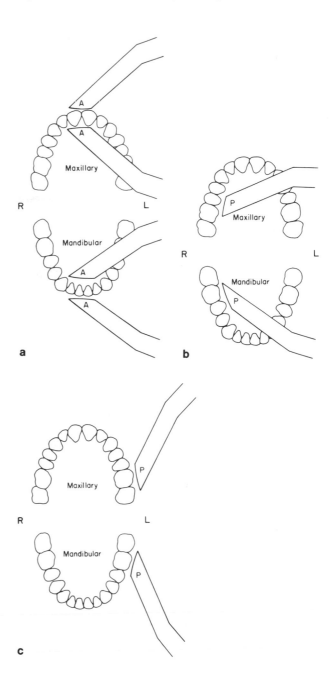

Figure 38.11
(a) Placement of evacuator tip in maxillary and mandibular anterior areas; (b) placement of evacuator tip in maxillary and mandibular right posterior areas; and (c) placement of evacuator tip in maxillary and mandibular left posterior area.

demonstrate this point. To further help you in selecting the correct end, hold the suction tip so that the arched side (convex) is toward the ceiling. When you do this, the end *P* that is angled upward is generally used for posterior teeth and the end *A* that is angled downward is generally used for anterior teeth.

a

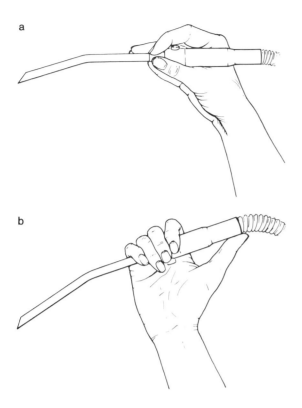

b

Figure 38.12
(a) The modified pen grasp; and (b) the thumb-to-nose grasp.

Control of the Evacuator Tip

Since the evacuator tip is primarily placed and operated intraorally, it is critical that the assistant maintain precise control of this device to prevent injury to the patient. Two methods of achieving control are to hold the tip in either (1) a modified pen grasp, or (2) a thumb-to-nose grasp (fig. 38.12a and b). The latter grasp provides more leverage when retraction is needed. When assisting a right-handed dentist, the evacuator tip is held in the assistant's right hand. The converse is true when assisting a left-handed dentist. Greater stability and control is achieved when the assistant's right arm is kept as close to her or his body as possible. The assistant's left hand must be kept free for retraction, manipulating the three-way syringe, and instrument transfers.

Tissue Retraction

To achieve effective evacuation, the assistant must often simultaneously retract the oral soft tissues with the evacuation tip. It is imperative to prevent bruising of the oral mucosa: (1) by poking, (2) by compressing the

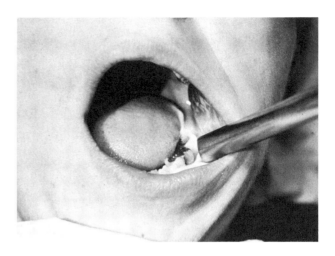

Figure 38.13
Placement of cotton roll to protect oral tissue.

tissue against the teeth, or (3) by inadvertently drawing the tissues into the evacuator tip. Bruising can be prevented in a variety of ways.

1. When using the tip to evacuate on the buccal surfaces, placement of cotton rolls in the buccal fold or sulcus will protect these tissues (fig. 38.13).
2. When evacuating in the posterior mandibular lingual areas, the assistant must retract the tongue and prevent damage to the tissues of the floor of the mouth. Cotton rolls placed between the tongue and mandibular arch may be sufficient. Often, however, an assistant will be unable to effectively retract an extremely muscular or active tongue with the evacuation tip alone. In these instances it is recommended that the assistant evacuate with the right hand and retract the tongue with either a mouth mirror or tongue blade held in the left hand (fig. 38.14). We prefer the tongue blade, because it retracts along the entire length of the tongue, permitting greater control and visibility.
3. When evacuating in the maxillary arch or in the posterior mandibular areas, the dental assistant must avoid compressing the lower lip between the mandibular anterior teeth and the evacuator tip (fig. 38.15). Careful placement of the evacuator tip and/or retraction of the lower lip with the index finger of the assistant's left hand eliminates the problem (fig. 38.16).

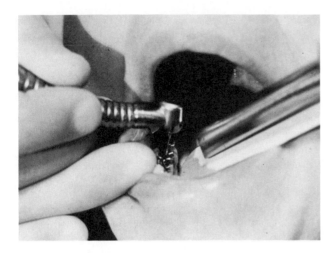

Figure 38.14
Placement of tongue blade to retract tongue. Note cotton roll to protect tissue of floor of mouth.

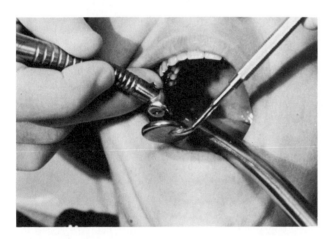

Figure 38.15
Compression of lip by evacuator tip.

Placement of the Evacuator Tip

Since both the patient's comfort and the dentist's visibility depend on the assistant's skill in evacuation techniques, it is important to develop a workable routine. The following sequence is suggested:

1. Select the appropriate end (*P* or *A*) for use in the quadrant of the mouth being treated.
2. Select that grasp (modified-pen or thumb-to-nose) which permits the greatest control of the tip and maximum retraction.
3. Activate the vacuum control to its most open position.
4. Place cotton rolls and/or retraction devices as necessary to protect the oral tissues.

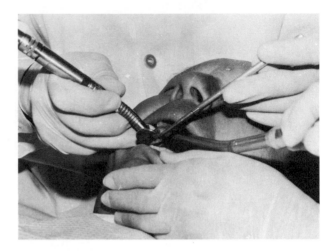

Figure 38.16
Retraction of lower lip by assistant during evacuation.

5. Place the evacuator tip in the oral cavity prior to the moment the dentist places the handpiece. This provides the dentist with a nonverbal signal that you are ready, and it minimizes the risk of blocking the dentist's view when a mirror is being used for indirect vision.
6. Place the bevel of the tip parallel to and slightly distal to the tooth being treated.
7. Place the tip just beyond the occlusal or incisal surface of the tooth.
8. Place the tip as close to the tooth as possible without touching the gingival tissues.

(Steps 6–8 insure maximum evacuation and assist in drawing the water coolant from the handpiece through the cavity preparation.)

9. As necessary, move the tip to the lowest point in the patient's mouth to evacuate accumulated fluids.
10. If access prevents placement of the tip as described in steps 5–8, evacuate in the lowest and most posterior position of the mouth. Most of the fluid will accumulate there.

Use of the Air-Water Syringe

During procedures requiring high volume evacuation, the assistant keeps the air-water syringe in the left hand and utilizes it for periodic rinsing of the operative field, and for keeping the mirror surface clean when it is in use.

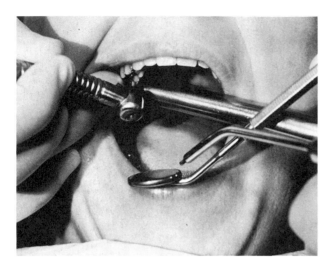

Figure 38.17
Placement of three-way syringe to keep mirror surface clean.

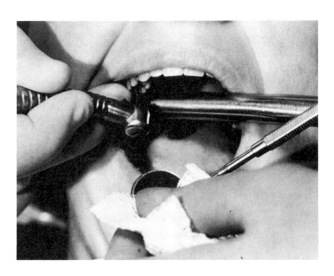

Figure 38.18
Assistant grasping and wiping mirror surface.

To keep the mirror surface clean, the assistant directs a steady stream of air across the mirror, while keeping the syringe tip from being reflected in the mirror's surface (fig. 38.17). The dentist can further minimize contamination of the mirror by positioning it at a distance from the tooth being prepared.

The assistant can periodically wipe the surface of the mirror with an alcoholed gauze kept in the left hand with the air-water syringe. The dentist need only turn the mirror away from the mouth. This serves as a nonverbal signal to the assistant, who can then easily and quickly wipe the mirror surface by grasping the mirror back with her or his middle finger and wiping the surface with the gauze held by the thumb (fig. 38.18). This technique enables the dentist to maintain his or her finger rests and eyes on the operative field.

Mastery of high volume evacuation techniques and coordination of these techniques with the dentist's operating activities require patience and practice on the part of the dental assistant. It represents one of the most essential and demanding aspects of four-handed dentistry. When mastered, it results in efficiency for the dental team and comfort for the patient.

Instrument Handling and Transfers

Dental instrument handling has benefitted greatly from the application of work simplification principles. Through the use of an assistant's mobile cabinet, pre-prepared trays, and effective instrument transfer techniques, treatment can be accomplished with savings in both time and energy.

Pre-prepared Trays

The use of pre-prepared trays to deliver sterile instruments for a specific clinical procedure has become a hallmark of four-handed dentistry. The emphasis is on *prior preparation, organization,* and *logical sequencing.*

Specific trays can be organized according to the individual dentist's working style. (Suggested tray set-ups for a wide range of clinical procedures can be found in the following chapter.) These trays can then be color-coded to indicate their particular use. For example, blue may indicate an amalgam procedure; red, a composite procedure; and gold, a crown and bridge procedure. There are numerous ways of coding both the trays and the instruments. One method is to place a strip of color-coding tape on the edge of the tray and bands of the same colored tape on all the instruments included on this tray (fig. 38.19).

These trays can be organized prior to the patient's arrival and stored in a central supply or sterilization area (fig. 38.20). Based on the treatment plan, a pre-prepared tray containing all the necessary instruments can be brought to the operatory.

Some practical suggestions governing the use of pre-prepared trays are as follows:

1. Include only those instruments and supplies routinely used in a given procedure.
2. Arrange the instruments from left to right in the sequence of their use.
3. After an instrument is used, return it to its proper location on the tray.

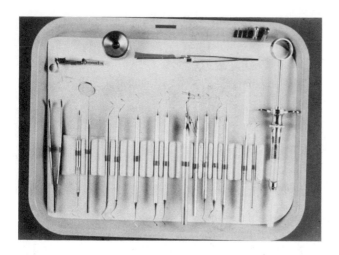

Figure 38.19
Pre-prepared tray demonstrating color-coded instruments and tray.

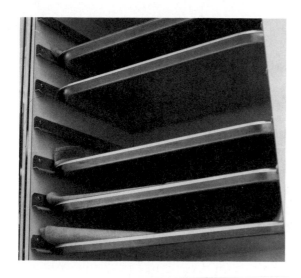

Figure 38.20
Pre-prepared trays stored in central supply.

4. Place the tray on the mobile cabinet in such a fashion that instrument transfers can be accomplished without resorting to Class IV and Class V motions (fig. 38.21).

The dentist must establish and maintain a specific working routine if the assistant is to meet with any degree of success with items numbered 1 and 2. Only then can the assistant correctly and quickly anticipate the dentist's instrument needs.

Additional items used during a procedure can be stored in the mobile cabinet and/or in fixed cabinetry or on counter-tops within the operatory. Location of these items should be determined by their priority of use. Frequently-used items may be stored on the mobile

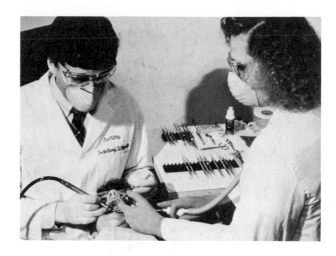

Figure 38.21
Proper position of pre-prepared tray on mobile cabinet.

cabinet top, in the well, and in upper drawers, whereas infrequently-used materials and supplies can be kept in the lower drawers and in other cabinetry. In addition, these materials and supplies should be arranged to allow the assistant easy visual identification and access (fig. 38.22).

All efforts at prior organization and arrangement of instruments and materials will not only enhance the flow of a given clinical procedure, but will result in a reduction of stress and a conservation of time.

Techniques of Instrument Transfer

The delivery and exchange of hand instruments and various dental materials require clear communication and careful coordination between the dentist and the dental assistant. Again, thoughtful application of work simplification techniques and the principles of motion economy will greatly facilitate the learning of effective instrument transfer methods.

Basic Instrument Grasps

Dental hand instruments, because of their design and function, will be held in different ways when in use. The most common of these positions are generally defined as:

Pen grasp: The instrument is held along the shaft by the index finger, third finger, and thumb (fig. 38.23a).
Reverse pen grasp: The instrument is held in the same manner as the pen grasp. However, the wrist is rotated in a clockwise direction (fig. 38.23b).
Palm grasp: The instrument is held in the palm of the hand with all fingers and the thumb grasping it (fig. 38.24a).

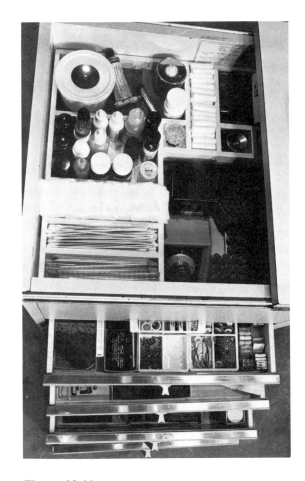

Figure 38.22
Organization of materials and supplies in well and drawers of mobile cabinet.

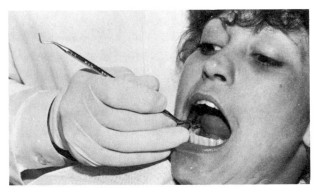

a

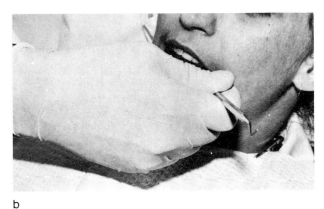

b

Figure 38.23
(a) Pen grasp; and (b) reverse pen grasp.

Palm-thumb grasp: The instrument is held along the shaft by all four fingers with the thumb extended and supporting the shank or working end of the instrument (fig. 38.24b).

Instrument Transfer

All instrument transfers occur at or just below the patient's mouth. The majority of transfers occur at the patient's mouth with the dentist maintaining a finger rest with the fourth finger. Instruments requiring a palm grasp (and oftentimes a palm-thumb grasp) are transferred just below the patient's mouth. By maintaining the transfer point at the mouth, the dentist is able to retain the finger rest position and to maintain eye fixation on the operative field. Instrument transfers are never made over the patient's face where a slipped instrument could result in serious injury to the patient. When transferred, instruments should have their working ends pointing in the direction of use.

The following step-by-step description of a one-handed instrument transfer technique assumes that both dentist and assistant are right handed. *All transfers are carried out with the assistant's left hand.* The right hand must be free for evacuation, retraction, or use of the air-water syringe.

1. The assistant lifts the desired instrument from the pre-prepared tray by grasping it with the thumb and first two fingers near the junction of the shaft and shank at the end opposite from the one the dentist will be using (fig. 38.25a). This action is facilitated by having the instruments slightly elevated rather than flat on the tray surface, allowing the assistant to get her or his fingers under the instrument for easy pick up.

2. The instrument is then held parallel to the instrument currently being held by the dentist, with the working end pointing in the direction of anticipated use (fig. 38.25b). If the dentist's working routine for various procedures is consistent, the assistant will be able to anticipate instrument usage and have each succeeding instrument in the parallel position without the need for frequent verbal direction from the dentist.

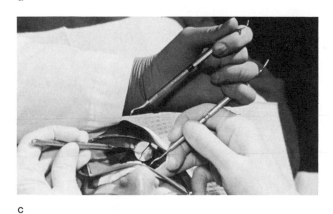
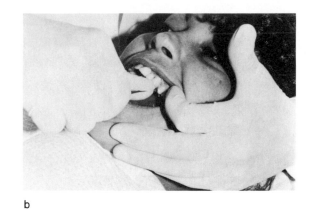
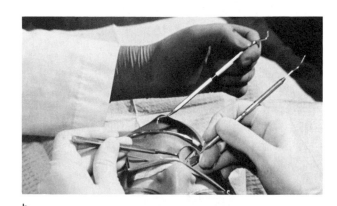
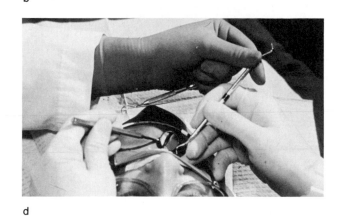
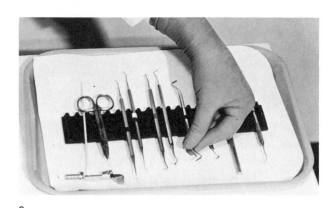

a   b

Figure 38.24
(a) Palm grasp; and (b) palm-thumb grasp.

a   b

c   d

Figure 38.25
(a) Instrument pick up; (b) paralleling instruments; (c) grasping unwanted instrument; and
(d) tucking retrieved instrument into palm and delivering desired instrument.

3. When the dentist indicates that he or she is ready to exchange instruments, the assistant grasps the used instrument at the nonworking end with her or his last two fingers (fig. 38.25c). (The signal to exchange instruments can be given nonverbally by the dentist who simply lifts the working end of the instrument from the tooth.)

4. The assistant immediately tucks the retrieved instrument back into the palm and in the same motion places the new instrument into the dentist's hand in the position in which it will be used (fig. 38.25d).

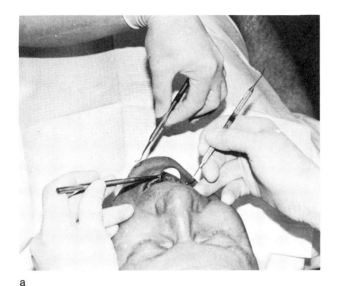

a

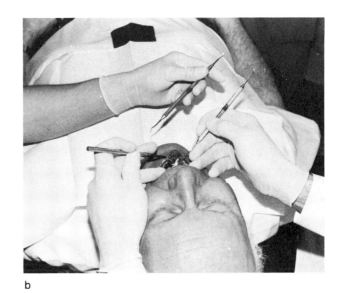

b

Figure 38.26
(a) Repositioning retrieved instrument; and
(b) repositioned instrument ready for transfer.

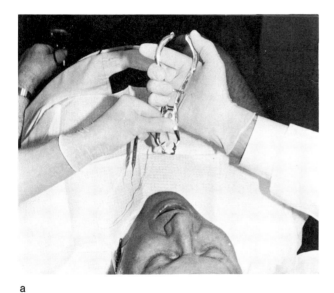

a

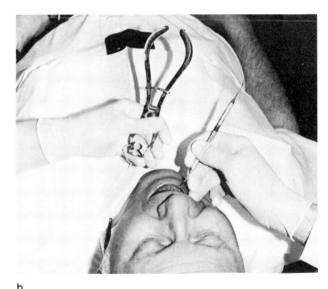

b

Figure 38.27
(a) Paralleling rubber dam clamp forceps; and (b) retrieval
of hand instrument and transfer of forceps.

At no time during this transfer is it necessary for the dentist to lose the finger rest or move his or her eyes from the operative field.

If the dentist wishes to reuse the instrument just retrieved, the assistant simply repositions it to the transfer position (fig. 38.26a and b).

The sequence described previously applies to the transfer of most hand instruments as well as dental handpieces.

Figures 38.27a and b and 38.28a and b demonstrate transfer techniques for the rubber dam forceps and dental handpiece. It should be noted that the principles of paralleling and delivering instruments with the working end toward the tooth are adhered to regardless of the dentist's grasp.

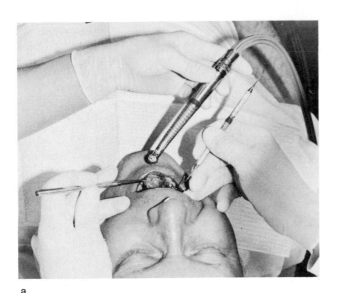

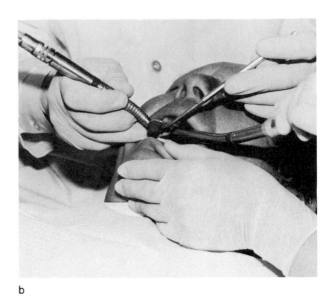

a   b

Figure 38.28
(a) Paralleling of handpiece; and (b) retrieval of hand instrument and transfer of handpiece.

Syringe Transfer

One of the most frequently transferred instruments in the dental office is the anesthetic syringe. For many patients the anticipation of this transfer may evoke feelings from mild to severe anxiety. Consequently, it is strongly recommended that the dental team establish a smooth and efficient routine for syringe transfer. The following sequence is offered as one way of accomplishing this task while minimizing discomfort to the patient. Contrary to the earlier discussion on instrument transfer, the syringe is delivered to and retrieved from the dentist by the assistant with the right hand. Also, during the sequence of syringe transfers and injection, it is helpful to distract the patient's attention from the syringe by appropriate light conversation.

1. While the dentist is applying topical anesthetic with his or her right hand, the fingers of the left hand serve as a screen to the patient's vision (fig. 38.29a).
2. The assistant holds the syringe by the barrel to the left of the patient's head and below the patient's line of vision.
3. The dentist removes the topical anesthetic applicator, which is retrieved by the assistant's left hand. The dentist's right hand is placed beneath the outstretched syringe.
4. The assistant places the thumb ring over the dentist's thumb and slides the needle cover off (fig. 38.29b).

5. The assistant rotates the syringe so that the needle bevel faces bone upon injection, and so that the anesthetic carpule is visible through the open side of the syringe barrel. This action permits proper orientation for injection and allows the dentist to observe any blood aspirated into the carpule during anesthesia administration (fig. 38.29c).
6. After the needle is oriented, the assistant's grasp on the syringe is released. This is a nonverbal signal to the dentist who can now begin the injection.
7. At the completion of the injection, the dentist carefully returns the syringe to the assistant's right hand in the same position as the original transfer (fig. 38.29d).

Summary

The main objective of four-handed dentistry is to provide a maximally efficient and effective work environment for both dental staff and dental patients. Much of four-handed dentistry is based on the principles of work-simplification and motion economy.

Eliminate, combine, rearrange, and simplify are the central components of work simplification. Classifying motions as Class I, II, III, IV, or V is used to analyze chairside activity in order to conserve time and

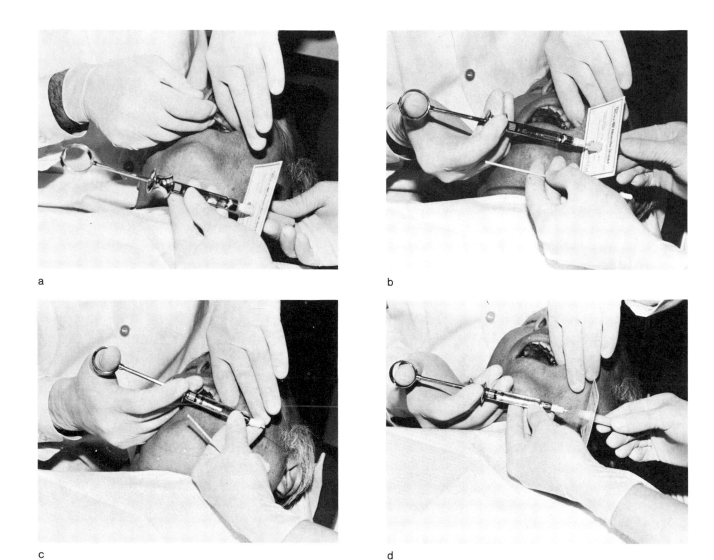

a

b

c

d

Figure 38.29
(a) Dentist applies topical anesthetic and screens patient's vision. Assistant holds syringe to the left of and below patient's face; (b) syringe placed over thumb of dentist and needle cover removed; (c) Assistant orients bevel of needle and syringe barrel; and (d) Dentist returns syringe to original transfer position.

reduce fatigue. Applying the principles of work-simplification and motion economy will enhance the effectiveness and efficiency of both the dentist and the dental assistant.

The functional operating position provides access and visibility to the work area, as well as comfort for the dental team and patient. Knowledge of proper patient positioning will assure that the functional operating position of the dental team is maintained.

The dental assistant must exercise continual caution in order to assure the safety and comfort of the patient.

Mastery of oral evacuation techniques prevents accumulation of debris and fluid in the patient's mouth and insures a clear operating field for the dentist. Proper retraction techniques and use of the three-way syringe will greatly enhance visibility and access. Correct instrument handling and transfer must be well-coordinated between the dentist and the assistant. Use of pre-prepared trays and establishment of a consistent work routine will result in saving time for patients and dental staff.

A well-developed method of transferring the anesthetic syringe will aid in reducing patient's fear.

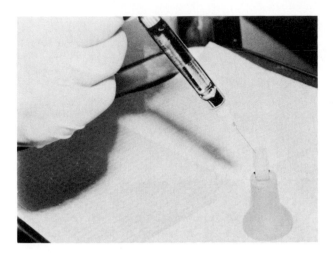

Figure 38.30
Use of a recapping device to prevent operator from accidentally puncturing self while disposing of a used needle.

Study Questions

1. Describe the four components of work-simplification and give an example of each.
2. What are the classifications of motions?
3. What is the "zones of activity" concept?
4. Describe the functional operating position for the dental assistant.
5. How does one identify the appropriate end of the evacuator tip for use in the posterior areas?
6. Describe the steps in effective instrument transfer.
7. Which hand is used for instrument transfers?
8. Which hand is used for transferring the anesthetic syringe?
9. In which direction is the needle bevel oriented before releasing the syringe?

Vocabulary

concave   hollowed inward, like a cave, arched in
contraindication   makes a treatment or procedure inadvisable
convex   arched up, the outside curve of a sphere or ball
critical   an important turning point, characterized by risk, uncertainty, being in a state of crisis, acute (also finding fault)
deviation   deflection, departure from accepted norms
dynamic   powerful, active, continuous productive activity
static   without motion, stationary

CHAPTER 39

Chairside Assisting

The Dental Assistant as Chair Assistant
Basic Setup for Nonoperative Procedures
New Patient Examination Procedure
   Adult
   Child
Bitewing X-ray Procedure
Complete X-ray Procedure
Panoramic X-ray Procedure
Toothbrushing Demonstration Procedure
Recall Prophylaxis and Examination Appointment
Basic Setup for Operative Procedures
Pulp-testing Procedures
Rubber Dam Application
Amalgam Filling Procedure
Polishing (Finishing) Amalgam Restorations
Direct Restorative Composite Resin Filling
     Procedure
Preparation of Zinc Oxide-Eugenol Cement
Preparation of Zinc Phosphate Cements
Gold-foil Filling Procedure
Temporary Crown Procedure
Orthodontic Procedures
   Placement of Bands and Direct Bonded Brackets
   Arch Wire Placement or Change
   Removal of Orthodontic Appliances
   Placement or Adjustment of Removable
     Appliances
Periodontic Procedures
   Diagnosis Tray
   Prophylaxis Tray
   Instrumentation Tray
   Occlusal Adjustment Tray
   Surgery Tray
   Postoperative Tray
   Pack Removal Tray
Endodontic Procedures
   Minimum Endodontic Setup for Intracanal
     Treatment

Endodontic Setup for Apicoectomy (or Apical
     Curettage)
   Periapical Surgery Tray
Oral and Maxillofacial Surgery Procedures
   Care and Medication Preliminary to Surgery with
     Local or General Anesthesia
     When General Anesthesia is Used
   Procedure for the Removal of Teeth
   Oral Surgery Basic Tray
   Oral Surgery Flap Tray
   Oral Surgery Soft Tissue/Biopsy Tray
   Oral Surgery Impaction Tray
Cast-gold Restoration Procedure (Inlay, Three-
     quarter Crown, or Full Crown)
Fixed Prosthodontic Procedures
   Bridge Procedure
   Setting Gold Prostheses
Impression Procedures
   Reversible Hydrocolloid Impression Procedure for
     Multiple Inlay or Bridge
   Compound Impression Procedure
   Alginate Impression Technique
   Hydrocolloid Impression Procedure for Partial
     Denture
Partial Denture Procedure
   Primary Impression
   Final Impression
   Interocclusal Records and Tooth Selection
   Try-in
   Insertion
   Adjustments
Complete Denture Procedure
   Primary Impression
   Final Impression
   Intermaxillary Records and Tooth Selection
   Try-in
   Insertion
Denture Adjustment Procedure or Denture Patient
     Recall Procedure

The Dental Assistant as Chair Assistant

This chapter presents basic setups for most of the routine dental operations with specific instructions for serving the dentist. These setups may not be exactly like the ones your dentist will use; and therefore, it is necessary to learn what your dentist utilizes. List on the pages of this text the materials your dentist wants that are omitted from the setups given and cross out any materials not used. No two dentists work exactly alike, and thus, the requirements vary from dentist to dentist. You can *begin* by learning the setups and procedures given in this chapter, and then vary them to suit your employer.

Remember that you are to be a second pair of hands in chairside assisting. If you can learn to anticipate your dentist's needs *in advance of the request,* you will be a superb assistant.

Basic Setup for Nonoperative Procedures

Armamentarium:

1. Mouth mirror
2. Explorer
3. Cotton pliers
4. Certain additional instruments or materials will be required for all specific procedures, such as removal of teeth, complete denture appointments, and postoperative treatments. (See lists under the appropriate headings in this chapter.)

New Patient Examination Procedure

Adult

Armamentarium:

1. The patient will have filled out an Acquaintance Form. Make available a complete set of patient records with the Acquaintance or Registration Form attached.
2. The basic setup for nonoperative procedures.
3. The material for a recall prophylaxis and examination.
4. Films for full-mouth and bitewing X rays are usually required.
5. Be prepared with the material for alginate impressions in case the patient has teeth missing or other conditions that require study models.
6. Pulp-testing equipment should be available.

Instructions:

Read "Oral Examination Technique" in chapter 37.

Child

Armamentarium:

1. Consult your dentist to know which films are to be used for children.
2. Bitewing X rays are the small No. 00 size for young children (under six years). The No. 0 size is often used from six to eleven years.

Instructions:

This procedure is similar to that used for adults. In many offices, however, full-mouth X rays of children are not taken until the child is approximately eight or nine; thus, it is necessary for the dentist to stipulate the correct films.

The dentist frequently has the parent present in the operatory for this appointment. It provides opportunity for parent education, provided the behavior of the child is good.

Bitewing X-ray Procedure

Armamentarium:

1. The required films
2. Bitewing tabs

Instructions:

For patients twelve years of age and older, four films are required, together with the paper bitewing tabs. The box of paper tabs may be kept with the film in the film storage box.

For children under twelve years, two of the small films are used if the child's mouth is small. As soon as possible, many dentists begin to use four adult-size films or regular adult bitewing films. Bite tabs are available that the assistant attaches to the small films to make them into bitewing X rays for the young child. Service to the child is expedited if you prepare these films in advance and keep them in the film storage box.

1. Seat the patient.
2. Protect the patient from X rays.
3. In some dental offices you are expected to take the X rays. If this is the case, always remember to wipe all moisture off each film packet immediately upon removal from the patient's mouth.

In offices where the dentist takes the X rays, you should be prepared to assist him or her with the following procedures:

4. The X-ray machine should be in operating readiness.
5. While the dentist is placing the film in the patient's mouth, swing the X-ray head near the patient so the dentist may reach it easily.
6. Take the timer or exposure button in your hands.
7. The sequence in which films are placed in the mouth will always be the same.

Exposures for these areas are:

Molar: _____ seconds
Premolar: _____ seconds

Bitewing X-ray Procedure—*Continued*

8. When two films are used for small children, the sequence will always be: first, left side; second, right side.
   Exposure for both is _____ seconds.
9. When making exposures, watch for a signal from your dentist, who will teach you the signal system.
10. Protect yourself and your dentist from X rays. Always be at least six feet away from the X-ray head when making exposures. Watch the dials of the X-ray machine to see that it is functioning properly. Your dentist will show you what these dials must indicate.
11. Upon completion of all exposures, hang up the timer and replace the X-ray extension arm and head in its customary out-of-the-way position.
12. Write the patient's name on the wrapper of the film immediately.
13. Place the rubber-banded bundle in the film storage box until time is available to develop them.

Complete X-ray Procedure

Armamentarium:

1. Correct films, protected in a film dispenser
2. X-ray machine

Instructions:

1. Seat the patient.
2. Protect the patient from X rays.
3. Preparation for filming:
   Fourteen films are used for a complete X ray—seven films for the upper arch and seven for the lower arch. The sequence of placing them in the mouth is always the same. The exposure time varies depending on the area of the mouth being X-rayed and the type of X ray used.
   The sequence of film placement, together with the space for your dentist to enter the correct exposure for the X ray, is:

Upper left molar area	_____ seconds
Upper left premolar area	_____ seconds
Upper left canine area	_____ seconds
Upper central area	_____ seconds
Upper right canine area	_____ seconds
Upper right premolar area	_____ seconds
Upper right molar area	_____ seconds
Lower right molar area	_____ seconds
Lower right premolar area	_____ seconds
Lower right canine area	_____ seconds
Lower central area	_____ seconds
Lower left canine area	_____ seconds
Lower left premolar area	_____ seconds
Lower left molar area	_____ seconds

4. Protect yourself and your dentist from X rays *before* you depress the timer button.
5. Wipe all moisture from film packets immediately after removal from mouth.
6. When all X rays have been taken, write the patient's name on the exposed film. Place the rubber-banded bundle in the film storage box.

Panoramic X-ray Procedure

Armamentarium:

1. Cassette
2. Two screens
3. Film sheet
4. Lead apron or other protection from X ray for patient

Instructions:

1. Insert film and screens in cassette prior to patient's arrival.
2. Protect the patient with proper shielding.
3. Insert the cassette in the machine.
4. Set the controls.
5. Protect yourself.
6. Expose the film.
7. Release patient.
8. Remove cassette from machine.

Toothbrushing Demonstration Procedure

Armamentarium:

1. Basic setup for nonoperative procedures
2. Large hand mirror—be sure that it is clean and free from fingerprints
3. Full denture for demonstration of brushing
4. Toothbrush for demonstrating on denture
5. Toothbrush for demonstrating in the patient's mouth and for presentation to the patient upon departure

This demonstration is often given to a new patient at the time of the initial appointment for examination as an aid in gauging the patient's interest in and appreciation of dental care. It is commonly performed at the final appointment of a patient who has undergone any major amount of operative or restorative work. Frequently, regular patients are taught proper brushing procedures on their recall prophylaxis and examination appointment. The demonstration may be given by the assistant. If this is the procedure in your office, you should understand fully just what the dentist wishes you to teach the patient. (See "Personal Oral Hygiene.")

Recall Prophylaxis and Examination Appointment

Armamentarium:

1. Basic setup for nonoperative procedures
2. Scalers
3. Dental tape
4. Bitewing films and tabs, if desired
5. Full-mouth films, if desired
6. Paper cup and mouth rinse
7. Dappen dish with prophylaxis paste
8. Prophylaxis right angle for handpiece, with rubber cup
9. Prophylaxis brush mounted in contra-angle, if desired
10. For the young child, the dappen dish with paste, the prophylaxis right angle with rubber cup, the child's size bitewing films with tabs

Instructions:

Seat the patient and place the bib or napkin.

Place the patient's last films, if any, on the viewbox, and his or her records convenient to the dentist.

When the oral examination is made upon completion of the prophylaxis, be prepared to note information required.

Before dismissing the patient, be sure that the patient's face is clean. If it is not, offer a disposable tissue. If a powder corner is not available, offer a hand mirror.

If dental work has been found necessary, see that the patient has an appointment for its completion. Some dental offices develop any X-ray films if taken while the patient is still present to complete the examination. Otherwise, if no dental work is found to be necessary, inform the patient that he or she will be notified if any work is found on examination of the X rays. If none is found, the patient will be notified when it is time for the next prophylaxis and examination.

The patient's recall control card is dated at this time for the month and year of his or her next recall and is placed properly in the recall file.

In many dental offices, complete denture patients are recalled once each year for examination. Adjustment of articulation is made if required or appointments are arranged for relining, rebasing, or new dentures if necessary. Material required for this type of recall will depend upon the dentist but may include carbon paper for occlusal marking, or disclosing wax for the same purpose, plus small mounted stones for adjustment of individual areas on the artificial teeth, and vulcanite burs for adjustment of the denture base, if required.

Basic Setup for Operative Procedures

Armamentarium:

1. Mouth mirror
2. Explorer
3. Cotton pliers
4. Air and water syringes
5. Medicaments available
6. Loaded anesthetic syringe
7. Air turbine prepared for use or contra-angle (miniature type for children)
8. Cotton rolls and cotton-roll holders or rubber dam
9. Burs and diamond instruments available as required (short-neck burs for miniature contra-angles)
10. A square of gauze or a disposable tissue inserted in the right-hand clip of the bib-holder for use by the dentist in removing debris from the instruments
11. Saliva ejector
12. High-volume evacuator prepared for use if needed
13. Topical anesthetic if needed

Pulp-testing Procedures

Armamentarium:

1. Basic setup for nonoperative procedures. At times, this procedure is required during an operative appointment, in which case the instrument setup is already complete.
2. Pulp tester. Some pulp testers are individual portable types. Others are part of the dental unit and require no assembly of components for use. The most recent type can be operated by the dentist alone.
3. Ice for pulp testing.

Instructions:

This procedure is used to gain information about the vitality of a tooth. In general, it is the application of a small electrical current to the tooth, increased slowly until the patient gives evidence of feeling the response in the tooth being tested. When the full degree of current is applied without response in the tooth, the tooth may be nonvital, or no longer alive.

The dentist applies the electrode to the tooth, using toothpaste as an electrolyte contact. The assistant gradually increases the amount of current through the tester, either by operation of a slide on the instrument or by rotation of a knob for that purpose on the dental unit. If the pulp tester used in your dental office is a separate unit, a manual is available that illustrates its assembly and correct use.

For a complete examination, the dentist will test each tooth in the mouth. The pulp tester may also be used in testing an individual tooth, in which case the dentist will usually test other teeth corresponding to the tooth in question in order to discover the usual range of response to be expected and then proceed to test the questionable tooth.

The patient will be instructed to raise a hand or give a signal of some kind to indicate that a response is felt. The dentist will tell you when it is time to test the tooth. As you increase the current *slowly,* watch or listen for the patient's signal. Note the figure at which the pointer rests at the moment the signal is made. Speak this number clearly to the dentist and return the slide or knob to zero.

The slide or knob controlling the degree of current should be carefully and slowly moved to increase the current at a rate that would cover the scale consistently in ten to fifteen seconds. *If a patient is highly sensitive, much care should be exercised in increasing the current very slowly. Too rapid increases in current are highly unpleasant to the patient.*

The pulp tester is returned to its case or its receptacle on the dental unit.

Electric pulp testers cannot be used through restorations, especially teeth with full metal or porcelain crowns. In such cases, ice is used to provide a thermal shock when contacting the tooth or restoration. Like the electric test, the response is positive or negative. No *degree of vitality* can be judged from either test.

Rubber Dam Application

Armamentarium:

1. Rubber dam
2. Rubber-dam frame
3. Rubber-dam punch
4. Assorted rubber-dam clamps
5. Rubber-dam clamp forceps
6. Dental floss
7. Plastic instrument
8. Saliva ejector
9. Vaseline or tissue lubricant

Amalgam Filling Procedure

Armamentarium:

1. Basic setup for operative procedures
2. Double-ended chisels
3. Double-ended hatchets, right and left
4. Double-ended gingival margin trimmers, right and left
5. Excavators, right and left, large and small
6. Amalgam carrier
7. Amalgam pluggers, hand type; automatic type, if used
8. Amalgam carvers
9. Amalgam burnishers
10. Matrix holders, Tofflemire or others
11. Matrix bands, molar medium and premolar medium
12. Wedge material, or separators
13. Curved crown and bridge scissors for adjusting bands when necessary

Instructions:

Be ready to assist at the chair by the time the dentist is ready to work on the preparation of the tooth. Some time may be available while the dentist is making the injection of local anesthetic or waiting for it to become effective. Make use of such minutes to perform other duties.

Keep used instruments and other items in position for reuse as the work progresses by keeping trays neat.

An appointment for finishing and polishing these fillings should be made. Twenty-four hours are required before an amalgam filling is considered ready for finishing and polishing.

Polishing (Finishing) Amalgam Restorations

Armamentarium:

1. Basic setup for nonoperative procedures
2. Prophylaxis right angle and rubber cup
3. Polishing brush on mandrel
4. Fine sandpaper discs and mandrels, straight and angle
5. Contra-angle for item 4
6. Finishing burs in bur block
7. Cotton rolls and left and right lower holders as required
8. Dappen dish of prophylactic paste for coarse polishing
9. Dappen dish of half-and-half dry tin oxide and whiting for final polish
10. Large hand mirror for patient's use

Direct Restorative Composite Resin Filling Procedure

Armamentarium:

1. Basic setup for operative procedures
2. Chisels
3. Cement-base materials
4. Mixing pad and spatula
5. Matrix retainer

In the *matrix method,* a resin strip or other means of containing the resin in the cavity is prepared, the mix is completed on the pad, the material is placed into the preparation, and the matrix positioned. When the material is set, the instructions that accompany the material used in your office should be read carefully and the recommended finishing procedure followed.

Preparation of Zinc Oxide-Eugenol Cement

Armamentarium:

1. Glass slab, parchment pad, or plastic pad
2. Steel spatula for mixing (one that is used only for this purpose)
3. Powder and liquid for zinc oxide-eugenol cement
4. Plastic instrument for placing the mixed zinc oxide cement

When used, this material will usually be called for as part of an operative procedure, in which case no separate setup is required.

Preparation of Zinc Phosphate Cements

Armamentarium:

1. Glass slab, cooled to between 65° and 75°F
2. Stainless-steel cement spatula
3. Selected bottle of cement powder
4. Bottle of corresponding cement liquid

Instructions:

Zinc phosphate cements are used for bases under fillings and for cementing inlays, crowns, bridges, and jacket crowns. The consistency for bases is usually heavier than that used for cementation. For use as a base, this type of cement is usually mixed to a molasseslike consistency. For cementation the consistency is usually similar to 30 percent cream; if the spatula is quickly raised from the finished mix of cement on the slab, the cement will follow the spatula in a thin line without breaking momentarily. Zinc phosphate cements are *not* mixed like synthetic porcelain.

Gold-foil Filling Procedure

Armamentarium:

1. Basic setup for operative procedures
2. Rubber dam
3. Rubber-dam holder
4. Rubber-dam retainers
5. Rubber-dam retainer forceps
6. Rubber-dam punch
7. Petrolatum to lubricate punched holes in dam
8. Napkin face mask for rubber dam
9. Red stick compound (to stabilize retainer)
10. Alcohol lamp filled with alcohol (or electric annealer)
11. Leather-faced mallet, long handle (or automatic mallet, if used)
12. Prepared gold foil, pellets, cylinders, or ropes, as desired
13. Gold-foil pluggers, trimming knives, trimming files, and holders
14. Chisels and excavators as required for cavity preparation
15. Polishing strips, discs, rubber cups, and fine-polishing abrasives

Instructions:

Your assistance is usually needed for a rapid application of the rubber dam to the required area of the patient's mouth.

Your direct and constant assistance is required in condensing and in annealing the gold foil into the cavity preparation when ready. Some dentists require the assistant to wield a mallet, applying the strokes to the end of a gold-foil condenser manipulated by the dentist on the foil in the cavity preparation. Other methods include the use of automatic malleting devices.

If you are using cohesive gold foil, it must be annealed. If you are using noncohesive gold foil, it is not annealed. However, restorations in which noncohesive gold foil is used are usually completed by the use of cohesive gold foil. Thus the entire setup of materials required, as listed above, is necessary for either type of restoration.

Practice alone will help the dental assistant understand and become adept at assisting with gold-foil work. It is one of the most exacting, precise operative procedures used in the dental office.

Temporary Crown Procedure

Armamentarium:

1. Basic setup for operative procedures
2. Diamond discs and mounted diamond wheels
3. Excavators, small, left and right
4. Zinc phosphate cement and liquid
5. Glass slab and stainless spatula for item 4
6. Plastic instrument
7. Set of contouring pliers for steel crowns
8. Crown and bridge scissors, curved

In cases involving extremely deep caries or pulp exposure, the following may be required by your dentist also.

9. Calcium hydroxide base material
10. Sterile glass slab for above item
11. Bottle of adrenalin
12. Sterile dappen dish for item 11
13. Sterile cotton pellets
14. Sterile No. 8 round burs for contra-angles
15. Other materials your dentist may use for pulp treatment
16. Rubber-dam setup

Instructions:

Temporary steel crowns are set at the same sitting that the preparation is made. No subsequent appointment for setting the crown is required.

The procedure involving treatment of the pulp requires extremely close assisting in the various steps, especially in the event that the patient is a very young child.

Orthodontic Procedures

Placement of Bands and Direct Bonded Brackets

Armamentarium:

1. Containers of bands for teeth to be banded
2. Set up of brackets to be bonded
3. Etching solution and applicators
4. Sealant and applicators
5. Bonding adhesive
6. Cement, slab, and spatula for bands
7. Amalgam plugger or band seating instrument
8. Aspirator tip and saliva ejector
9. Scaler
10. Mouth mirror
11. Cotton rolls
12. Cotton pledgets or balls
13. Warm air drier
14. Rubber prophylaxis cup and prophylaxis angle
15. Pumice

Orthodontic Procedures—*Continued*

Arch Wire Placement or Change

Armamentarium:

1. Ligature cutter
2. Scaler
3. Howe pliers
4. Bird beak pliers
5. Arch bending pliers
6. Mouth mirror
7. Arch marking pencil
8. Ligature wires
9. Ligature tying pliers
10. Amalgam plugger
11. Distal end cutting pliers

Orthodontic Procedures—*Continued*

Removal of Orthodontic Appliances

Armamentarium:

1. Ligature cutter
2. Mouth mirror
3. Scaler
4. Band removing pliers
5. Band cutting pliers
6. Bonding adhesive removal pliers
7. Prophylaxis angle and rubber cup
8. Pumice

Orthodontic Procedures—*Continued*

Placement or Adjustment of Removable Appliances

Armamentarium:

1. Acrylic bur
2. Mouth mirror
3. Three prong pliers
4. Bird beak pliers
5. Scaler

Periodontic Procedures

Diagnosis Tray

Armamentarium:

1. Basic kit
   a. Mirror
   b. Explorer
   c. Probe
2. U15 scaler and all curettes
3. Saliva ejector
4. Gauze sponges, two-by-two-inch
5. Disclosing tablets
6. Spool of dental floss
7. Toothbrush
8. Napkin chain
9. Handpiece
10. Proper contra-angle for prophylaxis

Periodontic Procedures—*Continued*

Prophylaxis Tray

Armamentarium:

1. Basic kit
   a. Mirror
   b. Explorer
   c. Probe
2. U15 scaler and all curettes
3. Sharpening stone
4. Disclosing tablets
5. Prophylaxis angle
6. Prophylaxis cup
7. Prophylaxis paste
8. Dental floss
9. Napkin chain
10. Handpiece
11. Saliva ejector
12. Topical anesthetic

Periodontic Occlusal Adjustment Tray

Armamentarium:

1. Mirror
2. Set of green stones for straight handpiece (Nos. 19, 22, 48, 23)
3. Burlew wheel
4. Midget or regular pumice-impregnated rubber polishing cups, tips, and points
5. Occlusal wax and pencil
6. Articulating paper holder (Miller)
7. Articulating paper
8. Two-by-two-inch gauze sponges
9. Napkin holder
10. Handpiece
11. Proper contra-angle prophylaxis
12. Saliva ejector

Periodontic Instrumentation Tray

Armamentarium:

1. Basic kit
   a. Mirror
   b. Explorer
   c. Probe
2. U15 scaler with curettes
   a. Gracey's 1 & 2, 9 & 10 (or 7 & 8), 13 & 14
   b. McCall's 13s & 14s, 17s & 18s
3. Two-by-two-inch gauze sponges
4. Sharpening stone
5. Napkin holder
6. Handpiece
7. Proper contra-angle for prophylaxis
8. Saliva ejector
9. Topical anesthetic

Periodontic Procedures—*Continued*

Surgery Tray

Armamentarium:

1. Mirror
2. Explorer
3. Probe
4. U15 scaler
5. Bard Parker handle and No. 15 blade
6. Knives
7. Periosteal elevator (No. 7 spatula)
8. Curettes—Gracey's 1 & 2, 9 & 10, 17s & 18s
9. Sharpening stone
10. Needle holder
11. Surture scissors
12. Burs
    a. No. 8 round, straight handpiece bur
    b. F1 and F3 diamond stones
13. Stainless-steel bowl
14. Water bulb
15. Topical anesthetic
16. Loaded anesthetic syringe with long and short needle
17. Two or three sterile cotton-tipped applicators
18. Aspirator handle and two tips
19. Jones clamp and sections of sterile rubber tubing with connector
20. Sterile napkin chain
21. Handpiece
22. Proper contra-angle for prophylaxis
23. Saliva ejector

Periodontic Postoperative Tray

Armamentarium:

1. Mirror
2. Explorer
3. Probe
4. Suture scissors
5. Cotton pliers
6. Handpiece
7. Proper contra-angle for prophylaxis
8. Saliva ejector

Periodontic Pack Removal Tray

Armamentarium:

1. Mirror
2. Probe
3. U15 scaler
4. Handpiece
5. Proper contra-angle for prophylaxis
6. Saliva ejector

Endodontic Procedures

Minimum Endodontic Setup for Intracanal Treatment

Armamentarium:

1. Mirror
2. Explorer
3. Excavator
4. Cotton pliers
5. Irrigation syringe (2 or 3 cc.) with needle
6. Scissors
7. Hemostat
8. Plastic instrument
9. Spreader
10. Measuring gauge

Also Available:

11. Two-by-two-inch gauze sponges
12. Two one-inch cotton rolls
13. Two applicator sticks
14. Topical anesthetic
15. Syringe with cartridge of local anesthetic
16. Reamers and files (standardized AAE sizes 10–140)
17. Gutta-percha points (standardized AAE sizes 25–140)
18. Broaches, smooth and barbed
19. Paper points
20. Rubber or silicone stops
21. Electric pulp tester
22. Endodontic cement (sealer)
23. Mixing slab and spatula
24. Cavit
25. Cements: zinc oxide-eugenol, zinc phosphate, and composite
26. Sodium hypochlorite
27. Eugenol
28. Camphorated paramonochlorophenol
29. Beechwood creosote
30. Tincture of Mercresin (untinted)
31. Eucalyptol
32. EDTAC
33. Rubber-dam squares
34. Rubber-dam punch
35. Rubber-dam clamp forceps
36. Rubber-dam holder

The purpose of this procedure is devitalization of the tooth involved, without apical surgery. A series of such treatments may be required.

Endodontic Setup for Apicoectomy (or Apical Curettage)

Armamentarium:

1. The complete Intracanal Tray
2. The Periapical Surgery Tray

Instructions:

All materials and instruments needed to perform the work should be arranged in an orderly fashion. For efficiency in operating, there must be no delay to search for instruments or prepare materials once the work is begun.

Endodontic Periapical Surgery Tray

Armamentarium:

1. Gilmore probe
2. Vehe carver
3. Scalpel (no. 15 blade)
4. Periosteotome
5. Burs (nos. 557 and 560 carbide)
6. Needle holder
7. Scissors
8. Bone chisel
9. Three periapical curettes
10. Tissue retractor
11. Needle (with silk suture)
12. Five two-by-two-inch gauze sponges
13. Two applicator sticks
14. Sterile water of saline
15. Topical anesthetic
16. Loaded anesthetic syringe

The purpose of this procedure is endodontic treatment of the tooth and removal of the periapical lesion.

Oral and Maxillofacial Surgery Procedures

(W. P. Frantzich, D.D.S., M.S.D.)

Care and Medication Preliminary to Surgery With Local or General Anesthesia

When the patient is brought to the operatory, the assistant should briefly review the medical history and note any abnormalities on a buck slip (figure 28.16). The buck slip should accompany the chart. Any physical problems, such as head cold, general illness, blueness of the lips (cyanosis), shortness of breath, or wheezing should be noted on the buck slip and then be called to the attention of the surgeon. The procedure to be performed should also be written on the buck slip. Any note from the referring doctor should be attached to the buck slip.

The patient should be properly seated in the dental chair in an upright position for X rays and a semi-upright position for surgery. (The position of the patient will vary according to the surgeon's preference.)

The anesthesia used may vary. Here is a list of the most commonly used anesthetics. They may be used singly or in combination.

1. Local anesthesia
2. Nitrous oxide and oxygen
3. Intravenous medications: Brevital, Versed, Valium, and narcotics

When General Anesthesia is Used

1. The patient must be monitored during surgery (blood pressure, blood oxygenation, pulse, respiration, color, and perspiration).
2. Therefore, bulky and excessive clothing should be removed.
3. An examining gown may be worn by the patient, if necessary.
4. The arms should be freely accessible for a blood pressure cuff and the placement of an I.V. needle.
5. There should be no clothing that is confining around the neck because a stethoscope may be used to monitor the airway or heart rate.
6. The patient should be properly draped and comfortably prepared for the procedures.
7. The blood pressure, percentage of oxygen saturation (oximeter), and pulse should be recorded on the chart.

8. Five items should be verified by the surgical assistant. The responses to the first two items should be noted on the buck slip. The surgical assistant is responsible for the patient's compliance with the third and fourth items. The fifth item indicates the surgical assistant's personal responsibility. These items are:
   a. The patient has had nothing to eat or drink for six hours.
   b. A responsible person is present to take the patient home.
   c. Removable dental appliances have been removed.
   d. The patient's bladder has just been emptied.
   e. Check the buck slip. Be sure you have accomplished all the appropriate items on the buck slip for which you are responsible.
9. During **local anesthesia** appropriate monitoring is necessary. This will vary according to the complexity of the procedure and the patient's medical status.
10. Present the patient with postoperative prescriptions and/or medication and any written instructions for postoperative care.
11. If the removal has been quite difficult, the patient may be asked to return in twenty-four hours for examination of the wound. If the removal has been quite routine, you may be asked to call the patient the day after the surgery. During such a call you indicate that your office is interested in the patient's comfort, therefore you have called to inquire. Any negative comments should be referred to the dentist.

Oral and Maxillofacial Surgery—
Continued

Procedure for the Removal of Teeth

1. Premedication, if required, given to the patient
2. Proper tray setup for procedures (with forceps)
3. Appropriate anesthesia (local, nitrous oxide, I.V.)
4. Postoperative information pamphlet; prepackaged, put-up medication or prescription
5. X rays on view box
6. The dentist will inform you of the need for other instruments

DUTIES

1. Both surgeon and surgical assistant should wear glasses and mask and scrub thoroughly, then glove. While maintenance of a truly sterile field in oral surgery is not generally possible in the office, every attempt should be made to prevent cross contamination with other patients.
2. Avoid contaminating objects (drawers, chairs, instrument trays) outside the operating field.
3. If general anethesia is used, the anesthesia assistant will properly support the jaw to insure a potent (open) airway.
4. A throat pack is placed to prevent secretions and debris from falling into the pharynx.
5. The surgical assistant should remove saliva, blood, and debris from the mouth and oropharynx during the procedures with the suction aspirator.
6. This assistant should be ready to irrigate the surgical site, assist the surgeon during suturing, and perform any other routine moves so the procedure is completed efficiently and smoothly.
7. No one considers the removal of a tooth a pleasant matter. Remain calm and poised at all times. Make no remarks that would indicate surprise at anything you may observe. Should either the assistant or the dentist inadvertently indicate surprise at some state of the proceedings, the patient will very quickly become alarmed. While the removal of teeth usually proceeds as expected, the only dentist who does not experience difficulty at times is the dentist who does not remove teeth.

8. Present the patient with the postoperative prescriptions and/or medication and any written instructions for post operative care.
9. If the removal has been quite difficult, the patient may be asked to return in twenty-four hours for examination of the wound.
10. For a routine removal, you may be asked to call the patient the day after the surgery. Explain that you have called because you are interested in the patient's comfort. Refer any negative comments to the dentist.

Oral and Maxillofacial Surgery—
Continued

Oral Surgery Basic Tray

Armamentarium:

1. Suction aspirator
2. Cheek retractor
3. Mouth mirror
4. Foil carrier
5. Double-ended curette
6. Periosteal elevator
7. Sponges

Additional Items to Add to the Tray:

8. Loaded anesthetic syringe
9. Loaded ligament injection syringe
10. Applicator sticks
11. Topical and antiseptic medications
12. General anesthetic (I.V. $+ N_2O/O_2$)
13. Mouth props
14. Throat packs
15. Bulb syringe and saline for irrigation
16. Burs and dental drill
17. Forceps and additional elevators as indicated

Oral and Maxillofacial Surgery— *Continued*

Oral Surgery Flap Tray

Armamentarium:

1. Oral Surgery Basic Tray
2. Scalpel
3. Root tip elevator
4. Gilmore probe
5. Bone file
6. End cutting rongeur
7. Side cutting rongeur
8. Hemostatic forceps (mosquito)
9. Suture
10. Suture scissors
11. Needle holder

Additional Items to Add to the Tray:

12. Loaded anesthetic syringe
13. Loaded ligament injection syringe
14. Applicator sticks
15. Topical and antiseptic medications
16. General anesthetic (I.V. + N_2O/O_2)
17. Mouth props
18. Throat packs
19. Bulb syringe and saline for irrigation
20. Burs and dental drill
21. Forceps and additional elevators as indicated

Oral and Maxillofacial Surgery— *Continued*

Oral Surgery Soft Tissue/Biopsy Tray

Armamentarium:

1. Oral Surgery Basic Tray
2. Scalpel
3. Allis forceps
4. Tissue forceps
5. Adson forceps with teeth
6. Sharp-pointed scissors
7. Hemostatic forceps, curved and straight
8. Suture
9. Suture scissors
10. Needle holder

Additional Items to Add to the Tray:

11. Loaded anesthetic syringe
12. Loaded ligament injection syringe
13. Applicator sticks
14. Topical and antiseptic medications
15. General anesthetic (I.V. + N_2O/O_2)
16. Mouth props
17. Throat packs
18. Bulb syringe and saline for irrigation
19. Burs and dental drill
20. Forceps and additional elevators as indicated

Oral and Maxillofacial Surgery—
Continued

Oral Surgery Impaction Tray

Armamentarium:

1. Oral Surgery Basic Tray
2. Scalpel
3. Root tip elevator
4. Gilmore probe
5. #46 straight elevator
6. #301 straight elevator
7. Pott's elevators
8. 190 and 191 elevators
9. Bone file
10. End rongeur
11. Hemostatic forcep
12. Suture
13. Suture scissors
14. Needle holder

Additional Items to Add to the Tray:

15. Loaded anesthetic syringe
16. Loaded ligament injection syringe
17. Applicator sticks
18. Topical and antiseptic medications
19. General anesthetic (I.V. + N_2O/O_2)
20. Mouth props
21. Throat packs
22. Bulb syringe and saline for irrigation
23. Burs and dental drill
24. Forceps and additional elevators as indicated

Cast-gold Restoration Procedure (Inlay, Three-quarter Crown, or Full Crown)

Armamentarium:

1. Basic setup for operative procedures
2. Block of diamond or carbide cutting instruments and handpieces
3. Double-ended Wedelstaedt chisels
4. Double-ended hatchets, one pair, right and left
5. Double-ended gingival margin trimmers, one pair, right and left
6. Excavators, one pair, right and left
7. Fine sandpaper discs and mandrels, straight and angle
8. Impression materials of choice
9. Impression trays or bands as indicated
10. Crown and bridge scissors
11. Dark red sheet wax to check clearance
12. Matrix holder, Tofflemire
13. Matrix bands, molar medium and bicuspid medium
14. Wedges
15. Stick of inlay wax
16. Plugger (Black No. 5)
17. Plastic instrument
18. Amalgam carver (Walls)

Also Available:

19. Sprue pins
20. Sprue base
21. Lighted gas burner or alcohol torch
22. Squares of hard gutta-percha for posterior temporary fillings; crown forms or resin forms with zinc oxide-eugenol paste for anterior teeth
23. Zinc oxide-eugenol cement
24. Cement slab and spatula
25. Peso pliers
26. Box of aluminum shells for temporary crowns (posterior only)
27. Box of crown forms or resin forms for temporary crowns (anterior only)

Cast-gold inlays are set at a subsequent appointment. Provide sufficient time between appointments for completion of the required laboratory work. For cementing inlays, see "Setting Gold Inlays, Crowns, Bridges, and Jacket Crowns."

Fixed Prosthodontic Procedures

Bridge Procedure

Armamentarium:

1. Basic setup for operative procedures
2. Bridges may be supported entirely on full crowns, on three-quarter crowns, on jacket crowns, inlays, or any combination of these. These are *abutments*. Instruments and materials should be prepared according to the types of support required for the particular bridge under construction.

In the Laboratory:

3. Impression trays as your dentist designates
4. Impression material as your dentist designates
5. Equipment for preparation of the impression material

Fixed Prosthodontic Procedures— *Continued*

Setting Gold Prostheses

Armamentarium:

1. Basic setup for operative procedure
2. Orangewood stick
3. Leather-faced mallet
4. Glass slab for cement preparation
5. Spatula for cement preparation
6. Silver cement for full gold crowns; regular zinc phosphate cement for three-quarter or veneer crowns, for inlays or jacket crowns
7. Finishing burs
8. Straight handpiece burs for carving
9. Roll of articulating paper (carbon paper)
10. Mounted stone, small, green Carborundum
11. Burlew disc on mandrel
12. Fine sandpaper discs and mandrels, straight and angle
13. Dappen dish with whiting-tin oxide mixture
14. Prophylactic contra-angle with rubber cup
15. Cotton-roll holder for lower arch

Impression Procedures

Reversible Hydrocolloid Impression Procedure for Multiple Inlay or Bridge

Armamentarium:

1. Basic setup for nonoperative procedures
2. Impression trays (the dentist will select)
3. Rubber hoses for connecting trays with cold-water outlet for cooling impression
4. Cold water for cooling. During the winter months, the water supply at the unit may be cold enough for this purpose, and in some areas the same may be true in summer. If the water at the unit is not sufficiently cold, at least two quarts of ice water for each impression should be made available at the chair.
5. Hydrocolloid conditioner for preparing the hydrocolloid and for storage of the prepared hydrocolloid
6. Two tubes or containers of hydrocolloid for one impression; three or four tubes or containers to be prepared for two impressions
7. (a) Hydrocolloid syringes, small, loaded with hydrocolloid material, or
   (b) Jar of hydrocolloid material diluted with water; brushes to apply
8. Glass of tepid salt water or mouthwash for rinsing to remove debris and saliva from the patient's mouth, used before your dentist prepares the mouth for the impression
9. Gum retraction kit
10. Wax (a high-melting-point variety) to build up trays as required

In the Laboratory:

11. Materials required to pour artificial stone casts
12. Materials required to pour die stone
13. A device for positioning brass dowel pins directly in the center of each die
14. Separating medium

The main point of difference between this procedure and that for a partial denture is the necessity to apply a thinner form of hydrocolloid in and around all recesses of the prepared teeth to eliminate trapping fine air bubbles in the impression. The small hydrocolloid syringe material can be used for this purpose, since the fine syringe needle permits squirting a thin, controlled layer of hydrocolloid material where the dentist desires.

Impression Procedures—*Continued*

Compound Impression Procedure

Armamentarium:

1. Basic setup for nonoperative procedures
2. Trays selected by the dentist
3. Two cakes of impression compound for each arch to be taken
4. Compound heater filled with water and set at the correct temperature to properly soften the impression compound used in your office (see the instructions for temperature packed with each box of compound)
5. Lighted gas burner or alcohol torch

This method of taking an impression is sometimes used in making study models of both arches, whether with or without teeth.

Impression Procedures—*Continued*

Alginate Impression Technique

Armamentarium:

1. Basic setup for nonoperative procedures
2. Paper cup or glass containing tepid salt water for mouth rinse
3. Stick of red boxing or carding wax for building up trays

In the Laboratory:

4. Alginate impression material
5. Measuring devices, if required. Some material is packaged in single units; some is available in bulk cans.
6. Plastic mixing bowl and plastic spatula
7. Sufficient water at the recommended temperature for the mix. If no temperature is specified, 70° may be satisfactory. Higher temperatures hasten setting. When the correct temperature has been decided upon, always use it exactly so that the material will react consistently.
8. The required trays (the dentist will usually select these)
9. Fixing solution prepared, if required, for immersion of the finished impressions prior to pouring the casts

Read the instructions for the alginate material used in your office. Comply with the manufacturer's recommendations exactly.

Impression Procedures—*Continued*

Hydrocolloid Impression Procedure For Partial Denture

Armamentarium:

1. Basic setup for nonoperative procedures
2. Impression trays (the dentist will select)
3. Rubber hoses for connecting trays with cold-water outlet for cooling impression
4. Cold water for cooling. During the winter months, the water supply at the unit may be cold enough for this purpose, and in some areas the same may be true in summer. If the water at the unit is not sufficiently cold, at least two quarts of ice water for each impression should be made available.
5. Hydrocolloid conditioner for preparing the hydrocolloid and for storing the prepared hydrocolloid
6. Prepare two tubes for one impression, three or four tubes for two impressions.
7. Glass of tepid salt water for rinsing (or a mouthwash) to remove debris and saliva from the patient's mouth; used immediately before impression is taken
8. Wax (a high-melting-point variety) to build up trays as required

In the Laboratory:

9. Materials required to pour artificial stone casts
10. Fixative for hydrocolloid, if required, or storage facilities. Hydrocolloid should be prepared exactly according to the directions for the specific brand used in your office.

Partial Denture Procedure

Primary Impression

Armamentarium:

1. Basic setup for nonoperative procedures
2. Alginate impression or other material of choice

The purpose of this appointment is to make impressions for study models. These study models are usually mounted in a simple articulator for preliminary study and are later placed on a "surveying" instrument to design the clasps that will hold the partial in the mouth.

If individualized impression trays are to be made, allow sufficient time for the laboratory procedures to be completed prior to the next appointment. If two partials, an upper and a lower, are to be constructed, both study models are poured in plaster. If but one partial is to be constructed, the *opposing* model is poured in artificial stone, not in plaster, since it may be used opposite the finished model of the arch that will have the partial.

Partial Denture Procedure—*Continued*

Final Impression

Armamentarium:

1. Basic setup for operative procedures
2. Hydrocolloid impression materials, or material of choice

The object of this appointment is to make an accurate impression to be used as the working model in constructing the partial or partials.

If but one partial is to be constructed, only this arch needs retaking for the final working impression. The previously made opposing cast poured in artificial stone is used.

Prior to the next appointment, time must be reserved for the construction of bite rims on the working models. In some cases, the partial dentures may be constructed at this point without making bite rims, etc., eliminating the next sitting. If so, the facebow transfer is accomplished at this sitting, and selection of mold of teeth and selection of shade are completed as well. The third sitting is thus combined with the second.

Partial Denture Procedure—*Continued*

Interocclusal Records and Tooth Selection

Armamentarium:

1. Basic setup for nonoperative procedures
2. Gas burner or alcohol torch
3. Heavy wax spatula
4. Tooth mold and shade-selecting equipment
5. Facebow and its auxiliary equipment, if used, or equipment of choice

The object of this appointment is to register the correct relationship of the upper and lower arches and to duplicate this relationship in mounting the casts in the articulator. The desired shape (mold) and color (shade) of the replacement teeth must also be selected at this time.

Partial Denture Procedure—*Continued*

Try-in

Armamentarium:

1. Disclosing paste
2. Mounted green stones
3. Articulating paper

The object of this appointment is to verify all preceding steps before final insertion. The cast framework is tried in and adjusted to fit accurately. The occlusion is checked to be sure the interocclusal records were accurate and the mounting correct. The mold and shade selection is checked to be certain no error was made in tooth selection.

Partial Denture Procedure—*Continued*

Insertion

Armamentarium:

1. Basic setup for operative procedures
2. Vulcanite burs for any necessary trimming of the partial denture base
3. Small mounted stones (S.S. White No. 48) for adjusting occlusion
4. Articulating paper

At this appointment the partial or partials are inserted in the patient's mouth. Any obvious adjustments are made at this time. The patient is usually given another appointment within one to three days for follow-up and as often as needed thereafter.

Partial Denture Procedure—*Continued*

Adjustments

Armamentarium:

1. Basic setup for operative procedures
2. Vulcanite burs for any necessary trimming of the partial denture base
3. Small mounted stone (S. S. White No. 48) for adjusting articulation
4. Articulating paper or sections of typewriter ribbon

These appointments are for the purpose of checking the progress and comfort of the patient. Since patients who wear partial dentures must have natural teeth present, their recall control cards are marked for the usual recall period.

Complete Denture Procedure

Primary Impression

Armamentarium:

1. Basic setup for nonoperative procedures
2. For full upper and lower dentures: impression material of choice
3. For single full denture: in addition, impression material of choice for impression of opposing arch

The object of this appointment is to make impressions for study models of the mouth for complete denture construction. If only one denture is to be constructed, an impression of the opposing arch or denture is made and poured in artificial stone. It then becomes the final opposing model.

Sufficient time will be required for the construction of a tray or trays for the final impression(s) between appointments.

Complete Denture Procedure—
Continued

Final Impression

Armamentarium:

1. Basic setup for nonoperative procedures
2. Previously prepared tray(s) for final impression(s)
3. Final impression material, with appropriate mixing pad and spatula
4. Cleansing agent for removing material from skin surfaces

The object of this appointment is to make final impressions of the complete denture area.

Complete Denture Procedure—
Continued

Intermaxillary Records and Tooth Selection

Armamentarium:

1. Basic setup for nonoperative procedures
2. Previously prepared bite rim(s)
3. Facebow and auxiliary equipment
4. Mold and shade guides

The object of this appointment is to register the relationship of the upper and lower arches, to duplicate this relationship in mounting the casts in the articulator, and to select the correct mold and shade of teeth to be used in the denture(s).

Complete Denture Procedure—
Continued

Try-in

Armamentarium:

1. Basic setup for nonoperative procedures
2. Previously prepared trial denture setup(s)
3. Compound heater, all trays removed, set at 120° to soften wax
4. Bite registration wax, if desired
5. Cold water for chilling bite registrations
6. Large scissors for cutting registration wax into strips
7. Large hand mirror
8. Spouse, relative, or friend of the patient

The object of this sitting is to register the *condylar inclinations* of the patient; also, and by no means incidentally, to verify the appearance of the teeth by having a close relative of the patient express an opinion, in addition to the patient's personal reaction.

Complete Denture Procedure—
Continued

Insertion

Armamentarium:

1. Basic setup for nonoperative procedures
2. Previously processed denture(s)
3. Articulating paper or piece of typewriter ribbon to check articulation of teeth
4. Disclosing wax, if desired
5. Mounting records retained from previous work
6. Compound heater, all trays removed, water at 120° for wax softening
7. Bite-registration wax
8. Scissors, large
9. Cold water for chilling registrations

The object of this appointment is to insert the denture(s) and to instruct the patient in their care. Sometimes a **checkbite** is taken at this time, and the dentures are remounted in the articulator to further refine the occlusion and to look for premature occlusal contacts.

Be sure to retain the mounting records to facilitate remounting the dentures at the next sitting. In some offices, these records are kept permanently.

The patient's recall control card is dated for recall one year from this appointment, unless natural teeth are present.

Denture Adjustment Procedure or Denture Patient Recall Procedure

Armamentarium:

1. Basic setup for nonoperative procedures
2. Vulcanite burs for trimming denture bases
3. Articulating paper
4. Small mounted stones for adjusting articulation
5. Disclosing wax, if desired

The purpose of these appointments is to relieve denture soreness or improper function when it occurs.

Denture recall appointments require the same materials as listed under denture adjustment procedures. Should the dentures require it, they are cleaned and polished on the laboratory lathe. If calculus has collected on the dentures, it is removed by using an ultrasonic cleaning mechanism.

Summary

This chapter presents suggested setups for many of the routine dental operations. Space is provided so that the lists of materials included in each setup may be altered to suit the individual dentist. One of the objectives for which a dental assistant should strive is to learn to anticipate the dentist's needs and have material or instruments ready *in advance of the dentist's request*.

Eventually, the dental assistant should have memorized the materials necessary for any specific operation; but in the beginning, the lists in this chapter will be of assistance in preparing the materials for each setup.

Study Questions
1. What is a basic setup for nonoperative dentistry?
2. What is meant by nonoperative dentistry?
3. What is a basic setup for operative dentistry?
4. What is meant by operative dentistry?
5. Pick two or three setups and list the materials required for each. Do this several times. It will help you memorize the necessary materials for each setup.

Appendices

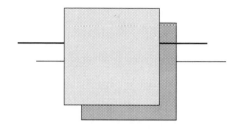

Tables of Weights and Measures
564

Table of the More Common Latin
or Greek Terms and
Abbreviations Used in
Prescription Writing *567*

Table of Thermometric
Equivalents *568*

Table of Certain Diseases *570*

Improving Your Speaking Ability
574

564

TABLES OF WEIGHTS AND MEASURES

Avoirdupois Weight

1 pound = 1.2153 pounds troy

Grains gr.	Drachms dr.	Ounces oz.	Pound lb.
27.34375 =	1		
437.5 =	16 =	1	
7000 =	256 =	16 =	1

Apothecaries' Weight

Grains gr.	Scruples ℈	Drachms ℨ	Ounces ℥	Pound lb.
20 =	1			
60 =	3 =	1		
480 =	24 =	8 =	1	
5760 =	288 =	96 =	12 =	1

Apothecaries' Measure

Minims ♏	Fluidrachms fℨ	Fluidounces f℥	Pints O.	Gallon C.
60 =	1			
480 =	8 =	1		
7,680 =	128 =	16 =	1	
61,440 =	1024 =	128 =	8 =	1

Comparative Values of Standard and Metric Measures of Length

Inches	Centimeters	Inches	Millimeters
1	2.54	1/25	1.00
2	5.08	1/12	2.12
3	7.62	1/8	3.18
4	10.16	1/4	6.35
5	12.70	1/3	8.47
6	15.24	1/2	12.70
7	17.78	5/8	15.88
8	20.32	2/3	16.93
9	22.86	3/4	19.05
10	25.40	5/6	21.16
11	27.94	7/8	22.22
12	30.48	11/12	23.28

Metric Weights

1 gram = 1 cubic centimeter of distilled water at 4° C.

		Grams	Grains	Av. Ounces
Milligram	=	0.001	= 0.01543	
Centigram	=	0.01	= 0.15432	
Decigram	=	0.1	= 1.54324	
Gram	=	1.	= 15.43248 =	.03528
Decagram	=	10.	=	.3528
Hectogram	=	100.	=	3.52758
Kilogram	=	1,000.	=	35.2758

Comparative Values of Apothecaries' and Metric Liquid Measures

Minims	Cubic Centimeters	Fluidrachms	Cubic Centimeters	Fluidounces	Cubic Centimeters
1	0.06	1	3.70	1	29.57
2	0.12	2	7.39	2	59.15
3	0.19	3	11.09	3	88.72
4	0.25	4	14.79	4	118.29
5	0.31	5	18.48	5	147.87
6	0.37	6	22.18	6	177.44
7	0.43	7	25.88	7	207.01
8	0.49			8	236.58
9	0.55			9	266.16
10	0.62			10	295.73
11	0.68			11	325.30
12	0.74			12	354.88
13	0.80			13	384.45
14	0.86			14	414.02
15	0.92			15	443.59
16	0.99			16	473.17
17	1.05			17	502.74
18	1.11			18	532.31
19	1.17			19	561.89
20	1.23			20	591.46
25	1.54			21	621.03
30	1.85			22	650.60
35	2.16			23	680.18
40	2.46			24	709.75
45	2.77			25	739.32
50	3.08			26	768.90
55	3.39			27	798.47
				28	828.04
				29	857.61
				30	887.19
				31	916.76
				32	946.33

Metric Linear Measure

		Meter	U. S. Inches	Feet	Yards	Miles
Millimeter	=	.001	= .03937 =	.00328		
Centimeter	=	.01	= .3937 =	.03280		
Decimeter	=	.1	= 3.937 =	.32808 =	.10936	
Meter	=	1.	= 39.37 =	3.2808 =	1.0936	
Decameter	=	10.	=	32.808	10.936	
Hectometer	=	100.	=	328.08 =	109.36	= .062137
Kilometer	=	1,000.	=	3,280.8 =	1,093.6	= .62137

TABLES OF WEIGHTS AND MEASURES—(Continued)

Table for Converting Metric Weights into Apothecaries' Weights

Grams	Exact Equivalents in Grains	Grams	Exact Equivalents in Grains
0.01	0.1543	12.0	185.189
0.02	0.3086	13.0	200.621
0.03	0.4630	14.0	216.054
0.04	0.6173	15.0	231.486
0.05	0.7716	16.0	246.918
0.06	0.9259	17.0	262.351
0.07	1.0803	18.0	277.783
0.08	1.2346	19.0	293.216
0.09	1.3889	20.0	308.648
0.1	1.543	21.0	324.080
0.2	3.086	22.0	339.513
0.3	4.630	23.0	354.945
0.4	6.173	24.0	370.378
0.5	7.716	25.0	385.810
0.6	9.259	26.0	401.242
0.7	10.803	27.0	416.674
0.8	12.346	28.0	432.107
0.9	13.889	29.0	447.538
1.0	15.432	30.0	462.971
2.0	30.865	31.0	478.403
3.0	46.297	32.0	493.835
4.0	61.730	40.0	617.294
5.0	77.162	45.0	694.456
6.0	92.594	50.0	771.618
7.0	108.027	60.0	925.942
8.0	123.459	70.0	1080.265
9.0	138.892	80.0	1234.589
10.0	154.324	90.0	1388.912
11.0	169.756	100.0	1543.236

Table for Converting Apothecaries' Weights into Metric Weights

Grains	Grams	Grains	Grams
1/50	0.00130	50	3.240
1/32	0.00202	51	3.305
1/20	0.00324	52	3.370
1/18	0.00360	53	3.434
1/16	0.00405	54	3.499
1/15	0.00432	55	3.564
1/12	0.00540	56	3.629
1/10	0.00648	57	3.694
1/8	0.00810	58	3.758
1/6	0.01080	59	3.823
1/5	0.01296	60	3.888
1/4	0.01620	61	3.953
1/3	0.02160	62	4.018
1/2	0.03240	63	4.082
3/4	0.04860	64	4.147
1	0.0648	65	4.212
2	0.1296	66	4.277
3	0.1944	67	4.342
4	0.2592	68	4.406
5	0.3240	69	4.471
6	0.3888	70	4.536
7	0.4536	71	4.601
8	0.5184	72	4.666
9	0.5832	73	4.730
10	0.6480	74	4.795
11	0.7128	75	4.860
12	0.7776	76	4.925
13	0.8424	77	4.990
14	0.9072	78	5.054
15	0.9720	79	5.119
16	1.037	80	5.184
17	1.102	81	5.249
18	1.166	82	5.314
19	1.231	83	5.378
20	1.296	84	5.443
21	1.361	85	5.508
22	1.426	86	5.573
23	1.490	87	5.638
24	1.555	88	5.702
25	1.620	89	5.767
26	1.685	90	5.832
27	1.749	91	5.897
28	1.814	92	5.962
29	1.879	93	6.026
30	1.944	94	6.091
31	2.009	95	6.156
32	2.074	96	6.221
33	2.138	97	6.286
34	2.203	98	6.350
35	2.268	99	6.415
36	2.333	100	6.480
37	2.398	120	7.776
38	2.462	150	9.720
39	2.527	180	11.664
40	2.592	200	12.958
41	2.657	480	31.103
42	2.722	500	32.396
43	2.786	600	38.875
44	2.851	700	45.354
45	2.916	800	51.833
46	2.981	900	58.313
47	3.046	960	62.207
48	3.110	1000	64.799
49	3.175		

TABLES OF WEIGHTS AND MEASURES—(Continued)

Metric Doses with Approximate Apothecary Equivalents

The approximate dose equivalents in the following table represent the quantities that would be prescribed, under identical conditions, by physicians trained, respectively, in the metric or in the apothecary system of weights and measures.

When prepared dosage forms such as tablets, capsules, pills, etc., are prescribed in the metric system, the pharmacist may dispense the corresponding approximate equivalent in the apothecary system, and vice versa. However, this does not authorize the alternative use of the approximate dose equivalents given below for specific quantities on a prescription that requires compounding, nor in converting a pharmaceutical formula from one system of weights or measures to the other system; for such purposes exact equivalents must be used.

LIQUID MEASURES		WEIGHTS	
Metric	*Approximate Apothecary Equivalents*	*Metric*	*Approximate Apothecary Equivalents*
1000 cc.	1 quart	30 Gm.	1 ounce
750 cc.	1½ pints	15 Gm.	4 drachms
500 cc.	1 pint	10 Gm.	2½ drachms
250 cc.	8 fluidounces	7.5 Gm.	2 drachms
200 cc.	7 fluidounces	6 Gm.	90 grains
100 cc.	3½ fluidounces	5 Gm.	75 grains
50 cc.	1¾ fluidounces	4 Gm.	60 grains (1 drachm)
30 cc.	1 fluidounce	3 Gm.	45 grains
15 cc.	½ fluidounce (4 fluidrachms)	2 Gm.	30 grains (½ drachm)
10 cc.	2½ fluidrachms	1.5 Gm.	22 grains
8 cc.	2 fluidrachms	1 Gm.	15 grains
5 cc.	75 minims (1¼ fluidrachms)	0.75 Gm.	12 grains
4 cc.	1 fluidrachm	0.6 Gm.	10 grains
3 cc.	45 minims	0.5 Gm.	7½ grains
2 cc.	30 minims	0.45 Gm.	7 grains
1 cc.	15 minims	0.4 Gm.	6 grains
0.75 cc.	12 minims	0.3 Gm.	5 grains
0.6 cc.	10 minims	0.25 Gm.	4 grains
0.5 cc.	8 minims	0.2 Gm.	3 grains
0.3 cc.	5 minims	0.15 Gm.	2½ grains
0.25 cc.	4 minims	0.12 Gm.	2 grains
0.2 cc.	3 minims	0.1 Gm.	1½ grains
0.1 cc.	1½ minims	75 mg.	1¼ grains
0.06 cc.	1 minim	60 mg.	1 grain
		50 mg.	¾ grain
		40 mg.	⅔ grain
		30 mg.	½ grain
		25 mg.	⅜ grain
		20 mg.	⅓ grain
		15 mg.	¼ grain
		12 mg.	⅕ grain
		10 mg.	⅙ grain
		8 mg.	⅛ grain
		6 mg.	1/10 grain
		5 mg.	1/12 grain
		4 mg.	1/15 grain
		3 mg.	1/20 grain
		2 mg.	1/30 grain
		1.5 mg.	1/40 grain
		1.2 mg.	1/50 grain
		1 mg.	1/60 grain
		0.8 mg.	1/80 grain
		0.6 mg.	1/100 grain
		0.5 mg.	1/120 grain
		0.4 mg.	1/150 grain
		0.3 mg.	1/200 grain
		0.25 mg.	1/250 grain
		0.2 mg.	1/300 grain
		0.15 mg.	1/400 grain
		0.1 mg.	1/600 grain

NOTE: A cubic centimeter (cc.) is the approximate equivalent of a milliliter (ml.).

Source: "Blakiston's New Gould Medical Dictionary," 2d ed., McGraw-Hill Book Company, Inc., Blakiston Division, New York, 1956.

TABLE OF THE MORE COMMON LATIN OR GREEK TERMS AND ABBREVIATIONS USED IN PRESCRIPTION WRITING

Term or Abbreviation	Latin or Greek	Translation
a.c.	ante cibum	before meals
ad	ad	to, up to
ad lib.	ad libitum	at pleasure
alternis horis	alternis horis	every other hour
ante	ante	before
aq.	aqua	water
b.i.d.	bis in die, bis in dies	twice daily
bis	bis	twice
caps.	capsula	a capsule
d.t.d. No. iv	dentur tales doses No. iv	let 4 such doses be given
et	et	and
H.	hora	an hour
hor. som., H.S.	hora somni	at bedtime
in d.	in dies	from day to day, daily
m.	minimum	a minim
min.	minimum	a minim
no.	numero, numerus	number
noctis	noctis	of the night
non	non	not
non rep.	non repetatur	do not repeat
omn. hor.	omni hora	every hour
omni nocte	omni nocte	every night
p.c.	post cibos; post cibum	after eating; after food
p.r.n.	pro re nata	as occasion arises, occasionally
q.h.	quaque hora	each hour, every hour
q.i.d.	quater in die	4 times a day
q.s.	quantum sufficit; quantum sufficiat; quantum satis	a sufficient quantity; as much as is sufficient
sig.	signa; signetur	write (thou); let it be written; label (thou)
sine	sine	without
ss, $\overline{ss}$	semis	a half
tabel.	tabella (dim. of *tabula*, a table)	a lozenge
t.i.d.	ter in die	3 times a day

Source: "Blakiston's Illustrated Pocket Medical Dictionary," 2d ed., McGraw-Hill Book Company, Inc., Blakiston Division, New York, 1960.

TABLE OF THERMOMETRIC EQUIVALENTS*

Centigrade to Fahrenheit Scales

$$\tfrac{9}{5}\,\text{C.}^\circ + 32 = \text{F.}^\circ$$

C. °	F. °	C. °	F. °	C. °	F. °	C. °	F. °	C. °	F. °
−20	−4.0	21	69.8	61	141.8	101	213.8	141	285.8
−19	−2.2	22	71.6	62	143.6	102	215.6	142	287.6
−18	−0.4	23	73.4	63	145.4	103	217.4	143	289.4
−17	1.4	24	75.2	64	147.2	104	219.2	144	291.2
−16	3.2	25	77.	65	149.	105	221.	145	293.
−15	5.	26	78.8	66	150.8	106	222.8	146	294.8
−14	6.8	27	80.6	67	152.6	107	224.6	147	296.6
−13	8.6	28	82.4	68	154.4	108	226.4	148	298.4
−12	10.4	29	84.2	69	156.2	109	228.2	149	300.2
−11	12.2	30	86.	70	158.	110	230.	150	302.
−10	14.	31	87.8	71	159.8	111	231.8	151	303.8
− 9	15.8	32	89.6	72	161.6	112	233.6	152	305.6
− 8	17.6	33	91.4	73	163.4	113	235.4	153	307.4
− 7	19.4	34	93.2	74	165.2	114	237.2	154	309.2
− 6	21.2	35	95.	75	167.	115	239.	155	311.
− 5	23.	36	96.8	76	168.8	116	240.8	156	312.8
− 4	24.8	37	98.6	77	170.6	117	242.6	157	314.6
− 3	26.6	38	100.4	78	172.4	118	244.4	158	316.4
− 2	28.4	39	102.2	79	174.2	119	246.2	159	318.2
− 1	30.2	40	104.	80	176.	120	248.	160	320.
0	32.	41	105.8	81	177.8	121	249.8	161	321.8
1	33.8	42	107.6	82	179.6	122	251.6	162	323.6
2	35.6	43	109.4	83	181.4	123	253.4	163	325.4
3	37.4	44	111.2	84	183.2	124	255.2	164	327.2
4	39.2	45	113.	85	185.	125	257.	165	329.
5	41.	46	114.8	86	186.8	126	258.8	166	330.8
6	42.8	47	116.6	87	188.6	127	260.6	167	332.6
7	44.6	48	118.4	88	190.4	128	262.4	168	334.4
8	46.4	49	120.2	89	192.2	129	264.2	169	336.2
9	48.2	50	122.	90	194.	130	266.	170	338.
10	50.	51	123.8	91	195.8	131	267.8	171	339.8
11	51.8	52	125.6	92	197.6	132	269.6	172	341.6
12	53.6	53	127.4	93	199.4	133	271.4	173	343.4
13	55.4	54	129.2	94	201.2	134	273.2	174	345.2
14	57.2	55	131.	95	203.	135	275.	175	347.
15	59.	56	132.8	96	204.8	136	276.8	176	348.8
16	60.8	57	134.6	97	206.6	137	278.6	177	350.6
17	62.6	58	136.4	98	208.4	138	280.4	178	352.4
18	64.4	59	138.2	99	210.2	139	282.2	179	354.2
19	66.2	60	140.	100	212.	140	284.	180	356.
20	68.								

* Courtesy, *The Pharmacopeia of the United States of America.*

TABLE OF THERMOMETRIC EQUIVALENTS - (Continued)

Fahrenheit to Centigrade Scales

$$(F.° - 32) \times {}^5\!/_9 = C.°$$

F. °	C. °	F. °	C. °	F. °	C. °	F. °	C. °	F. °	C. °
0	−17.78	51	10.56	101	38.33	151	66.11	201	93.89
1	−17.22	52	11.11	102	38.89	152	66.67	202	94.44
2	−16.67	53	11.67	103	39.44	153	67.22	203	95.
3	−16.11	54	12.22	104	40.	154	67.78	204	95.56
4	−15.56	55	12.78	105	40.56	155	68.33	205	96.11
5	−15.	56	13.33	106	41.11	156	68.89	206	96.67
6	−14.44	57	13.89	107	41.67	157	69.44	207	97.22
7	−13.89	58	14.44	108	42.22	158	70.	208	97.78
8	−13.33	59	15.	109	42.78	159	70.56	209	98.33
9	−12.78	60	15.56	110	43.33	160	71.11	210	98.89
10	−12.22	61	16.11	111	43.89	161	71.67	211	99.44
11	−11.67	62	16.67	112	44.44	162	72.22	212	100.
12	−11.11	63	17.22	113	45.	163	72.78	213	100.56
13	−10.56	64	17.78	114	45.56	164	73.33	214	101.11
14	−10.	65	18.33	115	46.11	165	73.89	215	101.67
15	−9.44	66	18.89	116	46.67	166	74.44	216	102.22
16	−8.89	67	19.44	117	47.22	167	75.	217	102.78
17	−8.33	68	20.	118	47.78	168	75.56	218	103.33
18	−7.78	69	20.56	119	48.33	169	76.11	219	103.89
19	−7.22	70	21.11	120	48.89	170	76.67	220	104.44
20	−6.67	71	21.67	121	49.44	171	77.22	221	105.
21	−6.11	72	22.22	122	50.	172	77.78	222	105.56
22	−5.56	73	22.78	123	50.56	173	78.33	223	106.11
23	−5.	74	23.33	124	51.11	174	78.89	224	106.67
24	−4.44	75	23.89	125	51.67	175	79.44	225	107.22
25	−3.89	76	24.44	126	52.22	176	80.	226	107.78
26	−3.33	77	25.	127	52.78	177	80.56	227	108.33
27	−2.78	78	25.56	128	53.33	178	81.11	228	108.89
28	−2.22	79	26.11	129	53.89	179	81.67	229	109.44
29	−1.67	80	26.67	130	54.44	180	82.22	230	110.
30	−1.11	81	27.22	131	55.	181	82.78	231	110.56
31	−0.56	82	27.78	132	55.56	182	83.33	232	111.11
32	0.	83	28.33	133	56.11	183	83.89	233	111.67
33	0.56	84	28.89	134	56.67	184	84.44	234	112.22
34	1.11	85	29.44	135	57.22	185	85.	235	112.78
35	1.67	86	30.	136	57.78	186	85.56	236	113.33
36	2.22	87	30.56	137	58.33	187	86.11	237	113.89
37	2.78	88	31.11	138	58.89	188	86.67	238	114.44
38	3.33	89	31.67	139	59.44	189	87.22	239	115.
39	3.89	90	32.22	140	60.	190	87.78	240	115.56
40	4.44	91	32.78	141	60.56	191	88.33	241	116.11
41	5.	92	33.33	142	61.11	192	88.89	242	116.67
42	5.56	93	33.89	143	61.67	193	89.44	243	117.22
43	6.11	94	34.44	144	62.22	194	90.	244	117.78
44	6.67	95	35.	145	62.78	195	90.56	245	118.33
45	7.22	96	35.56	146	63.33	196	91.11	246	118.89
46	7.78	97	36.11	147	63.89	197	91.67	247	119.44
47	8.33	98	36.67	148	64.44	198	92.22	248	120.
48	8.89	99	37.22	149	65.	199	92.78	249	120.56
49	9.44	100	37.78	150	65.56	200	93.33	250	121.11
50	10.								

TABLE OF CERTAIN DISEASES

Disease	Age	Transmission	Incubation
Bacterial Meningitis	Any age, but younger more susceptible.	Direct or indirect contact with patient.	Variable.
Chickenpox	2 to 8 years.	Air-borne spread, contact with discharges from skin lesions or nose or throat of patient.	10 to 21 days. More commonly 14 to 16 days.
Diarrheal Diseases	Birth to 5 years most common.	Direct contact fecal contamination.	Variable. 2 to 4 days.
Diphtheria	1 to 14 years.	Direct contact with nose or throat discharges of carrier or patient.	1 to 6 days.
German Measles	2 to 15 years.	Air-borne spread, and direct contact with nose or throat discharges of patient.	10 to 28 days. More commonly 14 to 21 days.
Impetigo	Any age.	Contact with lesions or infected articles, especially found on face.	2-5 days.
Infectious Hepatitis	Any age.	Contact with patient, or contaminated water or food or fecal contamination.	Usually 3 to 4 weeks, but can be 2 to 7 weeks.
Infectious Mononucleosis	2 to 20 years.	Believed to be direct contact with nose and throat discharges of infected patient. Also air-borne spread.	Believed to be 2 to 6 weeks. Really unknown.
Influenza	Any age.	Air-borne spread possible. Direct or indirect contact with nose or throat discharges of patient.	1 to 2 days.
Measles	2 to 8 years.	Air-borne spread. Direct and indirect contact with nose and throat discharges of patient.	10 to 12 days usually, but 7 to 14 days possible.
Mumps	Usually 2 to 14 years.	Nose and throat discharges of patient.	Usually 16 to 20 days, but 12 to 28 days possible.
Poliomyelitis	Any age; more common among infants and children.	Focal contamination. Direct or indirect contact with nose and throat discharges of patient.	Usually 7 to 12 days, but 3 to 28 days possible.

Early Symptoms	Length of Illness	Length of Contagion	Permanent Aftereffects
Headache, irritability, fever, nausea, muscular rigidity.	Variable, usually 1 to 3 weeks.	Variable. Probably less than one day after beginning of treatment.	Brain damage is frequent. Death occurs in about 10% of the cases.
Characteristic eruption, with slight fever.	9 to 14 days.	One day before ill until skin lesions scab.	Rare.
Nausea, vomiting, fever, abdominal pain, prostration.	Variable. Usually 2 to 5 days, but sometimes longer.	Shortly before onset until 5 days after onset usually.	Variable.
Sore throat, running nose, mild fever.	Variable. Possibly several weeks.	Usually 3 days before to 10 days after onset.	Possible heart or nervous system damage. Up to 10% of the cases may die.
Rash, swelling of lymph glands, slight fever.	1 to 4 days.	One week before to disappearance of rash.	Rare. However, damage to fetus early in pregnancy if a pregnant woman contracts the disease.
Circular raised lesion, usually on face, becomes crusted.	Varies.	Until sores heal.	None.
Mild headache, chilliness, jaundice, fever.	Variable. 2 to 4 weeks.	Unknown.	Rarely. Death and chronic liver disease do occur.
Sore throat, fatigue, enlarged lymph nodes, fever, possibly rash.	1 week to several months. Highly variable.	Unknown.	Rare.
Muscular pain, dry cough, sudden fever, marked prostration.	3 to 10 days.	1 day before to 4 days after onset.	Very rare.
Cold, severe cough, gradually increasing fever, running nose, conjunctivitis.	6 to 12 days.	4 days before to end of rash.	Occasionally death or brain damage.
Fever, swelling of salivary glands.	4 to 10 days.	1 week before onset to end of swelling.	Very rarely there is brain damage.
Fever, sore throat, headache, nausea, vomiting, muscle pain, and weakness.	Highly variable. Some possibility of several months.	Usually 3 days before to 10 days after onset.	Death in 5% to 10% of paralytic cases. Some paralysis may be permanent.

TABLE OF CERTAIN DISEASES—(Continued)

Disease	Age	Transmission	Incubation
Roseola	6 months to 3 years.	Unknown, probably air-borne spread, or contact with nose and throat discharges of infected patient.	Unknown. Believed to be 10 to 15 days.
Scarlet Fever or Scarlatina	1 to 9 years.	Direct or indirect contact with a carrier or a patient.	1 to 5 days.
Smallpox	Any age.	Air-borne spread. Contact with throat or skin discharges of patient.	7 to 16 days.
"Strep Throat," (acute pharyngitis)	Any age.	Droplet infection, infected milk.	Varies.
Syphilis	Usually post-puberty.	Contact with lesion.	Usually 21 days.
Tetanus (lockjaw)	Any age.	Puncture wound.	4-21 days.
Vincent's Disease (Trench mouth)	Any age.	Direct contact and contaminated articles.	Undetermined.
Whooping Cough	Birth to 8 years.	Direct contact with discharges of nose or throat from a carrier or patient.	Usually 7 to 10 days, but 5 to 16 days possible.

Early Symptoms	Length of Illness	Length of Contagion	Permanent Aftereffects
High fever for 3 to 5 days. Rash appears after temperature returns to normal.	4 to 6 days.	Unknown.	Rare.
Vomiting, sore throat, fever, nausea.	4 to 10 days.	Highly variable. Usually 1 to 2 weeks, but can be several months.	Kidney disease. Rheumatic heart disease.
High fever, characteristic eruption, prostration.	1 to 7 weeks.	4 to 5 days before rash until scabs disappear.	Blindness, brain damage, pox scars. 1% to 40% cases may die.
Severe sore throat, high fever, general aches.	Varies.	Until antibiotics take effect.	Not dangerous unless complications occur, such as rheumatic fever.
Running sore is usually a primary sore.	Varies.	Until antibiotics take effect.	Varies, depending on when treatment is begun. Early treatment can leave no aftereffects.
Muscle spasms, first local, then general paralysis.	Varies.		Highly fatal.
Painful ulcers of gums and mouth tissues, sore throat, slight fever.	Varies, depending on care.	As long as disease is present.	None if properly cared for.
Cold, with a gradually increasing intermittent dry cough.	Usually 4 to 6 weeks, but 2 to 10 possible.	Variable. Usually first 2 weeks.	In infants death and brain damage.

Improving Your Speaking Ability

This appendix is a brief, practical résumé of the process of speech and how an individual can apply it. Should you desire to improve your speaking ability, study this short section and practice the exercises given.

Skillful Use of the Speech Mechanism

Whenever one speaks, the resulting sounds should be pleasing to the audience—whether that audience is one person or a hundred persons. Effective use of the body to produce pleasant speech is something that can be accomplished by anyone who wishes to do so. It is a matter of understanding how good voice control is accomplished and then working with exercises to produce the desired results.

If you need to improve your voice production (and most of us do), perhaps you can take a speech course at your nearby college or night school. If this is impossible, the following discussion, with exercises, will be of help to you.

Good Voice Production

Four sections of the body are involved in good voice production. Based on the work they perform in the speech process, they are referred to as the bellows, the vibrators, the resonators, and the articulators.

The bellows: Good speech begins with good breath control. Technically, good breath control is attained by diaphragmatic breathing. The diaphragm is a large muscle that divides the thorax (chest cavity) from the abdomen. When the lungs fill with air in diaphragmatic breathing, the diaphragm is pushed down, thus enlarging the thorax to make room for air.

The other method of breathing—frequently called upper chest breathing—enlarges the thorax by lifting the ribs and sternum. In upper chest breathing there is very little control over the airstream used in speech. The resulting voice is usually referred to as thin, high, weak, or ineffective. If it is necessary to speak for any length of time, the speaker's throat is aching and tired from the strain.

Diaphragmatic breathing produces a strong, steady stream of air, which in turn produces a good voice tone and leaves the throat relaxed and able to work for hours.

It is important to check on your own method of breathing and to discover diaphragmatic breathing for yourself.

It is important for you to use diaphragmatic breathing. If you will lie down, relax, and breathe naturally, you will soon discover that you are breathing

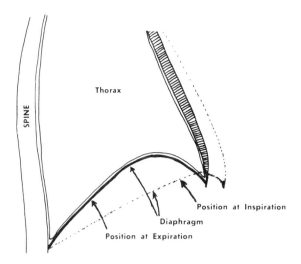

Figure A.1
Schematic drawing showing action of the diaphragm.

diaphragmatically. (The diaphragm area just below the ribs will be rising with each inhalation and falling with each exhalation.) Inhale, and as you exhale, laugh, *ha, ha, ha.* Continue to practice the *feel* of diaphragmatic breathing at intervals until you are using it for your speech. Nothing will make your voice more pleasing than a steady stream of air through a relaxed throat. This can be attained only through diaphragmatic breathing. Practice the following exercises to develop this method of breathing:

1. Work at inhaling and exhaling while standing and while sitting, until you can breathe diaphragmatically at will.
2. Put your hands on your diaphragm. Inhale slowly. Exhale and laugh, saying, *ha, ha, ha* through a complete exhalation. Notice the kick of the diaphragm.
3. Inhale and slowly exhale. Inhale. Say the letters of the alphabet until all the air has been exhaled. Repeat once or twice daily. You will gradually be able to increase the number of letters you can say during the length of one exhalation.
4. Try consciously to use diaphragmatic breathing whenever you speak.

The vibrators: The air coming from the lungs passes through the "voice box," or larynx. (See fig. A.2.) The larynx is located at the top of the trachea. Inside the larynx are two vocal chords, or bands. The air must pass between these two bands. When we speak, the bands tense; as the air escapes between them, the bands vibrate—producing sound which we then form into words with other parts of our speech mechanism.

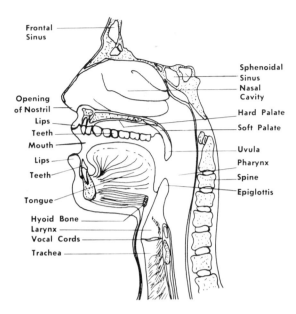

Figure A.2
Schematic drawing of head and neck.

To have a pleasing voice, only enough air should be sent through the larynx to vibrate the vocal bands. Too much air produces a breathy quality due to air escaping and practically hissing as it leaves the throat. Practice the following exercises:

1. Practice the third exercise given for diaphragmatic breathing, making sure that no air hisses as you recite the alphabet.
2. Inhale and exhale, slowly saying *a—e—i—o—u*. Be sure you are breathing correctly and that the tone is clear—not breathy.

The resonators: Once the air becomes "voiced" by causing the vocal bands to vibrate, it must be increased in volume—or resonated. Whistle softly into a bottle. The sound is increased many times by the walls of the bottle. This is a simple illustration of a resonator.

In speech, resonance is produced primarily by the cavity at the back of the throat, known as the pharynx, and by the mouth, the nasal passages, and the sinuses.

The articulators: The air that has been vibrated by the vocal bands and resonated by the resonators must be formed into words—or articulated. The articulators include the lips, teeth, tongue, hard palate, soft palate, uvula, pharyngeal walls, and jaws.

Careful use of the articulators results in beautiful diction. Most frequently the sounds in our language are produced automatically—with no thought about the placement of the tongue, lips, etc. If you will listen to yourself and place the articulators carefully when you speak, you will be amazed at the change in diction. Listen to yourself speak—in front of a mirror.

Do you say *doncha* or *don't you*? Can you hear the difference? Listen to your speech and eradicate as many of the slurs as you can. (Some examples are: *d'ya* for *do you*, *git* for *get*, *cuz* for *cause*, *jist* for *just*, *cancha* for *can't you*, and *wudja* for *would you*.) Also, try to eliminate the slang expressions you use. Check the dictionary for the correct pronunciation of words with which you are unfamiliar. Be sure that you know how to correctly pronounce simple words such as *Italian*.

To improve your diction, practice the following exercises daily, until you are conscious of how you use your articulators. Then a drill once a week should be sufficient to remind you of beautiful speech.

1. Open your jaws as wide as you can. Put the three middle fingers of your right hand between your teeth. The index finger should touch the upper teeth; the ring finger the lower teeth. If you cannot open your mouth this wide—and many people can't—exercise your jaws until you can. Open and close them several times, stretching them as far as possible. After several days of practice, some progress should be evident. Work until your mouth opens easily to a three-finger width.

   Clear speech depends, to a great extent, on a mouth that opens so that the articulated sounds can be released. The jaw must be relaxed and must move freely. Your lower jaw will feel as if you are exaggerating its use if you are speaking correctly and clearly.

2. Try to say as rapidly as possible all the tongue twisters you know. Here are a few examples:

She sells sea shells by the seashore.
Theophilus Thistle, the successful thistle sifter, thrust three thousand thistles through the thick of his thumb.
Peter Piper picked a peck of pickled peppers.
Rubber baby buggy bumpers.

These four sections of the body, then, *produce* the voice; but what kind of voice—pleasant or unpleasant, loud or soft, . . . or just right?

Four Characteristics of a Pleasing Voice

Let us think of the characteristics of a pleasing voice. It takes more than mechanics to make people enjoy hearing you speak. There are four characteristics of a pleasing voice: pitch, force, quality, and time.

The **pitch** of your voice is its relative highness or lowness. Your own pitch may be pleasing without effort.

If so, you are fortunate. Medium pitch is usually considered most pleasing. If someone who will tell you the truth says that your voice sounds high, perhaps you need to lower your pitch. Use a piano for accompaniment. Sing up and down the scales, finding the highest and lowest notes you can sing. The note midpoint between the high and low extremes is the normal pitch of your voice. If you have been speaking above that pitch, practice using the new note as your "home base." Practice these exercises:

1. Inhale; repeat *a-e-i-o-u* on your key pitch as you exhale.
2. If your new pitch is lower than your former speaking voice, get a copy of Alfred Tennyson's "Crossing of the Bar" or "Break, Break, Break" and read aloud, keeping your pitch low. It will help you express the meaning of the poems and allow practice in your new speaking range.
3. If you need to raise your pitch, use Lew Sarett's "Hollyhocks" and A. A. Milne's "The King's Breakfast."

With your new home-base pitch in mind, develop a wide range of pitch in speaking so that you do not speak in a monotone (on one note only). Practice reading selections you like—to be sure that you use a wide range of notes to make your voice interesting.

The **force** or **energy** with which you express yourself is another factor in attaining a pleasing voice. When you speak intensely, you are using much force. It may not be loud because a whisper can be intense. It depends on how hard and how suddenly you allow air to hit the vocal cords. For office work, force should not be applied, generally speaking. Keep the airstream well controlled without sudden bursts of vigor. You will sound relaxed and agreeable.

Most office speech occurs among two, three, or four persons and can be conducted quietly. Any intensity of tone tends to arouse emotion in listeners and may disturb some patients unpleasantly.

The normal **quality** of voice is largely determined by the resonators. It is important to use them correctly in pronouncing vowels in order to have full vocal quality. A round, open mouth when you say *ah* returns a beautiful sound. A partially closed mouth with a tense throat does not produce a quality enjoyed by your listener.

There are vocal qualities with technical names such as nasal quality, pectoral quality, oral quality, and orotund quality. While these are effective when portraying characters in a play, they have no place in a business office.

For improvement of vocal quality, exercise to relax, then exercise to add tone:

1. Drop the head to the chest, roll it to the right, and let it drop back; roll it to the left and let it drop forward. This makes a complete circle. Repeat several times.
2. Yawn to relax the throat and jaw. (Open your mouth wide enough, hold it, and you will yawn!)
3. Inhale, exhale, saying *mee-mee-ah*. Repeat until no air is left. Keep one tone for the exercise and listen to the quality. Make it as rich as you can. Repeat the exercise, using the vowels *o* as in *low, oo* as in *soon,* and *i* as in *high. Mee-mee-o, mee-mee-oo, mee-mee-i.*
4. Repeat the chorus of "John Brown's Body."

The final element is **time.** Our speech rate is determined by how long we hold sounds and by pauses between words or phrases. How cheerful you feel at the moment affects how rapidly or slowly you speak. Most of us tend to speak too rapidly. Speak reasonably slowly. Too fast a rate of speech causes poor diction and thus interferes with understanding. It also builds tensions in the listener who tends to feel hurried.

Practice reading aloud selections of poetry which have a slow pace, as "O, Captain! My Captain!" by Walt Whitman, and selections needing pauses for emphasis, such as Lew Sarett's "Wind in the Pines" and John Masefield's "Sea Fever."

Glossary

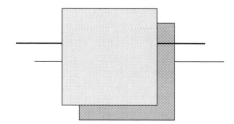

This glossary is not intended to be a technical dictionary. It is an attempt to explain commonly used words in language that can be understood by the beginner. This guide has been compiled as an aid to pronunciation without conforming to standard dictionary methods. The long sound of vowels is indicated by the symbol (¯) above the vowel. We suggest that after becoming familiar with the words in this section, the dental assistant consult *Boucher's Current Clinical Dental Terminology,* edited by Zweemer and published by the C. V. Mosby Company, St. Louis. In addition, it may be helpful to use *The American Illustrated Medical Dictionary* by W. A. Newman Dorland, published by Saunders Company, Philadelphia, or the *New Gould Medical Dictionary,* published by the Blakiston Company, Toronto and Philadelphia. These medical dictionaries give technical definitions of these words in language commonly used by dentists and physicians.

Not included in this glossary: the list of computer terms defined in chapter 17 and the list of insurance terms defined in chapter 18.

A special section of the glossary for the word elements included in chapters 3 through 30 will be found at the end of this word glossary. The word elements are alphabetized and defined.

A

abnormal (ab-nor′-mal) Markedly irregular. Deviating from the normal; not conforming with the general rule.

abrasion (uh-brā′-zhun) The wearing away of a tooth by mechanical means. Example: A person who chews tobacco markedly wears away his teeth over many years.

abscess (ab′-ses) Pus formation that is localized and limited in extent in any part of the body.

absorption (ab-sorp′-shun) 1. A substance passes into the interior of another by penetration or by solution. This process is called absorption. (Definition for Anesthesiology) 2. Skin, mucous surfaces, dental materials, etc., take up fluids or other substances. The process is called absorption. (Definition for Prosthodontology) 3. Radiation imparts energy to any material through which it passes by absorption. (Definition for Radiography)

abutment (a-but′-ment) Support. The natural tooth that is nearest the space left by a missing tooth when it has been crowned (or fitted with an inlay) and becomes one end of a bridge. An abutment is also a natural tooth to which the clasp of a partial denture is fitted.

accelerator (ak-sel′-er-a-ter) In dentistry it is a chemical that causes a reaction to happen faster than it would happen without the chemical.

account (uh-kount′) A formal record of the charges, payments, and balance of the patient whose name is at the top of the card or sheet.

acholic (ā kōl′-ik) Without bile.

aciculae (ā-sik′-ūl-ī) Needle-form crystals found in general-purpose artificial-stone preparations.

acrylic (uh-kril′-ik) One of a group of synthetic thermoplastic substances resembling clear glass but lighter in weight. It can be colored as desired. It is used in making both partial and full dentures and is colored pink to resemble natural gum color. It is also used for individual tooth restorations and colored the desired shade for the individual tooth. Methyl methacrylate resin is most commonly used in dentures at present.

acute (uh-kūt′) Severe, coming quickly to a crisis. It is therefore different from a chronic ailment that lasts over a long period of time.

adaptation (ad-ap-tā′-shun) Modification to fit the conditions of the environment.

adenopathy (ad-en-ahp′-uh-thē) Enlargement in size of glandular organs; any disease of a gland, especially a lymph gland.

adhesion (ad-hē′-zhun) Molecular binding.

aerobe (ay-ur-ōb′) A microorganism that must have oxygen to live.

aerobic (ay-ur-ō′-bik) Growing in free oxygen.

aesthetic (es-the′-tik) Appreciation of the beautiful in nature and art.

aesthetic dentistry Pleasing and beautiful dental operations aside from the purely practical function of replacement.

aesthetics The study of those components which make up beauty—color, form, etc. Applied to dentistry, it refers to the qualities involved in the appearance of a restoration—whether it is pleasing to the viewer.

aesthetic try-ins A trial fitting of artificial teeth to check appearance before final processing.

afebrile (ā-feb′-rīl) Without fever.

AIDS Acquired Immune Deficiency Syndrome.

alcohol (al′-kuh-hol) A transparent, colorless, volatile, mobile liquid that is most effectively used as a disinfectant at 70 percent strength. It can precipitate a protective coat around bacteria contained in blood, pus, and mucus, and should be used only after the instruments are thoroughly cleaned. Any residue of blood, etc., left on the instrument can cause infection on the next use even if alcohol has been used to disinfect it.

alkali (al′-kuh-lī) A strong, water-soluble chemical base, obtained from the ashes of plants. It is largely potassium or sodium carbonate. When in solution, it dissociates, forming hydroxyl (OH) ions. The term is used in Anesthesiology.

alkaline (al′-kuh-līn) Having the properties of an alkali, commonly having a pH of more than 7.

alkaloid (al′-kuh′loid) A bitter, alkaline, organic derivative of plants that is highly active physiologically.

synthetic alkaloid A synthetically prepared compound that has the chemical characteristics of alkaloids. (These terms are used in Oral Medicine and Pharmacology.)

allergy (al′-er-jē) A hypersensitive (exaggerated) reaction of the body to a substance that is harmless in most other persons. In the affected individual it produces asthma, hay fever and other respiratory disturbances, eczema, dermatitis, stomatitis, migraine headaches, edema, erythema, and other reactions. Some of the common allergies are allergies to dust, weeds, pollen, and certain foods and drugs.

alloy (a′-loi) Two or more metals are "fused" (melted together) to form a new metal called an "alloy." In dentistry the amalgam used for filling cavities is made of a silver alloy combined with mercury.

alveolar (al-vē′-ō-lar) Pertaining to the alveolus or the tooth socket.

alveolar process (al-vē′-ō-lar prah′-ses) *Process* in anatomy means an outgrowth or projecting part. The alveolar process is the part of the bone that projects from the maxilla (upper jaw) and mandible (lower jaw) and supports the roots of the teeth. It forms their sockets (alveoli).

alveolus (al-vē′-ō-lus) (pl., alveoli) The tooth socket in the alveolar process.

amalgam (uh-mal′-gam) A mixture of mercury with any other metal or metals.

dental amalgam A compound of mercury, silver, tin, and other metals for filling teeth. ADA Specification No. 1 for dental amalgam alloys requires the chemical composition to be within these limits: silver, 65 percent minimum; copper, 6 percent maximum; zinc, 2 percent maximum; and tin, 25 percent minimum.

ambidextrous (am-bih-dex′-trus) A person who performs manual skills with either hand equally well is said to be ambidextrous, whereas other persons are either right handed or left handed.

ameloblast (am-el'-ō-blast) A dental-enamel-forming cell. One of a group of cells from which the enamel on teeth is formed.

ammeter (am'-ēt-er) A contraction of the word *amperemeter*. It is an electrical device that measures the flow of electricity. An ammeter is used on dental X-ray machines to measure the current flowing through the X-ray tube. The higher the ammeter reading, the greater the amount of current flowing through the tube and the less time needed to record a satisfactory image on the film.

amorphous (uh-mor'-fus) Shapeless. A substance having no specific form in space. The molecules are distributed at random.

ampere (am'-peer) A unit of electrical current. It is the amount of electrical current produced by one volt acting through a resistance of one ohm. The measurement in dental X ray is usually in milliamperes, which is 1/1000 of one ampere.

ampul, ampule (am'-pūl) A small container, usually glass, that can be perfectly sealed (hermetically sealed). It is used to keep its contents sterile until needed. Local anesthetic comes in ampules in the dental office. Ampules are used for many types of hypodermic solutions.

anaerobe (an-ay'-ur-ōb) A microorganism that grows where there is no oxygen. If these microorganisms are exposed to air for any length of time, they are usually destroyed.

analgesic (an''-al-jēs'-ik) A mild remedy for relieving pain, such as aspirin, Anacin, Bufferin, ASA.

anaphylaxis (an''-uh-fuh-lak'-sus) A dangerous, violent reaction characterized by respiratory and circulatory failure or a sudden collapse or shock. It can occur following an injection. It is an allergic reaction following the injection of an allergen. A patient so reacting requires *immediate*, prompt treatment to prevent death.

anatomy (ah-nat'-ō-mē) The science that studies the way the parts of the body are formed and how the parts are related to each other. Anatomy applies to all plant and animal life, but we are interested in it only as it refers to human anatomy.

androgenic (an-drō-jen'-ik) Producing masculine characteristics.

anemia (uh-nē'-mē-uh) A decrease in the number of red blood cells or in the amount of hemoglobin they contain. Anemia is referred to as a quantitative or qualitative deficiency of the blood. The result is that the blood is unable to carry oxygen in sufficient amount for use by the body.

anesthesia (an''-es-thē'-sē-a) Loss of bodily feeling due to receiving an anesthetic or to disease. Thus, you do not feel pain when you are given an anesthetic.

anesthetic (an''-es-thet'-ik) A drug or gas that takes away the sense of feeling.

> **general** A drug or gas that produces unconsciousness (and, thus, the loss of feeling) either by inhalation or by injection.

> **local** A drug that, when injected into the tissues and absorbed into a nerve, will temporarily cause loss of feeling in the area supplied by that nerve. It is called local (to differentiate from general) because the area so anesthetized is only a part of the patient's body.

> **topical** A drug that is applied to the surface of tissues and produces the loss of feeling in that tissue area. It is used prior to the insertion of a hypodermic needle, preparatory to injection, to prevent pain.

angina (an-jī'-nuh) Derived from the Latin *angere*, which means "to strangle"; thus any disease accompanied by a spasmodic, choking pain or suffocation is called angina. There are other words added to differentiate the kind of angina, such as angina pectoris.

angiology (an-jē-ahl'-ō jē) Study of blood vessels.

animation (an-ih-mā'-shun) State of being alive.

anisocytosis (an''-ih-sō-sī-tō'-sis) Inequality in size of cells, especially red blood cells.

anneal (uh-nēl') To toughen, temper, or make glass or metal more lasting. This is accomplished by heating the metal or glass and slowly cooling it so that it is less brittle, relieving internal strain.

anode (an'-ōd) The target of the roentgen-ray tube. It is a tungsten block set at an angle of either 20 degrees or 45 degrees to the cathode.

The electronic stream from the cathode strikes the target; and since the anode is the positive terminal, it emits roentgen rays at this point, which are then directed through the opening in the tube head and are used for oral radiography.

anodontia (an''-ō-don'-shē-ah) Without teeth. Teeth may not have erupted. Teeth may be missing from lack of care or old age, or may never have formed.

anomaly (uh-nom'-uh-lē) Any noticeable change from the normal form, abnormal or irregular.

anoxia (an-oks'-ē-ah) An insufficient supply of oxygen in the body. The disturbance of bodily functions due to insufficient oxygen.

anterior (an-tē'-rē-or) Front or in the front or forward part of. Anterior teeth are the six front teeth in both the upper and lower arches.

anteroclusion (an-teer''-oh-klū'-zhun) Malocclusion of teeth in which the mandibular teeth are in front of their normal position.

anthropology (an-thrō-pahl'-ō-jē) Science that studies man and his origins.

antibiotic (an''-te-bī-ot'-ik) A medication made from certain microorganisms and given to a patient to prevent or fight an infection.

antibody (an'-ti-bah-dē) A specific substance produced by an animal as a reaction to the presence of an antigen (a toxin or enzyme). It reacts specifically with the antigen. It neutralizes the toxins, precipitates the antigen invaders, or gathers the bacteria cells into a mass.

antidote (an'-te-dōt) Medicine given to counteract a poison.

antigen (ant'-i-jen) A substance that, when introduced into an individual to which it is foreign, stimulates the formation of antibodies which react with it. It is usually a protein or carbohydrate (as a toxin or enzyme).

antipyretic (an-te-pi-ret'-ik) A medicine used to reduce a fever.

antiseptic (an-te-sep'-tik) A substance that is used to arrest the growth of disease germs (bacteria) or prevent putrefaction. It does not necessarily kill the bacteria.

anti-sialagogue, antisialogog (an-te-sī-al'-a-gog) A medication that reduces the flow of saliva.

apex (ā'-peks) (pl., apices) Tip. In dentistry it refers to the tip of the root of a tooth.

aphthous ulcer, aphtha stomatitis (af'-thoos-ul-sir) Commonly called the canker sore. An ulcer of unknown origin that appears on the mucous membrane, similar to herpes simplex lesion that appears on skin, but not of viral origin as is herpes lesion.

apical (ap'-i-kal) At or pertaining to the tip or apex.

apical foramen (ap'-i-kal for-ā'-men) The tiny opening of the pulp canal at the tip end of the root of the tooth. The vessels and nerves of the dental pulp pass through the apical foramen.

apoplexy (ap'-up-plek-sē) Sudden loss of consciousness, voluntary motion, and sensation caused by rupturing or obstruction of an artery of the brain. Commonly called a stroke. Also called a cerebrovascular accident.

apposition (ap-pō-zih'-shun) The placement or position of adjacent structures or parts so that they oppose each other and can come into contact.

arch, dental (*See* dental arch)

armamentarium (ar''-mah-men-tā'-rē-um) All the materials, equipment, books, journals, and supplies owned by a dentist and used for the practice of dentistry. (It also applies to a physician or hospital.) Also, the materials, equipment, supplies, etc., required to complete a specific operation.

aromatic (ar-ō-mat'-ik) Fragrant, spicy, smelling.

arteriosclerosis (ar-teer-ē-ō-skler-ō'-sis) Hardening of the arteries.

arthralgia (ar-thral'-jē-ah) Pain in a joint.

articulate (ar-tik'-ū-lāt) 1. To adjust the relationship of natural or artificial teeth so that they work properly for the mastication of food and for proper distribution of stresses. 2. To unite by means of a joint; e.g., bones of the skull articulate at sutures. 3. To form sound into words.

articulator (ar-tik'-ū-lā-tor) 1. An instrument that holds models or casts of a patient's dental arches in a given relative position while work is done on occlusion and articulation for either natural or artificial teeth. The patient's mandibular movements (lower jaw) may or may not be duplicated depending on the complexity of the articulator. 2. The articulators of the speech mechanism are the lips, teeth, jaw, tongue, soft palate, uvula, and pharyngeal wall.

artifact (ar'-te-fakt) An apparently diseased area visible in dental X ray that is caused by faulty manipulation of film developer or foreign matter.

artificial stone. (*See* stone, artificial.)

artificial teeth (ar-ti-fish'-al) A full or partial denture, or bridgework.

asepsis (ah-sep'-sis) Freedom from living germs of disease and decay (without decay).

aseptic (ah-sep'-tik) Surgically clean; free of all microorganisms.

asphyxia (as-fiks'-ē-ah) Suspension of breathing and animation because the body is deprived of oxygen, as in drowning or suffocation.

aspirate (as'-pi-rāt) To withdraw by suction.

aspiration (as-pir-ā'-shun) Using the aspirator or low-pressure evacuator to suck fluids and gases from the oral cavity (patient's mouth).

aspirator (as'-pir-ā-tor) A piece of equipment that has a hose and nozzle that the dental assistant holds at the patient's mouth during the preparation of a tooth. The aspirator is a vacuum, and all debris and water from the patient's mouth are sucked up by the aspirator nozzle and carried away.

aspirin (as'-pir-in) A mild pain-relieving drug; also reduces above-normal body temperature.

astringent (as-trin'-jent) A medication that tends to contract body tissue.

ataxia (uh-tax'-ē-uh) Failure of muscular coordination.

atom (at'-um) The smallest unit of an element that can exist either alone or in combination.

atrofe, atrophy (at'-rō-fē) The wasting away of tissue or parts through lack of use or disease.

attrition (ah-trish'-un) Normal wearing away by friction. In dentistry it refers to wearing down the surfaces of the teeth by mastication of food.

auricle (aw'-rih-kl) Part of ear not contained within the head.

autoclave (aw'-tō-clāv) A device for sterilizing instruments by steam under pressure.

autolysis (aw-tahl'-i-sis) Self-dissolution of a cell.

auxiliary personnel *See* personnel.

axial (ak'-sē-al) The axis of a tooth is an imaginary line passing through the center of the tooth the long way (from apex to occlusal or incisal surface). *Axial* refers to all lines, angles, and surfaces of a tooth that are parallel to this line.

B

bacillus (bah-sil'-us) (pl., bacilli) A group of bacteria that are shaped like rods and frequently appear in chains.

backing (bak'-ing) The metal back of a bridge or pontic to which the tooth or facing is attached.

bacteremia (bak-te-rē'-mē-ah) Bacteria in the blood.

bacterial plaque (bak-te'-rē-al) A filmlike covering on the teeth that is often very difficult to see in a well-kept mouth.

bacterial spore (bak-tē'-rē-al spor) The rough, resistant reproductive cell enabling some bacteria to remain alive under adverse conditions. A spore has a thick cell wall and the spore can remain dormant until conditions are favorable for bacteria to reproduce. This dormant stage of bacterial life is highly resistant to sterilizing procedures.

bactericide (bak-ter'-i-sīd) A substance (usually in liquid form) that kills bacteria.

bacteriostatic (bak-ter'-ē-ō-stat'-ik) Inhibits or arrests the growth of bacteria.

bacterium (bak-tē'-rē-um) Singular of bacteria. Any one of an important group of microscopic one-celled vegetable organisms, some of which are harmless, some of which produce disease. They were discovered by L. Pasteur, who found that they were responsible for producing disease. They are spherical, rod-shaped, or spiral. They live on organic matter, dead or alive.

band, orthodontic A thin strip of metal used to encircle the crown of a tooth closely. It wraps around the tooth horizontally. A band is used in orthodontic treatment to bodily move a tooth to its new position.

barbiturate (bar-bich'-a-rit) Any of the derivatives of barbituric acid. Its use is as a sedative.

base for filling A cement or other protective material placed over the pulpal area of the tooth to reduce thermal shock and irritation when a restoration is large.

bell-crowned (bel-krownd') A tooth whose dimensions as viewed from the facial or lingual aspect has a greater measurement at the incisal or occlusal than at the cervix.

benign (bē-nīn') Usually refers to a tumor that is not malignant and will not kill.

bicuspid (bī-kus'-pid) *Bi* means two, *cusp* means a prominent shape of a tooth; so a bicuspid is a tooth with two cusps, or rounded parts. A synonym is *premolar*. Man has eight bicuspids, two on each side of the upper and lower arches.

bifurcate (bī-fur'-kāt) Divided into two branches or forks.

bile (bīl') A viscid, alkaline fluid secreted by the liver that aids in the digestion and absorption of fats. It is yellow or greenish.

biology (bī-ahl'-uh-jē) The science of living matter in all its forms.

biopsy (bī-ahp'-sē) The removal of tissue from a living person and examination of this tissue by microscope for diagnosis. There are several methods of securing the tissue. When possible, part of a lesion and some of the normal tissue beside it are removed so that a comparison can be made.

bite fork Part of the mechanism used in facebow transfer.

bite rims A temporary wax shape to hold an initial setup of artificial teeth for checking.

bookkeeper One who maintains the business records of a dental practice or business firm.

boxing of an impression The process of enclosing an impression with wax, clay, or wet asbestos to shape the base of the cast while it hardens.

bridgework (brij-work) A missing tooth is replaced by a *bridge*.

Sometimes two or three teeth may be replaced by a bridge. The bridge consists of pontics (name of artificial tooth or teeth replacing the missing natural tooth or teeth) and the crowns or inlays that are cemented to the teeth on either side of the missing tooth or teeth. These crowns are called abutments. The entire bridge (pontics and abutment crowns) is a one-piece appliance, either cast as a whole unit or soldered together. It is "fixed" or cemented in place.

bruxism (bruk'-sizm) Grinding the teeth. Usually a person does this unconsciously in sleep or when under nervous strain.

buccal (buk'-al) *Bucca* is the Latin word for "cheek." Buccal in dentistry means the side of the tooth that is next to the cheek.

bur A cutting instrument used by the dentist in preparing a tooth for a restoration. Burs come in many shapes and sizes and of various materials.

C

cc Abbreviation for cubic centimeter.

CP Chemically pure; this abbreviation is used for chemicals that meet the U.S. Government standards for chemical purity.

calcarious deposit *See* calculus.

calcification (kal''-si-fi-kā'-shun) The deposit of calcium in the tissues of the body.

calcining (kal-sīn'-ing) Removing water by heat in the manufacture of artificial stone and plaster from gypsum.

calculus (kal'-kū-lus) The technical name for tartar. It is a hard calcium deposit on the tooth—usually near the gum line or where teeth overlap—places that are hard to brush clean. The dentist or dental hygienist removes this deposit with a scaler during prophylaxis.

canal (ka-nal') A narrow channel between two larger spaces (as Panama Canal). In dentistry it refers to tiny tubes or ducts such as the salivary ducts that permit the flow of saliva to the mouth from the salivary glands or the root canal of the tooth through which the nerves and blood supply pass.

cancer (kan'-ser) A malignant tumor. Malignant means capable of causing death.

canine (kā'-nīn) Preferred term for tooth with one cusp. Also called "cuspid."

canine eminence (kā'-nīn em'-ih-nens) A bony prominence on the anterior surfaces of the maxilla that overlies the root of the cuspid tooth, forming a noticeable bulge over the cuspid tooth on the upper jaw, just below and to the outside of the nose.

canker (kang'-ker) A shallow ulcer of the oral mucosa; characterized by a gray-yellow base and erythematous halo; the result of local minor trauma or the rupture of vesicles of apthous stomatitis.

capsule (kap'sūl) 1. A shell found around certain bacteria that protects the bacteria from destruction. 2. A tiny container of gelatin that holds medicine and may be swallowed.

Carborundum (kar-bō-run'-dum) An abrasive that is extremely hard (harder than emery). It is a registered trade name for silicon carbide.

Carborundum stones and wheels are used in dentistry to polish restorations and teeth. They mount in the handpiece, and the unit motor makes them spin as a bur spins.

carcinoma (kar''-si-nō'-mah) From the Greek *karkinoma,* which means "cancer." A malignant tumor. It originates in the epithelium.

cardiac (kar'-dē-ak) Refers to the heart. A patient with cardiac disease frequently requires special attention in the dental office.

cardiovascular (kar''-dē-ō-vas'-kū-lar) *Cardio* comes from the Greek, meaning "heart." Vascular comes from the Latin meaning "vessel." Thus, cardiovascular refers to the heart and blood systems; the carrying of the blood throughout the body.

caries (kār'-ēz) (dental caries) Decay. A disease process that attacks the hard tissues of the teeth, demineralizing and eventually destroying these hard tissues through loss of both organic and inorganic elements. Referred to as a localized, progressive, destruction and disintegration of enamel, dentin, and cementum.

> **interproximal caries** The interproximal surface of the tooth is that surface that touches another tooth. Thus, interproximal caries is decay found on the surfaces of the teeth that are in contact with other teeth.

carious (kār'-ē-us) Refers to caries or decay.

carotene (kār'-ō-tēn) An orange pigment that may be converted to vitamin A by digestive process within the body. It is found in leafy vegetables, carrots, and other vegetables. Our bodies need both carotene, which can be *converted* to vitamin A, and vitamin A, which does not have to be converted.

carpule (kar'-pūl) A glass cartridge containing local anesthetic ready for use.

carrier (care'-ē-er) One who harbors or carries a disease and transmits it to other people but does not necessarily have the disease. A typhoid "carrier" can infect anyone with whom he or she has contact, but that carrier does not have typhoid.

case history All the information your dentist is able to gather about a patient that will help in diagnosing and treating that patient. This information is strictly confidential.

cassette (kah-set') A holder for extraoral X-ray film or plates.

cast A positive reproduction made from an impression (or negative), usually of a dental arch.

casting Noun: A metallic object formed by using a wax replica, melting out the wax, and replacing it with molten metal that then hardens in the mold. Verb: The process of making the casting in the mold.

catalyst (kat'-ah-list) A chemical that accelerates a chemical reaction between two other chemicals but does not permanently combine with either of these chemicals and does not permanently change itself; provides a pathway that requires less energy for the chemical reaction to occur.

cathode (kath'-ōd) The negative terminal of the roentgen-ray tube. It is a spiral of tungsten wire that focuses the electron stream at the anode.

caustic (kaws'-tik) A chemical that eats away tissue. It is very irritating, and it can burn.

cauterize (kaw'-ter-īz) To destroy tissue by application of an agent, such as a caustic substance or electric current.

cavity (kav'-i-tē) The hollow space in a tooth made by dental caries.

incipient interproximal cavity Decay that is just beginning in the area where two teeth are in contact with each other.

cavity liner Material used to line the preparation in a tooth before the tooth is fitted or crowned or has an inlay placed, usually a varnish.

cement (se-ment') Any variety of substances that are used to lute inlays, crowns, bridges and acrylic fillings. It may also be used as a temporary filling. For example:

zinc phosphate cement (zink as'-id fos'-fāt se-ment') Used as a base under metallic fillings and for luting gold inlays and crowns.

zinc oxide-eugenol cement (zink ox'-īd ū-jen-ōl se-ment') When a tooth needs to be soothed, this "sedative" cement is used. It may be used as a temporary filling or as a base when sedation is required.

cementoblasts (sē-ment'-ō-blasts) One of the specialized osteoblasts that is involved in the production of cementum of the root of a tooth.

cementum (se-men'-tum) A thin, bonelike tissue covering the root of a tooth.

centigrade (sen'-ti-grād) Having 100 equal grades or gradients. The freezing point is 0 degrees and the boiling point is 100 degrees. To change centigrade to Fahrenheit: F = 9/5C + 32.

centimeter (sen'-ti-mē''-ter) The 100th part of a meter. It equals about 2/5 of an inch or 0.3937. The abbreviation is cm.

cubic centimeter (cc) 1/1000 part of a liter.

centric relation Objectionable as a noun. *See* occlusion, centric.

cephalalgia (sef''-ah-lahl'-jē-uh) Headache.

cephalometry (sef-ah-lōm'-eh-trē) Measurement of bone structure of the head by use of lateral and anteroposterior radiographs, which can be reproduced.

cervical (ser'-vi-kal) Pertaining to the neck or cervix.

cervical line The line at which the cementum meets the enamel on a tooth.

cervix (ser'-viks) Latin for *neck*. Neck of a tooth. The neck of the tooth is located where the root of the tooth and the crown of the tooth join.

cheilitis (kī-lī'-tis) Inflammation of the lip or lips.

cheilosis (kī-lō-sis) Fissuring at the corners of the mouth caused by vitamin B complex deficiency, drooling, decreased vertical measurements, or infection. The lips do not show inflammation but can be chapped.

chemotherapy (ke-mō-ther'-uh-pē) The use of chemicals to cure or arrest the process of diseases.

chondroseptum (kahn-drō-sep'-tum) The cartilaginous part of the nasal septum.

chronic (kron'-ik) Continuing for a long time and the opposite of acute; habitual. A chronic ailment is one that is not acute and is long established.

chronological (krahn-uh-lahg'-i-kal) An arrangement of events in the order in which they occur.

cingulum (sing'-gū-lum) The lingual prominence of enamel on the maxillary and mandibular anterior teeth, rising incisally from the cervical line.

circulation (sir-kyū-lā'-shun) Orderly movement through a circuit, as blood moving through the vessels.

cleft palate (kleft pal'-at) The dictionary defines cleft as a crack or split. The palate is the roof of the mouth. A cleft palate is one that has a crack or split in it because the two sides of the palate did not grow together along the midline of the roof of the mouth prior to birth. It may be a partial cleft with a small split only in the soft palate, or it may be a complete cleft and extend from the uvula through the soft and hard palates, the nose and upper lip. *See* oral pathology, chapter 25, for a nontechnical explanation.

coccus (kok'-us) (pl., cocci) A form of bacteria (see bacterium). Cocci are spherical in shape.

codeine (ko'-dēn) One of the stronger pain relievers. It is made from opium, hence is a narcotic and may only be prescribed by a dentist or physician holding a narcotic license.

colloid (kuh'-loid) A suspension of particles in a dispersion medium. The particles are somewhat larger than the molecules of material found in a solution. Dental example: hydrocolloid impression material.

colloidal (kuh-loi´-dal) Pertaining to colloid.

coma (kō´-ma) Prolonged loss of consciousness.

comminution (kom-in-ū´-shun) The act of breaking or crushing something into small pieces.

complication (kahm-plih-kā´-shun) A change (or twist) not always expected that makes a situation more difficult.

composite filling material A material composed of two distinct phases (plastic and filler) that are bonded together. The dispersed phase (or filler) complements the physical properties of the continuous phase (plastic) matrix material.

compound (kom´-pound) A material used in dentistry that can be shaped when warm. It is often used for preliminary impressions in prosthetics.

conductivity (kon-duk-tiv´-i-tē) Ability to convey or carry. In electricity or radiography, the ability to carry electric current.

conductor (kon-duk´-tor) Certain substances transmit electricity, heat, cold, or sound. That is, they pass the heat or electricity along. Copper is a good conductor of electricity so it is used as a wire to pass electricity from the power station to your light. Gold is a good conductor of heat and cold so crowned teeth may allow the person to notice more temperature change when masticating food.

condyle (kon´-dīl) A knoblike part on the end of a bone. In dentistry it refers to that part of the mandible that *articulates* with the rest of the skull.

congenital (kon-jen´-i-tal) Any condition that was present when the person was born is referred to as congenital.

connector (kuh-nek´-tor) There are several types of connectors used in dentistry. A connector is usually a device to unite two parts of a dental prosthesis.

consultation (kon-sul-tā´-shun) If two or more dentists, or a dentist and a physician, examine a patient and together decide on a diagnosis and treatment, it is called a consultation.

contact (kahn´-takt) The touching of two surfaces.

   c. area: Refers to the part of a tooth that touches the tooth next to it.

   c. point: Refers to the point of the proximate surface of a tooth that touches an adjacent tooth.

   occlusal or incisal c. The touching of the incisal or occlusal surfaces of opposing teeth.

contaminate (kon-tam´-i-nāt) To soil, dirty, or make impure by improper handling. Example: A sterile instrument is no longer sterile when you have touched it with your bare hands. It has been contaminated with microorganisms.

contour, height of (kon´-tour) A contour is an outline of a curve. The height of contour is the point where the curve has "bulged" the farthest.

contra-angle (kon´-trah-ang´-l) The dentist can use the contra-angle handpiece with burs, diamond stones, and discs at an angle to the shaft, thus enabling him or her to reach areas not readily accessible to the straight handpiece.

contraindication (kahn´´-trah-in´´-dih-kā´-shun) Any symptom or circumstance suggesting that a form of treatment is inadvisable although otherwise the treatment would be appropriate.

convulsion (kon-vul´-shun) An involuntary, irregular, intermittent, and variable muscular contraction, often accompanied by loss of consciousness.

coronal (kor-ō´-nal) Referring to the crown or visible portion of a tooth as seen in the mouth.

coronoid (kor´-ō-noid) The protuberance (swelling out) of the upper forward portion of the ramus of the mandible to which a large part of the temporal muscle is attached. (*See* anatomy.)

corrode (kuh-rōd´) A chemical or electrolytic action that wears away the surface of metal, such as rusting or tarnishing.

corrosion (kuh-rō´-zhun) A disintegration of a metallic surface by attack of electrolytic or chemical process.

craniofacial (krā-nē-ō-fā´-shul) Pertaining to the upper part of the head and the face.

crown (krown) The part of the tooth that is visible in the mouth, under normal circumstances. It is covered with enamel.

   anatomical crown (an-uh-tom´-i-kal) That portion of a tooth that is covered with enamel, whether visible or not.

   artificial crown (ar-ti-fish´-al) A dental substitute for the natural crown.

   clinical crown (klin´-i-kal) That portion of the tooth which is visible upon examination.

   full veneer crown A complete shell replacement of the outer portion of the natural crown.

   three-quarter crown A shell replacement, except for labial or buccal surface of the outer portion of the natural crown.

crucible (kroo´-si-bl) A container that withstands high heat. It is used for melting or holding material.

crucible former (sprue base) A stand into which a sprued pattern is placed. It controls the shape or form of the hollowed-out end of the investment in the casting ring, which receives molten metal through the sprue hole.

crystal (kris´-tal) A solid that is produced by nature. The final units of the substance from which it is formed are arranged systematically.

cubic centimeter (ku-bik sen´-ti-mē-ter) 1/1000 part of a liter. Abbreviation: cc. Used to measure liquids.

culture (kul´-chur) Propagation of microorganisms or living tissue cells in a special media.

   culture medium A liquid, semi-solid, or solid in which the microorganisms are grown.

   pure culture A bacterial colony that contains only one kind of bacteria.

cusp (kusp) A pointed or rounded part of a tooth, usually on the occlusal surface.

cuspid (kus´-pid) A tooth having one cusp (the canine tooth, the eye tooth, the stomach tooth).

cutaneous (kew-tā´-nē-us) Refers to the skin.

cyst (sist) A sac with a distinct epithelial wall containing fluid and at times other material such as hair, serum, or blood, or abnormally developed teeth, found in the body tissues.

cytology (sih-tahl′-ō-jē) Study of cells.

D

DDS Abbreviation for Doctor of Dental Surgery, the degree a dentist receives from a dental college.

DMD Abbreviation for Doctor of Dental Medicine, a degree granted by some dental colleges, similar to Doctor of Dental Surgery (DDS).

debris (de-brē′) Tissue fragments or foreign material found on the outer surface or within the root canal of a tooth.

decalcification (dē″-kal-si-fi-kā′-shun) The removal of calcium from the tooth surface by acid. Beginning of formation of cavity.

deciduous (dē-sid′-ū-us) That which is liable to shed, such as teeth.

   d. teeth: The twenty teeth of childhood that are normally replaced by permanent dentition; synonym: baby teeth.

delirium (di-lear′-ē-um) A state of mental excitement, usually including hallucinations, illusions, delusions, or confusion. The delirium is usually brought on by toxicity produced by disease or drugs.

density (den′si-tē) The ratio of mass to volume; such as the less air remaining in investment after mixing, the more solid is the finished material; its density has been increased.

dental arch The horseshoe-shaped curve made by the bony projection, gums, and teeth of either the upper or lower jaw.

dental hygienist *See* hygienist, dental.

dentifrice (den′-ti-fris) A cleanser used for brushing the teeth. It may be a powder or paste. It is usually flavored and may contain medicaments for specific purposes in mouth care. (For example, caries preventives, oxygenating agents, antiseptics, etc.)

dentin, dentine (den′-tin) Calcified hard tissue forming the main body of the tooth. The dentin has

innumerable tiny canals, many fibers that make the junction of the enamel with the dentin a very sensitive area. Dentin is slightly elastic, although not visibly so, and is very strong.

dentinocemental junction (den′-ti-nō-se-men′-tal) That junction of the inner surface of the cementum with the dentin.

dentition (den-ti′-shun) 1. The natural teeth in their normal position in the dental arches. 2. The process of eruption of the teeth through the alveolar ridge and gum.

   dentition, deciduous (*also* primary dentition) (dē-sid′ū-us) The twenty teeth of childhood that are normally replaced by permanent teeth (second dentition). Syn: deciduous teeth, primary teeth, milk teeth, baby teeth.

   dentition, mixed The teeth found in the dental arch after some of the permanent teeth have erupted but while some of the deciduous teeth are still present.

   dentition, permanent (Secondary dentition, permanent teeth) The teeth of adulthood that erupt as the primary teeth are shed and that replace or add to the dentition. (There are thirty-two teeth in a complete set.)

dentoenamel junction That junction of the inner surface of the enamel crown with the dentin. Syn: amelodentinal junction.

denture (den′-tūr) An entire set of teeth—either natural or artificial, deciduous or permanent.

   artificial denture Substitute for natural teeth.

   immediate denture Substitute for natural teeth inserted at time of extraction of remaining natural teeth.

   partial denture Substitute for part of natural dentition of either arch.

dermatitis (der-ma-tī′-tis) Inflammation of the skin.

dermatosis (der-ma-tō′-sis) (pl. dermatoses [sēz]) Any disease of the skin can be called dermatosis.

desquamation (des-kwam-ā′-shun) Shedding of the superficial epithelium as of the skin, mucous membranes, and renal tubules.

detergent (dē-ter′-gent) A surface cleanser.

diagnose (dī-ag-nōs) To recognize the nature of a disease, to make a diagnosis of.

diagnosis (dī″-ag-nō′-sis) 1. The art of determining one disease from another. 2. The conclusions arrived at.

diaphoretic (dī″-uh-for-ret′ik) A drug or medicine that increases perspiration.

diastema (dī″-uh-stē′-mah) A spacing between two adjacent teeth.

die An exact reproduction regardless of material used, of an original object. In dentistry it commonly refers to the reproduction of an individual tooth (die) on which a restoration may be constructed (such as a wax pattern).

diet (dī′-et) The food and drink consumed by a person. It is not the same as nutrition. Some of the diet may not be utilized by the body.

diplococcus (dip″-lō-kok′-us) Gram positive, elongated bacteria cells growing in pairs or short chains. They are usually parasitic.

direct technique *See* technique, direct.

discrete (dis-krēt′) Made up of separate parts.

disease (di-zēz) Illness or sickness; any state other than that of good health.

   acute disease Illness that appears suddenly and lasts a short time.

   chronic disease Illness that progresses slowly and continues over a long period of time.

disinfectant (dis″-in-fek′-tant) An agent, usually a chemical substance, that inhibits the microorganisms causing disease.

dislocation (dis-lō-kā′-shun) The displacement of any part of the body (especially bones) from the normal position. (Out of location.)

distal (dis′-tal) Away from the median line or center—thus, the distal side of a tooth is that which is away from the median line of the face or the back surface of a posterior tooth.

diuretic (dī″-ū-ret′-ik) An agent that increases the secretion of urine.

dorsal (dor′-suhl) Pertaining to the back or posterior part of an organ.

dram, drachm (dram) A unit of weight. It equals ⅛ part of an apothecaries' ounce, or 60 grains. Symbol 3.

drug Any chemical compound that may be used as an aid in the diagnosis, treatment, or prevention of diseases or pain.

duct (dukt) A passage with well-defined walls such as a tube for saliva to flow from the salivary gland to the mouth.

ductile (duk'-tal) Capable of being drawn out thinly into a wire, such as copper or gold.

dysfunction (dis-funk'-shun) Malfunction. Any impairment or abnormality of the normal working of a part of the body.

dysphagia (dis-fāj'-ē-uh) Difficulty in swallowing or inability to swallow.

dyspnea (disp'-nē-ah) Difficult or labored breathing.

dystrophy (dis'-trō-fē) Any condition arising from defective or faulty nutrition.

E

eccentric (eks-sen'-trik) Out of center or away from center.

ecchymosis (ek-i-mō'-sis) Bleeding into the tissues under the skin. The skin is discolored to purple, which gradually changes to brown, green, and yellow—such as a "black" eye or "black and blue" mark.

ectoderm (ek'-tō-derm) The outer layer of the skin.

edema (i-dē'-mah) When tissue fluid collects in a large amount in one place in the body there is a swelling known as edema.

edematous (i-dem'-ah-tus) Affected by edema.

edentulous (ē-den'-tū-lus) Without teeth.

elastic (ē-las'-tik) Adjective: Capable of being stretched and then returning to its original shape.

elastic (orthodontics) A rubber band used to apply force to teeth for orthodontic purposes.

elastic limit When any material is stretched beyond the point where it will return to its original shape, that point is known as the elastic limit.

elastic memory Capacity of a material to return to its original shape. The material is warmed, shaped, cooled, and then rewarmed.

Upon rewarming, it returns to its original shape.

electron (ē-lek'-tron) More frequently it is a unit of negatively charged electricity called a negatron. It is a necessary part of all atoms. It is sometimes a positively charged unit of electricity called a positron.

embolus (em'-buh-lus) A blood clot or other foreign matter that travels in a bloodstream, lodges in some blood vessel, and obstructs the flow of blood.

embrasure (em-brā'-zhur) The opening with sloping sides formed by the adjacent surfaces of teeth.

empyema (em''-pī-ē'-ma) The presence of pus in a cavity, space, or hollow organ.

emulsion (ē-mul'-zhun) Two liquids are mixed, but they will not blend. For example, oil and milk will not blend when poured in the same container. The oil remains in small particles.

emulsion, photographic A suspension of silver halide salts impregnated in gelatin and used to make radiographic film.

enamel (ē-nam'-l) The visible surface of the crown of a tooth is enamel, the hardest material in the body. The enamel forms a shell, covering the crown or coronal portion of the tooth. It varies in thickness, being heaviest on the chewing or biting surface of the tooth, and becoming thin toward that part of the crown which is farthest from the chewing or biting surface. The enamel consists of microscopic "rods." Calcium and phosphorus make up approximately 90 percent of the enamel. The rest is made up of other materials, plus a small amount of organic matter.

encephalic (en-seh-fal'-ik) Within the skull.

encyst (en-sist') Enclose in a cyst.

endocrine glands (en'-du-krin) Glands that secrete hormones directly into the bloodstream. The known endocrine glands are pituitary, adrenals, parathyroids, thyroid, pineal body, and gonads.

endodontics (en''-dō-don'-tiks) Branch of dentistry concerned with the prevention, diagnosis, and therapy of diseases and injuries of the dental pulp and pariapical tissue.

enzyme (en'zīm) An organic compound, a protein, that can by catalytic action promote a chemical change.

epidemiology (ehp-ih-dē-mē-ahl'-ō-jē) Science of epidemics and epidemic diseases involving the whole population, not just an individual.

epilepsy (ep'-ih-lep-sē) A chronic disease in which the patient has convulsive seizures with loss of consciousness; a seizure may last from five to twenty minutes.

epistaxis (ep-ih-staks'-is) Nosebleed; bleeding from the nose.

epithelium (ep''-ih-thē'-lē-um) The covering of the skin and mucous membranes.

epulis (ep-ū'-lis) Any benign neoplasm of the gingiva, usually pedunculated and raised.

erosion (ē-rō'-zhun) In dentistry, the destruction of surfaces, usually at the cervical area, beginning with the enamel and working inward. It is probably due to a combination of chemical action and abrasion. The cavities have dense and polished surfaces.

eruption (ē-rup'-shun) The process of a new tooth entering the mouth from its place of formation.

erythema (er-uh-thē'-ma) Abnormal redness of the skin. An acute inflammatory reaction seen in the skin and sometimes in mucous membranes.

esthetic (ez-thet'-ik) Pertaining to beauty or improvement of appearance.

ether (ē-ther) An inhalation anesthetic used for general anesthesia.

ethical (eth'-i-kal) In accordance with the rules governing the conduct of a specific group. Ethical conduct for dental assistants would mean observing the correct standards of conduct set for the profession. One example would be keeping as confidential all information learned about a patient.

ethics (eth'-iks) The science of right conduct.

etiology (ē-tē-ol'-ō-gē) The study or science related to the cause of any disease.

examination (eks-am-i-nā'-shun) In dentistry, a careful inspection to determine (or diagnose) the conditions that exist in a patient's mouth.

excision (ek-sih'-zhun) Removal by cutting.

exfoliation (eks-fo-le-a'-shun) Shedding. Thus, in dentistry, the shedding of a tooth.

exfoliation time Refers to the proper age at which the shedding of primary dentition should occur.

exodontia sponge A folded square of sterile gauze, usually two-by-two inches.

exodontics, exodontia (eks''-o-don'-tiks, eks''-o-don'-she-ah) The art and science of the removal of teeth.

exostosis (eks-os-to'-sis) Overgrowth of bone projecting outward from the usual surface; the most common are the tori, bony protuberances occurring along the midline of the hard palate in about 20 percent of the population (this protuberance is called a torus palatinus), and the bilateral or unilateral protuberances occurring on the lingual surface of the mandible in the premolar region in about 7 percent of the population (torus mandibularis).

expectorate (eks-pek'-to-rat) To spit.

expiration (eks'-pir-a-shun) The act of expelling air from the lungs.

expire (eks-pir) Cessation. A person is said to expire when he or she dies.

explorer (eks-plor'-er) An instrument with a sharp point, in various shapes, used to test the surface of the tooth for cavity formation.

extracoronal (eks''-trah-kor'-uh-nahl) Outside the body of the coronal portion of a tooth.

extrusion (eks-tru'-zhun) The projection of a tooth beyond the occlusal plane.

exudate (eks'-u'dat) Material, such as fluid, cells, or cellular debris, that has escaped from blood vessels and been deposited in tissues or on tissue surfaces; usually as a result of inflammation.

eye tooth The canine tooth of the upper arch.

F

facebow A mechanism used together with an articulator to construct dentures that will work together in the same relationship as do the patient's dental arches.

facial (fa'-shal) Referring to the face. Refers to those surfaces of the upper and lower teeth toward the lips and cheeks.

facial surface *See* surface.

facing (fa-sing) A piece of plastic or porcelain shaped to replace the outer surface of a tooth. It may be reinforced by gold and restores the full form and aesthetics of the natural tooth.

Fahrenheit scale (fah'-ren-hit) A method of scaling temperatures. The scale has 180 degrees between the freezing and boiling points of water. Freezing is 32 degrees and boiling 212 degrees. To change F to C: C = (F − 32) × 5/9.

faint *See* syncopé.

false teeth Correctly called dentures.

febrile (feb'-ril) Relating to fever or feverish. A synonym for fever.

fibroma (fi-bro'-mah) A benign neoplasm of fibrous connective tissue.

fibrosis (fi-bros'-is) The process of forming fibrous tissue.

file, numeric (fil', new-mare'-ik) A file using numbers for identification of the stored materials.

fissure (fish'-ur) A long, narrow fault in the surface of a tooth caused by imperfect joining of the enamel of different lobes.

fistula (fis'-tu-lah) An abnormal communication or canal between two areas of the body. In dentistry, it is usually an abnormal communication between a jaw abscess and the gum, or between the antrum and the mouth.

flora (flo'-ruh) Bacteria living in various parts of the digestive tract. Also plant life of a particular region or environment.

floss (dental) Nylon or silk cord, waxed or unwaxed used to clean between the teeth. Dental tape is the same as floss except that tape is wider and more ribbonlike.

flow Continuous movement. The change in shape of a material when placed under a given load, such as wax.

fluoridation (flur''-i-da'-shun) Adding fluorides to the water supply of any community to aid in control of dental caries. The recommended concentration is one part fluoride per million parts of water.

fluorosis (flur-o'-sus) When an individual consumes excessive fluorides in drinking water during the development of teeth, pitting occurs on the enamel surface, which is easily stained by foods. This pitting is called mottling of the enamel. This condition is called fluorosis.

follicle (fol'-li-kl) A small sac enclosing a developing tooth.

foramen (for-a'-men) A natural opening or passage, such as the foramen at the end of the roots of teeth where the nerves and blood vessels enter.

> **mental foramen** A foramen in the lower jaw for the mental nerve and vessels.

forceps (for'-seps) An instrument with two blades and two handles, like pliers, used to remove teeth.

fordyce's spots (for'-dis-es) Harmless, brownish, slightly raised spots on the oral mucosa or lips, found in more than 70 percent of the population. Erroneously called Fordyce's disease.

formation (for-ma'-shun) Process of giving shape or form.

fossa (fos'-sah) A round or angular depression, pit, or hollow on the surface of a tooth, usually in the lingual surfaces of the anterior teeth and in the occlusal surfaces of the bicuspids and molars.

fracture (frak'-chur) The breaking of a part, especially with reference to bone.

free gum margin That portion of the unattached gum encircling the neck of a tooth. Somewhat like a short cuff, usually not more than 1/16 inch in height. Also called free gingiva.

frenum (fre'-num) (pl., frena) A weblike fold of integument of mucous membrane that limits the movements of an organ or part. There are frenii inside the middle of each lip connecting the lips to the gum and one under the tongue connecting the tongue to the floor of the mouth, called the lingual frenum. Frena contain no muscle tissue.

fulcrum (ful'-krum) A point at which an action of balance or movement occurs. Therefore, the jaw pivot is a fulcrum.

fusion (fu'-zhun) The act of melting; uniting as by melting together.

G

gastrointestinal (gas'-tro-in-tes'-ti-nal) *Gastro* means "stomach," and thus gastrointestinal refers to both the stomach and the intestines.

germicidal Destructive to germs.

germicide An agent that destroys germs. Same as bactericide.

gingiva (jin'-ji-vah) (pl., gingivae) The part of the oral mucous membrane that is located nearest the neck of the tooth and covers the alveolar process; pale pink color when healthy; and when wiped dry, appears to be finely stippled, somewhat like a very fine sandpaper.

gingival crevice The space between the cervical enamel of a tooth and the free gum margin (or the overlying unattached gingiva). Also called subgingival space.

gingival line (jin'-ji-val) The line that marks the limit of the gingival crest around the tooth. It gradually moves from a position above the cervical line of the tooth crownwise toward the root of the tooth as age advances.

gingival papillae Projections of gum tissue that fill or nearly fill the interproximal spaces.

gingivitis Any inflammation of the gingiva (gum).

gingivitis, necrotizing ulcerative Also known as fusospirochetal gingivitis, trench mouth, ulcerative gingivitis, ulceromembranous gingivitis, Vincent's gingivitis, Vincent's infection. An inflammation of the gingivae characterized by death of the interdental papillae (the pointed area of the gum that rises between teeth), ulceration of the gingival margins, and in cases of more severe infection by the appearance of a false or pseudomembrane, the entire mouth painful and tender, with a foul odor.

gland An organ that manufactures and secretes a specific product—as salivary glands manufacture and secrete saliva or a sweat gland manufactures and secretes sweat.

glossitis (glos-ī'-tis) Inflammation of the tongue.

gold foil Gold foil is basically in the same physical form as you associate with aluminum foil except that it is the thinnest sheet of metal made, about 1/10 the thickness of the average human hair.

graduated (grad'-ū-āt-ed) Marked by a succession of degrees, lines, or steps, as a graduated measure.

gram A unit of weight in the metric system. One pound contains 454 grams. One kilogram is 1,000 grams.

granulation tissue (gran-ū-lā'-shun) New tissue found in the early stages of healing.

granuloma (gran-ū-lō'-mah) A dental granuloma may be found on the root of a tooth as a small mass of granulation tissue containing bacterial deposits.

groove A shallow, elongated depression in a tooth or bone. (Also called a sulcus.)

   developmental g A fine depressed line in the enamel of the tooth. When the tooth was developing, the lobes developed separately and joined when they had grown large enough. This fine line marks the union of the lobes of the crown.

H

hard palate An area forming the roof of the mouth that has a hard, bony support. It also forms the floor of the nasal passages.

harelip A split or cleft in the upper lip. An individual may have one or two. The cleft is congenital (present at birth).

hematoma (hē-mah-tō'-mah) A mass of blood in the tissue as a result of trauma or other factors, which cause the rupture of blood vessels (a tumor containing effused blood).

hemihydrate (hem-i-hī'-drāt) The chemical form of plaster or artificial stone before being mixed with water.

hemoglobin (hē'-muh-glō-bin) The oxygen-carrying red pigment of the red blood cells. It is an iron-containing protein.

hemorrhage (hem'-or-āj) In Greek: *blood* plus *to burst forth*. Bleeding.

hemostasis (hē-mo-stā'-sis) Stopping or arresting blood circulation.

hemostat (hē'-mo-stat) An instrument used to check hemorrhage. The instrument somewhat resembles a scissors, with flat serrated beaks, and can be locked in closed position over a cut or bleeding capillary, artery, or vein.

hemostatic agent Any drug used to arrest hemorrhage.

hepatitis, infectious (hep-uh-tī'-tus, in-fek'-shus) Hepatitis is inflammation of the liver. Infectious hepatitis is a viral hepatitis that can be epidemic, has an incubation period of seven through twenty-eight days, and even fifty days. It may be transmitted by human serum through transfusions and hypodermic injections. Autoclaving is the only safe method of sterilizing instruments to guard against transmitting this disease.

herpes simplex (her'-pēz sim-plex) An infection caused by the virus of the same name. When it occurs on the lips, it is a cold sore; when it occurs on the mucosa, it is called herpetic gingivostomatitis, which may become acute.

heterograft (het'-er-ō-graft) A graft of tissue taken from one species and used in a member of another species (vocabulary for Oral Surgery).

histology (hiss-tahl'-uh-gē) A branch of anatomy that studies the minute structure and composition of plant and animal tissues that are discernible with the microscope.

homogeneity (hō-mō-gi-nē'-i-tē) The quality or state of being uniform in structure or composition throughout.

homogeneous (hō-mō-jē'-nē-us) Greek: *Same kind.* Uniform, similar in makeup throughout.

hormone (hor'-mōn) A biochemical secretion of the endocrine glands that partially regulates the functional activity of organs, tissues, other glands, or the nervous system. The blood carries the hormones from the gland that produces them to the parts of the body that need them.

horn, pulpal A small projection of pulp tissue that lies directly under a cusp or lobe of a tooth.

hydrated (hī'-dra-ted) Combined with water, forming a hydrate or a hydroxide.

hydrocal (hī'-drō-kal) A trade name for artificial stone made from gypsum and used for making casts.

hydrocolloid A material used in dentistry for making an accurate impression (negative) for certain types of dental restorations such as partial dentures, inlays, crowns, bridgework. It is liquefied by heating to the temperature of boiling water and is solidified by cooling the tray that holds it while taking the impression (water-cooled trays).

hygiene (hī'-jēn) The science of health and how to preserve it.

hygienist, dental (hī-jen'-ist) A person trained and licensed by the state to practice dental prophylaxis under the direction of a licensed dentist.

hygroscopic (hī-gruh-skahp'-ik) Able to absorb moisture. Such a material has so strong an affinity for water that it absorbs moisture from the air to an unusual degree.

hyoid (hī-oyd) The U-shaped hyoid bone in the neck to which some muscles of mastication are attached.

hypercementosis (hī''-per-cē''-men-tō'-sis) An excessive formation of cementum usually at the apical portion of the root of a tooth, giving a bulbous appearance to the root tip.

hyperemia (hī-per-ē'-mē-uh) Excessive amount of blood in the vessels in any part of the body; congestion.

hyperplasia (hī-per-plā'-zhē-uh) An abnormal increase in the *number* of cells in normal arrangement in tissue. The tissue thickens or enlarges. One of the possible reactions of tissue to irritation, injury, or drugs; for example, continued long-term intake of Dilantin to control epileptic seizure may cause the formation of hyperplastic gingival tissue (Dilantin enlargement).

hypersecretion (hī-per-sē-krē'-shun) *Hyper* means "increase," thus increased secretion or excessive secretion. Excessive discharge of the liquid that the gland manufactures or stores.

hypersensitive (hī-per-sen'-si-tiv) Abnormally sensitive, i.e., more sensitive than average.

hypertrophy (hī''-per'-trō-fē) Greek: *overnutrition.* The abnormal increase in the *size* of the cells of a tissue, resulting in an enlargement or thickening of the tissue. True or physiologic hypertrophy results from excessive activity of muscle: for example, exercise makes a muscle larger.

hypnosis (hip-nō'-sis) The science of artificially induced sleep, or a trance induced by drugs, psychology, or both.

hypnotic (hip-not'-ik) 1. Inducing sleep. 2. Pertaining to hypnotism. 3. Sleep may be induced by certain drugs that produce normal sleep.

hypo- (hī'-pō) Beneath, under, insufficient.

hypodontia (hī''-pō-dahn'-tchē-uh) Fewer teeth than normal.

hypoplasia (hī-pō-plā'-zē-ah) Greek: *hypo* means "under" and *plasia* means "formation." Incomplete or defective development of any tissue. In dentistry, mostly associated with enamel hypoplasia: pits or ringlike grooves left in enamel due to interference with the function of the ameloblasts (enamel-forming cells) at the particular time this area was being formed. Hypoplasia is often associated with a highly infectious illness with high temperature. The age at which this occurred can be estimated quite accurately by the position of the defect.

hypothyroidism (hī-pō-thī'-roid-izm) Insufficient secretion from the thyroid gland. It lowers the basal metabolism rate, reduces growth, produces lethargy and a tendency to obesity. In children it may produce cretinism. Teeth may erupt late. In adults it may produce myxedema.

hysterical (hiss-tare'-ik-uhl) Lack of control over acts and emotions.

I

idiosyncrasy (id-ē-ō-sin'-krah-sē) A characteristic that is peculiar to an individual. An abnormal response to a drug, food, or cosmetic. This reaction may be quite violent.

immune (im-ūn') Latin: *safe.* Protected against a specific disease. It may be "natural" immunity or produced by vaccination or inoculation.

impaction (im-pak'-shun) Confinement of a tooth in the jaw so that its eruption is prevented. May be complete or partial.

impression (im-presh'-un) A metal band for a single tooth, or a tray full of "impression material" is placed over the teeth and ridges of either dental arch and allowed to "set." The hollows and grooves so formed (a negative) are called an impression or mold, and this may be filled with a stone mixture to form a cast, or positive.

impulse (im'-puls) An uncontrollable wave of excitation transmitted through tissues, especially nerve fibers and muscles following a stimulus. The result is physiological activity or inhibition of an activity.

incisal (in-sī'-zal) Cutting.

incisal edge The cutting edge of an anterior tooth formed where the labial and lingual enamel plates join. Synonym: cutting edge.

incisal papilla or palatine papilla The hump in the median line behind the two central incisors forming the front part of the hard palate that forms a pad protecting the anterior palatine foramen.

incisor A tooth with an incisal (cutting) edge. Man has four incisors in each dental arch. They are "anterior" teeth.

inclination (in-kli-nā'-shun) Tilting. To say, "A tooth is mesially inclined," means it is tilted to the mesial.

indirect (in-duh-rekt') Not direct (as in "indirect inlay impression").

infection (in-fek'-shun) Invasion of tissues by pathogenic microorganisms followed by a typical reaction in the area of invasion.

inferior (in-fē'-rē-or) Below or lower.

infiltration (in-fil-trā'-shun) To pass through or into by filtering or permeating. To permeate by penetrating.

inflammation (in-fluh-mā'-shun) The cellular and vascular response to any injury; characterized by pain, redness, swelling, heat, and disturbance of function, may be acute or chronic.

infraorbital (in-frah-or'-bih-tuhl) Below the eye.

injection (in-jek'shun) Introducing (forcing) liquid into tissue.

inlay (in'-lay) A filling made outside the mouth in the shape of the preparation cut in the tooth. When it has been finished, it is cemented into the tooth.

inspect (in-spekt') To look at critically, as the dentist inspects the oral cavity critically to aid in diagnosis.

insulator (in-sah-lā'-tor) Any material that will prevent the transfer of heat, electricity, or sound. In dentistry, cements may be used as insulators against extreme changes in temperature.

interdental space The space between two neighboring approximating teeth.

intermaxillary (in-tur-macks'-ihl-ary) Situated between the upper and lower jaws.

internal Within or inside.

interproximal space (in-ter-proks'-i''-mul) Situated between the proximal surfaces of adjoining teeth of the same arch. Same as interdental space.

intramuscular (in-trah-mus'-kū-lar) Latin: *within muscle.* Inside the substance of a muscle.

intrapulpal (in-trah-pulp'-uhl) Within the pulp.

intravenous (in-trah-vay'-nus) Into the vein, in the vein, or from within the vein.

introvert (in'-trō-vert) To turn inward or in on itself.

investing The process of placing investment material; of covering or enveloping an object to be cast, cured, or soldered.

investment 1. Material enclosing the wax pattern for crowns, inlays, and dentures while they are being cast or processed. 2. Material enclosing parts to be soldered. It is usually some form of plaster.

ion (ī'-on) An atom that carries a positive or negative electrical charge because it has lost or gained one or more electrons.

ionization (ī''-un-ī-zā'-shun) This refers to the process of being ionized.

ionize (ī'-un-īz) To convert partly or wholly into ions.

J

juxtaposition (juhx''-tuh-po-zih'-shun) Placed side by side.

K

kilovolt (kil'-uh-volt) A thousand volts. Refers to the quality of penetration of the X-radiation.

L

labial (lā'-bē-al) Pertaining to the lips.

labial commissure The thin connecting fold at the corners of the lips. It is quite tender. Protect during dental operations with a very light coating of vaseline to prevent soreness.

labial surface The surface of an anterior tooth which is next to the lips.

labiomental groove (lā-bē-ō-men'-tal) A groove running parallel to the lower lip and slightly below it.

laboratory stone *See* artificial stone.

lactobacillus (lak-tō-buh-sil'-us) Bacteria that forms lactic acid.

lancet (lan'-set) A small, two-edged, pointed surgical knife.

laryngitis (lair-in-jī'-tuhs) Inflammation of the larynx.

laryngoscope (lair-ing'-gō-skōp) An instrument to examine the larynx.

lateral (lat'-er-uhl) To the side.

lesion (lē-zhun) Latin: *to hurt.* Any change in continuity of a tissue due to disease or injury, or the loss of function of a part.

leukemia (lū-kē'-mē-ah) Greek: *white blood.* A fatal disease of the blood-forming organs, showing as a severe increase in the number of white blood cells and an increase in size or activity of the blood-forming organs.

leukocyte (lew'-kō-sīt) White blood cells.

leukocytosis (lew-kō-sī-tō'-sis) An increase in the leukocytes in the blood: may be defensive reaction of the body as inflammation or may be due to abnormal blood cell formation as in leukemia.

leukoplakia (lō-ko-plā'-kē-uh) A white, opaque, leathery plaque formed on the oral mucous membrane; considered premalignant; resembles lichen planus in appearance; differentiated by biopsy.

levorotation (lē-vō-rō-tā'-shun) Turning to the left.

lichen planus (lī'-ken plan-us) A disease of unknown etiology affecting either skin or oral mucous membranes, sometimes both together. The oral lesion appears on the buccal mucous membrane most commonly, a lacy pattern of raised bluish-white or white porcelain-like fine lines or dots. Painless and harmless. Distinguished from leukoplakia by biopsy (the removal of a small tissue sample from the suspect area for the purpose of microscopic examination).

ligature (lig'-uh-chur) A cord, thread, or wire used to tie off or bind. One type is used to hold rubber dam in place. Another type is used in an orthodontic appliance.

ligature wire (ortho) Steel filaments of several diameters are used to bind teeth together. The size of the filament is determined by the orthodontist for the particular work he or she wishes to accomplish. The purpose of binding the teeth together is to stabilize and immobilize or to produce minor movements.

linear (lin'-ē-er) Straight, or involving a single dimension. Thus a straight line is linear.

lingual (lin'-gual) Refers to the tongue.

lingual frenum A weblike fold of mucosa from the under surface of the tongue to the floor of the mouth near the lower front teeth, along the midline, restricting extension of the tongue.

lingual surface The surface of any tooth that is next to the tongue. All teeth have a lingual surface.

lipidema (lip-ih-dē'-mah) An excess of liquid and fat in the subcutaneous tissue.

liter (lē'-tur) A measure that equals 1.0567 quarts.

lithotomy (lith-aht'-ō-mē) Incision of a duct or organ.

lobe (lōb) A somewhat rounded projection or division of an organ of the body or a gland.

local Restricted to one spot or area. Not general.

local anesthetic *See* anesthetic.

M

malaise (ma-lāz') This is the French word for *illness.* Any indisposition, discomfort, or distress.

malar (mā'-lar) Referring to the cheek or cheek bone.

malignant (mah-lig'-nant) A term used to describe a neoplasm in the human body that will kill the human. Most people use the term as "a malignant tumor"—meaning a cancer that must be completely removed if the individual is to continue living.

malleable (mal'-ē-ah-bl) Latin: *to hammer.* Susceptible to being beaten or hammered out into a thin plate or sheet. Gold is extremely malleable.

malocclusion (mal''-ō-klū'-shun) *Mal* in Latin means "ill." Poor positioning of the teeth so that they interfere with best efficiency during mastication. Malocclusion can usually be corrected by correcting the articulation of the teeth through orthodontic procedures.

malpractice Latin: *bad* plus *practice.* Unskillful or faulty medical or dental treatment.

mamelon, mammelon (mam'-e-lon) One of the three rounded prominences on the incisal edge of a newly erupted incisor.

mandible The horseshoe-shaped bone forming the lower jaw. It provides support for lower teeth and provides places for attachment of various muscles that make it possible to chew. Also called the inferior maxilla.

mandrel A shaft that holds a tool for rotation.

margin The bounding line or border of a surface of a tooth or a cavity.

marginal ridge An elevation of enamel known as the margin of a surface of a tooth.

masticate Chew.

mastication The act of chewing food.

materia alba Soft white matter often found on the necks of teeth when not properly cleansed.

materia medica Latin: *medical material.* A branch of medical study dealing with the sources, uses, and preparation of drugs.

matrix (mā′-tricks) In *biomaterials:* the matrix refers to the continuous phase of the material that holds, and in amalgam, silicate, or composites, bonds to the dispersed phase (unreacted particles or filler). In *restorative dentistry:* a matrix is an instrument or device used to replace the missing walls of the cavity, provide form and contour, and retain the restorative material as it is being placed and allowed to harden in the cavity.

maturation (mach-uh-rā′-shun) The time or point at which something is fully developed—or fully grown.

maxilla One of a pair of bones forming the upper jaw (superior maxilla).

median (mē′-dē-an) In the middle—dividing into two equal halves.

median line An imaginary line dividing the body into right and left halves.

medication (med-i-kā′-shun) A drug or substance used to treat a disease. Also, the process of medicating.

medicine 1. Any drug or substance used to treat or prevent disease. 2. The art of healing.

medicine, oral The specialty in dentistry that concerns itself with the significance and relationship of oral and systemic diseases.

melanoglossia (mel-an-ō-glahs′-ē-uh) Black tongue.

mental Latin: *mind* and *chin.* 1. Refers to the chin. 2. Refers to the mind.

mental foramen (men-tal for-rā′-men) *See* foramen.

mercury (mer′-kur-ē) (quicksilver) A liquid metallic element. It is combined with silver alloy to make silver amalgam for filling teeth.

mesial (mē′-zē-al) Greek: *middle.* Toward the median line following the curve of the dental arch.

mesial surface Surface of the tooth following the dental arch nearest the median line.

metabolism (me-tab′-ō-lizm) Greek: *change.* The process by which the body changes food into material which can be used by the body to rebuild tissue or to provide energy.

metal An elementary crystalline substance that is opaque, fusible, malleable, ductile, and is capable of conducting electricity and heat. It is characterized by a lustrous surface on fracture.

metastasis (meh-tas′-tuh-sis) The transfer of disease from one organ or one place in the body to another organ or another place by diseased cells or pathogenic organisms via the blood or lymph streams.

method, indirect The formation of a wax pattern by taking an impression in the patient's mouth and working up the wax pattern *outside* the mouth (indirect) as opposed to direct method when the pattern is made in the mouth on the patient's tooth.

microorganisms (mı-kro-or′-ga-nizms) Tiny (or minute) living organisms, including bacteria, viruses, rickettsiae, yeasts, algae, and fungi. They may be part of the normal flora without producing disease, but they may also overgrow and produce disease. It is possible that organisms that are foreign to the individual may produce disease.

microscope (mī-kro-skōp) An instrument through which objects too small to be seen with the naked eye can be viewed.

microscopic (mī-krō-skop′-ik) Something so small that it can be seen only by assisting normal vision with magnifying lenses. Very tiny in size.

milleroentgen (mil-ē-rahnt′-gen) One one-thousandth of a roentgen.

milliammeter (mil-ē-am′-i-ter) A meter that indicates the milliamperes flowing in an X-ray tube.

milliampere (mil-ē-am′-per) One one-thousandth of an ampere. In X ray it is used to indicate the amount of current flowing in the X-ray circuit. When combined with seconds (time measurement), it is an indication of the quantity of roentgen ray.

mineral (min′-er-al) A substance not derived from plant or animal life, usually a solid.

model (mah′-del) A positive reproduction of any part of a tooth or dental arch made by filling an impression with a molding material. *See* cast and impression.

molar (mō′-lar) One of the grinding teeth found in the back of the mouth. They have three or more cusps. There are twelve molars in the upper and lower dental arches—first, second, and third molars in each quadrant. The first molar refers to the six-year molar. The second molar is the twelve-year molar. The third molar is the wisdom tooth. The terms first, second, and third molar are preferred terminology.

mold guide A group of porcelain or plastic teeth supplied by a manufacturer of artificial teeth. There is a tooth in each size and shape variation made by that firm. The dentist (and his patient) can select the correct tooth size and shape for the appliance or replacements to be made.

molecule (mahl′-i-kyul) The smallest part of an element or compound that is capable of keeping its chemical identity with the substance in mass.

morphology (mor-fol′-ō-jē) The science that deals with structure and form of organic beings in all their variations and in all stages. (*See* microbiology.)

mottled enamel. Due to excessive intake of fluoride during tooth development. *See* fluorosis.

mucin (mū′-sin) From mucous membranes originate various proteins that are called mucin.

mucobuccal fold The space or troughlike area between the gums and cheek. The little trough between the gingivae and the inner surface of the cheek.

mucocele (mū'-kō-sēl) A dilated gland or duct filled with mucous secretion.

mucosa (mū-kō'-sah) The mucous membrane.

mucous gland Glands occurring in all mucous membrane.

mucous membrane Pink to red tissue lining the mouth and other areas. It contains many tiny glands that secrete mucus, a viscid, watery secretion.

mucus (mū'-kus) A viscid, watery secretion that covers all mucous membranes.

myofunction (my-oh-funk'-shun) Normal muscle function.

myology (my-ahl'-ō-jē) Study of muscles.

N

narcotic (nar-kot'-ik) A drug that relieves pain while it tends to produce stupor or sleep at the same time, depending on the dosage.

nasal Refers to the nose.

nausea (naw'-sē-ah) Latin: *seasickness.* Sickness at the stomach, together with a tendency to vomit.

necrosis (nē-krō'-sis) Greek: *deadness of a certain portion of tissue,* not the entire body. Pulpal necrosis is death of the pulp of the tooth.

necrotic (nē-krot'-ik) Referring to (or affected with) necrosis.

neoplasm (ne'-ō-plasm) Greek: *new formation.* Any abnormal new growth, such as a tumor.

nephritis (neh-frī'-tus) Inflammation of the kidney.

neuralgia (ner-al'-jē-uh) Pain that extends along a nerve.

neuritis (nur-ī'-tis) Inflammation of a nerve.

neurotropism (ner-ō-trōp'-izm) 1. Having a special affinity for nerve fibers. 2. A tendency of nerve fibers to grow towards certain portions of the periphery.

nevus (nē'-vus) A congenital malformation seen occasionally on the oral mucosa; can be vascular (similar to a birthmark) or nonvascular with pigmentation. Some types can develop into malignancies.

nitrogen (nī-trō-gen) An odorless, tasteless, colorless gaseous element that constitutes 78 percent of the atmosphere by volume. It is a constituent of all living tissues.

nitrous oxide (nī-trus ox'-īd) A colorless gas (N_2O) with a sweet taste and pleasant odor. It is used for minor surgery. It produces unconsciousness by temporary asphyxiation. It is also called laughing gas.

nomenclature (nō'-men-klā-tur) Latin: *name* plus *to call.* Terminology. A system of names in a particular science, art, or field of knowledge.

normal flora *See* flora.

notation (nō-tā'-shun) A system of designating teeth by figures, letters, and/or signs. (*See* notating teeth for the various systems of notation.)

O

obesity (ō-bē'-sih-tē) Overweight.

occlude (ok-lūd') To fit close together. To shut.

occlusal (ok-lū'-sal) Refers to closing or shutting the masticating surfaces of the teeth (the occlusal surfaces).

occlusal surface The masticating surface of a premolar or molar tooth. This surface is in contact with the opposing dental arch when the jaws are closed.

occlusion The contact of the teeth of both jaws when closed or during the movements of the mandible in mastication.

   balanced occlusion An ideal relationship of the teeth in both dental arches to each other during all the movements of the mandible as well as in centric closure.

   centric occlusion Contact relationships of the teeth when the jaws are closed in normal position (subject to various interpretations).

   malocclusion Any variation from the so-called normal relationships of the teeth (see malocclusion).

   traumatic occlusion Malocclusion of the teeth that results in injury to the teeth, or the tissue either surrounding or underlying the teeth.

odontalgia (ō-don-tal'-jē-ah) Greek: *tooth* plus *pain.* Toothache.

odontectomy (oh-dont-ek'-tō-mē) Removal of a tooth.

odontoblast (ō-don'-tō-blast) Greek: *tooth* plus *germ.* A dentin-forming cell. Specialized connective tissue cells that develop the dentin and maintain its nutrition and translucency.

odontoma (ō-don-tō'-mah) Greek: *tooth* plus *tumor.* A tumor that is toothlike in structure. Some form at the time the tooth is developing. Some attack the tooth later. There are several types, each attacking a different part of the tooth.

odontophobia (oh-dont''-oh-fō'-bē-ah) An abnormal or morbid dread of dental operations.

odontotomy, prophylactic (oh-don-tōt'-ō-mē, prō-fi-lak'-tik) Cutting into a tooth for preventive treatment.

opaque (ō-pāk') That which blocks light. Light rays cannot penetrate.

   radiopaque That which blocks X ray (*See* radiolucent).

operation An act performed with the hands or instruments. In the dental office it usually refers to surgical procedures.

operatory A room in which dental treatment is performed.

ophthalmology (ahf-thal-mahl'ō-jē) Branch of medicine dealing with the eye: anatomy, physiology, and pathology.

opisthognathism (ō-pis-thō-nath'-izm) Receding jaws.

optimum (op'-ti-mum) The most favorable conditions for any activity or function.

oral Refers to the mouth.

oral cavity The space that is enclosed by the lips in front, the cheeks on either side, the palate above, and the floor of the mouth below. Restricted sense: space enclosed by the teeth, when closed together, with the palate above, and the floor of the mouth below.

oral hygiene The science of health and its preservation, as related to the mouth.

oral medicine *See* medicine, oral.

oral pathology The study of diseases of the mouth.

oral surgery Surgery of the mouth (a special field of surgery or dentistry).

oral vestibule *See* mucobuccal fold.

organism (or'-gan-izm) An individual constituted to live by means of organs which are separate in function but mutually dependent.

orolingual (or-ō-ling'-gwal) Pertaining to the mouth and tongue.

orthodontics (or''-thō-don'-tiks) That branch of dentistry which deals with the causes, prevention, and treatment of the irregularities or malocclusion of the teeth and arches.

osmosis (ah-smō'-sis) When two solutions are separated by a membrane, the solvents from the lesser pass to the greater concentration. This movement of the solvent is called osmosis.

osteoblasts (os'-tē-ō-blasts) Greek: *bone* plus *germ*. Bone-forming cells. Any cell active in producing bone or any cell that develops into bone.

osteoclast (os'-tē-ō-klast) Greek: *bone* plus *break*. A large, multinuclei which absorbs and destroys bone.

osteology (ahs-tē-ahl'-uh-gē) The scientific study of bones and their structures.

otogenous (ō-toj'-eh-nus) Originating within the ear.

otology (ah-tahl'-ō-jē) Branch of medicine specializing in the ear, its anatomy, physiology, pathology, and treatment.

oxidation (oxs-i-dā'-shun) The act of oxidizing or combining with oxygen.

oxidizing agent Anything that produces oxidation (such as the excess of oxygen in the flame of a blowtorch applied to casting gold).

oxygen A colorless, odorless, gaseous element that combines readily with most elements. It is necessary to all animal and vegetable life and for combustion. It makes up 20 percent by weight of the atmosphere and about 88 percent of water.

P

palatal (pal'-ah-tal) Refers to the roof of the mouth.

palate (pal'-at) Roof of the mouth.

   hard palate The front and larger portion of the roof of the mouth is hard because it is formed by a bony arch.

   soft palate That smaller portion toward the throat from which the uvula is suspended.

palatine (pal'-uh-tīn) Refers to the palate.

palliative treatment (pal'-ē-ā-tiv) Giving relief, but not curing a disease.

pallor Paleness, lack of color.

pantomography (pan-tō-mahg'-rah-fē) An X ray of all the dental arches accomplished on one film.

papilloma (pap-il-ō'-mah) An epithelial tumor, mushroomlike or fingerlike in appearance, found in other epithelial tissue: example, a wart is a papilloma.

paradental (pair-uh-den'-tuhl) Beside the teeth.

paralgesia (pair-ahl-jē'-zē-uh) Any condition marked by abnormal pain.

paralysis (pah-rahl'-uh-sis) Loss or impairment of motor function.

paraplegia (pair''-uh-pla'-jē''-uh) Paralysis of the legs and lower part of the body.

parotid gland (pah-rot'-id) Greek: *near* plus *ear*. A gland in front and below the ear that produces saliva, entering the mouth through Stenson's duct in the cheek just across from the first or second molar of the upper arch.

parulis (pah-roo'-lis) Technical name for a gum boil.

pathogenic (path-ō-jen'-ik) Greek: *disease* plus *to produce*. Capable of causing disease.

pathology (pah-thol'-ō-jē) Greek: *disease* plus *discourse*. That science that studies the nature of disease, its causes, effects, and the changes produced by disease.

pediatrics (pēd-ē-at'-riks) Medical specialty that treats only children.

pedodontics (pē''-dō-don'-tiks) Greek: *child* plus *tooth*. That branch of dentistry which studies and cares for children's dental needs (Syn. pedodontia).

perforate (per'-fuh-rāt) Latin: *through* plus *to bore*. To puncture, bore, or pierce through.

periapical (per-ē-ā'-pi-kal) Surrounding the root or apex of the tooth.

pericoronitis (per''-ē-ko-ron-ī'-tis) Inflammation (*itis*) of the gingiva around the crown of a tooth, especially a newly erupting tooth.

periodontal (per''-ē-ō-don'-tal) Greek: *around* plus *tooth*. Around the tooth, especially refers to the periodontal membrane.

periodontal membrane The fibrous and connective tissue running from the cementum to the tooth socket, supporting the tooth in its socket.

periodontics Specialty of dentistry that deals with the treatment and prevention of diseases of the soft tissue and bone surrounding the teeth.

periodontitis (per-ē-ō-don-tī'-tis) Inflammation of the tissues that surround and support the teeth—the gingivae, the cementum of the tooth, the periodontal membrane, and the alveolar and supporting bone.

periodontosis (diffuse alveolar atrophy) (per-ē-ō-don-tō'-sis) A noninflammatory condition affecting the tissues listed under periodontitis, in which the fibers of the periodontal membranes degenerate, alveolar bone is resorbed, and the epithelial attachment is proliferated along the root surfaces. The end result of the process is the loosening and moving of teeth.

periosteum (per''-ē-os'-tē-um) Greek: *around* plus *bone*. Dental periosteum is another name for the periodontal membrane. It is also tough membrane around bones and adhering to their surfaces.

peripheral (per-if'-er-al) Situated near the periphery (external boundary of a surface or area).

permanent Lasting; intended to last indefinitely.

personnel, auxiliary The dental office staff hired by the dentist to assist with the production of dentistry. It includes dental assistants, dental hygienists, dental laboratory technicians, and any other classification the dentist deems essential in assistant personnel.

pH The concentration of hydrogen ions expressed as the negative logarithm of base 10. It is used in expressing both acidity and alkalinity on a scale whose values run from 0–14 with 7 representing neutrality, acid below 7 and alkalinity above 7.

phagocyte (fag'-ō-sīt) A cell that engulfs or devours microorganisms, cells, debris, and other substances.

phagocytosis (fag-ō-si-tō'-sis) The engulfing and destruction of microorganisms, cells, or other substances by a cell called a phagocyte.

pharmacology (fahr-mah-kol'-ō-jē) Greek: *medicine* plus *discourse*. The science of drugs, their uses and actions.

pharyngitis (fair-in-jī'-tis) Inflammation of the pharynx.

phonetics (fō-net'-iks) The study of the production and understanding of speech sounds including variations by individuals and groups. Phonetics also includes the classification of the sounds produced.

photography (fō-tah'-grah'-fē) Making images on sensitized material by exposing the material to light or other radiation source.

physician (fi-zish'-un) A person holding the degree of doctor of medicine (MD), legally qualified to practice medicine.

physiological (fi-zē-ō-loj'-i-kal) Refers to normal functions of an organism.

pit A small, sharp depression in the enamel surface of the tooth.

plaster A roasted (calcined) calcium sulfate powder that is mixed with water to make casts and impressions for dental use.

plastic (plas'-tik) Greek: *to mold*. Material that can be shaped or molded.

plasticizer (plas'-ti-sī''-zer) One of several substances added to a plastic material to give a soft, viscous property to the finished product.

pleomorphic (plē-ō-mor'-fik) More than one distinct form occurs in the life cycle of a plant.

pleurisy (ploo'-rih-sē) Inflammation of the pleura with exudation into the cavity and on its surface.

plexus (pleks'-us) An interwoven combination of parts of a structure, thus, a network of nerves, veins, or lymphatics.

pneumatic (new-mat'-ik) Pertaining to air or gases in general; operated by air pressure.

pontic (pon'-tik) That part of a bridge or partial which replaces a missing tooth. Patients often refer to the pontic as the "false tooth."

posterior (pos-tē'-rē-or) Situated behind; to the back.

premature (prē-ma-tūr') Latin: *before* plus *ripe*. Something that occurs too soon or before the proper time.

premolar (prē'-mō-lar) preferred term for bicuspid tooth.

prescribe (prē-skrīb') To designate or indicate the directions for giving or using remedy or treatment.

prescription (prē-skrip'-shun) The written directions for the preparation and use of a drug, treatment, or remedy.

primary tooth *Primary* means first in order of time or any series, thus primary teeth means first teeth—those which are first seen in the child's mouth and are later replaced with permanent dentition. Synonyms: Deciduous dentition, baby tooth.

procedure (prō-sē'-dure) The manner of proceeding, a certain course of action.

process (pros'-es) A projecting part of bone.

> **alveolar process** A ridge in which the sockets of the teeth are found.

profession (prō-fesh'-un) A vocation for which specific study is necessary, usually requiring examination and licensing by the state in which the person wishes to practice the profession. (Examples: law, teaching, dentistry, medicine.)

professional Appropriate to a profession; in keeping with ethics.

prognosis (prahg-nō'-sis) A forecast as to the probable result of a disease or condition. Thus, in dentistry, an opinion about the probable success of a restoration.

proliferation (prō-lif''-er-ā'-shun) Latin: *offspring* plus *to bear*. To grow by reproduction or multiplication, referring especially to cells.

prophylactic (prō-fi-lak'-tik) A remedy that helps prevention of a disease.

prophylaxis (prō-fi-lax'-is) 1. The prevention of disease. 2. A procedure for removing substances from the surfaces of the teeth. Scaling and polishing techniques are used. The purpose of this procedure is the prevention of disease of the oral cavity.

prosthesis (pros'-thē-sis) Replacement of a natural part of the body with an artificial substitute.

> **dental prosthesis** Any replacement for natural dentition, as a bridge, denture, partial denture, etc.

prosthetic (pros-thet'-ik) Refers to prostheses.

prosthodontics (pros-thō-don'-tiks) The branch of dentistry concerned with making replacements for missing teeth.

protoplasm (prō-to-plazm) Greek: *first* plus *form*. A mixture of complex chemical compounds, mostly proteins and water, in a cell. The living matter of all vegetable and animal cells.

proximal (prok'-si-mal) Latin: *next*. Nearest to the chosen point or place.

> **interproximal** The area between two adjacent teeth; bounded by the contact point above and extending gingivally between the two curving surfaces.

> **proximal surface** One of the surfaces of a tooth, either mesial or distal, that is next to an adjacent tooth.

psychology (sī-kahl'-uh-gē) The science that studies the mental processes and the behavior of the individual. Modern psychology studies all the interactions between living organisms and their environment.

psychopathic (sī-kō-path'-ik) A mental illness creating antisocial behavior.

ptyalin (tī'-al-in) Greek: *spittle*. An enzyme found in the saliva of man and some of the lower animals that changes starch into dextrin, maltose, and glucose.

pulp The soft tissue found in the root canal and chamber of a tooth. It contains arteries, veins, lymphatic and nerve tissue—all of which connect to the rest of the body and supply the tooth its means of sensation and nutrition.

pulp canal The part of the pulp cavity found within the root or roots of the teeth.

pulp chamber That portion of the central cavity of the tooth which lies within the crown of the tooth. It has canals that form a passageway for blood vessels and nerve fibers to the tip of the root, the apex, and thence to the circulatory and nerve structures of the rest of the body.

pulpectomy (pulp-ehk-toe-mē) An operation in which all of the pulp is removed from a tooth.

pulpitis (pulp-ī'-tis) Inflammation of the dental pulp. Toothache.

pulpless tooth A tooth from which the pulp has been removed. A devitalized tooth.

pulpotomy (pulp-ot'-ō-mē) An operation in which part of the pulp is removed from a tooth.

pulse (puhls) Rhythmical beating; for example, that caused by the heart action which is felt in the expansion of the arteries. May be felt in various locations in the body.

pumice (pum'-is) Spongy volcanic lava used in powdered form to clean and polish teeth and other dental materials such as dentures.

pus A liquid made up of white blood cells (leukocytes) and a thin fluid called liquor puris. It is the product of inflammation.

pyogenic (pī-ō-jen'-ik) Refers to the production of pus.

pyorrhea (pī-or-rē'-uh) Term designating periodontal disease, means flow of pus.

pyrexia (pī-reks'-ē-uh) Fever: elevation of the body temperature.

pyrotoxin (pī-rō-toks'-in) A poison produced during a fever.

R

radiant energy The energy that travels as a wave motion; specifically, the energy of electromagnetic waves is called radiant energy. The waves are called roentgen rays.

radiation (rā-dē-ā'-shun) The processes of emission, transmission, and absorption of radiant energy combined.

radiation necrosis (rā-dē-ā'-shun ni-krō'-sis) Death of tissue caused by radiation. If treatment of carcinoma (cancer) of the throat, mouth, or lip is undertaken by means of X rays or cobalt, heavy destruction of bone and teeth with formation of a sequestrum (piece of dead bone, usually being expelled from the body) is generally one result. The destruction is apparently more easily controlled when teeth, if present in the area of treatment, are removed prior to exposure if possible.

radioactivity Some elements are capable of spontaneously emitting alpha, beta, or gamma rays by disintegration of the nuclei of atoms. This ability is called radioactivity.

radiodontics (rā''-dē-ō-don'-tiks) The specialty in dentistry that devotes itself to making and interpreting radiographs (X rays) of teeth and mouth.

radiograph (rā'-dē-ō-graf) X ray or roentgenogram.

radiography (rā-dē-ah'-graf-ē) Photography with X rays or roentgen rays.

radiology (rā-dē-ol'-uh-gē) A name for the branch of medical science that uses radiant energy in diagnosis and treatment. (Radiographs are made for diagnosis of conditions. Radioactive substances and roentgen rays are used to treat certain diseases.)

radiolucent (rā-dē-ō-lū'-sent) That which permits X rays to pass through, yet has some resistance to their passage.

radiopaque (rā-dē-ō-pāk') Highly resistant to penetration by X ray oentgen   ray); the image of radiopaque material appears within the range of gray to white—very light in color.

ramus (rā-mus) Latin: *a branch*. In dentistry, especially that part of the lower jaw which articulates with the skull.

record (rek'-ord) Usually a written recounting of facts to be kept for future reference. The record may include X rays and study models as well as written history.

rehabilitation (rē-hab-il-i-tā'-shun) Restoring a person to useful activity who has been physically or emotionally injured.

> **oral rehabilitation** The restoration of the mouth to normal in all respects through dental work.

repel (rē-pel') To drive or force away.

resection (rē-sek'-shun) Removal of a considerable part of an organ: for example, a tooth or one of the roots of a tooth.

residual cyst (rē-zid'-ū-l sist) An odontogenic cyst that remains within the jaw after the tooth with which it was associated has been removed.

residual ridge (rē-zid'-ū-l) Means *remainder*. The portion of the alveolar ridge that remains after the alveoli (sockets for the teeth) have disappeared from the alveolar process (the bone that surrounds and supports the teeth) following extraction of teeth.

resorption (rē-sorp'-shun) Latin: *to suck up*. The removal or loss of tissue by absorption. The gradual disappearance of the root of a primary tooth is due to resorption.

restoration (res-tō-rā'-shun) A general term often used to designate the filling, crown, bridge, partial, or full denture used to restore part or all of the dentition to normal function.

rest position A position of the lower jaw, usually with the teeth slightly apart, though the lips remain closed.

resuscitate (rē-sus'-i-tāt) To restore to life or consciousness an individual who is apparently dead or unable to breathe.

retainer (rē-tān'-er) An appliance designed to stabilize teeth after orthodontic treatment.

retarders (re-tard'-ers) *Retard:* to hold back, to slow down. A chemical is added to a substance to slow the chemical reaction. It prolongs the setting time of the material and provides more working time.

retraction (rē-trak'-shun) A shrinking of tissues, also a laying back of tissues to reveal or expose a given part.

retromolar (reht'-trō-mōl-er) Behind the molars.

rhinoanemometer (rī-nō-an-ē-mom'-uh-ter) An apparatus for measuring the air passing through the nose during respiration.

rickets (rik'-its) A disease found in children and infants caused by vitamin D deficiency. It causes defective ossification of bone because the body is unable to properly utilize calcium and phosphorus without adequate vitamin D intake.

ridge 1. Remainder of alveolar process (bone surrounding and supporting teeth) after teeth are removed. 2. A long elevation or crest of enamel on the surface of a tooth.

> **cervical r.** (serv'-ih-kl) Any prominent ridge of enamel immediately adjacent to the cervical line.

risk management 1. Minimizing the risk of cross contamination by wearing protective eye wear, masks, and gloves. 2. Adhering to practices that eliminate or lessen the possibility of professional liability claims.

roentgen (rent'-gen) The international unit of quantity or dose of roentgen (or X) ray and gamma rays. It shall be called the "roentgen" and be designated by the symbol *r*.

roentgenogram (rent-gen'-ō-gram) A photograph made with roentgen rays or more technically, a shadow image of radiopaque anatomic structures that are recorded on film sensitized to roentgen rays.

roentgenology (rent-gen-ahl'-uh-gē) The study and use of roentgen ray in diagnostic and therapeutic areas in medicine and dentistry.

root That portion of the dentin that lies beyond the enamel-covered coronal part of each tooth. It is covered with cementum.

root canal A passageway for nerves and blood vessels to the pulp chamber of the tooth.

rouge An iron oxide in cake or stick form used for polishing gold on a muslin wheel. (Jeweler's rouge.)

rubber dam A thin sheet of very lively rubber that the dentist perforates in such a manner as to fit over a tooth or group of teeth preventing saliva from wetting that portion of the tooth exposed through the rubber.

rupture (ruhp'tcher) A tearing apart, a breaking.

S

saccharide (sak'-uh-rīd) A simple sugar, carbohydrate.

sacrodynia (sā-krō-dī'-ne-uh) Pain in the sacro region of the back.

saddle That part of a partial denture which distributes the stresses of mastication over the ridge area, usually carrying the replacement teeth, where natural teeth have been removed.

sagittal (saj'-ih-tuhl) Refers to the midplane of the body. (See illustration in chapter 20.)

saliva (sah-lī'-vuh) A clear liquid secreted by the salivary glands into the oral cavity through various ducts; aids in the digestion of foods; contains ptyalin. Salivary glands are the sublingual, submaxillary, and parotid.

sanguine (sang'-gwen) Abounding in blood, ardent, hopeful.

sanitary (san'-ih-tare-ē) Relating to health, hygienic; relating to keeping something clean.

sarcoma (sar-kō'-mah) A malignant neoplasm found in bone, striated muscle, cartilage, or connective tissue.

sclerosis (skler-oh'-sis) Hardening, thickening, or increased density of tissue.

secretion (se-krē'-shun) 1. The process of separating and releasing some material, 2. The material that is released. Thus, saliva is the secretion secreted by the salivary glands.

sedative (sed'-uh-tiv) A remedy that reduces activity or excitement.

senility (seh-nil'-i-tē) The physical and mental infirmity of old age.

sensitive (sen'-sih-tiv) Able to feel; capable of sending or receiving a feeling or sensation.

sensitivity (sehn-sih-tiv'-ih-tē) A state of responsiveness to things felt, as heat.

sepsis (sep'-sus) A disease condition found in the mouth or adjacent areas that may affect the general health of the individual as well as the parts of the body adjacent to the diseased area because sepsis disseminates toxins. Sepsis may also be found in other areas of the body, but we are concerned with the term as it applies to dentistry.

septicemia (sep''-ti-cē'-mē-ah) Greek: *putrid* plus *blood*. A disease condition caused by the presence of microorganisms and their poisons in the blood.

septum (sep'-tum) A dividing wall or membrane. Interdental: the alveolar process (bone surrounding the teeth) extending between the roots of the teeth. Nasal: The membrane dividing the left and right nostrils.

sequence (sē'-kwenc) Order of performance.

shade guide A group of teeth furnished by a manufacturer of artificial teeth or filling material showing each color in which the product is manufactured. The dentist and patient are able to select the shades most suited to the patient's mouth for any artificial teeth or filling to be used.

shock A condition brought about by physical or emotional injury, consisting mainly of circulatory disturbances. Shock can lead to death if not successfully treated in time. An individual suffering from shock is pale, skin is clammy, pulse weak and rapid.

shoulder A term used in reference to a definite ledge or step in a dental preparation in the tooth structure.

sialadentitis (sī-al-uh-den-tī-tus) Inflammation of a salivary gland.

sialogogue (sī-ahl'-uh''-gohg) An agent that promotes the flow of saliva.

sialolith (sī-ahl'-ō-lith) A salivary stone.

sialolithiasis (sī''-ah-lō-lih-thī'-uh-sis) The formation of salivary calculi within the ducts of the salivary glands or the condition or infection caused by such formation.

sialorrhea (sī-ahl-or-rē'-uh) Excessive flow of saliva.

solder (sod'-er) An alloy that is used to join together other metal surfaces, requiring heat in its application.

soldering (sod'-er-ing) (ortho) The process of joining two pieces of metal by using an alloy that melts at a lower temperature than the metals to be joined. The alloy is melted and dripped on the joint, then allowed to harden.

solubility (sahl-ū-bil'-i-tē) Possible to dissolve.

solute (sahl-yūt') The dissolved member of a solution (usually the less abundant part). Thus, in sugary syrup, the sugar is the solute—it has been dissolved in the water.

solution (sō-lū'-shun) A liquid consisting of a mixture of two or more substances dispersed through one another uniformly.

solvent (sol'-vent) A chemical used to dissolve other substances.

spasm (spa'-zm) A sudden, violent temporary, involuntary contraction of a muscle group when referring to physical spasms. There is also an emotional spasm that is a sudden, violent effort.

spatulation (spat-ū-lā'-shun) Mixing by use of a flat, blunt instrument.

specialist (spesh'-ul-ist) In dentistry, a dentist who limits practice to a certain type of treatment, such as orthodontics or pedodontics.

spirillum (spi-ril′-um) Spiral-shaped bacteria. Spirilla may have many forms—a single curve, coiled, many curves, or coiled and curved at the same time.

spirochete (spī-rō-kēt′) An organism that is elongated and flexible, twisted spirally around its long axis. It exhibits motility without possessing flagella.

spondylitis (spahn-duh-lī′-tus) Inflammation of the vertebrae.

spores A form of bacteria especially difficult to destroy.

sprue In dentistry, the piece of metal or plastic attaching the wax pattern to the base; the hole through which the molten metal enters the mold; or the waste piece of the casting that filled this hole.

staphylococcus (staf″-i-lō-kok′-us) The bacteria commonly found in abscesses and other pus-forming conditions.

stenosis (steh-nō′sis) A narrowing or stricture of a duct, canal, or vessel.

sterilize The act of removing or destroying all microorganisms.

hot-water sterilization Sanitizing.

pasteurization Partial sterilization of a fluid at a temperature that destroys objectionable organisms without chemical alteration of the subject.

stomatitis (stō″-mah-tī′-tus) A general term for inflammation of the oral cavity that may occur from bacterial, viral, mechanical, chemical, electrical, thermal, or radiation injury, from allergens, and as a secondary (in sequence of time or development) manifestation of a systemic disease. May also occur as a reaction to medications or irritants, or systemic changes such as pregnancy. In the case of pregnancy it is often referred to as *pregnancy stomatitis,* and at this time a patient may also exhibit a gingivitis with hypertrophy of the gums, and occasionally develop a *pregnancy tumor* on the gingiva. Such pregnancy tumors are easily removed.

stomatology (stō-ma-tahl′-uh-ge) A branch of medical science that studies structures, functions, and diseases of the mouth.

stone A tool or instrument used for abrading.

Arkansas stone A fine-grained stone used in the final sharpening of instruments.

Carborundum stone is made of silicon carbide. It is an abrasive, handpiece-mounted instrument. There are several sizes, shapes, and degrees of abrasiveness. They are used to shape (or contour) tooth structure.

stone, artificial A special calcined gypsum derivative similar to plaster. Its grains are nonporous, and therefore artificial stone is stronger than plaster.

streptococcus (strep″-tuh-kok′-us) A genus of microorganisms found in many pathologic conditions, occurring as chains of cells.

study model A duplication of the dental arch of a patient, used for treatment planning, as opposed to a "working" model on which a denture may be constructed, for example.

styptic (stip′-tik) An astringent agent used to stop bleeding.

sublingual (sub-ling′-gwal) Beneath the tongue.

submaxillary (sub-max′-i-lary) Beneath the mandible.

submucosa (sub-mew-kō′-sah) The layer of tissue beneath the mucous membrane.

succedaneous (suk-suh-dā′-nē-us) Substituted or serving as a substitute (or following after).

sulcus, gingival (sul-kus) *Sulcus* means "groove." The gingival sulcus is the shallow groove between the gingiva and the surface of the tooth. It extends around the circumference of the tooth.

superior Above or upper.

supernumerary teeth (soo-per-noo′-mer-air-rē) Teeth in excess of the normal number.

supraclusion (soo-prah-klū′-zhun) Abnormally deep overlap of a dental arch or group of teeth.

surface, facial Surface means the external portion of an object, thus *facial surface* is the external side of a tooth which faces the lips and cheeks (the buccal and labial surfaces).

suture (sū′-chur) 1. A surgical stitch. 2. The line of junction of bones in the head. 3. The material used to sew up a wound.

symmetry (sim′-ih-trī) Similar arrangement on each side.

sympathy (sim′-puhth-ē) Having common feelings between persons so that what affects one also is felt by the other.

syncopé (sin′-kō-pay) The act of fainting. It is directly caused by an insufficient supply of blood to the brain.

synthesis (sin′-thuh-sis) The combination of parts to form a whole.

synthetic (sin-thet′-ik) Produced artificially.

syringe An instrument for injecting liquids.

system (sis′-tum) A set or series of parts that unite to function as a whole (as in *body system*).

T

target In radiography, the target is the tungsten button in the anode at which the electrons produced by the cathode are directed.

tartar A hard deposit on the surfaces of the teeth; more properly called "salivary calculus." Usually most heavily formed on those surfaces nearest the salivary ducts.

taxonomy (tax-ahn′-ō-me) Orderly classification.

technique, direct Preparation of a crown wax pattern in the patient's mouth.

technique, indirect Preparation of the wax pattern outside the patient's mouth on a die.

temporary stopping A material containing gutta-percha, capable of being softened by low heat and immediately placed in a cavity preparation in the tooth.

temporomandibular joints The joints, just ahead of each ear, upon which the lower jaw swings open and shut and can also slide forward.

terminology (ter-mi-nol′-ah-jē) The complete system of scientific or technical words applying to a science, art, or subject.

therapeutics (ther-uh-pew′-tiks) Branch of medicine that deals with the treatment of disease. (*Therapeutic* is Greek for treatment.)

therapy Remedial treatment of disease or bodily disorder.

thermoplastic A material that is rigid at normal temperatures but becomes soft when heated. The material can be softened by applying heat any number of times.

thrush (moniliasis) A disease caused by the yeastlike *Candida albicans*, characterized by white, curdy, raised patches that can be scraped off leaving a base which bleeds.

thyroid The endocrine gland that lies at the base of the neck. It produces a hormone containing iodine.

tincture (tink'-chur) An alcoholic solution of a medicinal substance.

tooth An organ of mastication. One of the hard bodies designed for the mastication of food. It is located in the oral cavity, attached to the alveolar process of the maxilla or mandible.

> **deciduous tooth** (dē-sid'-ū-us) A tooth that is shed; primary, baby, or milk tooth.

> **impacted tooth** (im-pak'-ted) A tooth that is in such a position within the jaws that it cannot erupt into complete visibility of the crown. A tooth may be partially or completely impacted.

> **nonvital tooth** (non-vī'-tal) A tooth that does not give a response to a stimulus because of a loss of vitality of the pulp.

> **permanent tooth** The tooth that replaces the primary tooth when it is shed.

> **supernumerary tooth** (sū-per-nū'-mer-ary) A tooth that is in excess of the usual or normally occurring number.

> **unerupted tooth** (un-ē-rup'-ted) A normal tooth before eruption into the mouth. Occasionally a tooth that lacks the physiologic impulse or erupting stimulus and therefore remains embedded. Not to be confused with "impacted."

> **vital tooth** (vī'-tal) A tooth with a normal, live pulp that gives a response to an irritating stimulus, much as you would expect a person whose skin is pricked to say "ouch!"

topical (top'-i-kal) On the surface, locally.

toxicity (tox-is'-i-tē) Usually used as a measure of the kind and amount of toxin (poison) produced by a given microorganism.

toxin (tox'-in) A secretion of cells that is poisonous to animals or man, resulting in the formation of resisting substances called antibodies. Bacteria produce most of the toxins with which we are concerned.

trachea (trā'-kē-uh) The windpipe, extending from the lower part of the larynx to the point of division into two bronchi.

tracheostomy (trā-kē-ahs'-tō-mē) An artificial opening into the trachea to provide airway to lungs when the normal passage is blocked.

tracheotomy (trā-kē-ot'-ō-mē) The act of cutting into the trachea to provide a patient with an airway when the airway has been blocked, creating a tracheostomy.

transformer A device used to convert variations of current in a primary circuit into variations of voltage and current in a secondary circuit. The principle of mutual induction is used for the conversion.

transfusion (trans-fū'-zhun) The process of passing from one to another, that is, transferring blood or saline solution into the vein or artery of a human.

transient (tran'-shent) Of short duration.

transilluminate (trans''-il-lū'-min-āt'') To pass strong light through an area or organ in order to examine its condition.

transverse (trans-vers') Placed crosswise, at right angles to the long axis.

trauma (trow'-ma) General: A hurt or wound to living tissue.

> **dental t.** An actual alteration of tissues produced by dental disharmony.

traumatic (trow-mat'-ik) Referring to that which has been caused by injury.

treatment (trēt'-ment) The actual process of treating anything. The management of an illness by any means in an effort to bring relief or aid in a cure.

trituration (trit-ur-ā'-shun) To mix by grinding and rubbing.

tuberosity (tū-ber-os'-it-ē) A large, rough prominence on a bone. It is also used to refer in specific cases to a prominence made up of soft tissues (flesh).

tumor (tū'-mōr) An abnormal mass of tissue cells in the body with no physiological function, a neoplasm.

tungsten (tung'-sten) An element used especially for electrical purposes and in hardening alloys. It is gray-white, heavy, high-melting, ductile, hard, polyvalent, metallic, and resembles chromium and molybdenum.

U

USP An abbreviation for "United States Pharmacopeia," the authority for all drug standards.

ulcer (ul'-cer) An open sore, whether on an external or internal surface of the body.

ultraviolet (ul''-trah-vī'-ō-let) Beyond the violet end of the color spectrum.

V

vascular (vas'-qū-lar) Relating to a channel for the conveyance of a body fluid, such as blood, or to a system of these channels, such as blood vessels.

vasoconstrictor (vā''-zō-kon-strik'-tor) A nerve or a drug that causes a blood vessel to become smaller in diameter, thus permitting less blood to flow through the blood vessel.

vasodilator (vā''-zo-dī'-lā-tor) A drug or nerve action that causes enlargement of a blood vessel, thus permitting more blood to flow through the blood vessel.

ventrolateral (ven-trō-lat'-er-uhl) Both to the front and to the side.

vestibule of the mouth (ves-ti-būl) The corridor or space between the alveolar gingiva and the lips and the cheeks.

virulent (vir'-yū-lent) Able to overcome bodily defenses, marked by a severe, extremely poisonous course.

virus (vī'-rus) An ultramicroscopic pathogen responsible for many diseases in man.

vitamin (vī'-tah-min) A protein substance that is essential to the metabolic processes and closely associated with enzyme function. Vitamins are not produced by the human body but must come from plant sources and be injested in the diet.

volatilize (vol'-uh-til-īz) To cause to pass off as a vapor; evaporate.

volt The electromotive force necessary to cause one ampere of current to flow against one ohm of resistance.

voltmeter A meter that registers the volts being used in operating the machine to which the meter is attached.

W

wax A substance of complex chemical form, used in dentistry in many variations for various purposes. In general, waxes become soft and plastic when warmed, more resistant to molding when chilled or cold, are not soluble in water, are soluble in ether or chloroform.

weld To unite two or more pieces by the application of heat along the joint.

X

xanthoma (zan-thō'-mah) Small yellow nodules, usually found in subcutaneous tissue.

X ray (roentgen ray) Electromagnetic radiation when electrons strike a target in a vacuum tube. X ray is preferred when speaking with lay personnel. Roentgen ray is preferred in scientific communication.

Z

zygomatic arch (zi'h-gō-mat-ik) An arch of bone commonly known as the "cheek bone." It begins just in front of the ear, arches slightly outward, forward, and then curves slightly inward to an area just below the outer corner of the eye. The *arch* portion of this bone is just above the ramus of the mandible. You can't get your finger under the arch because it is blocked by muscles.

Word Element Glossary

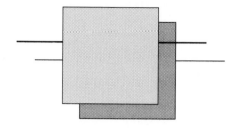

A

a, an prefix: without, not

ab, abs prefix: away, away from

acro prefix: extremity

ad prefix: to, toward, addition to, intensification

ad suffix: to, toward

aden combining form: relationship to gland

aer combining form: air

agogue, agig root word: lead, drive, make

al suffix: of, like, pertaining to

algia, alg suffix: pain

ambi prefix: on both sides

amphi prefix: both, doubly

ana prefix: upward, backward, excessive, again

and, andro combining form: relationship to man, male

angio combining form: relationship to a vessel

anim prefix: life, mind

aniso prefix: unequal, dissimilar

ante prefix: before, preceding in time, in front of

antero prefix: front

anthrop combining form: relationship to man, mankind

anti, ant prefix: against or over against

artero combining form: relationship to an artery

arthr, arthro combining form: relationship to a joint

aur combining form: ear

auto, aut prefix: self, relationship to self

B

bi prefix: two

bi combining form: life

bi, bis, bin prefix: two

bio combining form: relationship to life

blast combining form: root, germ cell

brachy combining form: short

bronch, broncho root word: windpipe

C

cale, calor combining form: heat

cardio, card combining form: heart

cata prefix: down, lower, under

cau prefix: burn

centi combining form: one one hundredth, indicates fraction in the metric system

cephalo, cephal combining form: relationship to the head

cerebro root word: brain

cerv root word: neck

cheilo, cheil root word: lip

chemo combining form: relating to chemistry

chole suffix: bile

chondr, chondro, chondri, chondrio combining form: relationship to cartilage

chron combining form: relationship to time

cid, cis combining form: relationship to kill, cut

circum combining form: around

clus, clud combining form: relationship to close, shut

co, com, con combining form: together with

contra prefix: against, counter

cranio combining form: relationship to the skull

cret combining form: distinguish, separate off

cyt combining form: relationship to cell

D

de prefix: down, from

dec, deca combining form: ten, ten times the root with which it is combined

dent, dento combining form: tooth

derm root word: skin

dextro combining form: relationship to the right

di prefix: two, twice

dia, di prefix: through, apart

diplo prefix: double

dis, di prefix: apart, away from

dorsi, dorso combining form: relating to the back, back

dys combining form: bad, improper

E

e, ec combining form: without

ec prefix: out of

ecto prefix: outside

ectomy suffix: surgical removal

emesis suffix: vomit

emia suffix: blood

en, em prefix: in

encephal combining form: brain

endo, end prefix: inward situation, within

ento prefix: within, inner

epi prefix: on, upon, over

er suffix: one who belongs to or is connected with

erythro combining form: red

esthes combining form: perceive, feel

ex, exo prefix: beyond, out of, without, from

exo prefix: beyond, out of, without, from, off, outward, outside

extra prefix: outside of, beyond

F

form prefix: shape

G

gastr root word: stomach

gen suffix: to produce

genous suffix: arising or resulting from

gingiva root words: gums

glosso root word: tongue

gnatho root word: jaw

gno combining form: know

grad, gress, gred combining form: go, step, walk, degree

gram suffix: tracing, picture

gram root word: a unit of weight in the metric system

graph suffix: to write, record, describe

gyn, gyne, gyneco combining form: relationship to woman

H

hect combining form: 100 times the unit of measurement, indicates multiple in the metric system

hem, hema, hemo, hemat root word: blood

hemi prefix: half

hepato root word: liver

hept combining form: seven

hetero combining form: relationship to others

hex, hexa, hexyl combining form: six

homo, homeo combining form: same, similar

hydro, hyd combining form: relationship to water, hydrogen

hyper prefix: excessive

hypo prefix: deficient

hypo combining form: insufficient, defective, under, deficient

hystero combining form: denoting relationship to hysteria (also to the uterus)

I

iatr combining form: heal, treatment

ics suffix: practice, skill, characteristic qualities

im prefix: in, within

in prefix: 1. not; 2. in, within

infra prefix: below or beneath the stem word

inter prefix: between

intra, intr prefix: situated or formed within

intro prefix: into or within

ism suffix: state of being, process, result of action

iso prefix or combining form: equal, alike, same

itis suffix: inflammation of

ize suffix: subject to action of the root word to which it is attached

J

ject combining form: throw, cast

juxta prefix: near

K

kilo combining form: 1000 times the unit of measure (indicates multiple in the metric system)

L

labi combining form: lip

lact combining form: denoting a relationship to milk

laryn combining form: relationship to the larynx

latero, lati combining form: relationship to the side

leuc, leuk prefix and combining form: white

levo combining form: to the left

lip combining form: fat

lith prefix or suffix: stone

logy suffix: the study of

lysis suffix: decomposition, destruction, dissolution

M

macro prefix or combining form: long, large

mal combining form: bad, abnormal

megalo, mega combining form: large, of great size

megaly suffix: enlargement

melano combining form: black

meso, mes combining form: middle

meter suffix: measure, especially an instrument used in measurement

micro combining form: small size

milli prefix or combining form: one one thousandth (indicates fraction in the metric system)

mon, mono prefix: one

morph combining form: form

multi combining form: many, much

my combining form: relationship to muscle

myo prefix: muscle

myx prefix: mucus

N

narco combining form: relationship to numb, stupor

necr combining form: death

neo combining form: new, strange

nephr root word: kidney

neur, neuro combining form: relationship to the nerves, nervous system

nomo combining form: relationship to law, custom

non, nona prefix: nine

O

ob prefix: over, to, against

octa combining form: eight

odonto combining form: relationship to a tooth

oid suffix: resemblance, form of the thing specified

oligo, olig combining form: few, less than normal

oma suffix: tumor

op, ops, opt prefix: vision, view, eye

ophthalm combining form: relationship to the eye

opistho combining form: backward

oro combining form: relationship to mouth

ortho prefix: normal, straight, right

os, osteo root word: bone

osis suffix: abnormal increase in a process

osteo prefix: bone

oto combining form: relationship to the ear

otomy suffix: incision

P

pan prefix: all, every

para prefix: beyond, beside, accessory to, against

path combining form: disease, feeling

patho combining form: relationship to disease

pathy suffix: disease, of feeling

pedo combining form: relationship to child

pel combining form: drive, force

pent, penta combining form: five

per prefix: throughout space or time

peri prefix: around

phage combining form and suffix: to eat, devour, relationship to eating, swallowing

pharyngo combining form: relationship to the pharynx

philia combining form: affinity for

phlebo, phleb combining form: relationship to the veins

phobia suffix: fear of

phono combining form: sound

phot combining form: relationship to light

phylac combining form: guard, defense

plas, plast prefix: mold, shape

plasia suffix: to form

plegia suffix: paralysis

pleura combining form: relationship to the side, rib or pleura

plex combining form: strike

plic combining form: fold or twist

pnea suffix: breath

pneum, pnea, pnoe root word: lung, air

pod combining form: relationship to the foot

poly combining form: much, many

pond combining form: weigh

pont combining form: bridge

post prefix: behind, after

pre prefix: before

pro prefix: forward, forth, for, before, in front of

pros prefix: toward

psych combining form: mind

puls combining form: beat

pyo combining form: pus

pyr, pyro combining form: fire, heat

pyre combining form: fever

Q

quadr combining form: four

R

radio combining form: relationship to ray or radiation

re prefix: back, again

retro prefix: backward, back of

rhea, rrhea suffix: abnormal or excessive flow

rhin combining form: relationship to the nose

rube, rubi combining form: red

rupt combining form: break

S

sacchar combining form: sugar

sacro combining form: relationship to the sacrum

sangui combining form: relationship to the blood

sarco combining form: relationship to flesh

sclero combining form: hard

scop suffix: an instrument to examine or view

sect combining form: cut

semi prefix: half, partly

sens combining form: to perceive, to feel

sep prefix: rot

sept combining form: seven

septi prefix: disease produced by microorganisms and their poisonous products

sequ, secu, sue combining form: follow

sex combining form: six

sialo combining form: relationship to saliva, salivary glands

son combining form: sound

spect, spic, spis combining form: look

spondylo combining form: relationship to vertebrae, spinal column

stasis suffix: standing still

steno combining form: contracted, narrow

stereo combining form: firm, solid, having three dimensions

stom combining form: mouth, orifice

stomy suffix: artificial mouth

sub prefix: under, below, deficient

super prefix: above, or implying excess

super, supr combining form: above, beyond, extreme

supra prefix: above or over

syn prefix: union, association

sys prefix: with, together

T

tax combining form: order, arrange

tetra combining form: four

therm combining form: heat

thermo combining form: relationship to heat

tomy, tome suffix: cut, an instrument for cutting

toxi prefix: poison

trachelo combining form: relationship to the neck or a necklike structure

tracheo combining form: relationship to the trachea

trans prefix: through, across

tri prefix: three

trophy suffix: nourish

tropism suffix: a growth response in a motile organism elicited either toward or away from the stimulus

U

ultra prefix: beyond excess

uni prefix: one

V

ventro combining form: in the front, abdomen

viscero combining form: relationship to organs of the body

X

xantho prefix: yellow

Z

zoo combining form: relationship to animal

Notes by Chapter

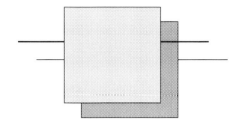

Chapter 1

1. W. A. Price, *Nutrition and Physical Degeneration* (Santa Monica: Price-Pottenger Foundation, 1970), chapter 8.

2. Zweemer, T. J. *Boucher's Clinical Dental Terminology* (St. Louis: C. V. Mosby Company, 1982).

Chapter 2

1. Vincenzo Guerini, *A History of Dentistry* (Philadelphia: Lea & Febiger, 1909), pp. 108–13.

2. Ibid.

3. Herman Prinz, *Dental Chronology* (Philadelphia: Lea & Febiger, 1945), p. 96.

4. Ibid.

5. Delta Dental of Minnesota statistical records, researched by Lori Johnson of Delta Dental.

Chapter 7

1. *Teletraining (Effective Use of the Telephone),* published by the Bell Telephone System for use within the system in training employees.

Chapter 12

1. Adapted from *Medical Radiography and Photography.* Courtesy of Roscoe E. Miller, M.D.

Chapter 16

1. Recommended by Andrew Froelich, C.P.A., medical and dental accountant, Minneapolis, MN.

Chapter 19

1. Permission granted by the International Consumer Credit Association and the American Collectors Association to include material supplied by them with modifications and additions by the authors.

2. Courtesy Dr. James Kershaw, with modification by the authors.

Chapter 20

1. Shirley P. Schwarzrock and Donovan F. Ward, *Effective Medical Assisting,* 2d ed., (Dubuque, Iowa: Wm. C. Brown Company Publishers, 1976). The material for this chapter is condensed from *Effective Medical Assisting,* Chapters 28–30, pages 343–401, with permission of the publisher and authors.

Chapter 23

1. A. Keys, et al., *The Biology of Human Starvation* (Minneapolis, Mn.: University of Minnesota Press, 1950), p. 36.

2. W. W. Tuttle, et al., "Effect on School Boys of Omitting Breakfast," *J. Am. Dietet. Assoc.* 30 (July 1954): 674–77.

3. Keys, *The Biology of Human Starvation*, p. 36.

4. R. M. Peel and M. L. Dodds, "Nutritive Intake of Women Factory Employees," *J. Am. Dietet. Assoc.* 33 (Nov. 1957): 1150–53.

5. N. S. Scrimshaw, et al. "Interactions of Nutrition and Infection," *The Am. J. Medical Sciences* 237 (March 1959): 367–403.

6. G. Toverud, "The Influence of War and Post War Conditions on the Teeth of Norwegian School Children—Eruption of Permanent Teeth and Status of Deciduous Dentition," *The Milbank Memorial Fund Quarterly* 34 (Oct. 1956): 354–450; "Caries in the Permanent Teeth of Children Aged 7–8 and 12–13," 35 (April 1957): 127–96; "Discussion of Food Supply and Dental Condition in Norway and Other European Countries," 35 (Oct. 1957): 373–459.

Chapter 24

1. *Accepted Dental Therapeutics* (Chicago: American Dental Association, 1984).

2. N. B. Williams, "Microbial Ecology of the Oral Cavity," *Journal of Dental Research* 42 (1963): 509–20. Supplement to No. 1.

Chapter 25

1. Maury Massler and Isaac Schour. *Atlas of the Mouth.* (Chicago: American Dental Association) page facing page 19.

2. James R. Jensen and Thomas Serene. *Fundamentals of Clinical Endodontics.* (Dubuque, Iowa: Kendall/Hunt Publishing Company, 1984).

Chapter 26

1. *Dorland's Illustrated Medical Dictionary,* 25th ed., (Philadelphia: Saunders, 1981), p. 476.

2. Ibid.

Chapter 27

1. Courtesy Lactona Products Division, Morris Plains, NJ, with adaptation by the authors.

Chapter 28

1. Henry B. Clark, Jr. *Practical Oral Surgery*, 2d ed. (Philadelphia: Lea and Febiger, 1959), pp. 150–58.

Chapter 31

1. Phillips, R. W. *Skinner's Science of Dental Materials*, 8th ed. Philadelphia: W. B. Saunders, 1982.

Chapter 33

1. This section adapted from materials supplied through the courtesy of Coe Laboratories, Chicago, IL.

2. Photos for this section through the courtesy of Dr. L. W. McIver, Minneapolis, MN.

Chapter 34

1. This section, "Successful Casting Technique," through the courtesy of J. M. Ney Co., Hartford, CT, with modifications.

Chapter 35

1. Zweemer, T. J. *Boucher's Clinical Dental Terminology* (St. Louis: C. V. Mosby Co., 1982).

Chapter 36

1. S. S. White Dental Health Products are to be credited with the description of the automatic processor. Adapted from their *Auveloper Catalogue* No. 2459.

2. This section, "X-ray Processing Solutions," through the courtesy of A. Porter, S. Sweet, D.D.S., F.A.A.O.R., formerly with X-ray Division, Eastman Kodak Company, Rochester, N.Y.

Photo Credits

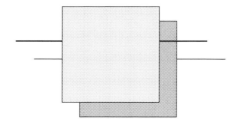

We wish to give credit for the illustrations furnished through the courtesy of the following firms and individuals.

Chapter 2

Figure 2.4: Univ. of Minnesota Dental Photo Lab

Chapter 5

Figure 5.2: ADEC

Chapter 7

Figure 7.1: Univ. of Minnesota Dental Photo Lab

Chapter 12

Figures 12.3 through 12.5: Roscoe Miller, M.D., Medical Radiography and Photography

Chapter 21

Figure 21.18: Univ. of Minnesota Dental Photo Lab; 21.19: Porter Instrument Company, Hatfield, Pennsylvania; 21.20: Univ. of Minnesota Dental Photo Lab

Chapter 24

Figures 24.2 and 24.3: Univ. of Minnesota Dental Photo Lab; 24.4: Courtesy Bard-Parker Co., Inc. Danbury, Connecticut; 24.5: Courtesy Ritter Equipment Co., Rochester, New York; 24.6: Courtesy Bard-Parker Co., Inc.; 24.7 and 24.8: Courtesy Dri-Clave Co., Westbury, New York; 24.9: Courtesy Harvey Dental Specialty Co., Gardena, California; 24.10: Univ. of Minnesota Dental Photo Lab

Chapter 25

Figures 25.1 through 25.19: Univ. of Minnesota Dental Photo Lab; 25.21: Univ. of Minnesota Dental Photo Lab; 25.23 through 25.26: Univ. of Minnesota Dental Photo Lab; 25.28: Univ. of Minnesota Dental Photo Lab

Chapter 26

Figures 26.3 through 26.8: Univ. of Minnesota Dental Photo Lab

Chapter 27

Figure 27.1: Reprinted from Hussen A. Zaki, *Clean Teeth Bright Your Smile* (Univ. of Minnesota, 1971); 27.2 through 27.4: Univ. of Minnesota Dental Photo Lab; 27.15: Univ. of Minnesota Dental Photo Lab

Chapter 28

Figures 28.10 through 28.14: Univ. of Minnesota Dental Photo Lab; 28.15: W. P. Frantzich, D.D.S., M.S.D.; 28.18: W. P. Frantzich, D.D.S., M.S.D.; 28.19 and 28.20: Courtesy L. M. McIver, D.D.S., M.S.; 28.22: Courtesy L. M. McIver, D.D.S., M.S.; 28.23 through 28.28: Univ. of Minnesota Dental Photo Lab; 28.29: Boos Dental Laboratory, Minneapolis, Minnesota; 28.30: Univ. of Minnesota Dental Photo Lab; 28.31 and 28.32: Boos Dental Laboratory, Minneapolis, Minnesota

Chapter 29

Figure 29.1 (both): Courtesy B. D. Fenchel, D.D.S.; 29.2a: Courtesy B. D. Fenchel, D.D.S.; 29.2b: Courtesy Siemens Corporation; 29.3 and 29.4: ADEC, Newberg, Oregon; 29.5 through 29.10: Univ. of Minnesota Dental Photo Lab

Chapter 30

Figure 30.1: Courtesy S. S. White Co.; 30.2: Kerr Mfg. Co.; 30.3 and 30.4: Univ. of Minnesota Dental Photo Lab; 30.6 (both): Univ. of Minnesota Dental Photo Lab; 30.8: Univ. of Minnesota Dental Photo Lab; 30.10: S. S. White Co.; 30.12: Courtesy Hu-Friedy Mfg. Co., Inc.; 30.15: Courtesy Clev-Dent, Denver, Colorado; 30.18: Courtesy Johnson and Johnson; 30.19: Courtesy Garmers Mfg. Co.; 30.20: Courtesy Ritter Dental Mfg. Co.; 30.21 and 30.22: Univ. of Minnesota Dental Photo Lab; 30.33: Courtesy Hu-Friedy Mfg. Co., Inc.; 30.36 through 30.45: Courtesy Hu-Friedy Mfg. Co., Inc.; 30.46: Courtesy Clev-Dent, Denver, Colorado; 30.47: Courtesy Hu-Friedy Mfg. Co., Inc.; 30.51: Courtesy Hu-Friedy Mfg. Co., Inc.; 30.53: Univ. of Minnesota Dental Photo Lab; 30.54: Courtesy Hu-Friedy Mfg. Co., Inc.; 30.56: Courtesy Hu-Friedy Mfg. Co., Inc.; 30.57: Courtesy Davol, Inc.; 30.58 and 30.59: Courtesy Hu-Friedy Mfg. Co., Inc.; 30.60: Courtesy Hu-Friedy Mfg. Co., Inc. and Univ. of Minnesota Dental Photo Lab; 30.65: Courtesy Hu-Friedy Mfg. Co., Inc.; 30.66: W. P. Frantzich, D.D.S., M.S.; 30.67 and 30.68: Courtesy Hu-Friedy Mfg. Co., Inc.; 30.70 and 30.71: Courtesy Hu-Friedy Mfg. Co., Inc.; 30.72 (both): Univ. of Minnesota Dental Photo Lab; 30.73 through 30.76: Courtesy Hu-Friedy Mfg. Co., Inc.; 30.77: Courtesy Johnson and Johnson; 30.80: Courtesy Unitek Corporation/3M; 30.82: Courtesy Hu-Friedy Mfg. Co., Inc.; 30.86: Courtesy Clev-Dent, Denver, Colorado; 30.87: Courtesy L. D. Caulk Co.; 30.88 and 30.89: Courtesy Kramer Dental Studio; 30.90 through 30.92: Courtesy Coe Labs, Inc.; 30.94: Courtesy Kerr Mfg. Co.; 30.95: Courtesy Hanau Engineering Co.; 30.96: Univ. of Minnesota Dental Photo Lab

Chapter 31

Figure 31.1: Univ. of Minnesota Dental Photo Lab; 31.3 through 31.5: Univ. of Minnesota Dental Photo Lab; 31.8: Joan Dako, Univ. of Minnesota Dental School; 31.9 through 31.17: Univ. of Minnesota

Dental Photo Lab; 31.18: Courtesy Morgan-Hastings and Co.; 31.20 and 31.21: Univ. of Minnesota Dental Photo Lab

Chapter 32

Figure 32.1: Courtesy Coe Labs, Inc.; 32.2: Courtesy Kerr Mfg. Co.; 32.3: Courtesy Hanau Engineering Co.

Chapter 33

Figures 33.1 and 33.2: Courtesy Coe Labs, Inc.; 33.3: Cristobalite; 33.5 through 33.8: Courtesy Kerr Mfg. Co.; 33.9 through 33.11: Univ. of Minnesota Dental Photo Lab; 33.13 through 33.16: L. M. McIver, D.D.S., M.S.; 33.20 through 33.21: L. M. McIver, D.D.S., M.S.; 33.22 through 33.68: Kerr Mfg. Co.; 33.69 through 33.72: Courtesy Coe Labs, Inc.; 33.73 and 33.74: S. S. White Co.; 33.75: Courtesy L. D. Caulk Co.

Chapter 34

Figures 34.8 through 34.10: Courtesy J. M. Ney Co.; 34.11: Courtesy Torit Mfg. Co.; 34.12: Courtesy Whip-Mix Corporation; 34.13: Courtesy J. M. Ney Co.; 34.14: Kerr Mfg. Co.; 34.15: Courtesy J. M. Ney Co.; 34.17: Kerr Mfg. Co.

Chapter 35

Figure 35.3 (both): Courtesy General Electric Co.; 35.5: Rinn Corporation; 35.6: Nuclear Corporation; 35.9 and 35.10: Courtesy Siemens Corporation; 35.11: Courtesy General Electric Co.; 35.12: Courtesy Eastman Kodak Co.; 35.13: Univ. of Minnesota Dental Photo Lab

Chapter 36

Figures 36.1 and 36.2 (photo): Courtesy Eastman Kodak Co.; 36.3b through 36.5: Courtesy Eastman Kodak Co.; 36.6a: Courtesy S. S. White Co.; 36.6b: Courtesy Siemens Corporation; 36.8 through 36.10: Courtesy Rinn Corporation

Chapter 37

Figure 37.1: Univ. of Minnesota Dental Photo Lab

Chapter 38

Figure 38.1: Univ. of Minnesota Dental Photo Lab; 38.4 through 38.9: Univ. of Minnesota Dental Photo Lab; 38.13 through 38.30: Univ. of Minnesota Dental Photo Lab

Line Art Credits

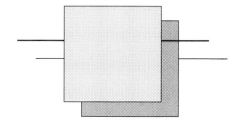

We wish to give credit for the illustrations furnished through the courtesy of the following firms and individuals.

Chapter 2
Figures 2.1 through 2.3: Univ. of Minnesota Dental Photo Lab; 2.5: Univ. of Minnesota Dental Photo Lab

Chapter 5
Figure 5.1: William S. Howell, Ph.D., Univ. of Minnesota

Chapter 6
Figure 6.1: From "You Always Communicate Something" Schwarzrock, Shirley P., American Guidance Service, Circle Pines, Minnesota; 6.2: William S. Howell, Ph.D., Univ. of Minnesota

Chapter 7
Figure 7.2: "Teletraining (Effective Use of the Telephone)," published by Bell Telephone System

Chapter 8
Figure 8.3: Spillanes, Inc., Minneapolis, Minnesota

Chapter 9
Figure 9.6: Spillanes, Inc., Minneapolis, Minnesota

Chapter 11
Figure 11.5: John Marcus Dental Supply Co., Minneapolis, Minnesota

Chapter 13
Figure 13.6: Herbert Gustavson, D.D.S., Skokie, Illinois and Delta Air Lines

Chapter 15
Figure 15.1: Spillanes, Inc., Minneapolis, Minnesota; 15.3: Spillanes, Inc., Minneapolis, Minnesota

Chapter 16
Figures 16.1 through 16.3: Spillanes, Inc., Minneapolis, Minnesota; 16.7 and 16.8: Spillanes, Inc., Minneapolis, Minnesota

Chapter 17
Figure 17.2: John Marcus Dental Supply Co.; 17.3: Little Press, Inc., Minneapolis, Minnesota; 17.9 through 17.12: Little Press, Inc.; 17.13 and 17.14: Wm. P. Frantzich, D.D.S., M.S.D.

Chapter 18
Figure 18.8: Delta Dental of Minnesota, Minneapolis, Minnesota

Chapter 19
Figure 19.1: Spillanes, Inc., Minneapolis, Minnesota

Chapter 20
Figures 20.1 through 20.4: From *Effective Medical Assisting* by Schwarzrock and Ward, 1976, Wm. C. Brown Publishers, Dubuque, Iowa. All Rights Reserved; 20.5: Postgraduate Medicine, 1975; 20.6: From Benson and Gunstream, *Anatomy and Physiology Laboratory Textbook,* 2d ed. © 1975 Wm. C. Brown Publishers, Dubuque, Iowa. All Rights Reserved; 20.7: From J. E. Wodsedalek, *General Zoology.* © Wm. C. Brown Publishers, Dubuque, Iowa. All Rights Reserved; 20.8: Univ. of Minnesota Dental Photo Lab; 20.9 through 20.11: Kendall/Hunt Publishing Co.

Chapter 21
Figures 21.1 through 21.7: Joan Dako, Univ. of Minnesota Dental School; 21.8: Model by Densco, Inc.; 21.9 and 21.10: Joan Dako, Univ. of Minnesota Dental School; 21.12 through 21.14: Univ. of Minnesota Dental Photo Lab; 21.15 through 21.17: Joan Dako, Univ. of Minnesota Dental School

Chapter 22
Figures 22.3 and 22.4: Univ. of Minnesota Dental Photo Lab

Chapter 24
Figure 24.1: Joan Dako, Univ. of Minnesota Dental School

Chapter 25
Figure 25.20: Univ. of Minnesota Dental Photo Lab; 25.22: Univ. of Minnesota Dental Photo Lab; 25.27: Univ. of Minnesota Dental Photo Lab

Chapter 26
Figures 26.1 and 26.2: Univ. of Minnesota Dental Photo Lab

Chapter 27
Figures 27.5 through 27.12: Lactona, Inc., St. Paul, Minnesota; 27.13: E. R. Squibb and Sons, New York; 27.14: Univ. of Minnesota Dental Photo Lab

Chapter 28
Figures 28.1 and 28.2: Univ. of Minnesota Dental Photo Lab; 28.3 through 28.9: Joan Dako, Univ. of Minnesota Dental School; 28.15 through 28.17: W. P. Frantzich, D.D.S., M.S.D.; 28.21: L. M. McIver, D.D.S., M.S.

Chapter 30
Figure 30.5: Univ. of Minnesota Dental Photo Lab; 30.7: Kerr Mfg. Co.; 30.9: S. S. White Co.; 30.11: Kerr Mfg. Co. and S. S. White Co.; 30.13 and 30.14: S. S. White Co.; 30.16 and 30.17: S. S. White Co.; 30.23 through 30.25: S. S. White Co.; 30.26: Astra Pharmaceutical Products, Worcester, Massachusetts; 30.27: Cook-Waite Labs, New York; 30.28: S. S. White Co.; 30.29 through 30.31: Courtesy Hu-Friedy Mfg. Co., Inc.; 30.34: S. S. White Co.; 30.35: Clev-Dent; 30.48: S. S.

White and Rocky Mountain Dental Products; 30.49 and 30.50: Star Dental Mfg. Co., Philadelphia, Pennsylvania; 30.52: Univ. of Minnesota Dental Photo Lab; 30.61 and 30.62: Courtesy Hu-Friedy Mfg. Co., Inc.; 30.63: S. S. White; 30.64: Bard-Parker; 30.69: Courtesy Hu-Friedy Mfg. Co., Inc.; 30.78: Courtesy Hu-Friedy Mfg. Co., Inc.; 30.79: S. S. White Co.; 30.81: Courtesy Hu-Friedy Mfg. Co., Inc.; 30.83: Courtesy Hu-Friedy Mfg. Co., Inc.; 30.84 and 30.85: S. S. White Co.; 30.93: S. S. White Co.

Chapter 31

Figure 31.2: Univ. of Minnesota Dental Photo Lab; 31.6 and 31.7: Joan Dako, Univ. of Minnesota Dental School; 31.19: Joan Dako, Univ. of Minnesota Dental School

Chapter 33

Figure 33.4: Univ. of Minnesota Dental Photo Lab; 33.12: L. M. McIver, D.D.S.; 33.17 through 33.19: L. M. McIver, D.D.S.

Chapter 34

Figures 34.1 through 34.5: Coe Labs, Inc.; 34.6: S. S. White Co.; 34.7: J. M. Ney; 34.16: Univ. of Minnesota Dental Photo Lab

Chapter 35

Figure 35.2: General Electric Co.; 35.4: General Electric Co.; 35.7: Rinn Corporation; 35.8: General Electric Co.

Chapter 36

Figure 36.3a: Eastman Kodak Co.; 36.7: Eastman Kodak Co.

Chapter 38

Figures 38.2 and 38.3: Univ. of Minnesota Dental Photo Lab; 38.10 through 38.12: Univ. of Minnesota Dental Photo Lab

Appendix

Figures A-1 and A-2: Drawings by the late L. H. Schwarzrock, D.D.S.

Color Plates

Plate 1: From Kent M. Van De Graaff, *Human Anatomy,* 2d ed. © 1988 Wm. C. Brown Publishers, Dubuque, Iowa. All Rights Reserved; Plate 2: From Kent M. Van De Graaff and Stuart Ira Fox, *Concepts of Human Anatomy and Physiology,* 2d ed. © 1989 Wm. C. Brown Publishers, Dubuque, Iowa. All Rights Reserved; Plate 3: From John W. Hole, Jr., *Human Anatomy and Physiology,* 5th ed. © 1990 Wm. C. Brown Publishers, Dubuque, Iowa. All Rights Reserved; Plate 4: From Kent M. Van De Graaff, *Human Anatomy,* 2d ed. © 1988 Wm. C. Brown Publishers, Dubuque, Iowa. All Rights Reserved; Plate 5: From John W. Hole, Jr., *Human Anatomy and Physiology,* 5th ed. © 1990 Wm. C. Brown Publishers, Dubuque, Iowa. All Rights Reserved; Plate 6: From Stuart Ira Fox, *Human Physiology,* 2d ed. © 1987 Wm. C. Brown Publishers, Dubuque, Iowa. All Rights Reserved; Plates 7 and 8: From John W. Hole, Jr., *Human Anatomy and Physiology,* 5th ed. © 1990 Wm. C. Brown Publishers, Dubuque, Iowa. All Rights Reserved; Plate 9: From John W. Hole, Jr., *Human Anatomy and Physiology,* 4th ed. © 1987 Wm. C. Brown Publishers, Dubuque, Iowa. All Rights Reserved; Plates 10, 11, 12, and 13: From John W. Hole, Jr., *Human Anatomy and Physiology,* 5th ed. © 1990 Wm. C. Brown Publishers, Dubuque, Iowa. All Rights Reserved

Bibliography/Recommended Reading List

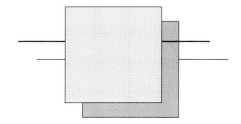

The following list of references has been prepared for the student who is interested in further information on subjects presented in this text.

Agard, Walter R. and Howe, Herbert M. *Medical Greek and Latin at a Glance*. New York: Hoeber-Harper, 1955.

American Dental Association. *Dentist's Desk Reference: Materials, Instruments and Equipment*. 2nd ed. Chicago: American Dental Association, 1983.

American Dental Association. *Accepted Dental Therapeutics*. 40th ed. Chicago: American Dental Association, 1984.

American Red Cross *First Aid Book*.

Anthony, C. P. and Thibodeau, G. A. *Textbook of Anatomy and Physiology*. 11th ed. St. Louis: C. V. Mosby, 1983.

Bennett, C. R. *Monheim's Local Anesthesia and Pain Control in Dental Practice*. 7th ed. St. Louis: C. V. Mosby, 1984.

Calisti, L. J. P. et al. *Handbook of Dental Specialties*. Wellesley, MA: Arandel Publishing, 1979.

Carranza, F. A. *Glickman's Clinical Periodontology*. 6th ed. Philadelphia: W. B. Saunders, 1984.

Castano, F. A. and Alden, B. A. *Handbook of Clinical Dental Auxiliary Practice*. Philadelphia: J. B. Lippincott, 1980.

Craig, R. F. *Restorative Dental Materials*. 7th ed. St. Louis: C. V. Mosby, 1985.

Craig, R. F.; O'Brian, W. J.; and Powers, J. M. *Dental Materials: Problems and Manipulation*. 4th ed. St. Louis: C. V. Mosby, 1987.

Davis, B. D. et al. *Microbiology*. 3rd ed. New York: Harper and Row, 1980.

Davis, F. W. and Solomon, E. *The World of Biology*. Orlando: Saunders College Publishers, 1986.

Diorio, L. P. *Clinical Preventive Dentistry*. Norwalk: Appleton-Century-Croft, 1983.

Dorland's *Illustrated Medical Dictionary*. 27th ed. Philadelphia: W. B. Saunders, 1988.

Dubril, E. L. *Sicher's Oral Anatomy*. 8th ed. Hazelwood, MO: Ishiyaku Euroamerica, 1988.

Dunn, M. J. and Shapiro, C. *Dental Anatomy: Head and Neck Anatomy*. Baltimore: Williams and Wilkins, 1975.

Freeman, B. A. *Burrow's Textbook of Microbiology*. 22nd ed. Philadelphia: W. B. Saunders, 1985.

Frenay, M. A. C. *Understanding Medical Terminology*. 7th ed. St. Louis: Catholic Health Association, 1984.

Golden, A.; Powell, D. E.; and Jennings, C. D. *Pathology: Understanding Human Disease*. 2nd ed. Baltimore: Williams and Wilkins, 1985.

Granath, L. and McHugh, W. D. *Systematized Prevention of Oral Diseases*. Boca Raton: CRC Press, 1986.

Grossman, L. I. *Endodontic Practice*. 10th ed. Philadelphia: Lea and Febiger, 1981.

Guerini, Vincenzo. *A History of Dentistry*. Philadelphia: Lea and Febiger, 1909.

Heartwell, C. M. and Rahn, A. O. *Syllabus of Complete Dentures*. 4th ed. Philadelphia: Lea and Febiger, 1986.

Henderson, D.; McGivney, G. P.; and Castleberry, D. J. *McCracken's Removable Partial Prosthodontics*. 7th ed. St. Louis: C. V. Mosby, 1985.

Hole, John W., Jr. *Human Anatomy and Physiology*. Dubuque, Iowa, Wm. C. Brown Company Publishers, 1987.

Holroyd, S. V.; Wynn, R. L.; and Requa-Clark, B. *Clinical Pharmacology in Dental Practice*. 4th ed. St. Louis: C. V. Mosby, 1988.

Howard, W. M. *Dental Practice Planning*. St. Louis: C. V. Mosby, 1975.

Jensen, J. R. and Serene, T. P. *Fundamentals of Clinical Endodontics*. 8th ed. Dubuque: Kendall/Hunt Publishing Co., 1984.

Langlais, R. P.; Bricker, S. L.; Coltone, J. A.; and Baker, B. R. *Oral Diagnosis, Oral Medicine, and Treatment Planning*. Philadelphia: W. B. Saunders, 1984.

Langland, O. E.; Sippy, F. H.; and Langlais, R. P. *Textbook of Dental Radiology*. 2nd ed. Springfield: C. C. Thomas, 1984.

Little, J. W. and Falace, D. A. *Dental Management of the Medically Compromised Patient*. 3rd ed. St. Louis: C. V. Mosby, 1988.

Lynch, M. et al. *Burket's Oral Medicine, Diagnosis and Treatment*. 8th ed. Philadelphia: Lippincott, 1984.

Malamed, S. F. *Handbook of Medical Emergencies in the Dental Office*. 3rd ed. St. Louis: C. V. Mosby, 1987.

Mathewson, R. J.; Primosch, R. E.; and Robertson, D. *Fundamentals of Pediatric Dentistry*. 2nd ed. Chicago: Quintessence Publishing Co., 1987.

National Academy of Science: *Recommended Dietary Allowances*. 10th ed. Washington, D.C. National Academy of Sciences, 1989.

Nester, E. W. et al. *Microbiology.* 3rd ed. New York: Holt, Rinehart and Winston, Inc., 1983.

Newman, M. G. and Nisengard, R. *Oral Microbiology and Immunology.* Philadelphia: W. B. Saunders, 1988.

Phillips, R. W. *Skinner's Science of Dental Materials.* 8th ed. Philadelphia: W. B. Saunders, 1982.

Price, W. A. *Nutrition and Physical Degeneration.* Santa Monica: Price-Pottenger Foundation, 1970.

Prinz, Herman. *Dental Chronology.* Philadelphia: Lea and Febiger, 1945.

Schwarzrock, Shirley P. *Perception of Communication in the Dental Office.* Doctoral Dissertation. Minneapolis, MN: University of Minnesota, 1974.

Schwarzrock, Shirley P. *Food as a Crutch.* Circle Pines, MN: American Guidance Service, 1984.

Schwarzrock, Shirley P. *You Always Communicate Something.* Circle Pines, MN: American Guidance Service, 1984.

Shillingburg, H. T.; Hobo, S.; and Whitsett, L. D. *Fundamentals of Fixed Prosthodontics.* 2nd ed. Chicago: Quintessence Publishing Co., 1981.

Smith, M. A. *A Short History of Dentistry.* New York: Roy Publishers, 1958.

Snyder, T. L. *Personalized Guide to Stress Evaluation.* St. Louis: C. V. Mosby, 1983.

Snyder, T. L. (ed). *Personalized Guide to Legal Issues.* St. Louis: C. V. Mosby, 1985.

Stallard, R. E. (ed). *A Textbook of Preventive Dentistry.* 2nd ed. Philadelphia: W. B. Saunders, 1982.

Stedmans Medical Dictionary. 24th ed. Baltimore: Williams and Wilkins, 1984.

Striffler, D. F.; Young, W. O.; and Burt, B. A. *Dentistry, Dental Practice and the Community.* 3rd ed. Philadelphia: W. B. Saunders, 1983.

Ten Cate, A. R. *Oral Histology: Development, Structure, and Function.* 2nd ed. St. Louis: C. V. Mosby, 1985.

Wolfson, E. *Four-Handed Dentistry for Dentists and Assistants.* St. Louis: C. V. Mosby, 1974.

Wood, N. K. *Review of Diagnosis, Oral Medicine, Radiology, and Treatment Planning.* 2nd ed. St. Louis: C. V. Mosby, 1987.

Zweemer, T. J. *Boucher's Clinical Dental Terminology.* St. Louis: C. V. Mosby Company, 1982.

Index of Instruments

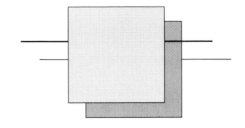

A

Amalgam
burnishers, fig. 30.44, **394**
carriers, fig. 30.33, **392**
condensers, fig. 30.34, **392**
die, fig. 30.89, **407**
mixed in disposable capsule, fig. 31.15b, **425**
pluggers, fig. 30.32, **392**
Angle formers, fig. 30.39, **394**
Articulating paper with holder, fig. 30.15, **386**
Articulator, Hanau, fig. 30.95, **410**
Articulator, Kerr Dentatus, fig. 30.94, **409**
Aspirator, Coupland, fig. 30.56, **398**

B

Band driver, for orthodontic use, fig. 30.79, **403**
Bands,
copper, fig. 30.86, **406**
2 "thimble" impressions (or copper bands), fig. 30.88, **407**
Bone file, Miller, fig. 30.68, **401**
Broaches, for Endodontics, fig. 30.50, **396**
Bur
assortment used in amalgam preparations, fig. 30.6a, **383**
scratch brush, fig. 30.6b, **383**
shapes, fig. 30.5, **382**

C

Capsule, disposable with preportioned alloy and mercury, fig. 31.15a, **425**
Carbon paper, fig. 30.15, **386**
Chisels,
for general dentistry, fig. 30.37, **393**
for oral surgery, bi-bevel, fig. 30.52a, **396**
for oral surgery, single bevel, fig. 30.52b, **396**
Cleoid-discoid, fig. 30.41, **394**
Composite instruments, fig. 30.47, **395**

Cone, Gracey Arkansas Sharpening, fig. 30.31, **391**
Contra-angle, Latch-type, fig. 30.3, **381**
Cotton holder, fig. 30.16, **386**
Cotton roll holders, fig. 30.19, **387**
Crown forms, fig. 30.87, **407**
Curettage for periodontists, fig. 30.83a, **406**
Curettes,
Gracey, fig. 30.81, **405**
Miller bone, fig. 30.58, **398**
for periodontists, figs. 30.83b, 30.83c, **406**
Cutting instruments,
angle formers, fig. 30.39, **394**
chisels, fig. 30.37, **393**
for oral surgery (bi-bevel), fig 30.52a; (single bevel), fig. 30.52, **396**
cleoid-discoid, fig. 30.41, **394**
hatchets, fig. 30.36, **393**
hoes, fig. 30.38, **393**; figs. 30.83d, 30.83e, **406**
knives, fig. 30.43, **394**
margin trimmers, fig. 30.40, **394**
spoon excavators, fig. 30.42, **394**

D

Dappen dish, fig. 30.17, **386**
Diamond instruments, fig. 30.7, **383**
Die, amalgam, fig. 30.89, **407**

E

Elevator,
Cryer root, fig. 30.76, **403**
Periosteal, M 4, fig. 30.59b, **399**
Periosteal, Molt 9, fig. 30.59a, **399**
Potts, fig. 30.73, **402**
Root tip, fig. 30.70, **401**
Schmeckebier Apexo, fig. 30.74a, **402**
Straight, fig. 30.75, **403**
Elevators, additional for 501 handle, fig. 30.74b, **402**
Evacuator tips, fig. 30.1a, **380**
Explorers, fig. 30.12, **385**

F

Facebow, Kerr, fig. 30.94, **409**; with bite fork and pointer, fig. 30.95, **410**
File, Miller bone, fig. 30.68, **401**
Files, Gracey Arkansas sharpening, fig. 30.30, **391**
Flexiboles, Hygienic, fig. 33.4, **440**
Forceps,
Adson tissue, fig. 30.62, **399**
Allison tissue, fig. 30.61, **399**
hemostatic, fig. 30.78, **403**
mandibular, incisors, canines, premolar, fig. 30.55a, **398**
mandibular, molar, fig. 30.55b, **398**
mandibular, third molar, fig. 30.55c, **398**
maxillary, anterior, figs. 30.54a, 30.54b, **397**
maxillary, right and left molar, fig. 30.54c, **397**
maxillary, right and left first molar, fig. 30.54e, **397**
maxillary, third molar, fig. 30.54d, **397**
rubber-dam clamp, fig. 30.24, **388**
tissue, (Adson), fig. 30.62, **399**
tissue, (Allison), fig. 30.61, **399**
transfer, fig. 24.6, **305**
Frahm's carvers, fig. 30.35, **393**

G

Gags,
Molt Universal, fig. 30.67b, **400**
mouth, McKesson, fig. 30.67a, **400**
Gauze, medicated sterile with radiopaque thread, fig. 30.72, **402**
Gauze packer, fig. 30.71, **401**

H

Handpiece,
ball bearing, fig. 30.2, **381**
contra-angle, fig. 30.3, **381**
ultraspeed, fig. 30.4, **381**

Hatchets, fig. 30.36, **393**
Hoe for periodontist, figs. 30.83d,
    30.83e, **406**
Hoes, fig. 30.38, **393**

I

Impression removed in superimposed
    plaster tray, fig. 30.88b, **407**

K

Knife,
    heavy-shanked, fig. 30.83f, **406**
    office, fig. 33.6, **440**
    spear-pointed, fig. 30.83, **406**
Knives, cutting instruments, fig.
    30.43, **394**

M

Mandrels, fig. 30.9, **384**
Margin trimmers, fig. 30.40, **394**
Matrix retainer, Tofflemire, fig.
    30.46, **395**
Mirrors, dental, fig. 30.11, **385**
Mouth gags,
    McKesson, fig. 30.68b, **400**
    Molt Universal, fig. 30.68a, **400**

N

Napkin holder, fig. 30.14, **386**
Needle,
    Holder, Mayo-Hegar fine, fig.
        30.65, **400**
    Huber dental, fig. 30.27, **389**
Needles, suture, fig. 30.66, **400**

P

Packer, gauze, fig. 30.71, **401**
Plastic filling instruments, fig. 30.47,
    395
Pliers
    alastik separator, fig. 30.80n, **404**
    arch-bending, fig. 30.80b, **404**
    band-removing, figs. 30.80e,
        30.80k, **404**
    band-slitter, fig. 30.80j, **404**
    bird-beak, fig. 30.80d, **404**

contouring, fig. 30.48, **395**
cotton, fig. 30.13, **385**
direct bond bracket removing,
    dual tips, fig. 30.80f, **404**
direct bond bracket removing,
    single chisel tip, fig. 30.80g,
    404
dressing, figure 30.13, **385**
end cutter, fig. 30.80h, **404**
hard wire cutter, fig. 30.80i, **404**
Howe, fig. 30.80a, **404**
ligature-tying, fig. 30.80m, **404**
pin and ligature cutter, fig. 30.80l,
    404
three-jaw wire-bender, fig. 30.80c,
    404
Pocket markers, fig. 30.82a, **405**
Pocket probe, fig. 30.82b, **405**
Prophylaxis right angle and cups, fig.
    30.8, **383**
Pulp tester, fig. 30.20, **387**

R

Reamers, for endodontics, fig. 30.49,
    396
Retractor,
    Austin, fig. 30.60b, **399**
    triangular tissue, fig. 30.83h, **406**
    University of Minnesota, fig.
        30.60a, **399**
Rongeur,
    end cutting, fig. 30.63a, **399**
    side cutting, fig. 30.63b, **399**
Root canal spreaders, fig. 30.51, **396**
Rubber-dam,
    clamp forceps, fig. 30.24, **388**
    clamps, fig. 30.25, **389**
    frame (Young's), fig. 30.22, **388**
    punch, fig. 30.23, **388**

S

Saliva ejector, fig. 30.1c, **380**
Scalers,
    a selection, fig. 30.45, **395**
    universal, fig. 30.81c, **405**
Scalpels, fig. 30.64, **400**

Scissors,
    curved collar and crown, fig.
        30.84, **406**
    Dean surgical, fig. 30.69b, **401**
    Metzenbaum curved-blunt, fig.
        30.69a, **401**
    straight crown, fig. 30.85, **406**
Sharpening stones,
    Bates Arkansas, fig. 30.29, **391**
    Gracey Arkansas cone, fig. 30.31,
        391
    Gracey Arkansas file, fig. 30.30,
        391
Spatulas,
    cement, fig. 30.28, **390**
    plaster, fig. 33.7, **440**
    wax, fig. 34.6, **467**
Sponge, exodontia, fig. 30.77, **403**
Spoon excavator, fig. 30.42, **394**
Stones, mounted, fig. 30.10, **384**
Suture, disposable swedged-on and
    needles, fig. 30.66, **400**
Syringe
    aspirating, fig. 30.26, **389**
    dry socket, fig. 30.72a, **402**
    for elastic impression materials,
        fig. 33.22a, **448**
    Ligmaject, fig. 30.53, **397**
    water-air, fig. 30.1b, **380**

T

Tissue retractor (triangular), fig.
    30.83h, **406**
Tonsil suction, disposable, fig. 30.57,
    398
Trays,
    impression, Frigidtrays, fig.
        30.90a, **408**
    impression, for partials, fig.
        30.90b, **408**
    impression, perforated, partial, fig.
        30.92, **408**
    impression, perforated, upper and
        lower, fig. 30.91, **408**
    water-cooled with rubber tubing,
        fig. 30.93, **408**

Index

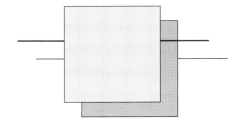

A

Abrasion, 311
Abscess, 311
  acute, 318
  lancing, 318
  periapical, 318
Account, payments on, (*See* Records, financial)
Account record, patient's, 171
Accounts receivable, **216**
  age analysis of, 215
  control, 227
  depreciation of, 215
Acquaintance form, 158, **159**
ADA, Council on Dental Health, 25
Administration of the office,
  administrator, 93
    succeeding as, 97
  advance record preparation, 99
  birthday control card, 104–105, **105**
  come-up card files, 101
  commercial communication services, 96
  coordinating office staff, 93–94
  current invoices, 101
  dentist's personal reminder service, 96
  functions in dental office organization, **93**
  information sources, 96
  laboratory schedule, 99, **101**
  office task control, 102–104, **103**
  orderly office routines, 99
  procedure manual, 94–95
  recall control card, **97, 102**
  recall control file, 101
  staff conference, 95
  thank-you notes, 101
  understanding patient recall philosophy, 97
  verification of information, 100
  work schedule, successful operation of, 99
Adolescent behavior characteristics, 59–60
Adult behavior, 60–62

Age analysis, 215
  of accounts receivable, **216**
Agenda, 155
Air turbine, 26
Alginate impression technique, 557
Allergic reaction, first aid for, 330
Alloy, spherical amalgam, 26
Amalgam,
  dental, **423–426**
    excess, **426**
    manipulation of, 425
  filling procedure, 544
  instruments, 392
  restorations, polishing (finishing) procedure, 544
American Dental Assistants' Association, 11
Analgesia, 275
Anatomical landmarks, 266
Anatomy of the head, 255–277, **255–259, 263, 264, 266, 267, 269, 272, 273, plates 9–13**
  blood supply to dental area, 270, **plates 5, 6**
  myology, 261–265
    facial muscles, 265
    infrahyoid muscles, 365
    muscles of mastication, 261, **262–264, plate 9**
    suprahyoid muscles, 265
  nerve supply to dental area, 270–274, **271–273**
  osteology, 255–261
    facial landmarks, **255**
    hyoid bone, 269, **plate 12**
    mandible, **259**
    maxilla, 259
    other bones of skull, 260
    skull, 255–259, **256–258**
    temporomandibular joint, 261
  salivary glands, 265–266, **266**
    parotid, 266
    sublingual, 266
    submandibular, 266
Anatomy of the teeth, 268–270, **269, plates 10, 11**

Anesthesia, 25, 274, **275**
  general, 275
  local, **276**
  motor and sensory nerves, 274
  prevention of pain, 274
  topical, 276
Anesthetic,
  syringes and needles, **389, 390**
Angle, Edward Hartley, 24
Angle's classifications, 362
Antibiotics, 26
Antiseptic, 301
Aphthous ulcer, **311**
Apical curettage, 550
Appointment book, 108–118, **114, 115, 116, 117**
  emergencies, 111
  entries, 111, **113**
  judging time allotment, 109
  management of, 109
  planning appointments, 109
  preparing, 108
  scheduling, 110–115
Appointment card, 116, **117**
Appointment failures, reducing, 116
Arrangements for meetings for dentists, (*See* Dentist)
Articulation, (joints), (*See* Systems of the body)
Articulators, 26, 408–411, **409, 410**
Artificial stone, 438–440, **438**
  mixing, 439
Aspirin burn, **312**
Assistant,
  certified, 9
  chairside, 9
  coordinating, 9
  laboratory, 9
Assisting
  with children, 517
  new patients who telephone, 98
  with preparations, 516
Attrition, **311**

B

Bacteriology, 298–299, **298**
Basic setup for nonoperative procedures, 539

Basic setup for operative procedures, 542
Basic setups, 384, **385**
Behavior characteristics
of adolescents, 59–60
of adults, 60–62
of children, 57–58
Bib or napkin holder, **386**
Biomaterials, 415
Bitewing X-ray procedure, 540
Black, Greene Vardiman, 24
Bleeding, (hemorrhage), first aid for, 334
Blood supply to the dental area, 211–212
Body structure, **226**
cavities, 227
cells, 226
organs, 227
planes, **228, 229**
surfaces, 229
tissues, 227
Bookkeeping systems,
double entry, 168
write-it-once, or pegboard, **181–191**
Bridge procedure, 555
Burns, 311
Burs,
dental, **382, 383**
tungsten carbide, 26
Business,
letters, **144, 145**
records, (*See* Records)
supplies, (*See* Supplies)

C

Calculus, **340**
Carbon paper (for dentistry), **386**
Caries,
control of, **294**
dental, 316
Case history, 160
presentation of, 162–164
Cast gold restoration
impressions for, 433–436, **434, 435**
procedure (inlay, ¾ crown, full crown), 554
Casting to dimension, 460–476
burning out the mold, **471–474**
casting, **474**
casting technique, 460–466, **462–466**
finishing and polishing, 475
investing methods, 469–471, **470, 471**
mounting pattern on crucible former, 468
pickling, 475
removing crucible former and sprue, 470
spruing the pattern, 467
wax patterns, 466–467, **467**

Casts and dies, 438–458
artificial stone and plaster, **438–441**
basic instructions, 458
boxing, **441**
denture, 455–456
dies or positives, 447
indirect inlay technique, (*See* Indirect inlay technique)
orthodontic, **443–446**
pouring, **442**
restorations, 446–447
separating, 443
trimming, 443
Cavity classification, 281
Cells, 226
Cements, dental,
zinc-oxide-eugenol, 545
zinc-phosphate, 545
Cement slabs and spatulas, 380–381, **380**
Chairside assisting, 538–561
Chairside dental assistant, 9, 513, 539
Chairside dental health team, 513–519
Charting, 282
Cheilitis, 311
Cheilosis, 311, **312**
Chest pain, first aid for, 330
Children, assisting with, 517–518
Children, behavior characteristics, 57–59
Children's teeth, identification of, 281–282
Circulatory reaction, first aid for, **331, 332**
Cleanliness, 302–303, 307
cleansing the environment, 303
routines for, 373
Cleft palate, 312
Clinical records, (*See* Records, clinical)
Come-up card files, 101
birthday control, 104, **105**
office task control, 101, **102**
recall control, 97, **102**
Communication,
basis for understanding, 69
component parts of, **70**
coworkers and communication, 76
feedback, 74
inadvertent, 14
interacting with people, 75
message transfer, 74
misinterpreted silences, **72**
other writing, 148
process of, 73–74, **73**
typing reports, 147
ways we communicate, 69–73
written communications, 142–149
by dental assistant, 145–147, **147–149**

Computers in the dental office, 192–193
computer routing slip, **193**
magic box concept, 192
Contouring pliers, **395**
Conversation, office technique, 76
Convulsions, first aid for, 332
Cotton holder, **386**
Cotton pliers, 385, **384**
Cotton roll holder, **387**
Credit, 213
collection advice from American Credit Association, 222
collection ratio, 216
consumer, 213
control, 219
dental, 213
federal regulation of, 214
follow-up procedure, 219–222
good management of, 216
how patient pays, 214
truth-in-lending laws, **214**
Credit and collections, 212–223
Cutting instruments, **393–394**
Cyst, residual, 319

D

DAU, 10, 25
da Vinci, Leonardo, 20
Dappen dish, **386**
Day sheet, daily record, 171, **172, 173**
Day's work schedule, 100
Death in the office, 333
Decalcification of enamel, 316
Delta Dental Plan, 207, **208**
Dental assistant
chairside, 9
coordinating, 9
duties of, 10
ethics for, 11–12
laboratory, 9
personal impression created by, 13–14
professional, 11
role of, 9
secretarial, 13
work opportunities for, 10
Dental cabinet, **25**
Dental caries, **310**
control of, 321
four stages of, **317**
schematic illustration of progress, **316**
Dental chairs, 26, **371**
Dental disease, **310**
Dental engine, 26
Dental equipment, care of, 374, **374–377**
autoclave, 377
dental cabinet, 371
dental unit, 26, 374
manufacturers of, 9
ultrasonic cleaner, 377
Dental floss and tape dispenser, **386**

Dental health team, 8
  assisting with preparations, 516
  chairside dental health team, 513–539
  color coding instruments, **515**
  creating confidence in, 56
  dismissing the patient, 517
  general rules for conduct in the operatory, 514
  oral examination technique, 518
  preparing the patient, 515
  tray setups, 515
Dental implants, 26
Dental instruments, 380–411
Dental insurance programs, 206
Dental law, (*See* Jurisprudence)
Dental mirrors, 384, **385**
Dental office, 371, **371–374**
  atmosphere, **373**
  cleanliness routines, 373
  components, 372
  daily routines, 372
  housekeeping and maintenance, 31
  laboratory, care of, 372
Dental office purchases, 122
Dental prophylaxis, 343–346, **340–346**
  right angles, brushes and cups, **383**
Dental public health, 5
Dental services, need and demand for, 4
Dental specialties, 5, 349–368, **349–354, 356–359, 361–362, 364–367**
Dental supply salespersons, 9
  detail persons, 9
Dental terminology, 28
Dental-medical vocabulary, 29
  aids, 29
  sound-alike, look alike words, 31
  technical vs. layman's language, 29
  using your knowledge, 30
  word study, 31
Dentifrice, 342
Dentist,
  arrangements for meetings, 152–155
    agenda, 155
  arrangements for meetings and conferences, 154
    itinerary, **153**
    reservations, 152–153
    return preparation, 154
    travel necessities, 153
  business services for, 167
  personal reminder service, 96
  role of, 4
Dentistry,
  four-handed, 521–557, **523–557**
  general, 4
  past, 18–27
  today, 3

Denture,
  adjustment procedure, 561
  casts, 455–457, **456, 457**
  complete procedure, 560–561
  emergency repair, **457**
  partial procedure, 558–559
Diabetes mellitus, 312
Diabetic shock (insulin shock), first aid for, 335
Diamond instruments, 26, 382–383, **383**
Dictation, 143–144
Dies or positives of the impression, 447
Diet and nutrition, 285–295, **289–291, 294**
  for control of caries, **294**
  diet, 286–287
  oral cavity, 294
  recommended dietary allowances, 292
Direct restorative composite resins, 544
Disinfectant, 301
Disposables, 26
Drugs, 324–328
  controlled, 327
  dispensing or administering to patient, 324–325, **325**
  food-drug reactions, 324
  generic, proprietary, 326
  incompatible, 324
  liquids, 325
  poison to panacea, 324
  prescriptions, 329
  solids, 326
  terminology, 325
  types of, 326
  use in office, 338

E

Emergencies, 328–336, **329–336**
Emergency care, 330
  allergies, 330
  chest pain (hypertension), 330, **313–332**
  circulatory reactions, 331
  convulsions, 332
  death, 333
  epistaxis, 334
  fainting (syncope), **332, 333**
  hemorrhage, 334
  insulin shock, 335
  mouth-to-mouth resuscitation, 331
  preparation for action, 328
  psychosis, 335
  respiratory reaction, 335
  shock, 336
Emergency denture repair, 457
Empathic response, favorable, 56
Endocrine system, (*See* Systems of the body)
Endodontic armamentarium, **396**
  procedures,
    endodontic setup for apicoectomy, 550

minimum endodontic setup for intracanal treatment, 550
Endodontics, 5, 349–353, **349, 350**
Epistaxis, first aid for, 334–345
Epulis, **312**
Erosion, **312**
Ethics, principles of, 6, 11, 12
Exostosis, 312, **313**
Expanded duties personnel, 9
Ethylene oxide gas sterilizer, **306**

F

Fainting, first aid for, **333, 334**
Fibroma, 312
Filing, 133–140
  account records file, 133
  accounts receivable, 137
  accuracy in recording, 135
  active file, 137
  caption for file folder, **133**
  chargeout methods, 135
  clinical records file, 133
  cross-reference index card, **134**
  dead file, 138
  dental office filing, 133, **139**
  files for patient account records, 138
  filing color slides, **139**
  general, 133
  grouping of patient records, 137
  inactive file, 138
  master cross index file, **138, 139**
  numeric file, 137
  open shelf files, 137
  process of, 133
  records search, 136
  shelf filing with numeric system, 137
  steps in filing, 134
  subject files, 133
  terminal digit filing, 137
  transfer file, 138
Financial records, (*See* Records, financial)
Fistula, 312, **313, 319**
Fixed prosthodontic procedures, 555
  bridge procedure, 555
  setting gold prostheses, 555
Flossing, **345**
Fluoride, 341
Foot engine, **23**
Fordyce's spots, **313**
Fountain spitoon, **23**
Four-handed dentistry, applied principles, 520–537, **523–537**
  concepts of motion economy, 522
  dimensions of four-handed dentistry, 521
  functional operating positions, 522–523, **523, 526**
  general precautions in patient care, 526, **527**
  instrument handling and transfers, 530
    basic instrument grasps, 531, **532, 533**

instrument transfer, 531–532, **533–535**
oral evacuation 527, 527–529
pre-prepared trays, **531**
principles of work simplification, 521–522
seating and positioning the patient, 523–524, **524**
syringe transfer, 535, **536, 537**
use of the air-water syringe, 529, **530**
zones of activity, 524, **525**
Fundamental human needs, 54

G
Germicide, 301
Glass Inomer cement, 422
Gold and gold alloys, 426–430, **427–429**
Gold-foil filling procedure, 545
instruments, 395
Gold, melting, 473
Granuloma, 319–320, **320**
Group practice, 6

H
Hand bit and drill, 23
Handpiece, **381**
accessories for, **382–384**
Heart, schematic drawing, **271**
Hemic or blood system, (*See* Systems of the body)
Hemorrhage (bleeding), first aid for, **334**
Herpes simplex, 313
Histological section of reparative dentin, **318**
History, 8,
ancient, 19–20
anesthesia, 22, 25
dentistry, 18–27
education and publication, 21
eighteenth century, 20
innovators and progression, 21
material and equipment for dentistry, 25
Middle Ages, 20
nineteenth century, 21
preventive dentistry, growth of, 24
professional advances, 25
twentieth century, 33
Hobbs, Lucy, 21
Human needs, fundamental, 545
Hydrocolloid impression procedure, multiple inlay or bridge, 556
Hygienist, 8
Hyperplasia, 314
Hypertension, first aid for, 330
Hypertrophy, 314
Hypoplasia, **314**

I
Impression materials, 26, 433–436
hydrocolloid impression materials, **436**

impressions for cast gold restorations, 433, **434**
rubber-base materials, 434
Impression procedures, 556
alginate impression technique, 557
compound impression procedure, 556
hydrocolloid impression procedure for partial denture, 557
reversible hydrocolloid impression procedure for multiple inlay or bridge, 556
Indirect inlay technique, 447–454, **448–454**
copper band impressions, 454, **455**
cutting the removable dies and completing the castings, **452–454**
fixed prostheses impression technique, **454**
making the impression in the custom-made tray, **449–451**
pouring the model, **451–452**
removable prostheses, 455–457, **456, 457**
denture casts, 455
emergency denture repair, **457**
occlusal rims, 456, **457**
trial bases, 456, **457**
tray impression for single or multiple inlays, 447–449, **448, 449**
Inlay procedure, 554
Instruments, **380–411**
dental unit and accessories, **382–384**
diamond stones, **383**
general instructions, 380
hand instruments, 391–411, **391–410**
handpieces, 381, **382**
accessories for, **382–384**
numbering, 392
sharpening devices, **391**
Insulin shock, first aid for, 335
Insurance,
cases, procedure for managing, 207
forms, 123
Delta Dental, 207, **208**
dental programs, 206
determination of reasonable charges, 209
plans, 207
principle of, 206
terminology, 209
types, 207
Insurance and prepaid care programs, 206–211
Integumentary system (*See* Systems of the body)
Investing, **469–470**
Invoices for dental office purchases, 122, 180
Itinerary, **153**

J
Judge made law, 34
Judicial precedents, 34
Jurisprudence, 31–50
admissions, 43
American law, 33
assistant as agent, 36
assumption of risk, 45
authorization form for disclosure of information, **39**
auxiliary personnel, requirements, 35
avoiding liability claims, 44–49
breach of contract, 43
breach of duty, 41
burden of proof, 42
code, 34
common law, 34
contract, 36
contract, termination of, 38
contributory negligence, 45
criminal liabilities, 43
dental practice acts, 33–35
dentist's public duties, 40
doctrine of common knowledge, 43
duties of patients, 37
duties to patients, 36–37
expert testimony, 42
expert witness, 40
federal law, 34
financial responsibility, 36
form for refusal to permit X rays, **39**
insurance, professional liability, 43
laws regulating dentistry, 34
legal relationship of dentist and patient, 35–40
letter of confirmation, **39**
letter of withdrawal, **38**
letter to patient who refuses to follow advice, **39**
liabilities, professional and criminal, 40–44
malfeasance, 41
malpractice claims, 41
medical professional liability, 41
minimizing danger of unjustified claims, 45–49
misfeasance, 41
nonfeasance, 41
personal injury claims, 41
privileged communication, 48
proof of negligence, 42
proximate cause, 43
regulation, need for, 33
relationship of dentist to patients, 35–36
remuneration for dentist, 37
requirements for licensed dentists, 35
res ipsa loquitur, 42
revocation of license, 35
state law, 34
statutes of limitation, 45
tort liability, 43

L

Laboratory
   cases, 122
   schedule, 99, **101**
   technician, 9
Laundry, care of, 130
Law, dental, (*See* Jurisprudence)
Letter writing, 142–147, **144, 145, 147**
Leukoplakia, **314**
Lichen planus, 314
Local anesthesia, 276
Lymphatic system, (*See* Systems of the body)

M

Mail services and care of, 120–124
   classes of mail, 120–121
   during dentist's absence, 123
   incoming mail, 121
   metered postage, 120
   outgoing mail, 123
   permit postage, **120**
   when office is closed, 123
   working with mail, 122
Malignancy, **315**
Malignant neoplasms, 315
Mandrels, **384**
Manual, office procedure, 94–95
Matrix, matrix holders, **394**
Medicament bottles, **386**
Microbiology, 298–300
   bacteriology, **298**
   fungi, 300
   protozoa, 300
   rickettsia, 300
   understanding microbiology, 298–299
   viruses, 300
Minerals, 289–290, **290**
Motivation, ladder of deficit motives, **72**
Mottled enamel, **315**
Mouth, **267**
Muscular system, (*See* Systems of the body)

N

Napkin holder, **386**
Necrotizing ulcerative gingivitis, 315
Nerve supply to the dental area, 270, **272, 273**
Nervous system, (*See* Systems of the body)
Nevus, 315
New patient examination procedure, adult and child, 539
Nomenclature, 28–31
Nosebleed, first aid for, 334, 345
Nutrition, 288

O

Observation, 75
Occlusal rims, 456, **457**
Office administration, (*See* Administration of the office)

Operatory, conduct rules, 514
Oral examination technique, 518
Oral hygiene, **339–346**
   stains, 340
Oral and maxillofacial surgery, 5, 353–360, **354, 356–358**
   instruments for, **397–493**
   procedures for, 551–554
      care and medication
         preliminary to surgery with local or general anesthesia, 551
      oral surgery basic tray, 552
      oral surgery flap tray, 553
      oral surgery impaction tray, 554
      oral surgery soft tissue/biopsy tray, 553
      procedure for removal of teeth, 552
Oral pathology, 310
   control of dental caries, 321
   dental caries, 316–321, **320**
   granuloma, 319, 321, **320**
   inflammation, 310
   other tissue changes, **311–316**
   periapical abscess, 318–319, **318**
   periodontitis, 321
   pulp reaction, 317
Oral surgery armamentarium, **397–403**
   color coding of surgical instruments, 397
   definition, 353
   forceps, care of, 399
   sterile instruments, care of, 400
Oral surgery assistant, role of, 353–355
   efficient assisting, 358–360
   post operative duties, 359–360
Orderly office routines, 99
Orthodontic,
   appliance parts, 362
   armamentarium, **403–404**
   assistant, duties of, 363
      chairside, 363
      secretarial, 363
   bands, prefabricated and prewelded, 26
   casts, **443–445**
   instruments, 403–404
   procedures, 546–547
Orthodontics, 5, 360–363, **361**
Osteology, 255–261, **255–259**

P

Papuloma, 315
Partial denture procedure, 558–559
Pathology, 310
Patient,
   appointing children, 111
   appointing emergency, 111
   appointing new patient, 110
   appointing patient not on recall, 111

   appointing patient of another dentist, 111
   as a person, 226
   awareness of appointment time, 115
   care of patient's dental appliance, 515
   comfort, 56
   dismissing, 82, 517
   educator, 13
   how patient pays for services, 214
   preparation of, 515
   recall philosophy, 129
   registration, 217–219
      acquiring information, 218–219
Patient's ledger card, 172
Pedodontics, 5, 364
Pegboard bookkeeping system, 243–246
People, working with, 54
   ladder of deficit motives, 54
Periapical abscess, 318
   cyst of maxilla, **315**
Periapical armamentarium, 404, **405**
Periapical infection, **318**
Periodontic procedures, 547–549
   diagnosis tray, 547
   instrumentation tray, 548
   occlusal adjustment tray, 548
   pack removal tray, 549
   post-operative tray, 549
   prophylaxis tray, 548
   surgery tray, 549
Periodontics, 5, **364–366**
   assistant, duties of, 366
Periodontitis, 315, 321
Periodontosis, 315, 321
Plaque, 339–346, **339**
Plaster and artificial stone, **438–441**
Plastic filling instruments, **395**
POH (Personal Oral Hygiene), 25, 339–345
Polymerized acrylic resin, 26
Power of attorney, 195
Practice, types of, 6
Prepaid care programs and insurance, 206–210
Preparations, assisting with, 516, 517
Pre-prepared trays, 530, **531**
Preventive dentistry, 338–346
Primary teeth, 269
Problem solving, 98
   selling your dentist, 98
Procedure manual for dental office, 94, 95
Prophylaxis
   armamentarium for POH, **340**
   dental, 340, **340**
   right angle brushes and cups, **383**
   units, 26
Prosthodontics, 5, **366, 367**
   armamentarium, 405–411, **406–411**
   assistant, duties of, 367

Psychology in the dental office, 57
Psychosis, first aid for, 335
Public relations, 62–66
   communication, 69
   factors establishing, 65–66
Public, service to, 3
Purchases, dental office, 22
Pulp tester, **387**
Pulp testing procedure, 543

R

Radiation necrosis, 315
Radiographic techniques, 494–510
   intraoral and extraoral techniques,
      494–500, **496–500**
      bitewing technique, 499
      occlusal technique, **499**
      periapical long anode-film
         procedure, 498–499, **499**
      quality radiographs, 495
      relationship of patient to X-ray
         tube, 495–496, **496**
      seven steps for better X-ray
         exposures, 500
   processing of film, 501–506
      automatic film processing, **501**
      care of X-ray developing tank
         and solutions, 503–505
      darkroom or processing room,
         501–502, **502**
      hand processing of films, 501
      procedures for developing
         X rays, 505–506
      processing radiographs, 506
      X-ray processing solutions,
         503–505
   processed film, 507–510
      bitewing X rays,
         distinguishing, 508
      filing X rays and records, 508
      preserving radiographs, 509
      mounting radiographs, **507**
      panoramic X ray, 508
      periapical X-ray series,
         distinguishing, 508
Radiography, 479–493
   creation and use of X rays,
      480–482, **480–481**
   defined, 479
   film, intraoral and extraoral,
      490–491, **491, 492**
   safety, **486**
   theory, 479–484
      geometry of shadows, 482–483,
         483
      panoramic X ray, **489**
      recording the image, 483
   use of X-ray machine, 487–489,
      488–489
Recall
   card, **97**
   patient recall control file, 101, **102**
   philosophy, 97
   prophylaxis and examination
      appointment, 542
Receptionist, 8

Reception of patients, 80–90
   cordial reception, creation of, **80**
Reception room procedures, 81–90
   receiving new patients, 81
      previous patients, 81
      professional colleagues, 82
      salespersons, 82
      strangers, 81
      unidentified callers, 82
Records, clinical or professional,
      156–164
   acquaintance form, **159**
   case history, 160
   case presentations, 162
   color coding records of special
      patients, 160
   combination examination and
      estimate form, **163**
   new patient examination and
      diagnosis card, 162
   patient registration (acquaintance
      form), 158
   patient's individual record card,
      159
   purpose of clinical records, 158
   radiographs, 160
   radiography, 209
   slides, 161
   study models, 161
Records, financial, 166–196
   accounts receivable control, 175
   assets, 168
   banking procedures, 183
      check and stub, 185
      checkbook, 186–195
      checkbook reconciliation
         procedures, 186–188, **186,
         188**
      check register, 185
      deposit slip, 184
      services, 193, **194**
   basic requirements, 169
   computers in the dental office,
      192–193
   day sheet, 171, 172, **172, 173**
   dental office charge accounts, 180
   disbursement record, 180–183,
      181, 182
   discounts, 173
   double-entry bookkeeping, 168
   expenditures records, 178
   invoices for dental office
      purchases, 180
   liabilities, 168
   monthly record-keeping
      responsibilities, 188
   notary public, 195
   office change fund, 170
   patient's account record, **171**
   patient's records and government,
      third-party payments, 173
   patient's service and account
      record, 171
   patient's service record, 171, **172**
   payments by check from patients,
      174

   petty cash fund, **178**
   power of attorney, 195
   proprietorship, 168
   receipt book, 170
   source documents, 168
   statements for dental office
      purchases, 180, **179**
   statements for patients, **174**
   why keep records, 167
   write-it-once, or pegboard
      bookkeeping systems,
      189–192, **189–191**
   yearly summary, 183
Records for taxes, 199–205, **201–205**
   complete, accurate records, 199
   office salary and tax records, 199,
      200
   payments to IRS, 200
      state unemployment tax form,
      200
   tax forms, 199–200, **201–205**
Registration form, 158, **159**
Removable prostheses, **455–457**
Reproductive system, (*See* Systems
      of the body)
Reservations, 152
   hotel, 153
   travel and convention, 152
Residual cyst, 315
Respiratory reaction, first aid for,
      335
Respiratory system, (*See* Systems of
      the body)
Restorations, 446
Restorative materials, 9, 414–431
   biomaterials, 415
   cements, 419–422, **420, 421**
   dental amalgam, **423–426**
   esthetic restorative materials,
      422–423
   gold and gold alloys, 426
   ten tenets for, 415–418, **415–419**
Risk management, 27, 513
Roentgen ray, (*See* Radiography)
Roentgen, Wm. K., 24
Rubber dam, **388, 389**
   application of, 543
Running inventory, **127**

S

Salary and tax record, 199, **200**
Sales persons, appointing, 111
Scalers, 394
Schedules, laboratory, 99
Scrubbing procedures, 302
Secretarial assistant, 8
Setting gold prostheses, 555
Sharpening devices, instrument, **391**
Shock, first aid for, 336
Sialolithiasis, 316
Skeletal system, (See Systems of the
      body)
Solo practice, 6
Staff conference, 95
Statements for dental office
      purchases, 122

Sterilization and related processes, 301–307
   autoclave, **305, 306**
   chemical agents, **304**
   cleanliness, 302–303
   dry heat, **306**
   ethylene oxide sterilizers, **306**
   practical applications, 301
   preparation of materials for disinfecting and sanitizing, 303–304
   purposes in sterilizing, 305
   sanitizing and disinfecting, 304
   sanitizing by boiling in water, 304
   sterilization, purposes of, 305
Stomatitis, 316
Stone, artificial, **438–441**
Stones, mounted, **394**
Structure of the body
   body cavities, 227
   body planes, **228, 229**
   body surfaces, 229
   cells, 226
   organs, 227
   tissues, 227
Supplies
   back-ordered, 129
   care of, on delivery, 123, 128
   code label, **128**
   control card, **128**
   control of, 126
   damaged merchandise, 129
   dental supply invoice, back-order marking, **129**
   disposable, 126
   expendable, 126
   for business, 126
   inventory control card, 130
   inventory control system of Leo Hoffman, 127
   inventory, running, 126, **127**
   laundry, care of, 130
   methods for, 126
   nonexpendable supplies, 126
   professional supplies, 126
   proper storage of, 130
   selecting suppliers, 126
Surgery, (*See* Oral and maxillofacial surgery)
Syncope, first aid for, 333–334
Systems of the body, 230–251
   circulatory, 234–237, **235, plates 6, 7, 8**
      blood circulating, 236–237
   digestive, 246–248, **247**
   endocrine, 245–246, **245**
   genitourinary, 249–251, **249, 250**
      reproductive, 250–251

   hemic or blood, 237–239
   integumentary, 233–234, **plate 3**
   lymphatic, 237, **238**
   muscular, 233, **plate 2**
   nervous, 241–244, **242–244**
   respiratory, 239–241, **plate 4, 243–244**
   skeletal, 230–233, **231–232, plate 1**

T
Taxes, 119–205, **200–205**
   complete, accurate records, 119
   office salary and tax, 199, **200**
   payment to IRS, 200
   state unemployment tax forms, 200
   tax forms, 199, **200–205**
Team dentistry, 3, 10
   chairside dental health, 513–519
   cooperating with, 15
   desirable member, 15
Technical language vs. laypersons, 29
Teeth
   identification of, and cavity classification, 279–283
      cavity classification, 281, **282**
      charting, **283**
      identification of children's, 281, **282**
      names for, **279**
      terminology, 280
      written identification, 280
   supporting structures, 268
      cross section, **269**
      eruption table, 269
      functions of, 270
Telephone procedures, 83–89
   answering service, 89
   appointments for children, 88
   assisting new patients who call, 88
   difficult calls, 89
   holding phone correctly, **83**
   outgoing calls, 89
   professional telephone calls, 83
   recording calls, 84
   sample page of telephone notebook, 84
   suggestions, 85–88
   taking messages, 84
   technique in professional office, 83
Temporary crown procedure, 546
Third-party payment plans, 25, 173
Three quarter crown procedure, 554
Thrush, 316
Time allotment, judging for appointments, 109
Time management, importance of, 108

Tissue changes, 311
Tissues (body), 227
Toothbrushes and brushing technique, **343–345**
   electric toothbrushing technique, 343–345, **344**
Toothbrushing demonstration procedure, 541
Transfer forceps, 390, **305**
Trauma, 316
Traumatic injury, **315**
Travel arrangements, 152–154
   necessities, 153
   preparation for homecoming, 154
Tray setups, 515
Trial bases, **456**

U
Ultrasonic cleaners, 26
Ultraspeed handpieces, **381**

V
Vitamins, 290–292, **291**

W
Water jets, 345, **346**
Waste management, 513
Wax patterns, **466–468**
Welded gold restorations, 426–430, **427–429**
Word elements, 30, 51, 67, 78, 90, 106, 118, 124, 131, 140, 150, 155, 165, 176, 197, 211, 223, 253, 277, 296, 308, 322, 337, 347, 268, 378, 412
Word study, 31
Words, sound alike-look alike, 31
Written communications, 141–149

X
X ray, 479–510, (*See* Radiographic techniques and Radiography)

Y
Yearly summary, 183

Z
Zinc-oxide-eugenol cement, preparation of, 419, **420**
Zinc phosphate cement, preparation of, 420–422, **421**
Zinc polyacrylate (zinc polycarboxylate) cement, 422
Zinc silicophosphate cement, 422